D1710763

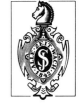

Preceding Symposia on Hearing:

I. 1969: Driebergen, The Netherlands, *Frequency Analysis and Periodicity Detection in Hearing.* (R. Plomp and G. F. Smoorenburg) A. W. Sijthoff, Leiden (1970).

II. 1972: Eindhoven, The Netherlands, *Hearing Theory.* (B. L. Cardozo) IPO, Eindhoven (1972).

III. 1974: Tutzing, Germany, *Facts and Models in Hearing.* (E. Zwicker and E. Terhardt) Springer-Verlag, Berlin, Heidelberg, New York (1974).

IV. 1977: Keele, Great Britain, *Psychophysics and Physiology of Hearing.* (E. F. Evans and J. P. Wilson) Academic Press, London, New York, San Francisco (1977).

V. 1980: Noordwijkerhout, The Netherlands, *Psychophysical, Physiological and Behavioural Studies in Hearing.* (G. van den Brink and F. A. Bilsen) Delft University Press, Delft (1980).

HEARING –
Physiological Bases and Psychophysics

Proceedings of the 6th International Symposium
on Hearing,
Bad Nauheim, Germany, April 5 – 9, 1983

Editors:

R. Klinke and R. Hartmann

With 211 Figures

Springer-Verlag
Berlin Heidelberg New York Tokyo 1983

Dr. Rainer Klinke
Dr. Rainer Hartmann

Zentrum der Physiologie
Theordor-Stern-Kai 7
D-6000 Frankfurt 70, FRG

Organizing Committee:

D.M. Caird, A.W. Gummer, R. Hartmann, M. Kaluza, R. Klinke,
U. Müller-Planitz, R. Plotz, H. Querfurth, R. Schmidt, J. Smolders,
and G. Topp

ISBN 3-540-12618-X Springer-Verlag Berlin Heidelberg New York Tokyo
ISBN 0-387-12618-X Springer-Verlag New York Heidelberg Berlin Tokyo

Offset printing: Beltz Offsetdruck, Hemsbach. Bookbinding: J. Schäffer OHG, Grünstadt
2153/3130-543210

PREFACE

The present book contains the original papers and essential points of the general discussion of a meeting organized in a series of tri-annual conferences, initiated by Dr. R. Plomp with the meeting in Driebergen, The Netherlands, 1969. These symposia have tried to bring together people from extreme fields in auditory research and to amalgamate their recent findings. This series of conferences has proven to be most successful and has attracted much attention by scientists in auditory research.

The organizers have tried to maintain the character of the meeting with emphasis on discussion by precirculation of the full text of the papers and by restricting the number of active contributions. Unfortunately, this forced us to reject a great number of submitted papers – in selection we attempted to compose a fair survey of certain fields of auditory research but leave others untreated. Because of the same reason the number of invited review papers had to be limited to three. The reader may decide whether or not this selection was adequate. We thank all those participants who attended the meeting inspite of the rejection of their paper.

The authors have been responsible for text and typing of their manuscripts. The editors have not attempted to standardize the spelling.

The general discussions were put down in concise form immediately after the sessions and all the printed remarks have been approved by the speakers before the end of the conference. Literature not quoted in the discussion can be found in the preceding paper.

The editors wish to thank the sponsors of the meeting, the Deutsche Forschungsgemeinschaft (4850/15/82), the Hessische Kultusminister and the US Air Force Office for Scientific Research (AFOSR-83-0130). Without this help the organization of the meeting would not have been possible. The authors are thanked for preparing their manuscripts according to the instructions; only a small number of manuscripts had to be retyped by our secretaries. We sincerely thank Ms. Renata Plotz and Ms. Mechthild Kaluza for reliably typing the discussions during the meeting and later for the edition of the book. Thanks have also to be extended to our technician Ms. Ursula Müller-Planitz, who did a marvelous job in collating the camera-ready version of the manuscripts. Finally the editors thank the Springer-Verlag, in particular Dr. Czeschlik for their understanding, their concessions and the quick printing.

Frankfurt/Main   Dr. Rainer Klinke
May 6, 1983   Dr. Rainer Hartmann

CONTENTS

SECTION III. BINAURAL INTERACTION

SECTION IV. PSYCHOPHYSICS

SECTION V.   PITCH PERCEPTION

SECTION VI.   SPEECH AND HEARING IMPAIRMENT

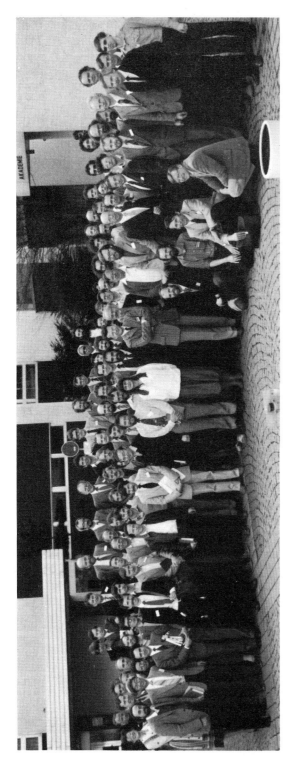

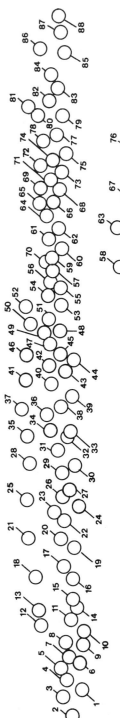

Identification numbers are found in the list of participants.

LIST OF PARTICIPANTS

ASHMORE, J.F., School of Biological Sciences, University of Sussex, Brighton
    BN1 9QG, Great Britain. (66)
BIALEK, W., Department of Biophysics, University of California, Berkeley CA 94720,
    USA. (61)
BILSEN, F.A., Applied Physics Department, University of Technology, Lorentzweg 1,
    Delft, The Netherlands. (7)
BLAUERT, J., Ruhr-Universität Bochum, Postfach 10 21 48, D-4630 Bochum 1,
    Germany.
BOCK, G.R., Institute of Hearing Research, University Park, Nottingham NG7 2RD,
    Great Britain. (71)
BOER, E. de, Academic Medical Centre, Meibergdreef 9, 1105 AZ Amsterdam, The
    Netherlands. (55)
BOTTE, M.-Ch., Laboratoire de Psychologie Expérimentale, 28 rue Serpente,
    75006 Paris, France. (9)
BRINK, G. van den, Department of Biol. and Med. Physics, Erasmus University,
    P.O. Box 1738, 3000 DR Rotterdam, The Netherlands. (68)
BROWNELL, W.E., Departments of Neuroscience and Surgery (ENT), University of
    Florida College of Medicine, Gainesville, Florida 32610, USA. (76)
BURNS, E.M., Department of Audiology and Speech Sciences, Purdue University,
    West Lafayette, IN 47907, USA. (69)
CAIRD, D.M., Zentrum der Physiologie, J.W.Goethe-Universität, Th.-Stern-Kai 7,
    D-6000 Frankfurt 70, Germany. (54)
COLBURN, H.S., Biomedical Engineering Department, Boston University,
    110 Cummington St., Boston MA 02215, USA. (39)
COSTALUPES, J.A., Johns Hopkins Univ. School of Medicine, 506 Traylor Research
    Building, 720 Rutland Avenue, Baltimore, Maryland 21205, USA. (82)
DALLOS, P., Frances Searle Building, Northwestern University, Evanston IL 60201,
    USA. (30)
DRESCHLER, W.A., Department of Clinical Audiology, Academic Medical Centre,
    Meibergdreef 9, 1105 AZ Amsterdam, The Netherlands. (37)
DUIFHUIS, H., Biophysics Department, Lab. Gen. Physics, R.U.G., Westersingel 34,
    9718 CM Groningen, The Netherlands. (26)
EGGERMONT, J.J., Department of Medical Physics and Biophysics, University of
    Nijmegen, Geert Grooteplein Noord 21, 6525 EZ Nijmegen, The Netherlands. (38)
EVANS, E.F., Dept. of Communication and Neuroscience, University of Keele, Keele,
    Staffordshire ST5 5BG, Great Britain. (13)
FAHEY, P., Department of Physics, University of Scranton, Scranton PA 18510, USA.
    (57)
FASTL, H., Institute of Electroacoustics, Technical University München, P.O. Box
    20 24 20, D-8000 München 2, Germany. (14)
FESTEN, J.M., Faculty of Medicine, Free University, van der Boechorststraat 7,
    1081 BT Amsterdam, The Netherlands.
FETTIPLACE, R., Physiological Laboratory, Downing Street, Cambridge CB2 3EG,
    Great Britain. (24)
FLOCK, Å., Department of Physiology II, Karolinska Institutet, S-104 01 Stock-
    holm, Sweden. (73)
FRITZE, W., II. HNO-Klinik Wien, A-1090 Garnisong. 13, Austria. (5)
GHITZA, O., Tel-Aviv University, School of Engineering, Dept. of Electronic
    Communications, Control and Computer Systems, Tel-Aviv 69978, Israel. (35)

GUMMER, A.W., Zentrum der Physiologie, J.W.Goethe-Universität, Th.-Stern-Kai 7, D-6000 Frankfurt 70, Germany. (41)

HAFTER, E.R., Department of Psychology, University of California, 3210 Tolman Hall, Berkeley 94720, USA. (48)

HAGGARD, M., MRC Institute of Hearing Research, University Park, Nottingham NG7 2RD, Great Britain. (49)

HARRISON, R.V., Laboratoire d' Audiologie Expérimentale, Hôpital Pellegrin, Place Amélie Raba Léon, F-33076 Bordeaux Cedex, France. (29)

HARTMANN, R., Zentrum der Physiologie, J.W.Goethe-Universität, Th.-Stern-Kai 7, D-6000 Frankfurt 70, Germany. (19)

HELLE, R., Siemens AG UBMed HE, Gebbertstr. 125, D-8520 Erlangen, Germany. (45)

HENNING, G.B., Department of Experimental Psychology, South Parks Road, Oxford OX1 3UD, Great Britain. (75)

HOEKSTRA, A., Audiologisch Centrum, Zangvogelweg 150, 3815 DP Amersfoort, The Netherlands. (88)

HOKE, M., Experimental Audiology Ear, Nose and Throat Clinic, University of Münster, Kardinal-von-Galen-Ring 10, D-4400 Münster, Germany. (85)

HORST, J.W., Institute of Audiology, University Hospital, P.O. Box 30 001, Groningen, The Netherlands. (16)

HOUTGAST, T., Institute for Perception TNO, Postbox 23, 3769 ZG Soesterberg, The Netherlands. (15)

JOHNSTONE, B.M., Department of Physiology, University of Western Australia, Nedlands, Australia. (74)

KATE, J.M. ten, Biophysics Group, Applied Physics Dept., Delft University of Technology, Lorentzweg 1, 2600 GA Delft, The Netherlands. (21)

KEMP, D.T., Institute of Laryngology and Otology, Gray's Inn Road, London WC1X 8EE, Great Britain. (79)

KIM, D.O., Dept. of Physiology and Biophysics, Washington University School of Medicine, St. Louis MO 63110, USA. (6)

KLINKE, R., Zentrum der Physiologie, J.W.Goethe-Universität, Th.-Stern-Kai 7, D-6000 Frankfurt 70, Germany. (53)

KLOPPENBURG, B., Institute for Perception TNO, Postbox 23, 3769 ZG Soesterberg, The Netherlands. (31)

KOHLLÖFFEL, L., Institut für Physiologie und Biokybernetik, Universitätsstr. 17, D-8520 Erlangen, Germany. (3)

KONISHI, T., Laboratory of Enviromental Biophysics, National Institute of Health, P.O. Box 12233, Research Triangle Park, N.C. 27709, USA. (50)

KROESE, A.B.A., Biophysics Department, Lab. General Physics, R.U.G., Westersingel 34, 9718 CM Groningen, The Netherlands. (64)

LAAT, J.A.P.M. de, Faculty of Medicine, Boechorststraat 7, 1081 BT Amsterdam, The Netherlands. (47)

LANGNER, G., Zoologisches Institut, Schnittspahnstr. 3, D-6100 Darmstadt, Germany. (62)

LEWIS, E.R., Department of EECS, University of California, Berkeley CA 94720, USA. (67)

LEWIS, R.S., California Institute of Technology, Division of Biology, Pasadena CA 91125, USA. (65)

LINDEMANN, W., Ruhr-Universität Bochum, Universitätsstr, 150, D-4630 Bochum, Germany. (42)

LONG, G.R., Kresge Hearing Research Lab. of the South, L.S.U. Medical Centre, 1100 Florida Ave., New Orleans, Louisiana 70115. (32)

O'LOUGHLIN, B.J., Department of Psychology, Monash University, Clayton, Victoria, 3168, Australia. (87)

LÜTKENHÖNER, B., Hals-Nasen-Ohrenklinik der Westf. Wilhelms-Universität, Experimentelle Audiologie, Kardinal-von-Galen-Ring 10, D-4400 Münster, Germany.

MANLEY, G.A., Institut für Zoologie, Technische Universität München, Lichtenbergstr. 4, D-8046 Garching, Germany.

MEHRGARDT, S., Drittes Physikalisches Institut, Universität Göttingen, Bürger-
    str. 42-44, D-3400 Göttingen, Germany. (51)
MERZENICH, M.M., Coleman Laboratory, HSE 863, University of California, San
    Francisco, CA 94143, USA. (60)
MILLER, M., Johns Hopkins School of Medicine, 506 Traylor Research Building,
    720 Rutland Ave., Baltimore, Maryland 21205, USA. (80)
MOORE, B.C.J., Dept. of Experimental Psychology, University of Cambridge,
    Downing Street, Cambridge CB2 3EB, Great Britain. (78)
NARINS, P.M., Department of Biology, University of California at Los Angeles,
    Los Angeles, CA 90024, USA. (58)
PALMER, A.R., National Institute for Medical Research, The Ridgeway, Mill Hill,
    London NW7 1AA, Great Britain. (27)
PATTERSON, R.D., MRC Applied Psychology Unit, 15 Chaucer Road, Cambridge, Great
    Britain. (43)
PICK, G., Dept. of Postgraduate Medicine, University of Keele, Keele, Stafford-
    shire ST5 5BG, Great Britain. (77)
PICKLES, J.O., Dept. of Physiology, Birmingham University, Birmingham B15 2TJ,
    Great Britain. (25)
PLASSMANN, W., Zoologisches Institut d. J.W.Goethe-Universität, Siesmayerstr. 50,
    D-6000 Frankfurt, Germany. (59)
PLOMP, R., Institute for Perception TNO, Kampweg 5, 3769 ZG Soesterberg, The
    Netherlands. (36)
PRIJS, V.F., Academisch Ziekenhuis, Afd. KNO, Rijnsburgerweg 10, 2333 AA Leiden,
    The Netherlands. (44)
QUERFURTH, H., Zentrum der Physiologie, J.W.Goethe-Universität, Th.-Stern-Kai 7,
    D-6000 Frankfurt 70, Germany.
RAATGEVER, J., Applied Physics Dept., Delft University of Technology, Lorentz-
    weg 1, 2628 CJ Delft, The Netherlands. (83)
RAKOWSKI, A., Frederic Chopin Academy of Music, Okólnik 2, 00-368 Warszawa,
    Poland. (4)
RITSMA, R.J., Institute of Audiology, University Hospital Groningen, P.O. Box
    30 001, 9700 RB Groningen, The Netherlands. (18)
RUSSELL, I.J., Ethology and Neurophysiology Group, School of Biology, University
    of Sussex, Brighton, Sussex, Great Britain. (33)
RUTTEN, W.L.C., ENT Dept. (KNO), University Hospital, 10 Rijnsburgerweg, 2333 AA
    Leiden, The Netherlands. (17)
SCHARF, B., Northeastern University, Boston MA 02115, USA. (8)
SCHMIDT, R., Zentrum der Physiologie, J.W.Goethe-Universität, Th.-Stern-Kai 7,
    D-6000 Frankfurt 70, Germany. (70)
SCHROEDER, M.R., Rieswartenweg 8, D-3400 Göttingen, Germany. (28)
SMITH, R.L., Institute for Sensory Research, Syracuse University, Syracuse NY
    13214, USA. (10)
SMOLDERS, J., Zentrum der Physiologie, J.W.Goethe-Universität, Th.-Stern-Kai 7,
    D-6000 Frankfurt 70, Germany. (63)
SMOORENBURG, G.F., Institute for Perception TNO, Postbox 23, 3769 ZG Soesterberg,
    The Netherlands. (31)
STERN, R.M., Dept. of Electrical Engineering, Carnegie-Mellon University,
    Pittsburgh, Pennsylvania 15213, USA. (1)
STOPP, P.E., Neurocommunications, The Medical School, University of Birmingham,
    Edgbaston, Birmingham B15 2TJ, Great Britain. (2)
SYKA, J., Institute of Experimental Medicine, Czechoslovak Academy of Sciences,
    U nemocnice 2, 128 08 Praha 2, Czechoslovakia. (46)
TERHARDT, E., Lehrstuhl für Elektroakustik der TU München, Arcisstr. 21,
    D-8000 München 2, Germany. (22)
TOPP, G., Zentrum der Physiologie, J.W.Goethe-Universität, Th.-Stern-Kai 7,
    D-6000 Frankfurt 70, Germany. (52)
TYLER, R.S., The University of Iowa Hospital, Dept. of Otolaryngology Speech and
    Hearing, Iowa City IA 52242, USA. (11)

URBAS, J.V., Max Plank Institut für Psychatrie, Kraepelinstr. 2, D-8000 München, Germany. (72)

VEEN, T.M. van, Institute for Perception, Kampweg 5, 3769 DE Soesterberg, The Netherlands. (12)

VERSCHUURE, J., Dept. of Otolaryngology, Erasmus University Rotterdam, P.O. Box 1738, 3000 DR Rotterdam, The Netherlands. (40)

WICKESBERG, R.E., HNO-Klinik, Experimentelle Audiologie, Kardinal-von-Galen-Ring 10, D-4400 Münster, Germany.

WILSON, J.P., Dept. of Communication and Neuroscience, University of Keele, Staffordshire ST5 5BG, Great Britain. (84)

WIT, H.P., Institute of Audiology, Postbox 30 001, 9700 RB Groningen, The Netherlands. (20)

YOUNG, E.D., Johns Hopkins School of Medicine, 506 Traylor Building, 720 Rutland Ave., Baltimore, Maryland 21205, USA. (86)

ZWICKER, E., Institut für Elektroakustik, Technische Universität München, Arcisstr. 21, D-8000 München 2, Germany. (23)

LIST OF AUTHORS

f refers to first page of main paper

Section I
Inner Ear Mechanisms and Cochlear Emissions

REVIEW PAPER: HAIR CELLS, RECEPTORS WITH A MOTOR CAPACITY?

Åke Flock

*Department of Physiology II, Karolinska institutet,
S-104-01 Stockholm 60, Sweden*

1. INTRODUCTION

This article is intended to serve two purposes, one is to fulfill a request by the organizers of this symposium to review hair cell mechanisms, the other is to present new experimental results of our own. As to the first aspect, the reviewing can only be brief in the allotted space. More extensive reviews are: for cochlear physiology Dallos (1981), for non-vertebrates Wiederhold (1976), for intracellular electrical responses Weiss (1983).

2. BASIC HAIR CELL MECHANISMS

a) *Electrical response*
i) *Ionic mechanisms*. The cellular membranes of all cell types have incorporated macromolecules of various types serving as receptors, ionic pumps, enzymes, antigens etc. Some of these serve the transport of ions responsible for the resting potential of the cell. Other ionic channels are sensitive to different types of stimuli, like transmitter substances, hormones, sensory stimuli. These channels respond to stimulation by changing their permeability for ions. In nerve fibres the channels are voltage dependent and open for sodium ions in response to a decrease in membrane potential (depolarization) this inward flow of positive current leads to further depolarization and accelerated sodium flow which in this nonlinear fashion gives rise to the nerve action potential. Mechano-receptors are equipped with channels which are sensitive to mechanical strain, the applied force leads to deformation of some sensitive spot at the molecular level, and ionic flow gives rise to depolarization or hyperpolarization of the membrane (the receptor potential). An example is the crustacean stretch receptor where the mechanisms involved have been studied in detail (Ottoson and Swerup, 1982). The ionic mechanisms involved appear to be fundamentally similar to those of the photoreceptor in the eye (Fain and Lissman, 1981).

Hair cells (HC) are specialized mechano-receptors which appear to utilize ionic mechanisms related to those of the crustacean stretch receptor and the eye. This has been elegantly elucidated by Corey and Hudspeth (1979). It appears that in vestibular HC the transduction channels are not selective to any particular ion species. Due to the high potassium content of endolymph the receptor potential is mainly carried by this ion. Calcium ions are a necessary co-factor. Voltage sensitive potassium channels exist in parallel and impart nonlinear properties to the HC membrane. In some HC types inductive properties are implied in the membrane, giving rise to resonating properties (Crawford and Fettiplace, 1981).

ii) *Mechanoelectrical transduction*. The stereocilia are the transducing elements of HC (Hudspeth and Jacobs, 1979), more specifically; the entry of current has been localized to the tip of the stereocilia (Hudspeth, 1982). At this site the membrane of each stereocilium is connected to its neighbours by cross-links (Flock, 1977). On the inside the membrane is connected by side arms to a core of parallel filaments of the protein actin (Flock and Cheung, 1977; Hirokawa and Tilney, 1982) packed in paracrystalline order (Tilney et al., 1981). At the top of the stereocilia the membrane is attached to the actin filaments end-on. The transduction channels are presumably located in this neighbourhood because this is where applied force will impinge on the membrane.

iii) *Synaptic mechanisms.* The receptor potential that results from ionic flow in the sensory region is spread throughout the cell and acts at the base of the cell to govern the release of transmitter substance at the afferent synapse (Sand et al., 1975). Lately it has been put to question whether the receptor potential is for the benefit of the synapse only, or if it may also interfere with mechanical events in the receptor region for reasons that will become clear later in this text. The same may be true for the efferent innervation; excitation of efferent fibres may interfere not only with afferent synaptic transmission but also with the mechanics of the HC system. Our attention will therefore turn next to the mechanical response of the HC.

b) *Mechanical response*
i) *Filter property of sensory hairs.* Sensory hair mechanics can now be studied by direct microscopic observation on several types isolated specimens. The mechanical filter characteristics of sensory hair bundles in the frog crista ampullaris has been found to be determined by the arrangement of the stereocilia in the bundle (Orman and Flock, 1981). Depending on their structure, bundles may be fast rapidly adapting, or slow with a long time constant. The reptilian auditory organ shows frequency selectivity in single nerve fibres although basilar membrane (BM) tuning is absent (Weiss et al., 1978). In this organ the sensory hairs are graded in length and studies of their motion pattern in stroboscopic illumination show frequency dependent amplitude maxima that agree with tonotopic localization (Frischkopf et al., 1982; Holton and Hudspeth, 1982). In this organ sensory hairs apparently contribute to frequency selectivity of the organ.

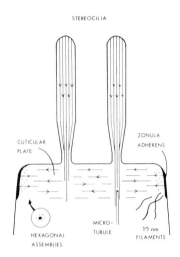

Fig. 1. Organization of actin filaments in hair cells (from Flock et al., 1981)

ii) *Active mechanisms.* Actin is one of the major components in muscle fibres. The finding of actin in the stereocilia, as well as in the cuticular plate where these are inserted by rootlets (Fig. 1), made it important to investigate if hair motion could be influenced by muscle-like mechanisms. In response to a brief jet of fluid the sensory hairs in the crista ampullaris describe a swing-away motion. This response became severely restricted in the presence of calcium ions and adenosinetriphosphate (ATP), conditions that would cause contraction in a muscle fibre (Orman and Flock, 1981). One may conclude that HC in the vestibular system have means of interacting with the mechanical properties of their sensory hairs.

3. COCHLEAR HAIR CELL MECHANISMS

a) *Electrical response*
     The ionic mechanisms of cochlear HC have not been investigation in detail. Experiments by Russell (personal communication) indicate that the receptor current of inner hair cells (IHC) is carried by potassium ions regulated by a pure resistance as suggested by Davis (1965). Mountain (1978) finds voltage resistive elements presumed to be a property of outer hair cells (OHC).
     The electrical responses from IHC (for ref. see Russell this volume) and OHC (Dallos et al., 1982) exhibit similar sharpness of tuning and show similar intensity thresholds for both the ac and the dc components. They also show the same phase at best frequency. They differ in that responses from IHC are approximately 3 times as large as those of OHC. The membrane potential of IHC is about half that of OHC. Both cell types show nonlinear behaviour above approximately 50 dB, with saturation, development of harmonic components and

dc components of the response. If the transduction channel is purely resistive as suggested for the IHC, such a nonlinear behaviour would not be expected. Mechanical factors could therefore be involved.

b) *Mechanical response*

The mechanical properties of single sensory hairs in isolated coils of guinea pig organ of Corti have been investigated with the aid of a probe of quartz glass used to measure the compliance of the sensory hairs (Strelioff and Flock, 1982). A stiffness gradient was found for OHC along the coil, IHC being of approximately equal stiffness for the different turns. The force needed to displace the tip of a hair 1 μm was 3.48±0.38 dyn/cm in turn 2 compared to 0.9±0.35 dyn/cm in turn 4 (values apply to first row OHC). This implies that cochlear HC may be tuned like those in the lizard auditory organ and contribute to the damping of the organ of Corti through their coupling to the tectorial membrane. There was also a radial gradient, OHC getting less stiff towards stria vascularis. The stiffness values are matched by differences in length for the different cell types as described by Lim (1980) but the relationship may not be linear.

An interesting finding was that the sensory hairs resist displacement in the excitatory direction with a force twice as large as that in the inhibitory direction. This again points to the possible existence of a contraction-like mechanism that can be activated in the sensory hair region. We shall therefore next consider the distribution of cytoskeletal proteins in the organ of Corti.

c) *Distribution of contractile and structural proteins*

A family of cytoplasmic proteins are responsible for the maintenance of cell shape and the generation of motion. Over the last few years immunofluorescence methods have been used to identify and localize several of these proteins in organ of Corti cells.

i) *Hair cells.* Of several proteins searched for in stereocilia only two have been clearly identified, actin as previously mentioned, and fimbrin which probably crosslinks actin filaments in the stereocilia to stiff cables (Flock et al., 1982). Conditions for contractility appear to be lacking in the stereociliary shaft. These two proteins are also present in the cuticular plate. Here is also found ✦ -actinin, an actin anchoring protein, and myosin the protein that reacts with actin in the contractile process (Drenkhahn et al., 1982). We have developed a method by which solitary HC (Fig. 2) can be attached to a glass slide and labelled with antibodies (Fig. 3). Such labelling demonstrates existence also of tropo-

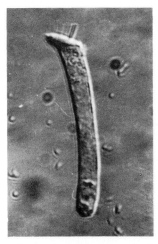

Fig. 2. Solitary OHC isolated from the organ of Corti

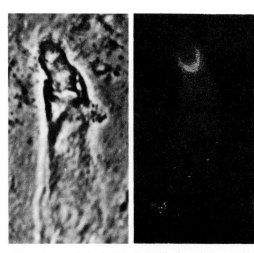

Fig. 3. Isolated OHC labelled with antibodies against tropomyosin. It is located at the level of the rootlets of the stereocilia in the W-shaped bundle

myosin in HC (Fig. 3). In muscle
fibres this protein controls the
interaction between myosin and actin.
It has an interesting location; namely corresponding to the rootlets of
the stereocilia entering into the
cuticular plate. The co-location of
actin, myosin and tropomyosin at the
stereocilium rootlet is highly sug-
gestive in terms of active mechanical events at this point.

ii) *Supporting cells.* In the supporting cells of Corti's organ other combinations of proteins are found
(Fig. 4). Here tubulin exists together
with actin forming stiff arcs inside
the pillar and Deiter's cells (Flock
et al., 1982; Slepecky et al., 1983).
These cables constitute a mechanical
framework conspicuously centering on
and encasing the three rows of OHC's,
the IHC being conspicuously discriminated (Fig. 4).

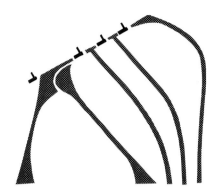

*Fig. 4. The pillar cells and the
Deiters cells contain rigid columns
of mixed microtubules and actin filaments connectin to the reticular
lamina*

4. DISCUSSION

It is interesting to consider a possible relationship between the following
observations:

1. HC transduction channels allow entry of calcium ions during the excitatory
   phase of hair displacement (vestibulal system).

2. Calcium ions cause a restriction of hair motion in the presence of energy donat-
   ing ATP (vestibular system).

3. Tropomyosin, part of a calcium sensitive regulatory protein complex for actomyosin interaction, is present in the rootlet region of the stereocilia. Actin
   and myosin are present at the same site (cochlear hair cells).

4. Sensory hairs in the organ of Corti resist motion in the excitatory direction
   more than in the inhibitory.

A causative relationship could be envisioned as follows: Calcium influx
during excitatory hair deflection, through tropomyosin promotes binding between
actin in the rootlets and myosin in the cuticular plate. This restricts motion of
the stereocilia, hence the mechanical nonlinearity seen in organ of Corti sensory
hairs. There are missing links; myosin and tropomyosin have not yet been demonstrated in vestibular hair cells, and a calcium-ATP effect has not been shown in the
cochlea. There is also evidence in support, such as the finding that stimulation
of efferent nerve fibres to OHC alters cochlear micromechanics (Mountain, 1980) including the mechanical nonlinearity (Siegel and Kim, 1981). If such a calcium dependent mechanism is operational in the organ of Corti it would probably be required to build up over a number of cycles, at least at high frequencies. It
would be interesting to know if the summating potential has any mechanical correlate in BM motion, as the saturating compression and the development of harmonic
components do.
It is quite possible that the design is different in the cochlea and in the
vestibular system having different demand on for example the speed of the system.
For instance, calcium ions need not be involved in the development of force in
an actomyosin system. In certain insect flight muscles myosin is permanently

attached to actin and force is generated in response to applied tension with a phase delay so that the wing and the body form an oscillating system determined by the relative masses (Pringle, 1977). Such systems operate well above 1000 Hz. In this context it is pertinent to point to the discovery of evoked (Kemp, 1978) as well as spontaneous acoustic emmissions from the ear (Züreck, 1981), and to the call for a mechanism that can impact negative damping in the cochlea (Kim et al., 1981).

The mechanical framework seen encasing OHC (Fig. 4) seems well suited to transmit BM motion to the sensory region in the reticular lamina. The OHC stereocilia are tightly connected to the tectorial membrane and therefore mechanical properties contributed by OHC would be transmitted equally well in the opposite direction, i.e. from the reticular lamina down to the BM. Recent data (Johnstone et al., 1981) show that BM tuning is as sharp as that of primary auditory nerve fibres. The OHC system appears to constitute a motor region, the sensing element being the inner hair cells with their abundant afferent innervation. Mechanical activity, be it passive or active, in the OHC region would be effectively transmitted to the IHC with their palisades of stereocilia sensing radial displacement in the subtectorial space.

Acknowledgement: I wish to thank Drs Mary Osborn and Klaus Weber for the gift of antibody and Britta Flock for patient work with isolated cells. Supported by grants from the Swedish Medical Research Council (No. 04X-02461), Karolinska Institutet, Söderbergs Foundation and the Foundation Tysta skolan.

REFERENCES

Corey, D.P., Hudspeth, A.J. (1979). Ionic basis of the receptor potential in a vertebrate hair cell. *Nature* 281, 675-677.

Crawford, A.C., Fettiplace, R. (1981). An electrical tuning mechanism in turtle cochlear hair cells. *J. Physiol.* 312, 377-412.

Dallos, P. (1981). Cochlear physiology. *Amer. Rev. Physiol.* 32, 153-190.

Dallos, P., Santos-Sacchi, J., Flock, Å. (1982). Intracellular recordings from cochlear outer hair cells. *Science* 218, 582-584.

Davis, H. (1965). A model for transducer action in the cochlea. *Coldspring Harbor Symposia on Quantitative Biology* 30, 181-190.

Drenkhahn, D., Keller, J., Mannherz, H.G., Groschel-Stewart, U., Kendrick-Jones, J., Scholey, J. (1982). Absence of myosin-like immunoreactivity in stereocilia of cochlear hair cells. *Nature* 300, 531-532.

Fain, G.L., Lissman, J.E. (1981). Membrane conductances of photoreceptors. *Progr. Biophys. Molec. Biol.* 37, 91-147.

Flock, Å., Flock, B., Murray, E. (1977). Studies on the sensory hairs of receptor cells in the inner ear. *Acta Otolaryngol.* 83, 85-91.

Flock, Å., Cheung, H. (1977). Actin filaments in sensory hairs of the inner ear receptor cells. *J. Cell. Biol.* 75, 339-343.

Flock, Å., Cheung, H.C., Flock, B., Utter, G. (1981). Three sets of actin filaments in sensory cells of the inner ear. Identification and functional orientation, determined by gel electrophoresis, immunofluorescence and electron microscopy. *J. Neurocytol.* 10, 133-147.

Flock, Å., Bretscher, A., Weber, K. (1982). Immunohistochemical localization of several cytoskeletal proteins in inner ear sensory and supporting cells. *Hearing Res.* 6, 75-89.

Frischkopf, L.S., De Rosier, D.J. and Engelman, E.H. (1982). Motion of basilar papilla and hair cell stereocilia in the excised cochlea of the alligator lizard: relation to frequency analysis. *Soc. Neurosci.* Abstr. 8, 40.

Hirokawa, N. Tilney, L. (1982). Interactions between actin filaments and between actin filaments and membrane in quick-frozen and deeply etched hair cells of the chick ear. *J. Cell. Biol.* 95, 249-261.

Holton, T., Hudspeth, A.J. (1982). Motion of hair cell stereocilia in the auditory receptor organ of the alligator lizard. *Soc. Neurosci.* Abstr. 8, 40.

Hudspeth, A.J., Jacobs, R. (1979). Stereocilia mediate transduction in vertebrate hair cells. *Proc. Natl. Acad. Sci.* USA. 76, 1506-1509.

Hudspeth, A.J. (1982). Extracellular current flow and the site of transduction by vertebrate hair cells. *J. Neurosci.* 2, 1-10.

Kemp, D.T. (1978). Stimulated acoustic emissions from within the human auditory system. *J. Acoust. Soc. Amer.* 64, 1386-1391.

Kim, D., Neely, S., Molnar, C., Matthews J.W. (1980). An active cochlear model with negative damping in the partition. Comparison with Rhodes ante- and post-mortem observations. In: Psychophysical, Physiological and Behavioural studies in Hearing. Ed. F.A. Bilsen, B. van den Brink. *Delft Univ. Press,* Delft. p 32.

Lim, D. (1980). Cochlear anatomy related to cochlear micromechanics. A review. *J. Acoust. Soc. Amer.* 67, 1686-1695.

Mountain, D.C. (1978). A comparison of electrical changes in the cochlea caused by stimulation of the crossed olivocochlear bundle and by DC polarization. *Thesis, Univ. of Wisconsin.* 1-119.

Mountain, D.C. (1980). Changes of endolymphatic potential and crossed olivocochlear bundle stimulation alter cochlear mechanics. *Science.* 210, 71-72.

Orman, S., Flock, Å. (1981 a). Micromechanics of the hair cell stereociliary bundles in the frog crista ampullaris. *Ass. Res. Otolaryngol.* Abstr. 4, 30-31.

Orman, S., Flock, Å. (1981 b). Stiffness measurements of stereociliary bundles in frog crista ampullaris. *Soc. Neurosci.* Abstr. 7, 536.

Ottoson, D., Swerup, C. (1982). Studies on the role of calcium in adaptation of the crustacean stretch receptor. *Brain Res.* 244, 337-341.

Pringle, J. (1978). Stretch activation of muscle: function and mechanism. *Proc. R. Soc. Lond.* B. 201, 107-130.

Sand, O., Ozawa, S., Hagiwara S. (1975). Electrical and mechanical stimulation of hair cells in the muduppy. *J. Comp. Physiol.* A. 102, 13-26

Sellick, P., Patuzzi, R., Johnstone, B.M. (1982). Measurement of basilar membrane motion in the guinea pig using the Mössbauer technique. *J. Acoust. Soc. Amer.* 72, 131-141.

Siegel, J., Kim, D. (1982). Efferent neural control of cochlear mechanics?; Olivo-cochlear bundle stimulation affects cochlear biomechanical nonlinearity. *Hearing Res.* 6, 171-182.

Slepecky, N. (1983). Distribution and polarity of actin in inner ear supporting cells. *Ass. Res. Otolaryngol.* Abstr. 5.

Strelioff, D., Flock, Å. (1982). Mechanical properties of hair bundles of receptor cells in the guinea pig cochlea. *Soc. Neurosci.* Abstr. 8, 40.

Tilney, L.G., De Rosier, D.J., Mulroy, M.J. (1980). The organization of actin filaments in the stereocilia of cochlear hair cells. *J. Cell. Biol.* 86, 244-259.

Weiss, T.F., Peake, W.T., Ling, A., Holton, T. (1978). Which structures determine frequency selectivity and tonotopic organization of vertebrate cochlear nerve fibres? In: Evoked electrical activity in the auditory nervous system. Ed. R. Naunton, C. Fernandez. *Academic Press, N.Y.* pp. 9.-112

Weiss, T. (1983). A review of hair cell electrical responses. *In press.*

Wiederhold, M. (1976). Mechanosensory transduction in "sensory" and "motile" cilia. *Ann. Rev. Biophys. Bioengin.* 5, 39-62.

Zurek, P.M. (1981). Spontaneous narrowband acoustic signals emitted by human ears. *J. Acoust. Soc. Amer.* 69, 514-523.

GENERAL DISCUSSION

PICKLES:
The question of the existence of myosin in the stereocilia themselves, as shown
by immunofluorescence techniques, has become controversial. We (Comis, Osborne and
Pickles) have therefore been looking for the associated ATPase by a technique
which involves the deposition of cobalt. X-ray micro-analysis shows the precipi-
tate to be present, in approximately equal concentrations, in the stereocilia as
well as in the cuticular plate. Controls and inhibitors suggested that the
ATPase was indeed actin-myosin ATPase. This confirms our previous suggestion
(McCartney et al., Nature 288, 491, 1980) as to the distribution of myosin in
hair cells.

R.S. LEWIS:
Concerning the suggestion made by Dr. Pickles that myosin is present in the stereocilia, why has there been no report of thick filaments in transmission EM
sections of stereocilia?

FLOCK:
If myosin were present as thick filaments in stereocilia they would have been
seen. However, myosin is present in the terminal web of brush border as thin
microfilaments but it is hard to see how even these could be housed within the
actin paracrystal. A perhaps possible location is at the periphery between the
actin cable and the membrane.

BIALEK:
Regarding the analogy to insect flight muscle:
The muscle can be extracted and held in solutions of fixed ionic concentration,
with the muscle membrane removed. In this condition, mechanical "tuning curves"
of the muscle show high Q's and slopes $\approx$60-100 dB/oct. This tuning is purely mechanical, and does not involve ionic or electrical effects.

KLINKE:
You gave a number of mechanisms working in different hair cells. I don't want to
debate these findings. I assume, however, that not all of them operate in one
type of hair cell. We assume major differences in the mode of action of different types of hair cells and even assume substantial differences in mechanisms of
mammalian and avian hearing. From the number of arguments we have gathered for
this assumption, let me briefly mention that the ototoxic drug Furosemide is ineffective on pigeon hearing in doses as high as 280 mg/kg (Wit and Bleeker,
Arch. Otolaryngol., in press; Schermuly, Göttl and Klinke, Hear. Res., in press).

DUIFHUIS:
I wonder whether you have any ideas on where we might find the basis for the directional sensitivity of the hair cells. Is the hypothesis that the transduction
channels are located at the tops of the cilia reconcilable with directional sensitivity, in view of the relatively isotropic properties of the single cilia?
Or is it conceivable that the transduction process originates in the cuticular
plate, possibly in relation to the orientation of actin and myosin molecules?

FLOCK:
An explanation to directional sensitivity could be in the gradation in length of
the stereocilia and the fact that the longest ones are the ones that are attached to the overlying membrane. A pull on these in the excitatory direction would
lead to separation and thus a pull through interciliary crosslinks on the membranes that could open transduction channels, opposite displacement would cause
closure and relieve membranes from strain. Orthogonal displacement would lead to
a net zero change in strain.

DUIFHUIS:
I do not quite see how that could lead to the marked insensitivity in the direction perpendicular to the sensitivity (the longitudinal direction in the cochlea).

JOHNSTONE:
What is the difference in protein composition between IHC and OHC?

FLOCK:
None that we have seen.

ASHMORE:
I would like to know whether you are able to quantify the concentration of actin
and myosin in cochlear hair cells. Since the rate constant for actomyosin cross-
bridge attachment is known, at least in skeletal muscle (e.g. Goldman et al.,
Nature 300, 701, 1982), the protein concentration would give information about
force of possible kinetics and generation.

FLOCK:
We are now developing techniques to do gel electrophoresis on purified fractions
of hair cells, until they give us the ratio I can only say that the brightness
for actin and myosin fluorescense is approximately equal.

DE BOER:
Over the length of the cochlea you find stiffness variations over a factor of
four. Do you believe that would be relevant for tuning?

FLOCK:
The factor of 4 is not for the entire coil but between turn 2 and 4 (see also
reply to Kim).

KIM:
Is myosin found in the rootlets? Following up the question of Brian Johnstone,
is there any difference noticeable between the OHC and the IHC regarding the
distributions of actin, myosin and related proteins or regarding any other aspects that may help assess the hypothesis that the OHC is specialized in producing negative damping by "reverse" transduction of electrochemical energy
into mechanical energy?

FLOCK:
For values of stiffness gradients (static force) see ref. Strelioff and Flock,
1982. We (Karlsson and Flock, unpublished) now study the threshold for detectability of motion of sensory hairs at 200 Hz in stroboscopic light. Under these
dynamic conditions the mechanical gradients are much more pronounced. Both
longitudinally and radially 30 dB differences can be seen for some cell types.
Depending on position along the coil, OHC can be 30 dB stiffer than IHC.

INNER HAIR CELL RECEPTOR POTENTIALS INVESTIGATED DURING
TRANSIENT ASPHYXIA: A MODEL FOR HAIR CELL COUPLING

I.J. Russell & J.F. Ashmore
Ethology and Neurophysiology Group,
School of Biology, University of Sussex, Brighton, BN1 9QG.

1. INTRODUCTION

    The sensitivity and frequency selectivity of inner hair cells (IHC) and their
afferent innervation are reversibly decreased when the cochlea is momentarily made
anoxic (Robertson and Manley, 1974; Brown, Nuttall, Masta and Lawrence, 1983). In
this paper we describe the changes which take place, during transient asphyxia, in
the waveform of the receptor potentials recorded from (IHCs) in the basal turn of
the guinea pig cochlea and suggest a possible mechanism producing the observed
receptor potential asymmetry changes.

2. METHODS

    The intracellular recording techniques and stimulus presentation used in these
experiments have been described in detail elsewhere (Sellick & Russell, 1980;
Russell & Sellick, 1983). Young guinea pigs 180-260gms in weight were used. They
were anaesthetized with pentabarbitol sodium, Droleptan and Operidine (Jansens)
according to a regime devised by Evans (1979). Heart rate was monitored
continuously and just before intracellular recordings were begun, about one hour
before the termination of the experiment, the animals were injected with the muscle
relaxent Flaxedil (M & B) (0.5mg/kg) and artificially respired with a gas mixture
of 95% O_2 and 5% CO_2 supplied by a constant pressure respirometer.
    IHCs were identified by their large asymmetrical voltage responses to low
frequency tones, their small resting potentials relative to those of supporting
cells (30-40mV cf.80-90mV), their phase lead of about 90° relative to CM for
frequencies below 70Hz, and the production of large DC receptor potentials in
response to tones close to their characteristic frequency (CF). A total of 23 cells
with these characteristics were studied in these experiments. When an IHC had been
impaled and its responses characterised, the respirator was switched off until the
heart rate dropped to 12 beats per minute when it was switched on again. This
criterion was chosen as a means of standardizing the experiments. It was found that
within a single preparation the endocochlear potential (EP) fell to about the same
level each time the heart rate fell to the criterion and that this effect was fully
reversible. In these experiments it was possible to make simultaneous measurements
of the intracellular and extracellular potentials with the exception of the EP. The
effects of transient asphyxia on this potential was measured separately after the
intracellular potentials.

3. RESULTS

    Transient asphyxia caused a large, slow decline in the EP recorded from the
scala media (SM) and a simultaneous, but much smaller, hyperpolarization of the IHC
receptor potential (Figure 1). These potentials reached minimum values 70-190 sec
after the respirator was switched off. The EP and IHC resting potentials changed
by 50%-80% and 5-10%, respectively, of their resting values. They quickly returned
to levels slightly above this when the respirator was switched on, and remained
there for periods between 1-5 minutes before slowly returning to normal. The time
course for the decline and recovery of the CM was similar to those of the EP and IHC
membrane potential. The decline of the compound action potential (CAP) and AC and
DC components of the receptor potential occurred with a shorter latency and
recovery was slower. For tones close to the CF of the IHC, and 25dB above the N_1

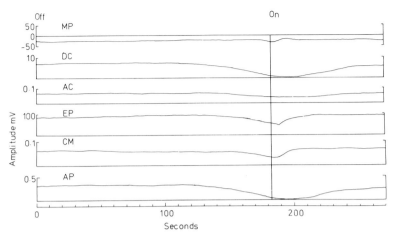

Fig. 1. *The effect of transient asphyxia on the membrane potential (MP),*
DC component (DC) and AC component (AC) of the IHC receptor potential.
Endocochlear potential (EP), cochlear microphonic (CM), and gross compound
action potential of the auditory nerve (AP) from a single preparation in
response to 60msec tone bursts at 15kHz and 55dBSPL presented every 100msec

threshold of the CAP, the CAP and DC components of the IHC receptor potential were
virtually abolished during asphyxia, while the AC component was reduced to 40-70%
of normal.

In an attempt to discover why the DC component of the receptor potential was
apparently more vulnerable than the AC component, the waveform of the IHC receptor
potential was measured in response to low frequency tones. At frequencies of a
few hundred Hz or less the phasic AC component is not attenuated by the low pass
filter characteristics of the IHC membrane time constant (Sellick & Russell, 1980;
Russell & Sellick, 1983). It is asymmetrical about the resting potential, with
the amplitude of the depolarizing phase exceeding the phase of hyperpolarization
by a factor of 2-5 (Figure 2A). During asphyxia the peak-to-peak amplitude of the
receptor potential is reduced by 40-70% and it becomes almost symmetrical.

These changes are also illustrated in the transfer characteristics of the IHC
receptor potentials (Figure 2B) which were plotted before and during asphyxia. It
can be seen that, during asphyxia, the transfer function becomes almost
symmetrical about zero.

It is possible that the increased symmetry of the IHC receptor potential
which occurs during brief periods of asphyxia is due to the changes in EP and the
resting potential, which together constitute the driving voltage across the apical
membrane of the IHC (Davis, 1958; Russell, 1983). To test this hypothesis, the
symmetry of the receptor potential (the ratio of the AC and DC components of the
receptor potential) was measured while the IHC membrane potential, was altered by
the injection of depolarizing and hyperpolarizing currents through the recording
electrode. It can be seen from Figure 3 that, over a wide range of membrane
potentials, this ratio was not altered.

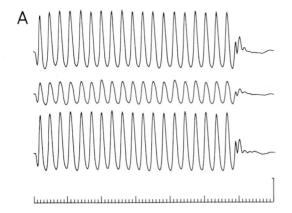

Fig. 2A. The voltage response of an IHC to a 340Hz tone burst at 93dBSPL, before (upper trace), during (middle trace) and after (lower trace) transient asphyxia when normal respiration had been restored. Horizontal scale; small division 1msec, large division 10msec; vertical scale 5mV. Each trace is an average of 8 sweeps

B. The relationship between the amplitude of the receptor potential recorded from an IHC, and SPL recorded at the tympanic membrane in response to a 180Hz tone at 90dBSPL during normal respiration (thick trace) and transient asphyxia (thin trace). Each curve is based on 192 samples of single cycle receptor potential and sound pressure waveforms. The amplitude of the receptor potential (vertical axis) is with reference to the membrane potential (-45mV), and the sign of the horizontal axis refers to the rarefaction phase of the sound pressure (positive) and its compression (negative). The phases of the acoustic waveform and receptor potentials were adjusted so that there was coincidence between their zero crossing phases during rarefaction. The curve measured during asphyxia (thin trace) is scaled up by a factor of 2. Inset: single traces of the receptor potential before (upper trace) and during (lower trace) transient asphyxia. Vertical bar: 10mV; Horizontal bar: 20msec

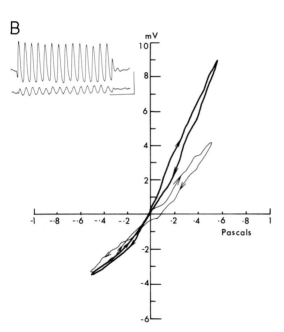

4. DISCUSSION

It is well known that transient asphyxia causes a reversible decrease in the EP, CM and CAP, and our findings that IHCs become slightly hyperpolarized is in agreement with those of Brown et.al. (1983). The relative size of the hyperpolarization may be an indication that the leakage conductance of the apical membrane of IHC is less than that of the lateral and basal membranes.

The decrease in driving voltage across the apical membranes of the IHCs during asphyxia, will presumably influence the post synaptic responses of the afferent fibres, resulting in a decrease in the N_1 component of the CAP. However, the close correlation, in time and amplitude, of the decline in the DC receptor potential and N_1 response, during transient asphyxia, reinforces the concept that the DC component is directly responsible for exciting the afferent nerve fibres during high frequency acoustic stimulation, presumably by providing the control voltage for the release of the afferent transmitter (Russell & Sellick, 1978;

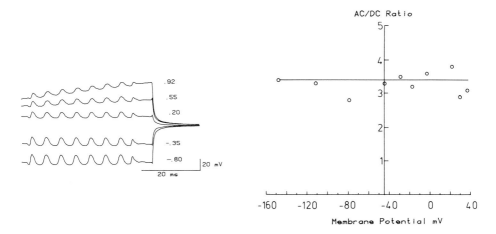

Fig. 3. *The relationship between the AC/DC ratio of the voltage response of an*
IHC to low frequency tones, and the membrane potential. The line is the mean
value of the points. The numbers adjacent to the records are the currents in
nA which were injected to produce the observed membrane potentials. Each trace
is a single sweep. Stimulus tone: 200Hz at 86dB

1983). The decline in the DC component is attributed to the increased symmetry of
the IHC receptor potential which was observed in response to low frequency tones
(Figure 2). The receptor potentials of the hair cells to tones close to their CF
were similarly effected during asphyxia in that the DC component was reduced to a
greater extent than the AC component, and it is tempting to suggest that this is
because the transduction process at high frequencies also becomes more symmetrical
during asphyxia.

The decrease in the amplitude of the IHC receptor potential might be expected
as a consequence of the drop in driving potential across the apical membrane of
the IHC membrane during asphyxia, but the increased symmetry of the IHC receptor
potential does not appear to be due to some voltage dependent property of the IHC
(Figure 3). Neither is it likely to be due to a redistribution of the transducer
conductances, because the resting potential of the IHC is changed only slightly
during asphyxia. Phase measurements reveal that, during asphyxia, the stereocilia
are still coupled to the viscous drag of fluid in the subtectorial space and
respond to basilar membrane velocity during low frequency tones (Russell,
unpublished). However, the change in symmetry of the waveform during asphyxia is
associated with a desensitization and loss of frequency selectivity in the IHCs
(Brown et.al. 1983), and there is evidence that the frequency selective properties
of IHCs are determined by their mechanical input (Russell & Sellick, 1978;
Sellick, Patuzzi and Johnstone, 1982). Thus it is proposed that the change in
symmetry of the IHC receptor potential is due to a change in their mechanical
input.

A mechanism producing the receptor potential asymmetry may arise from the
coupling of the outer hair cell (OHC) stereocilia to the tectorial membrane (TM).
According to Lim (1980), the OHC stereocilia may be embedded in the TM since
corresponding pits are seen in scanning electron microscopy of the underside of
the TM. The stereocilia of the IHC do not show the same coupling and may even be
velocity coupled up to at least 700Hz (Sellick & Russell, 1980; Russell & Sellick,
1983). Any resistance offered to relative motion of the TM by the OHC stereocilia
would be expected to modify the free motion of the TM required in the Davis's
classical model of cochlear excitation (Davis, 1958), and produce a force in the
radial direction tending to bend the TM when the basilar membrane moves towards
the SM. However when the basilar membrane moves away from SM, the geometry of the

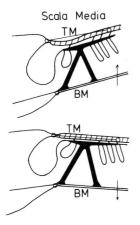
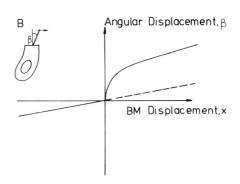

Fig. 4. *Proposed mechanism to explain symmetrization of the IHC receptor potentials during asphyxia. A, schematic organ of Corti showing bending of the TM when the BM is displaced towards the scala media. Thin line shows the position of the TM in the absence of a force produced by OHC coupling. B, angular displacement of the IHC stereocilia predicted by model. Dotted line shows effect of reducing the bending force to zero. The effect would produce a symmetrization of the IHC stimulus, and hence the receptor potentials*

shear displacement at the IHC would be that suggested by Davis, (Figure 4).
    Although little is now known about the mechanical parameters of the TM, each radial section of the membrane can be considered in the first approximation as a section undergoing Euler deformation and it may be noted that a significant asymmetry can be generated at least qualitatively. The midpoint of such a section would buckle and reduce the subtectorial spacing by an amount $d=kl^{\frac{1}{2}}x^{\frac{1}{2}}$ when the BM displacement towards SM is x, l is the width of the tectorial membrane and k is a geometric factor of order unity determined by the dimensions of the cochlear partition. The additional deflection angle of the IHC stereocilia would be - $(d/h)^{\frac{1}{2}}$ where h is the length of the stereocilia if the hairs were deflected so as to be accommodated in the subtectorial space. It might be expected that this geometric argument might be modified by taking into account viscous forces acting on the IHC during a stimulus cycle.
    Thus in this model, the angular displacement of the IHC stereocilia, β would be $x+Ax^{\frac{1}{4}}$ for motion towards the scala media, and x for displacement of the BM away from SM up to a numerical factor of close to 1 which depends on the lever advantage afforded by the geometry of the organ of Corti. $A=k(l/h)^{\frac{1}{2}}$ is a numerical factor equal to about 4 from measurements of the guinea pig cochlea. The predicted form of the transfer function is shown in Figure 4, where it is seen that the motion of the IHC stereocilia is essentially linear in the direction which leads to a hyperpolarization of the IHC. Although the three dimensional geometry of the organ of Corti would be expected to modify this behaviour, (in particular by smoothing the discontinuity in the angular displacement around the null point x=0), it is seen that bending of the tectorial membrane could give rise to the asymmetry of the inner hair cell receptor potentials.
    Any manipulations which reduced the bending force in the radial plane of the tectorial membrane would also tend to symmetrize the inner hair cell potentials, and produce a linear transfer characteristic of the type shown in Figure 4. It may be suggested that asphyxia reduces this force, possibly by reducing the stiffness of the stereocilia of the outer hair cells. No recordings have yet been reported from inner hair cells in animals that have been subjected to loud sounds or ototoxic drugs, both of which are known to produce damage to outer hair cells

(Spoendlin, 1971, Dallos, 1973), but it is probably that the observed loss of threshold observed in the auditory nerve may be associated with the same mechanism of symmetrization of the IHC receptor potentials as seen in the present studies.

Acknowledgement: We thank Mrs. E.M. Cowley for excellent technical assistance and Miss J. Harper for carefully typing the manuscript. This work was supported by grants from the M.R.C.

REFERENCES

Brown, M.C., Nuttall, A.L., Masta, R.I., Lawrence, M. (1983). Cochlear inner hair cells: effects of transient asphyxia on intracellular potentials. *Hearing Res.* (In press).
Dallos, P. (1973). Cochlear potentials and cochlear mechanics. In: *Basic Mechanisms in Hearing*, Ed. A. Møller, pp 335 - 372. Academic Press, New York and London.
Davis, H. (1958). Transmission and transduction in the cochlea. *Laryngoscope* 68, 359 - 382.
Evans, E.F. (1979). Neuroleptanaesthesia for guinea pigs. *Arch. Otolaringol.* 83, 85 - 91.
Lim, D.J. (1980). Cochlear anatomy related to cochlear micromechanics. A review. *J. Acoust. Soc. Am.* 67, 1686 - 1695.
Robertson, B., Manley, G.A. (1974). Manipulation of frequency analysis in the cochlear ganglion of the guinea pig. *J. Comp. Physiol.* 91, 363 - 375.
Russell, I.J. (1983). The origin of the receptor potential in inner hair cells of the mammalian cochlea. Evidence for Davis' theory. *Nature* 301, 334 - 336.
Russell, I.J., Sellick, P.M. (1978). Intracellular studies of hair cells in the mammalian cochlea. *J. Physiol. (Lond.).* 284, 261 - 290.
Russell, I.J., Sellick, P.M. (1983). Low frequency characteristics of intra-cellularly recorded receptor potentials in guinea pig cochlear hair cells. *J. Physiol. (Lond.).* (In press).
Sellick, P.M., Russell, I.J. (1980). The responses of inner hair cells to basilar membrane velocity during low frequency auditory stimulation in the guinea pig cochlea. *Hearing Res.* 2, 439 - 445.
Sellick, P.M., Patuzzi, R., Johnstone, B.M. (1982). Measurement of basilar membrane motion in the guinea pig using the Mössbauer technique. *J. acoust. soc. Am.* 72, 131 - 141.
Spoendlin, H. (1971). Primary structural changes in the organ of Corti after acoustic overstimulation. *Otolaryngol.* 71, 166 - 176.

GENERAL DISCUSSION

KLINKE:
As you know we have shown (Göttl and Klinke, INSERM 68, 103, 1977) that during anoxia positive and negative going portions of CM behave differentially in that CM^- disappears soon whereas CM^+ may initially even increase (thus leaving CM_{p-p} unchanged). Is there any correlate between this behaviour and your intra-cellular recordings?

RUSSELL:
We did not attempt to correlate our findings with your observation on the changes in CM^- and CM^+ during anoxia. Our observations were confined to the responses of inner hair cells, and not to those of the outer hair cells which are relevant to your studies.

PICKLES:
Your comments on the effects of hypoxia on the nonlinearity concern frequencies well below the characteristic frequency. Do you have any evidence on the effects near the CF, where the nonlinearity may be different and have a particularly in-teresting nature?

RUSSELL:
At very high frequencies, the properties of the transfer functions of cochlear hair cells cannot be measured with intracellular microelectrodes. We observed changes in response amplitude-stimulus intensity curves for AC and DC receptor potentials close to the characteristic frequencies of the inner hair cells. They were shifted to higher values along the intensity axis, their slopes increased from 1 to about 2 and they showed no tendency to saturate within the stimulus intensities used (30-80 dB SPL).

R.S. LEWIS:
As I am sure you are aware, measurements made on bullfrog saccular hair cells have shown that the displacement-response relation in these cells is inherently asymmetric and nonlinear. Do you have evidence that a similar relation does not apply for cochlear inner hair cells? If it does, a symmetric decrease in displacement acting on this asymmetric relation could produce an asymmetric change in the hyperpolarizing and depolarizing phases of the receptor potential which you observe under anoxic conditions, or anoxia could act on this relation directly.

RUSSELL:
We have no direct measurement of the displacement-response relationships for cochlear inner hair cells. However, at low stimulus frequencies the receptor potentials are symmetrical but become asymmetrical when the stimulus frequency exceeds about 120 Hz. Above this frequency, the asymmetry is apparent in low level responses where the amplitude scales with sound pressure level. Thus we propose that the asymmetry is produced by a mechanism which precedes movement of the inner hair cell stereocilia, and it is this, and not the inner hair cell displacement-response relationship which is changed by anoxia.

DALLOS:
The hyperpolarization of inner hair cells (IHC) during transient asphyxia was also seen by us, as well as by Brown et al. (Hear. Res. 9, 131, 1977). We have also observed a similar change in the membrane potentials of Hensen's cells. These alterations may be due, for the most part, to the reduction in the endocochlear potential, and are predicted by the model that I described during this conference. Thus assuming that EP is reduced to +30 mV, that E_1 is unchanged, and that the shape factor for IHC is 0.32, one predicts with the aid of Eq. 6 of my paper a hyperpolarization of approximately 10 mV. The model does not predict a linearization of the response which is likely due to alterations in micromechanics, as the authors suggest.

EVANS:
Can you further clarify the role played by changes in the EP caused by anoxia: could it have an indirect effect?

RUSSELL:
Changes in the EP are likely to have an indirect effect. For example, associated with a drop in the EP, changes in the ionic composition of the endolymph may alter the physical properties of the tectorial membrane. Alternatively the decline in the EP may influence the mechanical properties of the outer hair cell stereocilia and thereby cause a change in their coupling to the tectorial membrane.

JOHNSTONE:
Anoxia probably causes osmotic unbalance in scala media, as well as altering the endocochlear potential. There is certainly a sodium entry and although it is small, it is enough to cause a water entry into scala media and so a pressure increase. This in turn will alter basilar membrane mechanics. Unfortunately anoxia is a very poor tool to use to investigate the effects of EP change.

FREQUENCY TUNING AND IONIC CONDUCTANCES
IN HAIR CELLS OF THE BULLFROG'S SACCULUS

R. S. Lewis and A. J. Hudspeth

Division of Biology, California Institute of Technology
Pasadena, California 91125, USA

1. INTRODUCTION

An important function of the peripheral auditory system is the resolution of complex sounds into their constituent frequency components. The responses of individual nerve fibers and hair cells (Russell and Sellick, 1978; Crawford and Fettiplace, 1980) in the auditory organs of several species show extremely sharp selectivity for particular frequencies. There is currently much debate over the mechanisms that determine this selectivity, or tuning, particularly for frequencies close to the characteristic frequency, or CF (Dallos, 1981). In the cochleas of some species it appears that the sharpness of tuning results from processes that maximize mechanical input to the hair cells. In the turtle's cochlea, however, an electrical resonance in the hair cell may supplement the mechanical properties of the organ in conferring sharp frequency selectivity at the CF, by maximizing the cell's response to sound of frequencies near the resonant frequency (Crawford and Fettiplace, 1981).

We present here preliminary evidence that hair cells in the bullfrog's sacculus are also maximally sensitive to particular frequencies of mechanical input, and that the underlying mechanism is, as for the turtle, most likely electrical in nature. Using gigohm-seal-electrode recording techniques on hair cells enzymatically isolated from the sacculus, we have identified three voltage- and ion-dependent conductances that may contribute to the electrical tuning mechanism (Lewis, 1982).

2. METHODS

(a) Microelectrode recordings from hair cells in the excised sacculus. The saccular macula of the bullfrog, *Rana catesbeiana*, was dissected and mounted in an experimental chamber that allows independent superfusion of the two epithelial surfaces. The otolithic membrane was loosened by exposing the upper surface of the preparation for one hour at 25°C to 30 μg/ml subtilopeptidase BPN' in a solution containing (in mM) 110 Na, 2 K, 4 Ca, 118 Cl, 3 D-glucose, and 5 HEPES (pH 7.2). After the otolithic membrane was removed by gentle dissection, the preparation was maintained in an identical saline medium without enzyme. Stimuli were applied to each hair bundle by sucking the bulbous tip of its kinocilium into a heat-polished capillary approximately 1 μm in internal diameter. This probe was moved by a piezoelectric stimulator (Corey and Hudspeth, 1980) whose displacement output was essentially linear and flat with frequency up to 760 Hz. Intracellular recording was conducted at 20-22°C with microelectrodes having resistances greater than 300 megohms; cells impaled with lower-resistance electrodes in general produced oscillations of smaller amplitude, lower frequency, and more phasic character.

(b) Gigohm-seal-electrode recordings from solitary hair cells. Excised sacculi were treated with a solution containing papain and were scraped with a sharpened needle to dissociate individual hair cells, as described in detail elsewhere (Lewis and Hudspeth, 1983). Recordings were made at 20-22°C in a solution containing (in mM) 120 Na, 2 K, 4 Ca, 128 Cl, 3 D-glucose, and 5 HEPES (pH 7.2). In some experiments, tetraethylammonium ion (TEA) or 4-aminopyridine (4-AP) replaced an equal amount of Na, or Mg an equal amount of Ca. Whole-cell recordings were made using heat-polished glass pipettes which contained (in mM) 126 K or Cs, 1 Ca,

2 Mg, 120 aspartate, 6 Cl, 3 D-glucose, 2 EGTA, and 5 HEPES (pH 7.2), with 10^{-7} M free Ca. Isolated cells formed seals of 1-20 gigohms' shunt resistance with the pipette tips, which had internal diameters of 1-2 μm. Slight suction was applied to rupture the patch of membrane under the tip, and the cells were current- or voltage-clamped through the pipette (Hamill *et al.*, 1981). Data were digitized and averaged with a computer (Fig. 3) or were recorded and reproduced as single traces with an FM tape recorder (other Figures).

3. RESULTS

(a) Frequency selectivity and electrical oscillations in saccular hair cells.
Fig. 1A shows the receptor potential of a hair cell in response to constant-amplitude, sinusoidal deflections of the hair bundle, delivered as a linear frequency sweep from 13 to 163 Hz. The cell responded best at 120 Hz, its CF. Because the amplitude of hair-bundle motion was constant, the frequency selectivity observed in this experiment evidently arose from some mechanism other than a mechanical resonance in the sacculus.

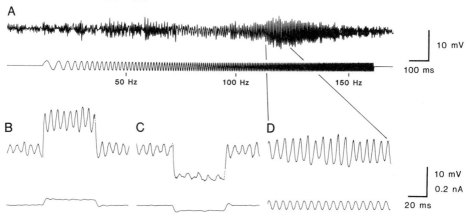

Fig. 1. Recordings from a hair cell in the excised saccular macula, made with a conventional intracellular microelectrode. A, Stimulation of the hair bundle with ±0.03-μm deflections in a frequency sweep (lower trace) evoked a maximal receptor potential (upper trace) at 120 Hz, with a secondary peak at about half that frequency. Note the spontaneous oscillations before and after the frequency sweep. B, Depolarization of the cell by injection of a constant-current pulse (lower trace) increased the frequency of voltage oscillations (upper trace) to 140 Hz from the spontaneous rate of 125 Hz at resting potential (-68 mV). C, Hyperpolarizing current conversely lowered the oscillation frequency to 91 Hz. D, A segment of the cell's response to the frequency sweep near the CF in A, displayed on a faster time scale. Note that the CF of the cell's response to mechanical stimulation is near the frequency of spontaneous oscillation in B and C

It seems likely instead that an electrical resonance in the hair cell forms the basis of the tuning mechanism. The resonance is manifested either as spontaneous voltage fluctuations at the resting potential (Figs. 1B and C) or as voltage oscillations evoked by the injection of small current pulses (Fig. 2B). Because similar oscillatory behavior occurred in cells lacking hair bundles entirely, this phenomenon is not dependent on the transduction process. The oscillation frequency is voltage-dependent, increasing with depolarization. This is shown in Figs. 1B and C, in which pulses of de- or hyperpolarizing current injected into the cell increased or decreased the oscillation frequency. The cell shown in Fig. 1 oscillated spontaneously at 125 Hz at a resting potential of -68 mV. This frequency is close to the CF of the cell measured during mechanical stimulation at the same potential (Fig. 1D), a result that would be expected if the electrical resonance were responsible for the frequency selectivity of the cell's response to mechanical stimuli. Moreover, the CF changed in parallel with the oscillation frequency when the cell was de- or hyperpolarized by injection of constant current. These observations support the hypothesis that an electrical mechanism determines the frequency selectivity to mechanical stimuli in these cells.

(b) Electrical oscillations in solitary saccular hair cells. The following experiments were designed to investigate the biophysical mechanism of the electrical resonance in hair cells. In order to achieve high temporal resolution in voltage-clamp experiments and to gain relatively unrestricted access of test solutions to the interior and exterior membrane surfaces of the cells, we employed gigohm-seal-electrode recording techniques to study enzymatically dissociated hair cells. A solitary cell is shown in contact with a recording pipette in Fig. 2A. Many of the isolated cells displayed oscillatory responses to current injection (Fig. 2B) similar to those recorded with microelectrodes from cells in the excised sacculus. In 20 cells that clearly showed such behavior, oscillation frequencies ranged from 80 to 160 Hz at resting potentials of -58 to -65 mV. Occasional cells that had lost their hair bundles during the isolation procedure also displayed an ability to oscillate, again demonstrating that an intact transduction apparatus is not necessary to produce this behavior.

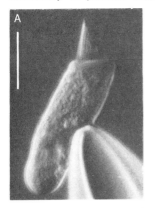

Fig. 2. Voltage oscillations in a solitary hair cell. A, Differential-interference-contrast micrograph of a solitary hair cell from the bullfrog's sacculus, in contact with the tip of a recording pipette. The bar represents 10 μm. B, Injecting a small depolarizing current (lower trace) evoked membrane-potential oscillations in a solitary cell (upper trace). Oscillation frequency increased with depolarization; here it was 195 Hz during the pulse and 137 Hz at the resting potential of -62 mV

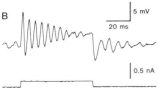

(c) Voltage- and ion-dependent conductances in solitary saccular hair cells. Under voltage-clamp conditions, three specific ionic currents could be elicited by depolarization in over 90% of the solitary hair cells that were studied. Each of these conductances was isolated and characterized by its ion and voltage dependences and its pharmacological sensitivity. The three conductance mechanisms are more completely described elsewhere (Lewis and Hudspeth, 1983); here we will emphasize their characteristics relevant to the issue of electrical resonance

I. Calcium current. The substitution of Cs for the cell's internal K blocks outward K currents that are produced by depolarization, leaving a sustained inward current that is activated at potentials more positive than -60 to -55 mV (Fig. 3A). Based on characteristics that it shares with the Ca currents of other preparations (Hagiwara and Byerly, 1981), we have identified this as a Ca current. A significant feature of the current is that it does not inactivate appreciably during prolonged depolarizations. This characteristic, together with its activity at potentials close the the resting potential, suggests that the Ca current functions in the tonic release of transmitter from hair cells onto afferent nerve fibers (Sand *et al.*, 1975).

II. Transient K current (A current). When hair cells are depolarized to potentials more positive than about -50 mV from holding potentials more negative than -60 mV, a transient, outward K current results which is similar in several respects to the A current described in molluscan neurons (Connor and Stevens, 1971). It is the only current we have observed routinely in hair cells that rapidly inactivates as a function of membrane voltage. This characteristic, along with the current's insensitivity to external TEA, can be used to isolate the A current from

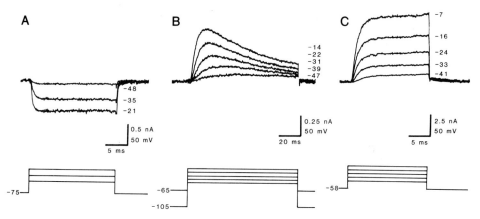

Fig. 3. *Voltage-clamp recordings from solitary hair cells, showing the three ionic currents. In each panel the upper set of traces shows membrane current and the lower set represents command voltage. To the right of each current trace is the corresponding command voltage in millivolts; the holding potential in milli- volts is to the left of the voltage command in each panel. A, Ca current, record- ed with 126 mM Cs in the pipette to block outward K currents. Averages of five presentations. B, Transient K current (A current). With 20 mM TEA blocking the Ca-activated K current, a series of voltage steps was applied to the cell from holding potentials of -65 or -105 mV. At -65 mV, about 95% of the A current is inactivated at steady-state, and the voltage steps elicited primarily Ca current. At -105 mV the A current's inactivation is removed, and the voltage steps elicited the sum of Ca and A currents. Subtracting the former set of currents from the latter isolated the A current from the Ca current. Averages of four presenta- tions. C, Ca-activated K current. These responses were obtained by subtracting the currents produced by voltage steps in the presence of 20 mM TEA (a fully blocking concentration) from those produced in its absence. Averages of two presentations. Note the different current scale used here*

the Ca and Ca-activated K currents (Fig. 3B). The A current is not abolished by divalent cations that block the Ca and Ca-activated K currents, but is blocked by 10 mM 4-AP.

III. Ca-activated K current. The largest current in the hair cell, occurring at potentials more positive than -60 to -45 mV, is an outward K current that is ac- tivated by intracellular Ca ions. It can be isolated using its sensitivity to TEA (Fig. 3C), which specifically blocks the Ca-dependent outward current in these cells. The Ca-activated K current is abolished by external agents or conditions that suppress the hair cell's Ca current, suggesting that this K current is depen- dent on Ca ions that have entered the cell through Ca channels. In addition, lowering external Ca from 4 to 0.5 mM (with Mg substitution) slows the kinetics and lowers the steady-state magnitude of this current.

(d) Effects on oscillatory behavior of conditions that alter the voltage- and ion- dependent currents. If the three currents described above interact to generate electrical resonance, then conditions that change the magnitude or kinetics of the currents should also affect resonant behavior. Fig. 4 shows the effects of sever- al such conditions on the voltage oscillations produced in a solitary hair cell by an applied current step. In normal saline, the cell's voltage oscillated during the step at a frequency of 196 Hz, with a maximum peak-to-peak amplitude of 10 mV (Fig. 4A). External TEA at 1 mM, a level that blocks about half of the Ca-activa- ted K current, partially suppressed the oscillations (Fig. 4B). Lowering external Ca to 0.5 mM, which diminishes the Ca current and slows and reduces the Ca-acti- vated K current, also decreased the amplitude of the oscillations (Fig. 4C). While the low-Ca condition depolarized this cell by 9 mV, similar results were obtained

in cells that were not depolarized by low Ca. In contrast, exposure to 10 mM 4-AP, a treatment that specifically blocks the A current, had little or no effect on oscillations (Fig. 4D). The changes produced by the different treatments were reversible (Fig. 4E).

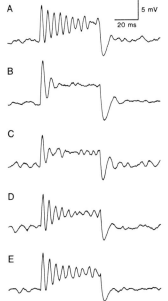

A

B

C

D

E

Fig. 4. Effects of various external conditions on voltage oscillations in a solitary hair cell. This cell was stimulated with a 50-ms, 0.17-nA current pulse in different external solutions in the order shown. Resting potentials (RP) are noted in parentheses. A, Control (saline containing 4 mM Ca). The current evoked large voltage oscillations in the cell (RP=-64 mV). B, 1 mM TEA, which blocks about half of the Ca-activated K current, partially suppressed the oscillations (RP=-61 mV). C, Lowering Ca to 0.5 mM, with 3.5 mM Mg added, also reduced oscillatory activity. This condition diminishes both the Ca and Ca-activated K currents (RP=-55 mV). D, 10 mM 4-AP, which blocks the A current, had little or no effect on the oscillations (RP=-62 mV). E, A normal oscillatory response was elicited after returning the cell to control conditions (RP=-64 mV)

4. DISCUSSION

We have shown that hair cells in the excised bullfrog's sacculus are selective for particular frequencies of controlled mechanical input. There are several reasons to suppose that the mechanism involved in this selectivity is electrical in nature. First, tuning was demonstrated by deflecting the hair bundles directly with a suction probe. This stimulation technique bypasses most of the mechanical components of the sacculus that might contribute to mechanical resonance in the system. Second, an electrical resonance tuned to the mechanical CF was observed in these hair cells as manifested by spontaneous or current-induced voltage oscillations at resting potential. This behavior resembles that observed in hair cells of the turtle's cochlea, whose tuning to auditory stimuli results in part from similar electrical properties (Crawford and Fettiplace, 1980, 1981). Third, membrane polarization induced by current injection increased or decreased the CF of cells in parallel with the frequency of electrical oscillations.

Solitary hair cells, which also display oscillatory behavior, possess three voltage- and ion-dependent conductance mechanisms: a noninactivating Ca conductance, an A conductance, and a Ca-activated K conductance. Although the A conductance is largely inactivated at resting potential and therefore may not contribute significantly to generating oscillations, there is evidence that the Ca and Ca-activated K currents play a role. First, they are activated in the same voltage range in which oscillations occur. In addition, their activation becomes more rapid with increasing levels of depolarization, which is consistent with the voltage dependence of oscillation frequency. Finally, conditions which interfere with the Ca and Ca-activated K currents suppress the oscillatory behavior.

Since oscillations occur in hair cells without hair bundles, modulation of the transduction conductance is not necessary to produce oscillatory activity. It remains possible, however, that frequency tuning is enhanced in intact preparations by interactions between the transducer and the electrical resonance mechanism (Weiss, 1982). While an intact efferent innervation is also not required for oscillations to occur in solitary hair cells, postsynaptic conductances associated with the efferent system may contribute to electrical resonance.

Several properties of the hair cell's Ca-activated K current are interesting in view of its probable role in the resonance mechanism. It is activated 10-100 times as rapidly as Ca-activated K currents in other preparations (Meech, 1978), which may permit its participation in oscillatory phenomena usually mediated by fast, voltage-dependent currents. Furthermore, the hair cell's Ca-activated K channel, like those in other preparations (Barrett *et al.*, 1982), may be sensitive to both voltage and the internal level of free Ca. If so, there are two partially independent means of controlling the current's activity in the cell. Such a dual control mechanism could have important consequences for determining the characteristic frequency of a hair cell and for regulating resonant properties in response to stimulation of the efferent innervation.

Acknowledgments: We thank R. Jacobs for technical assistance and R. A. Eatock and T. Holton for helpful comments on the manuscript. This work was supported by the System Development Foundation and by National Institutes of Health grants NS13154 and GM07737. The authors' present address is: Department of Physiology, University of California School of Medicine, San Francisco, California 94143, USA.

REFERENCES

Barrett, J. N., Magleby, K. L., Pallotta, B. S. (1982). Properties of single calcium-activated potassium channels in cultured rat muscle. *J. Physiol.* 331, 211-230.
Connor, J. A., Stevens, C. F. (1971). Voltage clamp studies of a transient outward membrane current in gastropod neural somata. *J. Physiol.* 213, 21-30.
Corey, D. P., Hudspeth, A. J. (1980). Mechanical stimulation and micromanipulation with piezoelectric bimorph elements. *J. Neurosci. Meth.* 3, 183-202.
Crawford, A. C., Fettiplace, R. (1980). The frequency selectivity of auditory nerve fibres and hair cells in the cochlea of the turtle. *J. Physiol.* 306, 79-125.
Crawford, A. C., Fettiplace, R. (1981). An electrical tuning mechanism in turtle cochlear hair cells. *J. Physiol.* 312, 377-412.
Dallos, P. (1981). Cochlear physiology. *Annu. Rev. Psychol.* 32, 153-190.
Hagiwara, S., Byerly, L. (1981). Calcium channel. *Annu. Rev. Neurosci.* 4, 69-125.
Hamill, O. P., Marty, A., Neher, E., Sakmann, B., Sigworth, F. J. (1981). Improved patch-clamp techniques for high-resolution current recording from cells and cell-free membrane patches. *Pflügers Arch.* 391, 85-100.
Lewis, R. S. (1982). Characterization of voltage- and ion-dependent conductances in vertebrate hair cells. *Soc. Neurosci. Abstr.* 8, 728.
Lewis, R. S., Hudspeth, A. J. (1983). Voltage- and ion-dependent conductances in solitary vertebrate hair cells. Submitted for publication.
Meech, R. W. (1978). Calcium-dependent potassium activation in nervous tissues. *Annu. Rev. Biophys. Bioeng.* 7, 1-18.
Russell, I. J., Sellick, P. M. (1978). Intracellular studies of hair cells in the mammalian cochlea. *J. Physiol.* 284, 261-290.
Sand, O., Ozawa, S., Hagiwara, S. (1975). Electrical and mechanical stimulation of hair cells in the mudpuppy. *J. Comp. Physiol. A* 102, 13-26.
Weiss, T. F. (1982). Bidirectional transduction in vertebrate hair cells: a mechanism for coupling mechanical and electrical processes. *Hearing Res.* 7, 353-360.

GENERAL DISCUSSION

ASHMORE:
Your finding of cells tuned to frequencies around 130 Hz differs from results I have reported in saccular hair cells of R. pipiens (J. Physiol. 336, 24P, 1983). The cells of this preparation show spontaneous oscillations in the range 11-59 Hz at the resting potential and ringing responses characteristic of an electrical resonance. I have also found that best frequencies of the cells are found in this frequency range and match a peak in the amplitude spectrum of the noise.

R.S. LEWIS:
There may not be a significant difference between the tuning properties of saccular hair cells of these two species. We have recorded from bullfrog hair cells that are tuned to mechanical stimuli of about 20 to 150 Hz at resting potential.

However, we cannot say at present whether this range of CFs corresponds to those that would be present in saccular hair cells in vivo, because we commonly found that measured CFs, as well as the frequency of spontaneous or current-evoked oscillations, decreased with time after the start of recordings and were in general lower when lower resistance (<300 Megohm) electrodes were used.

MANLEY:
Your finding of voltage oscillations in sacculus hair cells is interesting. I have reported the presence of preferred intervals in the spontaneous activity in bird cochlear ganglion units of CF below about 900 Hz which may be traceable to such voltage noise in hair cells (Naturwiss. 66, 582, 1979). We subsequently reported similar spontaneous activity patterns in lizard fibres (Eatock et al., J. Comp. Physiol. 142, 203, 1980).

ASHMORE:
Do you have information about whether use of the enzymes papain and subtilopeptidase to prepare the cells affects the membrane channels? It could be that reduction of a channel population enzyme digestion significantly alters the cell's tuning properties.

R.S. LEWIS:
Subtilopeptidase applied to apical and basal surfaces of the saccular macula may decrease the hair cell's Ca^{++} current, as it seems to reduce the occurrence of Ca^{++} action potentials produced under conditions of high external Ca^{++} in these cells. For this reason, and because the Ca^{++} channels are probably localized to the hair-cell basal membrane, we confined this treatment to the apical surface. It is possible that exposure to papain reduces ionic currents in hair cells, since isolated cells did not spontaneously oscillate as frequently as those in excised sacculus. On the other hand, mechanical stresses applied to the cell during the isolation procedure, as well as possible effects of internal perfusion through the gigohm-seal pipette, could produce this result. The important point for this study is that the isolated cells show resonant behaviour similar to that observed in cells in the sacculus and therefore can be used to investigate the biophysical basis of the electrical resonance.

WILSON:
Did I understand you correctly that you can find hair cell tuning under conditions where the possibility of mechanical feedback has been eliminated?

R.S. LEWIS:
Not exactly. Our stimulation technique controls hair bundle motion at the bulb of the kinocilium. If electromechanical feedback acts on the stereocilia to change their mechanical properties (Kim, Hear. Res. 2, 297, 1980; Weiss, Hear. Res. 7, 353, 1982; Flock, this volume) we may not be controlling the mechanical input to the transduction apparatus at a subcellular level. Our results do implicate an electrical resonance in determining the tuning to mechanical stimuli in these cells. However, the question remains as to whether this tuning can be accounted for quantitatively by an electrical resonance in series with the mechanical transduction process, or whether these two systems must also be coupled through electromechanical feedback.

KIM:
I have two questions and a comment. Is the spontaneous oscillation of HC membrane potential affected in any way when the end bulb of the kinocilium was sucked into the stimulating probe? I wonder whether rigidly holding the hair bundle, thereby preventing any possible mechanical oscillation, affects the electrical oscillation. This information should be helpful in evaluating the hypothesis of a bidirectional HC transduction (see comment of Kim on paper by Fuchs et al.). Is there any difference in the spontaneous oscillation behaviour depending upon the location of the HC within the saccule? My comment is that occurrence of spontaneous electrical oscillation in HC without the hair bundle is not evidence against the hypothesis of a bidirectional transduction. This is because an electrical oscillation signal, even if generated by an exclusively electrical mechanism, may still be reverse transduced in to a mechanical oscillation of the hair bundle in a normal HC.

R.S. LEWIS:
Although we have not analyzed this in detail, attaching the stimulating probe to
the hair bundle has no obvious effect on spontaneous voltage oscillations. An
example of this can be seen by comparing the oscillations occurring before the
frequency sweep in Fig. 1A (probe attached) with those occurring in the same
cell before current injection in Fig. 1B (probe removed). As I mentioned in the
talk, the observation of the electrical oscillations in cells lacking hair bundles does not absolutely rule out operation of a "bidirectional transduction"
mechanism (Weiss, 1982) in intact saccular hair cells. However, it does show
that spontaneous, sustained oscillations can result from an independent electrical resonance mechanism in the cell, and are not necessarily dependent on the
interaction of voltage- and mechano-sensitive systems as suggested by Weiss.
Furthermore, spontaneous oscillations in one cell lacking a hair bundle were
among the largest we have seen in any cell (12 mV peak-to-peak), which argues
against significant enhancement of oscillations by these proposed interactions
in saccular hair cells.
I cannot give a complete answer to your second question since in this report we
have studied only hair cells in the distal margin of the saccular macula, directly opposite the side of nerve insertion, or isolated hair cells whose original location in the macula was unknown, due to the dissociation procedure.

SYNAPTIC HYPERPOLARISATION AND LOSS OF
TUNING IN TURTLE COCHLEAR HAIR CELLS

P.A. Fuchs, R. Fettiplace, A.C. Crawford and J.J. Art

Physiological Laboratory, Cambridge CB2 3EG, U.K.

1. INTRODUCTION

Efferent inhibition of the vertebrate ear may provide an important clue to
the role of the hair cells in cochlear function. Via synapses on these cells,
the efferents are capable of both modifying auditory nerve tuning (Kiang *et al.*,
1970) and reducing acoustic distortion products attributed to changes in
cochlear mechanics (Mountain, 1980; Siegel & Kim, 1982). It is difficult to
interpret such complex effects without first understanding the post-synaptic
events in the hair cells. We describe here intracellular recordings from hair
cells in the turtle cochlea, where we have shown that efferent stimulation
generates hyperpolarising synaptic potentials and a concomitant loss of
frequency selectivity (Art *et al.*, 1982). The results to be presented indicate
that neither the synaptic hyperpolarisation nor the underlying conductance
change alone is the primary agent mediating efferent inhibition of tuning.

2. METHODS

The techniques for intracellular recording and current injection of cochlear
hair cells in the isolated half-head of adult *Pseudemys scripta elegans* were
similar to those employed previously (Crawford & Fettiplace, 1980). Sound stimuli
were generated by a dynamic earphone (Beyer DT48) connected through a coupler to
the external ear. After decapitation, the head was split in the midline, most of
the brain removed and the scala tympani opened from the cranial side. The
anterior and posterior roots of the VIIIth nerve were left attached to a piece of
medulla, but the remaining cranial nerves were severed at their foramina. The
efferent axons were stimulated with trains of constant current pulses (0.4 ms
duration, 20-200 μA) from platinum electrodes placed at the junction between the
two roots of the VIIIth nerve. It was possible to position the stimulating
electrodes so as to excite the efferents without simultaneous antidromic firing
of the afferents.
     Hair cell tuning curves were determined by measuring the fundamental compo-
nent of the receptor potential for continuous tones swept at constant intensity
from 20 Hz to 2 kHz (see Crawford & Fettiplace, 1980). Throughout alternate
frequency sweeps, the efferents were stimulated continually with single shocks
at 50/sec. For receptor potentials of a few millivolts, the form of the
isointensity tuning curve is independent of intensity (Crawford & Fettiplace,
1980); the frequency response of a hair cell may therefore be represented as a
linear sensitivity curve, where the amplitude of the receptor potential at each
frequency is scaled by the sound pressure.

3. RESULTS

(a) Synaptic hyperpolarisation and inhibition of the receptor potential. The
main features of efferent inhibition of a cochlear hair cell are shown in the
records of fig. 1. A train of eight shocks to the efferent axons generated a
slow hyperpolarisation of the membrane potential which had an average size of
15 mV for the cell illustrated. During a sequence of efferent stimuli, the
hyperpolarisation fluctuated in amplitude as might be expected from the probabilistic release of synaptic transmitter. Such fluctuations were most prominent
with stimulus trains comprising just a few shocks. The average hyperpolarisation

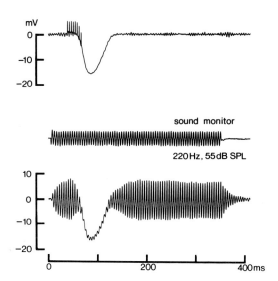

*Fig. 1. Average i.p.s.p.
resulting from 8 shocks
to efferents alone (top
trace) and in combination
with a CF tone burst
(bottom trace). Membrane
potentials on ordinates
are relative to resting
potential (-45 mV), and
timing of efferent
shocks indicated by
artefacts. About 55
responses were averaged
for each record but
this was insufficient
to remove narrow band CF
noise which is apparent
in top trace. Maximum
sound response 50 mV*

increased with shock number and in most cells attained a maximum value of 10 to
20 mV. Efferent hyperpolarising potentials of comparable size and shape have
also been recorded in hair cells of the lateral line (Flock & Russell, 1976) and
frog saccule (Ashmore & Russell, 1982).

The efferent hyperpolarisation could be reversed in polarity to become
depolarising with injection of steady currents which shifted the hair cell
membrane potential more negative than -80 mV (Art *et al.*, 1982). The reversal is
consistent with the efferents causing an increase in membrane conductance to ions
with an equilibrium potential negative to the resting potential. In this respect
the efferent hyperpolarisation resembles inhibitory post-synaptic potentials
(i.p.s.p.s) described in other neurones (Eccles, 1964).

Accompanying the i.p.s.p. was a reduction in the hair cell sensitivity for
tones at the cell's characteristic frequency (CF). With a CF tone of 220 Hz,
55 dB SPL, the hair cell of fig. 1 produced a receptor potential of 12 mV that was
attenuated by an order of magnitude to 1 mV at the tip of the i.p.s.p. The
desensitisation, maximal for low level CF tones, varied considerably in different
cells from a factor of 1.6 to 25. Such variation was related to the initial
sharpness of tuning of the receptor potential, and the largest efferent desensitisation achievable in a given cell was roughly proportional to the quality factor
(Q) of that cell's control tuning curve. This relationship between initial tuning
and loss of sensitivity is expected if the main action of the efferents is to
interfere with the hair cell tuning mechanism.

Two examples of efferent modification of hair cell tuning are illustrated in
fig. 2, the open symbols denoting the control curves. The efferents can be seen
to eliminate the most sensitive tip region and broaden the curves, so reducing the
quality factor of tuning. As an example, in the higher frequency cell, which had
a CF of 314 Hz, the initial Q_{3dB} of 25 was reduced during efferent stimulation to
about 1.0. The changes in the shape of the tuning curves induced by the efferents
can be summarised as follows: (i) around the CF a pronounced reduction in
sensitivity larger the more sharply tuned the cell; (ii) an enhancement of sensitivity at frequencies below about 0.7 CF; (iii) a superposition of the control
and inhibited curves in the high frequency region above CF. One further point
worth noting is that for all the tuning curves examined there was little change

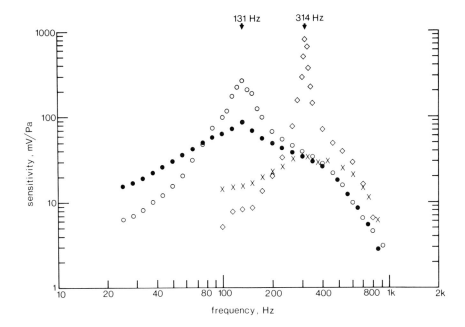

Fig. 2. Isointensity tuning curves for two hair cells in the same preparation in the absence (o,◇) and presence (●,×) of continual efferent stimulation at 50/sec. Sensitivity (r.m.s. voltage divided by sound pressure) is plotted against tone frequency for frequency sweeps at 45 dB SPL (controls) and 55 dB SPL (efferents). Mean synaptic hyperpolarisation in the lower and higher frequency cells was 5 mV and 8 mV respectively

in CF as far as this could be accurately measured. The lower frequency cell in fig. 2 provides a clear example, for the control and inhibited curves both have a CF at 131 Hz. The significance of the constancy of the hair cell's CF during efferent stimulation is discussed in the next section.

(b) Comparison of hyperpolarisation by efferents and current injection. A property of hair cell tuning in the turtle cochlea is that it can be modified by alterations in membrane potential (Crawford & Fettiplace, 1981). To examine whether membrane hyperpolarisation mediates the efferent inhibition, we compared the effects on tuning of current injection through the recording electrode and of efferent stimulation (fig. 3). To assay tuning, it was convenient to use brief acoustic clicks, the responses to which provide information about the tip of the tuning curve. The membrane potential change in a turtle hair cell to a low level click consists of an exponentially decaying oscillation at the CF of the cell. The quality factor (Q) of the tuning curve can be ascertained from the CF and the time constant of decay of these oscillations (Crawford & Fettiplace, 1980). The upper trace of fig. 3A illustrates the average click response of a hair cell with a CF of 328 Hz and a quality factor of 6.6. When the click was superimposed upon a current which hyperpolarised the membrane potential by about 11 mV (lower trace, fig. 3A), the oscillations of the click response were at a lower frequency and decayed more rapidly, indicating that the hyperpolarisation had reduced the tuning. The new CF and Q were 225 Hz and 2.3 respectively. Smaller hyperpolarising currents produced intermediate effects on the CF and Q, but it should be stressed that changes in membrane potential which gave a significant loss of tuning also substantially altered the CF.

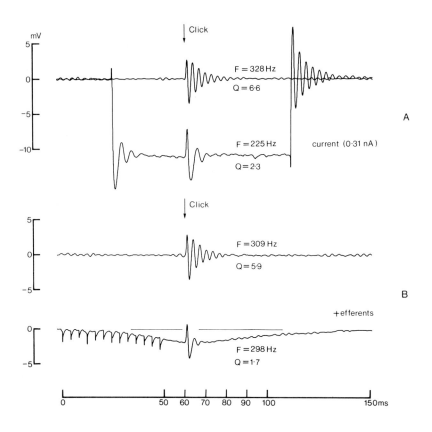

Fig. 3. *Efferent inhibition and extrinsic hyperpolarising current reduce hair cell tuning. A. Average click response in absence and presence of –0.31 nA current pulse, voltage drop in electrode balanced out. B. Click responses without and with efferent stimulation (shock artefacts filtered). Ordinate scales are relative to resting potential (–51 mV) and records are averages of 118–261 responses. Frequency (F) and quality factor (Q) of tuning given by each trace; during course of experiment, cell's control tuning deteriorated slightly. Click stimuli were rarefactions of intensity 7.8 × 10⁻⁵ Pa.s. Note that oscillations in the click response are slower with current than with efferents. Maximum i.p.s.p. in this cell was 12 mV*

The frequency selectivity of turtle hair cells is also revealed in the oscillations in membrane potential that occur at the beginning and end of a current pulse (Crawford & Fettiplace, 1981). From fig. 3, it may be noted that the oscillations at the current onset resemble the click response at the steady membrane potential during the current, whereas the oscillations at the termination of the current yield a CF and Q which are similar to those deduced from the control click. For a range of currents there was good agreement between the tuning characteristics derived from electrical and acoustic stimuli. This result confirms our previous conclusion that the tuning mechanism of turtle hair cells is intimately associated with their electrical properties (Crawford & Fettiplace, 1981).

The differential action of efferent inhibition and extrinsic current injection is emphasised in fig. 3B, which shows the inhibitory effect of a small

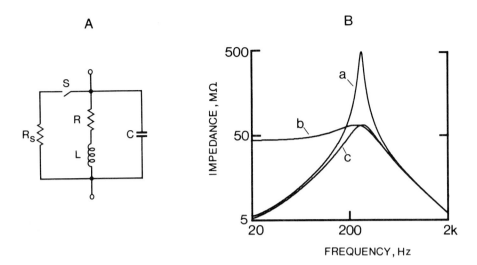

Fig. 4. A. *Equivalent circuit used to describe the electrical resonance in a
hair cell. With the switch, S, open, the circuit is tuned to a resonant
frequency, F, of $(4\pi^2 LC)^{-\frac{1}{2}}$ with a Q of $(L/R^2 C)^{\frac{1}{2}}$. The circuit may be damped
by increasing R or by switching in R_S, identified with the efferent synaptic
resistance.*
B. *Changes in the theoretical tuning curve produced by the two kinds of
damping. (a) Impedance of the equivalent circuit versus frequency in the
undamped condition with F = 263 Hz, Q = 10.9. Circuit parameters L = 27.8
kH, C = 13.2 pF, R = 4.2 MΩ. (b) The Q of the circuit is reduced to 1.0
by increasing R to 44.5 MΩ. Note the increase in low-frequency impedance.
(c) The Q is reduced from 10.9 to 1.5 by switching in a synaptic resistance
R_S of 78.5 MΩ. Note the impedance is reduced at all frequencies. The two
conditions of damping were chosen to yield the same suppression at the
resonant frequency*

efferent hyperpolarisation for the same cell as fig. 3A. Making use of the
fluctuations in response for a long series of efferent stimuli, we sorted the
i.p.s.p.s according to size and selected those hyperpolarisations of between 1
and 3 mV to produce the illustrated average. Although the mean hyperpolarisation
is only 2 mV, the alteration of tuning is dramatic: the Q is reduced from 5.9 to
1.7 by the i.p.s.p. while the change in CF is minimal (309 Hz to 298 Hz). In
similar experiments on four other cells, we found that an efferent hyperpolarisation of a few millivolts substantially reduced the quality factor of tuning
with less than ten percent reduction in CF. Comparison with extrinsic membrane
polarisation indicates that while both efferent and current hyperpolarisation
diminish the sharpness of tuning the processes involved are different. To achieve
a given reduction in quality factor, hyperpolarising current is associated with a
big drop in CF, and, in some cells, a relatively large change in membrane
potential. We conclude that the hyperpolarisation generated by stimulation of the
efferents is not primarily responsible for their ability to abolish hair cell
tuning.

4. DISCUSSION

The tuning mechanism of turtle cochlear hair cells can be approximately described as a simple resonance, which we have previously represented by an equivalent circuit composed of a capacitor in parallel with a series combination of an inductor and resistor (fig. 4A with the switch open). This circuit correctly predicts the form of the membrane potential change to both acoustic clicks and injected current steps if the maximum voltage excursions are only a few millivolts (Crawford & Fettiplace, 1981). The changes in hair cell tuning seen in fig. 2, which include loss of sensitivity at the CF and an augmentation at low frequencies, can be described solely by an increase in the series resistance of the equivalent circuit, causing a damping of the resonance. This single modification of the circuit cannot be simply equated with either the efferent synaptic hyperpolarisation or the underlying conductance change. As we have shown, direct hyperpolarisation is associated with a reduction in resonant frequency and would require an alteration in one of the circuit's reactive elements. The conductance alone may be eliminated by considering its effects on the circuit. If represented as a shunt conductance in parallel with the resonance (fig. 4A with the switch closed) it would result in a sensitivity loss at all frequencies, inconsistent with the observed low-frequency sensitisation. The theoretical effects of series and shunt damping on the tuning curve of a resonance with a CF of 263 Hz and a Q of 10.9 are illustrated in fig. 4B. Although some interaction between membrane voltage and conductance might still suffice to explain the inhibitory effects, it is clear that neither one alone can completely account for the efferent action on turtle cochlear hair cells.

Acknowledgements

This research was supported by a grant from the Medical Research Council and N.I.H. and NATO post-doctoral fellowships to J.J.A. and P.A.F. respectively.

REFERENCES

Art, J.J., Crawford, A.C., Fettiplace, R., Fuchs, P.A. (1982). Efferent regulation of hair cells in the turtle cochlea. *Proc. R. Soc. Lond B* 216, 377-384.

Ashmore, J.F., Russell, I.J. (1982). Effect of efferent nerve stimulation on hair cells of the frog sacculus. *J. Physiol.* 329, 25-26P.

Crawford, A.C., Fettiplace, R. (1980). The frequency selectivity of auditory nerve fibres and hair cells in the cochlea of the turtle. *J. Physiol.* 306, 79-125.

Crawford, A.C., Fettiplace, R. (1981). An electrical tuning mechanism in turtle cochlear hair cells. *J. Physiol.* 312, 377-412.

Eccles, J.C. (1964). *The Physiology of Synapses*. Berlin, Springer-Verlag.

Flock, A., Russell, I.J. (1976). Inhibition by efferent nerve fibres: action on hair cells and afferent synaptic transmission in the lateral line organ of the burbot, *Lota lota*. *J. Physiol.* 257, 45-62.

Kiang, N.Y.S., Moxon, E.C., Levine, R.A. (1970). Auditory nerve activity in cats with normal and abnormal cochleas. In: *Sensorineural Hearing Loss*. Eds. G.E.W. Wolstenholme and J. Knight, pp. 241-268, London, Churchill.

Mountain, D.C. (1980). Changes in endolymphatic potential and crossed olivo-cochlear bundle stimulation alter cochlear mechanics. *Science* 210, 71-72.

Siegel, J.H., Kim, D.O. (1982). Efferent neural control of cochlear mechanics? Olivocochlear bundle stimulation affects cochlear biomechanical non-linearity. *Hearing Res.* 6, 171-182.

GENERAL DISCUSSION

KIM:

The phenomenon of occurrence of lightly damped oscillations in the HC membrane potential in response to injections of electric currents (Fig. 3) does indeed indicate that "the tuning mechanism of turtle hair cells is intimately associated with their electrical properties". It is important to note, however, that this phenomenon is not evidence against the hypothesis of a bidirectional HC transduction (e.g. Kim, Hear. Res. 2, 297, 1980; Weiss, Hear. Res. 7, 353, 1982; Flock, this volume): stereocilia of a HC may indeed move when a HC is electrically stimulated, i.e. a "reverse" or electromechanical transduction may be present besides the familiar "forward" or mechano-electric transduction. In mammals, it has been demonstrated (Mountain, Siegel and Kim, Hear. Res. 6, 171, 1982) that stimulation of the efferent nerve exerts a mechanical influence in the cochlea most likely through activation of the efferent synapses at the outer hair cells. This supports the hypothesis of a bidirectional transduction. It appears that incorporation of a bidirectional HC transduction as a working hypothesis should be helpful in interpreting the turtle HC data as well as in comparing them with mammalian results.

Is it true that there is really no evidence against a bidirectional HC transduction?

Direct experimental determination whether HC stereocilia move in response to electrical stimulation is needed.

FETTIPLACE:

We have previously argued that the oscillations in hair cell membrane potential evoked by extrinsic current pulses are similar to the subthreshold excitation seen in the squid giant axon, and therefore could most simply be explained by a voltage-sensitive potassium conductance in the hair cell membrane (Crawford and Fettiplace, J. Physiol. 312, 377, 1981). The evidence in support of this explanation included the voltage dependence of the frequency of the oscillations and the fact that they were abolished by treatment with 10–15 mM TEA (Crawford and Fettiplace, J. Physiol. 315, 317, 1981). Similar observations have been made in bullfrog saccular hair cells (Lewis and Hudspeth, this volume). None of these observations eliminates the possibility that the hair cell membrane potential may also influence the mechanical properties of the stereocilia, but presently we have no evidence for or against this hypothesis.

MANLEY:

As stimulation of the efferent fibres would have affected all or most papilla hair cells, is it not possible that some of the effect observed in single cells under these conditions is due to, say, a general change in stiffness of all stereocilia and a concomitant positional change in the tectorial membrane?

FETTIPLACE:

We have attempted to explain the efferent effects on tuning in terms of a synaptic alteration of the electrical properties of single hair cells. While neither the synaptic conductance nor the hyperpolarisation is adequate on its own to explain the changes in shape of the tuning curve, it still seems possible that a combination of the two will suffice, the conductance being more important near the characteristic frequency and the membrane hyperpolarisation causing the low-frequency sensitisation. We feel it is important to determine to what extent these simple changes can account for efferent action before invoking more speculative and non-specific mechanisms such as the one you suggest.

COCHLEAR ELECTROANATOMY: INFLUENCE ON INFORMATION PROCESSING

Peter Dallos

Auditory Physiology Laboratory (Audiology) and Department
of Neurobiology and Physiology, Northwestern University
Evanston, Illinois 60201, USA

The term *electroanatomy* was introduced by von Békésy (1951) during his studies aimed at determining the resistance and capacitance patterns that corresponded to the structural features of the cochlea. Considerations of gross impedance configurations (studied by several groups in recent years: Kurokawa, 1965; Johnstone et al., 1966: Honrubia and Ward, 1969; Strelioff, 1973; Honrubia et al. 1976; Cannon, 1976; Geisler et al., 1977) may now be refined by incorporating individual hair cell characteristics. Recent intracellular recordings from mammalian hair cells (Russell and Sellick, 1978; Dallos et al., 1982) provide various electrical measures that describe the properties of these cells and highlight differences between inner (IHC) and outer hair cells (OHC). The purpose of this paper is to consider a simple circuit model of a cochlear cross-section and to investigate relationships between computed electrical quantities and those obtained experimentally. It is shown that several hitherto baffling differences between IHC and OHC electrical properties are a simple consequence of their impedance configurations. The results also suggest that electrical interactions between OHCs and IHCs are highly unlikely.

The circuit that is analyzed below is shown in Fig.1b which is a reduction of Fig.1a. The latter incorporates a single IHC and a single OHC for simplicity, as well as various bulk impedances representing the electrical environment of the cochlear scalae. It is assumed that the endolymph-contacting apical surface of the IHC has a resistance of R_a^I, whereas that of the OHC: R_a^O. The perilymphatic surfaces are represented by resistances R_b^I and R_b^O for IHC and OHC respectively. Davis' resistance-modulation scheme is adopted (Davis, 1965) and it is assumed that excitation is in the form of resistance changes in the apical cell surface:

$$R_a^I = R_1^I + \Delta R^I \;\; ; \qquad R_a^O = R_1^O + \Delta R^O \qquad \qquad 1.$$

In these equations R_1^I and R_1^O are the resting resistances, while ΔR^I and ΔR^O are controlled by the stimulus; these are some function of basilar membrane motion. Thus parametric excitation is assumed as in the earlier models of Strelioff (1973) and Dallos (1973). In order to keep our considerations entirely elementary, in the present

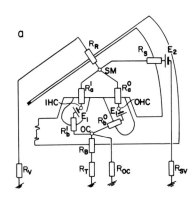

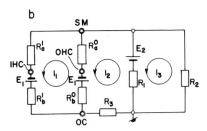

Fig. 1.a. Circuit diagram of cochlear cross-section including a single IHC and OHC in the organ of Corti. Voltage sources represent the following: E_1=Nernst potential of IHC and OHC cell membrane, E_2=stria vascularis source of EP. Association of resistance values with anatomical features is evident. b. Simplified circuit with the following relationships: $R_1 = R_S + R_{SV}$; $R_2 = R_R + R_V$; $R_3 = R_{OC}(R_B + R_T)/(R_{OC} + R_B + R_T)$. E_{SM} may be computed as $E_2 \approx R_2/(R_1 + R_2) = +70$ mV.

approximate treatment we ignore all reactive elements in the circuit. Moreover, it is assumed that the only variable elements are R_a^I and R_a^0, in other words, voltage-dependent conductances (associated with the basal cell membrane) are ignored as well. From measurements of various bulk resistances and hair cell input resistances (Johnstone et al., 1966; Cannon, 1976; Russell and Sellick, 1978; Dallos et al., 1982) it is clear that the former are much smaller than the latter, i.e. R_1, R_2, $R_3 << R_i^I$, R_i^0. One may note that input resistances can be approximated as follows:

$$R_i^I \approx \frac{R_a^I R_b^I}{R_a^I + R_b^I}; \qquad R_i^0 \approx \frac{R_a^0 R_b^0}{R_a^0 + R_b^0} \qquad\qquad 2.$$

By setting up Kirchoff's equations one may easily express both resting and stimulus-related potentials at various nodes of the circuit. Before such computations are performed, we introduce a quantity which is fundamental to the remainder of our arguments.

1. SHAPE FACTORS (α AND β)

As will become apparent below, in all expressions for electrical circuit quantities, the resting hair cell resistances appear only as ratios:

$$\alpha = \frac{R_b^0}{R_1^0}; \qquad\qquad \beta = \frac{R_b^I}{R_1^I} \qquad\qquad 3.$$

We will designate α and β as shape factors for the following reason. Assuming that the resting cell membrane has uniform specific resistance over its entire extent, and moreover, that the specific resistance of OHC and IHC membranes are the same, we can rewrite Eq.3 if we keep in mind that $R=R_s/S$ (R_s=specific membrane resistance, S=membrane surface area):

$$\alpha = \frac{S_a^0}{S_b^0}; \qquad\qquad \beta = \frac{S_a^I}{S_b^I} \qquad\qquad 4.$$

where S_a^0 and S_a^I are the areas of the endolymphatic surface of OHC and IHC, and S_b^0 and S_b^I are the areas of the basal, or perilymphatic, surfaces. We thus see that α and β are entirely determined by the cell configurations, hence the name: shape factor.

From radial sections of plastic-embedded guinea pig cochleas we determined α and β, using approximations for hair cell geometry as shown in Fig. 2. Computations were made for IHCs and OHCs located in the hook-region of the cochlea [where Russell and Sellick (1978) took their measurements] and in the third turn

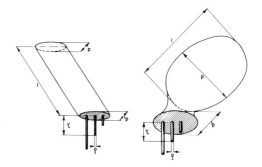

Fig. 2. *Computation of hair cell surfaces is obtained by assuming that OHCs are cylindrical, while IHC bodies are prolate spheroids. Cuticular plates are assumed circular. Cilia are taken to be cylinders with average length λ, and numbering 60 on IHCs and 100 on OHCs. Ciliary dimensions are obtained from Lim (1980). Apical cell surface is the sum of ciliary and cuticular surfaces while basal cell surface corresponds to that of the cell body. For third turn hair cells we obtained the following. For OHC: S_a=141.9, S_b=2,218, for IHC: S_a=223.9, S_b=720.9 (all values are in cm^2 times 10^{-8})*

where we obtained intracellular data (Dallos et al., 1982). The following numbers are computed:

	Turn one	Turn three
α =	0.156	0.0639
β =	0.320	0.311

A few comments are in order about the consequences of these numerical values. First, β is quite constant along the length of the cochlea, whereas α changes quite radically. In general, a much larger fraction of the total cell resistance is concentrated in the apical region for OHCs. Second, since circuit quantities depend on α and β, one may expect that IHC characteristics are less variable along the longitudinal cochlear dimension than those of OHCs. The latter change quite significantly, likely influencing the filter characteristics of the cell, as well as the properties of coupled mechano-electric transduction (Weiss, 1982).

2. RESTING POTENTIALS

One may express the node voltages representing the intracellular OHC and IHC potentials from Kirchoff's Laws:

$$E_{OHC} = E_{SM} + (I_1 - I_2) R_a^0 \quad \text{and} \quad E_{IHC} = E_{SM} - I_1 R_a^I \qquad 5.$$

After substitution of expressions for I_1 and I_2 and neglecting small terms in conformity with the relation: $R_1, R_2, R_3 << R_1^I, R_1^0, R_1^I, R_b^0, R_b^I, R_b^0$ one obtains the following for the resting potential:

$$E_{OHC} \approx \frac{\alpha E_{SM} - E_1}{1 + \alpha} \quad ; \quad E_{IHC} \approx \frac{\beta E_{SM} - E_1}{1 + \beta} \qquad 6.$$

Substituting numerical values for third turn α and β, as well as $E_{SM}=70$ mV and $E_1=80$ mV, one computes $E_{OHC}=-71.0$ mV and $E_{IHC}=-44.5$ mV. We reported a median value of -71 mV (highest -94 mV) for third turn OHC membrane potentials and a median of -20 mV (highest -47 mV) for third turn IHC resting potentials. Computations for turn one IHCs predict a value of -43.6 mV while Russell and Sellick (1978) found a median of -25.0 mV and a largest value of -45 mV. The computed and observed resting potentials show similar trends. Both indicate considerably higher membrane voltages for OHCs than for IHCs.

3. RECEPTOR POTENTIALS

a. *Magnitude of response.* By combining Eqs. 1 and 5 one can solve for the dynamic responses at the IHC and OHC circuit nodes:

$$\Delta E_{OHC} \approx \frac{-\alpha (E_1 + E_{SM}) y^0}{(1+\alpha)(1+\alpha+y^0)} \quad ; \quad \Delta E_{IHC} \approx \frac{-\beta (E_1 + E_{SM}) y^I}{(1+\beta)(1+\beta+y^I)} \qquad 7.$$

where we substituted the fractional resistance changes: $y^0 = \Delta R^0/R_1^0$ and $y^I = \Delta R^I/R_1^I$. For low levels of excitation (i.e. for y^0, $y^I << 1$) one may write the small-signal expressions for the receptor potentials:

$$e_{OHC} \approx \frac{-\alpha (E_1 + E_{SM}) y^0}{(1+\alpha)^2} \quad ; \quad e_{IHC} \approx \frac{\beta (E_1 + E_{SM}) y^I}{(1+\beta)^2} \qquad 8.$$

If one makes the simplifying assumption that the input excitation of the two types of cell is the same, $y^0 = y^I$, then the ratio of the receptor potentials assumes the particularly simple form:

$$\frac{e_{IHC}}{e_{OHC}} = \frac{\beta(1+\alpha)^2}{\alpha(1+\beta)^2} \qquad 9.$$

A substitution of the values of α and β, valid for the third turn location, yields the numerical ratio of 3.2. This number well represents the experimentally observed relationship between IHC and OHC receptor potentials (Dallos et al., 1982). Figure 3 shows tone burst-evoked responses from IHC and OHC to illustrate the relative magnitudes of these ac potentials at the cells' best frequency. The ratio is about three-to-one, not significantly different from the computed value. This agreement is surprising because one would not a priori expect y^0 and y^I to be equal. In fact, most authorities surmise much greater sensitivity for OHCs than for IHCs. It is possible that mechanical excitation of OHCs is indeed greater, but the above agreement would then suggest that the IHC transducer mechanism possesses higher gain.

A glance at the responses shown in Fig.3 indicates that both hair cells produce a pronounced dc receptor potential component. Around the cells' best frequency this dc response is depolarizing. We now examine how the circuit model accounts for these observations.

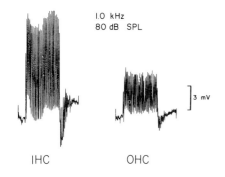

1.0 kHz
80 dB SPL

3 mV

IHC   OHC

Fig. 3. Receptor potentials from one IHC and one OHC from the same organ of Corti. Responses are averaged. Stimulation is with tone bursts at the cells' best frequency

b. *Nonlinearity of response.* Plots of Equations 7 are shown in Fig. 4. It is apparent that both ΔE_{OHC} and ΔE_{IHC} are highly nonlinear functions of the excitation, with the depolarizing phase rising much more steeply than the hyperpolarizing phase. A construction of sample waveforms is included in the figure, along with examples of actual recorded waveforms from IHC and OHC. There are many similarities between the computed and experimental response patterns. This resemblence is particularly interesting if one notes that *linear* excitation of the hair cells is assumed here. It is the fundamental nonlinearity of the parametrically excited circuit which is manifested in the computations above. This circuit nonlinearity may, in part, be responsible for the observed distortion of intracellular responses. Without a doubt, other nonlinearities in the system contribute (Rhode, 1971; Kim et al., 1980; Sellick et al., 1982) to the total distortion and may in fact dominate it. Nevertheless, the circuit nonlinearity should not be ignored. One may compute the dc receptor potential (Dallos, 1973). It is noted that with increasing input level the dc component rises with a slope of two (in agreement with experimental results) up to apical resistance modulation magnitudes of approximately 25%. For larger modulation depth the model predicts an accelerating dc response which exceeds the fundamental ac component at very large input. The ratio of IHC and OHC dc responses is predicted as 2.6, in reasonable agreement with our data. A very conspicuous nonlinearity seen in hair cell responses is saturation at high sound levels. This nonlinearity is not predicted by the circuit model, its causes are probably in the mechanical transformations preceding the transduction process and also in that process itself. Saturation affects both ac and dc response components (Russell and Sellick, 1978).

4. ELECTRICAL INTERACTIONS

It has been suggested that OHCs may exert some influence upon IHCs by field currents or potentials (Geisler, 1974; Honrubia et al, 1976: Manley, 1978: Brownell, 1982). The schemes generally envision that OHCs control the current flow through IHCs by shunting more or less current away from the IHC population. In Figure 5 our circuit is further simplified in showing a single OHC as a voltage source, in parallel with a passive IHC and the equivalent resistance of the

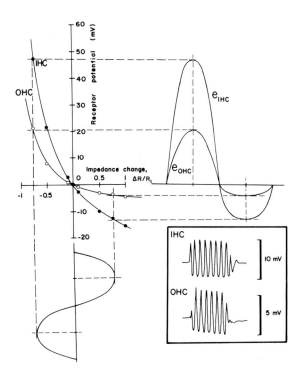

Fig. 4. Computed receptor potentials for both IHC and OHC as functions of fractional resistance changes ($\Delta R/R_i$) at the cell's apex. Computations are based on Eq. 7. Construction of response waveforms with sinusoidal resistance change is also shown. Insert: recorded responses from one IHC and one OHC at a stimulus frequency of 150 Hz and 70 dB SPL

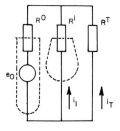

Fig. 5. Simplified circuit showing the OHC as the only signal source in parallel with an IHC (R^I) and another resistance (R^T) representing all other circuit elements

entire remaining cochlear circuit as "seen" by the OHC. One may compute $R^O = R^O_1 + R^O_b$ and $R^I = R^I_1 + R^I_b$ if the surface areas of the cells and the specific membrane resistance are available. We determined the former as described above. The latter may be obtained from the input impedance data of Russell and Sellick (1978) with the aid of Eq. 2, providing a value of $R_s \approx 337 \Omega cm^2$. Since R_s was assumed constant throughout the cochlea, we may now compute $R^I \approx 200$ MΩ, and $R^O \approx 250$ MΩ at the third turn location of interest. From various sources (Johnstone et al., 1966; Cannon, 1976) one may estimate the total bulk resistance in parallel with the hair cells as $R^T \approx 14$ kΩ. If the voltage generated by the "source" OHC is e , then the fraction of this voltage that appears across R^I is $R^T/R^O \approx 5.6 \times 10^{-5}$. It is apparent that due to the extreme impedance disparity between hair cells and their electrolyte fluid environment, extraneous current generated by a cell is shunted by the bulk resistance from other hair cells. One can compute that if *all* OHCs in the cochlea were to sum their currents, they could only produce a change in the voltage drop across an IHC which would be about one-tenth of that cell's own response to the stimulus. It appears therefore, that electrical interactions between hair cells are unlikely. If OHCs influence the environment of IHCs, they probably do so by altering cochlear micromechanics. The only possible exception to this argument is the situation where the IHC itself produces negligible response, say a high frequency hair cell at low stimulus frequencies. In such a case extracellular potentials conducted from highly excited cochlear segments could exceed the cell's own response and thus could control the transmembrane potential. It may not be likely that such field currents could be responsible for, or be of influence upon such fundamental response characteristics as frequency selectivity, two-tone suppression or efferent effects.

Acknowledgements. Supported by NINCDS Grant NS-08635. I thank Å. Flock, E. Relkin, J. Santos-Sacchi and J. Siegel for their contributions to this work. Figs. 1, 2 and 3 are included in a more complete description of this work (Dallos, 1983).

REFERENCES

Békésy, G. von (1951). The coarse pattern of the electrical resistance in the cochlea of the guinea pig (electro-anatomy of the cochlea). *J.Acoust.Soc.Am.* 23, 18-28.

Brownell, W.E. (1982). Cochlear transduction: an integrative model and review. *Hearing res.* 6, 335-360.

Cannon, M.W., Jr. (1976). Electrical impedances, current pathways, and voltage sources in the guinea pig cochlea. Rept. ISR-S-14, Inst. for Sensory Research, Syracuse University, Syracuse, NY.

Dallos, P. (1973). *The Auditory Periphery. Biophysics and Physiology.* 278-283, 428-431. New York, Academic Press.

Dallos, P. (1983). Some electrical circuit properties of the organ of Corti. I. Analysis without reactive elements. *Hearing Res.* to be published.

Dallos, P., Santos-Sacchi, J. and Flock, Å. (1982). Intracellular recordings from cochlear outer hair cells. *Science* 218, 582-584.

Davis, H. (1965). A model for transducer action in the cochlea. *Cold Spring Harbor Symp.Quant.Biol.* 30, 181-190.

Geisler, C.D. (1974). Model of crossed olivocochlear bundle effects. *J.Acoust. Soc.Am.* 56, 1910-1912.

Geisler, C.D., Mountain, D.C., Hubbard, A.E., Adrian, H.O. and Ravindran, A. (1977) Alternating electrical-resistance changes in the guinea-pig cochlea caused by acoustic stimulation. *J.Acoust.Soc.Am.* 61 1557-1566.

Honrubia, V. and Ward, P.H. (1969). Dependence of the cochlear microphonics and the summating potential on the endocochlear potential. *J.Acoust.Soc.Am.* 46, 388-392.

Honrubia, V., Strelioff, D. and Sitko, S.T. (1976). Physiological basis of cochlear transduction and sensitivity. *Ann.Otol.Rhinol.Laryngol.* 85, 697-710.

Johnstone, B.M., Johnstone, J.R. and Pugsley, T.D.(1966). Membrane resistance in endolymphatic walls of the first turn in the guinea pig cochlea. *J.Acoust. Soc.Am.* 40, 1398-1404.

Kim, D.O., Molnar, C.E. and Matthews, J.W. (1980). Cochlear mechanics: Nonlinear behavior in two-tone responses as reflected in cochlear-nerve-fiber responses and in earcanal sound pressure. *J.Acoust.Soc.Am.* 67, 1704-1721.

Kurokawa, S. (1965). Experimental study on electrical resistance of basilar membrane in guinea pig. *Jap.J.Oto-Rhino-Laryngol.* 68, 1177-1195.

Lim, D.J. (1980). Cochlear anatomy related to cochlear micromechanics. A review. *J.Acoust.Soc.Am.* 67, 1686-1695.

Manley, G.A. (1978). Cochlear frequency sharpening--a new synthesis. *Acta Otolaryngol.* 85, 167-176.

Rhode, W.S. (1971). Observations of the vibration of the basilar membrane in squirrel monkeys using the Mössbauer technique. *J.Acoust.Soc.Am.* 49, 1218-1231.

Russell, I.J. and Sellick, P.M. (1978). Intracellular studies of hair cells in the guinea pig cochlea. *J.Physiol. (London)* 284,261-290.

Sellick, P.M., Patuzzi, R. and Johnstone, B.M. (1982). Measurement of basilar membrane motion in the guinea pig using the Mössbauer technique. *J.Acoust. Soc.Am.* 72, 131-141.

Strelioff, D. (1973). A computer simulation of the generation and distribution of cochlear potentials. *J.Acoust.Soc.Am.* 54, 620-629.

Weiss, T.F. (1982). Bidirectional transduction in vertebrate hair cells: A mechanism for coupling mechanical and electrical processes. *Hearing Res.* 7, 353-360.

GENERAL DISCUSSION

R.S. LEWIS:
Would the asymmetry in the receptor potentials of IHC or OHC predicted by your
model be affected by changes in the shape factors, brought about, for example,
by changes in hair cell basal conductance?

DALLOS:
If from Eq. 7 one computes the ratio of the responses to the negative and positive maxima of a symmetrical stimulus then the following relationships are found:

$$\left|\frac{\Delta E^-_{OHC}}{\Delta E^+_{OHC}}\right| = \frac{1+\alpha+y^o}{1+\alpha-y^o} \quad ; \quad \left|\frac{\Delta E^-_{IHC}}{\Delta E^+_{IHC}}\right| = \frac{1+\beta+y^I}{1+\beta-y^I}$$

It is seen that these ratios become larger as the shape factor becomes smaller.
Thus the responses are expected to be more asymmetrical for cells with larger
base to apex resistance disparities.

MANLEY:
Due to the strong possibility that the subtectorial hair cell space is physically separated from the scala media proper, it seems hardly prudent to assume that
the hair cells are coupled directly into the bulk resistances out of scala media
(Kronester-Frei, Arch. Otol. Rhinol. Laryngol. 224, 3, 1979; Manley and
Kronester-Frei, in Psychophysical Physiological and Behavioural Studies in Hearing. Bilsen and v.d. Brink, Eds. pp. 24-31. Delft, 1980).

DALLOS:
It is probably fair to say that the matter of functional relationship between
subtectorial space and scala media proper is unresolved. Thus, for example, we
find that the resting potential and response characteristics within the inner
sulcus are the same as in scala media. Similarly we find that electrodes that
pass through the reticular lamina into the subtectorial space encounter the EP
immediately upon leaving the organ of Corti. These observations are consonant
with the notion that the potential barrier for EP is at the level of the reticular lamina (the basic assumption of the model) and are in contrast to the
findings of Manley and Kronester-Frei.

ELECTROCHEMICAL PROFILE FOR POTASSIUM IONS ACROSS
THE HAIR-CELL MEMBRANES

T. Konishi and A.N. Salt*

Laboratory of Environmental Biophysics
National Institute of Environmental Health Sciences
National Institutes of Health
Research Triangle Park, N.C. 27709 USA

1. INTRODUCTION

Since Davis (1954) first described the physiological relationship between the unique ionic environment surrounding the cochlear hair cells and generation of the cochlear microphonics (CM), extensive studies on the receptor potentials of the single hair cells have been reported. In spite of these studies the ionic mechanisms occuring in the cochlear hair cells, especially electrochemical profile for K^+ across the hair-cell membranes have not been fully elucidated. Utilizing K^+ selective liquid membrane electrodes, the present experiments were designed to estimate the electrochemical driving force for K^+ ions across the hair-cell membranes of normal guinea pigs. The preliminary report of these studies was presented to the 4th Midwinter Research Meeting of Association for Research in Otolaryngology (Konishi and Salt, 1981).

2. METHODS

(a) Animals and surgical preparation: Guinea pigs were anesthetized with pentobarbital sodium (30-35 mg/kg). After exposure of the right auditory bulla the round window membrane was ruptured and removed by a fine metal hook. In some cases the bony edge of the round window was gently thinned and removed before opening the round window. Microelectrodes were positioned so that, when advanced with a piezoelectric microdriver, they would penetrate the organ of Corti in the hook region of the cochlea. Animals were immobilized by intravenous injection of gallamine triethiodide and respired artificially.

(b) Microelectrode fabrication: Two segments of Pyrex capillaries with internal filaments were glued together and pulled into a double barreled electrode with an electrode puller. The inside surface of the ion barrel was silanized by exposing to dichlorodimethyl silane (Zeuthen et al., 1974). The capillaries were then baked in an oven. The shank of the ion barrel was filled with the ion exchanger (Corning 477317) and the shaft was filled with 160 mM KCl solution. The potential difference (PD) barrel was filled with 500 mM NaCl solution.

(c) Electrode calibrations: The electrodes were calibrated in isotonic mixtures of NaCl-KCl solutions (160 mM) maintained at 38.0 $\pm$ 0.5°C. The mean K^+ sensitivity was 37 mV/decade change of K^+ activity. The tip potential was less than 5 mV and the response time of the ion barrel was shorter than 3 sec. The selectivity coefficient, $k_{K \cdot Na}$ was tested in equimolar pure KCl and NaCl solution. For $a_{Na} = a_K = 117$ mEq/l the mean value of the calculated $k_{K \cdot Na}$ was 0.025.

(d) Intracellular recording: Each barrel of a double barreled K^+ electrode was connected to an electrometer ($R_{in} \sim 10^{15}$ Ω). A Ag-AgCl wire inserted into the neck muscles was used as a reference electrode. The potential recorded from the PD barrel was substracted from the potential recorded from the K^+ barrel to obtain K^+ dependent potential (K^+ potential). The dc potential recorded from a PD barrel and K^+ potential were measured by digital voltmeters and also recorded on a chart recorder. The CM and ac component of the intracellular responses to 500 Hz tone bursts were recorded from the PD barrel. Their waveform was displayed on an oscilloscope and photographed on running film.

*Inst. Sound and Vibration Res., Univ. Southampton, U.K.

The criteria for a successful impalement of cell membranes were a) an abrupt appearance of a negative dc potential plateau and an associated increase in K^+ activity with no more than 10% variation for at least 5 sec and c) return of the dc potential to the original level when the tip of the electrode was withdrawn to the perilymph of the scala tympani. Successful puncture of a hair-cell membrane, in addition to the above criteria, was accompanied by a sudden increase of ac component of the receptor potential and a return to the original level when the electrode was later withdrawn.

The electrochemical potential difference for K^+ across the cell membrane was calculated from the following equation;

$$\frac{\Delta \tilde{\mu}_K}{F} = \frac{RT}{F} \{ln[a_K^i/a_K^o] + \Delta \psi_m\}$$

where $\Delta \tilde{\mu}_K$ is the electrochemical potential difference between inside and outside of cell and a_K^i and a_K^o are K^+ activity of intracellular and extracellular fluid respectively. $\Delta \psi_m$ is a resting potential. R, T and F have their usual meanings. Data on the electrochemical potential difference were expressed in terms of mV and presented with respect to the extracellular fluid in the organ of Corti.

3. RESULTS

(a) Exploration of the organ of Corti with K^+ selective microelectrodes: One representative example of exploration of the organ of Corti with a double barrel-ed K^+ selective electrode is shown in Fig. 1. When the electrode pierced the basilar membrane, small changes in the dc potential were observed. The extracell-ular fluid in the organ of Corti showed similar dc potential and K^+ activity to those recorded in the perilymph of the scala tympani. The magnitude of CM record-ed from the extracellular space in the organ of Corti did not show a substantial increase. Further advancement of the electrode resulted in a sudden increase of the ac component of the receptor potential accompanied by sudden appearance of a stable negative potential. This steep rise in the membrane potential was accom-panied by a gradual rise in the K^+ potential. On the basis of the criteria de-scribed in the Methods this impaled cell could be categorized as a hair cell. When the electrode was again advanced in a stepwise fashion, a large positive potential (EP) and the phase reversal of the receptor potential were simultane-ously observed. The K^+ activity did not show a decrease but remained high.

A large and stable membrane potential without an increase of the ac response was frequently observed during penetration of the organ of Corti with microelec-trodes. There was an increase of the K^+ activity at the moment of appearance of the negative potential. These responses usually remained stable for a longer period than those accompanied by an increase of the ac receptor potential. It is probable that these responses originated from supporting cells.

(b) Determination of the electrochemical gradient for K^+ across the hair-cell membranes: Data were collected from 47 successful cell punctures. Out of these cells 9 cells could be categorized as hair cells on the basis of an amplitude increase of the ac component of the receptor potential.

The K^+ activity in the extracellular fluid in the organ of Corti was 1.98 $\pm$ 1.14 mEq/l. This value was similar to that measured in the perilymph of the scala tympani. The intracellular K^+ activity of hair cells was 64.8 $\pm$ 43.6 mEq/l and the resting potential was −82.4 $\pm$ 18.0 mV. The K^+ activity of the endo-lymph was 113.8 $\pm$ 6.7 mEq/l. If the activity coefficient of the endolymph is assumed to be similar to that of 150 mM KCl at 37°C (0.7273), the average K^+ concentration in the endolymph was 156.5 mM. The EP recorded in the subtectorial space was 84.7 $\pm$ 4.2 mV.

Fig. 2 represents a computed electrochemical potential profile for K^+ expressed as an equivalent electric potential relative to a zero potential in the extracellular fluid in the organ of Corti. The electrochemical gradient for K^+ across the basolateral hair cell membrane was 6.9 $\pm$ 21.5 mV. Thus K^+ ions are near electrochemical equilibrium distribution across the basolateral hair cell membrane. In contrast the electrochemical gradient for K^+ across the hair-bearing surface of hair cells was 196.4 $\pm$ 20.8 mV.

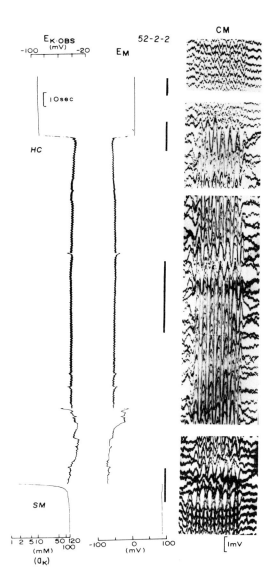

Fig. 1. Changes in the K^+ potential, E_{KOBS} (left column) and dc potential E_M, (middle column) and cochlear microphonics, CM, (right column) recorded during penetration of the organ of Corti with a double barreled K^+ selective microelectrode in a normal guinea pig. The K^+ and dc potentials were recorded on a chart recorder and CM was photographed on running film and approximate periods of CM recording are indicated by vertical bars. The thick traces with regular fluctuations appearing in the dc and K^+ potential records are artifacts caused by 60 Hz line voltage and animal's respiratory movement. Records are read from the top. The electrode was advanced from the scala tympani towards the scala media in stepwise fashion as described in the text. The scale at the left bottom is K^+ activity in mM/l. Notice a sudden increase in ac response amplitude accompanied by stable resting potential and increase of K^+ activity which indicate impalement of hair-cell membrane (HC) on the basis of criteria described in the text

(c) Determination of the electrochemical gradient for K^+ across supporting-cell membranes: The intracellular K^+ activity and the resting potential were 67.3 ± 31.0 mEq/l and -92.8 ± 13.5 mV respectively. The electrochemical potential difference between the cell interior and extracellular fluid of the organ of Corti was -3.6 ± 12.9 mV. The intracellular K^+ ions of supporting cells are in electrochemical equilibrium with respect to the K^+ ions in the extracellular fluid of organ of Corti. On the other hand, the electrochemical gradient between the cell interior and endolymph was 199.1 ± 11.6 mV. These values were comparable with those obtained in the hair cells (Fig. 2).

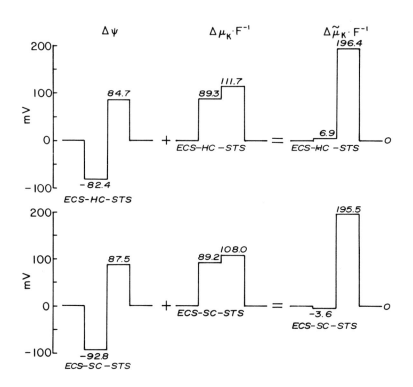

Fig. 2. Electrochemical profile for K^+ across the hair-cell membranes (top) and the supporting cell membranes (bottom). The mean values of potentials are expressed in mV and referred to the potential level of the extracellular fluid of the organ of Corti. $\Delta\psi$ electrical potential difference; $\Delta\mu_K F^{-1}$, chemical potential difference; $\Delta\tilde{\mu}_K F^{-1}$, electrochemical potential difference. ECS, extracellular space; HC, hair cell; STS, subtectorial space; SC, supporting cell

4.   DISCUSSION

Our results show that the dc potential in the extracellular fluid of the organ of Corti does not depart significantly from that in the perilymph of the scala tympani and that the K^+ activity in the extracellular fluid within the organ of Corti is comparable with that found in the perilymph. These findings exclude the possibility that a negative extracellular potential exists within the organ of Corti (Tasaki and Spyropoulos, 1959; Butler, 1965).

It is our consistent finding that when an electrode passed through the organ of Corti, the positive dc potential was in all cases accompanied by high K^+ activity. These findings indicate that the fluid in the subtectorial space is positively polarized and has high K^+ activity. These observations confirm results reported by Tasaki et al. (1954) who originally characterized the reticular lamina as a boundary between K^+ rich endolymph and Na^+ rich perilymph-like extracellular fluid in the organ of Corti. Utilizing X-ray microanalysis, Flock (1977) and Ryan et al. (1980) reported that the K^+ concentration in fluid in the subtectorial space was comparable with that found in endolymph. Using a dye marking technique Tanaka et al. (1977) clearly demonstrated the positive potential in the subtectorial space. Our data, together with reports described above imply that the subtectorial space communicates with the scala media through the open marginal net. However, conflicting results have been reported by other investigators. Manley and Kronester-Frei (1980) argued that the Ep was not

present in the inner sulcus and that the subtectorial space was separated from
the scala media proper and also from the inner sulcus. Burgio and Lawrence
(1980) proposed that the subtectorial space does not exist under normal conditions. A complication arising from these data is a substantial decrease of
the electrochemical gradient for K^+ across the apical hair-cell membrane.

Davis (1958) proposed that the mechano-electric transduction process in the
cochlear hair cells is the modulation of a resting current by a mechanically
induced change in the membrane permeability which takes place on the apical hair-
cell membranes. *In vivo* K^+ ions are the dominant cation in both endolymph and
cytoplasma of hair cells and it has been speculated that the transduction current
is predominately carried by K^+ ions. Recently Corey and Hudspeth (1979) reported
that the receptor current of 100 pA at the membrane potential of -60 mV could be
abolished by an inward current of 10 pA, when the hair cells were stimulated
mechanically. But the magnitude of the resting current flowing through the
hair cells has not been clearly understood. In the steady state the net ionic
current through the hair cells, I^{net}, is zero.

$$I^{net} = I^{in} + I^{out} = 0 \tag{1}$$

where I^{in} and I^{out} are the ionic current at the apical and basolateral membranes
of the hair cells respectively. I^{in} and I^{out} are characterized by

$$I^{in} = F \sum_i z_i J_i^{in}$$
$$I^{out} = F \sum_i z_i J_i^{out} \tag{2}$$

where J_i is the flux of ionic species, i and F and z have their usual meaning.
When there are no changes in cell volume (dV=0), J_i is a sum of the diffusional
flux and the active flux and can be expressed as follows

$$J_i = \omega_i \overline{C}_i \, \Delta\tilde{\mu}_i + J_i^{active} \tag{3}$$

where ω_i is the mobility of ionic species i in the membrane, $\Delta\tilde{\mu}_i$ the electrochemical potential for i ions, J_i^{active} the active flux for i ions and $\overline{C}_i$ the
mean concentration difference of i ions

$$\overline{C}_i = \frac{C_i^{1-2}}{ln\frac{C_i^1}{C_i^2}}$$

From eqs (2) and (3) the ionic current at the basolateral cell membrane is

$$I_i^{out} = F \sum_i z_i (\omega_i \overline{C}_i \Delta\tilde{\mu}_i + J_i^{active}) \tag{4}$$

Suppose that I^{out} is carried by K^+ Na^+ and Cl^- ions, then

$$I^{out} = (\omega_k \overline{C}_K \Delta\tilde{\mu}_K + \omega_{Na}\overline{C}_{Na} \Delta\tilde{\mu}_{Na} - \omega_{Cl}\overline{C}_{Cl} \Delta\tilde{\mu}_{Cl} + J_K^{active} + J_{Na}^{active}).F \tag{5}$$

From eq (5) it is obvious that a small electrochemical potential difference
across the basolateral membrane does not always result in a small resting current.
In fact, the magnitude of the K^+ current becomes substantial, if the basolateral
hair-cell membranes are highly permeable to K^+ ions. In addition, as shown in
eq (5), the resting current is affected by other terms involving Na^+ or Cl^- ions
and the resting current cannot be soley estimated by the electrochemical gradient for K^+ across the basolateral membrane. We are now studying the electrochemical gradients for Na^+ or Cl^- ions across the cochlear hair cell membranes.
These results together with the present findings will shed light on the ionic
mechanism for generation of the transduction current.

Finally, our data on the membrane potential recorded from the hair cells of
the basal turn are comparable with those recorded from the outer hair cells of

the third turn (Dallos et al., 1982). Russell and Sellick (1978) reported the smaller resting potential in the inner hair cells of the basal turn. Dallos et al. (1982) reported the similar findings in the third-turn inner hair cells. Although identification of the recording site could not be made in our present studies, it is most likely that the hair cells with the large resting potential belong to the outer hair cells. If this is the case, the membrane potential of the outer hair cells is mainly generated by the K^+ diffusion across the basolateral membrane and is not affected by the contact of the apical membrane with the K^+ rich endolymph. It is still uncertain whether the low resting potential of the inner hair cells can be attributed to electrical properties of the cell membranes. More experimental evidence is needed before differences in the electrophysiological properties of cell membranes between the two types of hair cells can be clearly defined.

Figures 1 and 2 are included in a paper accepted by Hearing Research (Konishi, T. and Salt, A.N.)

REFERENCES

Burgio, P.A. and Lawrence, M. (1980). A new technique to determine the attachments of tectorial membrane and chemical composition of the fluids of the inner sulcus and tunnel of Corti. In: *Assoc. for Res. in Otolaryngol: Abstracts of the third Midwinter Research Meeting,* (David, Lim, ed.) p. 22, St. Petersburg, Fla.

Butler, R.A. (1965). Some experimental observations on the dc resting potentials in the guinea pig cochlea. *J. Acoust. Soc. Amer.* 37, 429–433.

Corey, D.P. and Hudspeth, A.J. (1979). Ionic basis of the receptor potential in a vetebrate hair cell. *Nature* 281, 675–677.

Dallos, P., Santos-Sacchi, J. and Flock, Å. (1982). Intracellular recording from cochlear outer hair cells. *Science* 218, 582–584.

Davis, H. (1954). Mechanism of hearing. In: *Nerve Impulse.* Transactions of the 4th Conference. (D. Nachmansohn, ed.) pp. 58–139, New York, Josiah Macy Jr. Foundation.

Davis, H. (1958). A mechano-electrical theory of cochlear action. *Ann. Oto-Rhino-Laryngol.* 67, 789–801.

Flock, Å. (1977). Electron probe determination of relative ion distribution in the inner ear. *Acta Otolaryngol.* (Stockh) 83, 239–244.

Konishi, T. and Salt, A.N. (1981). Eelectrochemical profile for K^+ across the hair cell membrane of the organ of Corti. In: *Assoc. for Res. in Otolaryngol: Abstracts of the 4th Midwinter Research Meeting,* (David Lim, ed.) p. 56–57, St. Petersburg, Fla.

Manley, G.A. and Kronester-Frei, A. (1980). The electrophysiological profile of the organ of Corti. In: *Psychophysical, Physiological and Behavioural Studies in Hearing.* Proceedings of the 5th International Symposium on Hearing, (F.A. Bilsen and G van den Brink, eds.) pp. 24–31, Delft, Delft Univ. Press.

Russell, I.J. and Sellick, P.M. (1978). Intracellular studies of hair cells in the mammalian cochlea, *J. Physiol.* (Lond) 284, 261–290.

Ryan, A.F., Wickham, M.G. and Bine, R.C. (1980). Studies of ion distribution in the inner ear: Scanning electron microscopy and X-ray microanalysis of freeze-dried cochlear specimens. *Hearing Res.* 2, 1–20.

Tanaka, Y., Asanuma, A., Yanagisawa, K. and Katsuke, Y. (1977). Electrical potentials of the subtectorial space in the guinea pig cochlea. *Jpn. J. Physiol.* 27, 539–544.

Tasaki, I., Davis, H. and Eldredge, D.H. (1954). Exploration of cochlear potentials in guinea pig with a microelectrode. *J. Acoust. Soc. Amer.* 26, 765–773.

Tasaki, I. and Spyropoulos, C.S. (1959). Stria vascularis as source of endocochlear potential. *J. Neurophysiol.* 22, 149–155.

Zeuthen, T., Hiam, R.C. and Silver, I.A. (1974). Microelectrode recording of ion activity in brain. *Adv. Exp. Med. Biol.* 50, 145–156.

GENERAL DISCUSSION

SYKA:
To your interesting data I have a couple of questions: What is the diameter of tip of your double-barrell electrodes? What is the impedance of the potassium selective channel? Did you check impedance of the electrode during penetration through the structures of the organ of Corti? Finally, did you find any increase or accumulation of potassium in extracellular spaces of the organ of Corti during intensive acoustical stimulation? The question is because an accumulation of potassium in the CNS extracellular spaces is known to produce changes in polarisation of neurones.

KONISHI:
Judging from an electrode resistance of 30 to 50 megohms when blanks were filled with 3M KCl, the tip diameter of each barrel seems to be less than 1 μm: The input resistance of electrometers used was 10^{15} ohms. The resistance of the ion barrel ranged from 10^{12} to 10^{13} ohms. Impedance changes of the PD barrel were not measured during penetration of the organ of Corti. We have not used intense stimulation in these experiments. We are not certain whether or not the K^+ activity in extracellular space (especially in the tunnel of Corti) is altered under overstimulation conditions.

COMPARISON OF BASILAR MEMBRANE, HAIR CELL AND NEURAL RESPONSES

B.M. Johnstone, R. Patuzzi and P. Sellick

*Department of Physiology, The University of Western Australia,
Western Australia.*

For many years, the relationship between basilar membrane (BM) mechanics and auditory nerve responses have been a matter of great interest.

The major discrepancy, viz. sharp neural tuning versus broad BM tuning has been at least partially resolved by Khanna (1982) and Sellick et al. (1982a). Khanna presented results from cats using a laser system and Sellick et al. from guinea pigs using the Mössbauer technique. Some results from our Mössbauer measurements are presented in Fig. 1. This shows a comparison of some of our sharpest and most sensitive Mössbauer measurements with the range of 10 neural spiral ganglion recordings made opposite a similar BM position. There is evidently a great similarity. However, a close inspection of Fig. 1 shows a consistent discrepancy of up to 10 dB at about half an octave below CF.

Further experiments (Sellick et al., 1983) revealed that measurements made on the spiral ligament side of the BM showed similar sensitivity, but much broader tuning compared with measurements made nearer the spiral lamina. This dissonance is again particularly evident half an octave below CF (Fig. 1 solid curve). These results leave the possibility that some additional processing may take place, possibly in the sub-tectorial space, or that the presence of the source alters BM motion, making the tuning slightly broader.

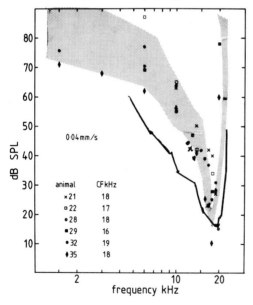

Fig. 1. Comparison of BM and neural tuning.
The hatched area defines the limits of 10 normal neural curves. The points are BM measurements (.04 mm/S) from 6 animals. The solid line is a BM tuning curve with the source near the spiral ligament.

animal	CF kHz
× 21	18
□ 22	17
● 28	18
■ 29	16
◆ 32	19
♦ 35	18

Other parameters of auditory nerve response can be compared with BM motion. These include input/output functions, and non linear responses (Patuzzi and Sellick, 1983a). A comparison of BM, inner hair cell and neural input/output responses at various frequencies are shown in Fig. 2. It is seen that at high frequencies, the slopes of the hair cell and neural input/output functions are dominated by BM non linearities. At frequencies close to CF the nerve response shows saturation at or below the same level as the BM whilst the hair cell receptor potential essentially mirrors the BM function. The closeness of the BM CF non linearity and the neural saturation suggests that sometimes the BM function may predominate, so that occasionally CF neurons may exhibit anomalous "saturation" behaviour. It appears that the different slopes of input/output functions can be ascribed to BM responses, suitably modified by the known passive properties of inner hair cells, and nerve and synapses.

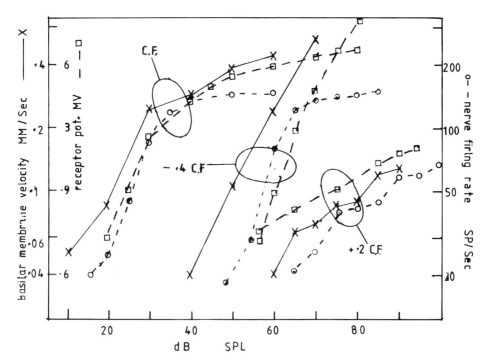

Fig. 2. _Neural, hair cell and BM input-output functions. The results are from various animals and have been normalized to the same CF. The circles are neural data, the squares hair cell and the crosses BM velocity. Three frequencies are presented, CF, +.2CF and -.4CF_

    Another non linear phenomenon that we have investigated is the modulation in the cochlea of high frequencies by low (Sellick et al., 1982b, and Patuzzi et al., 1983b). The psychophysical correlate of this paradigm has been described by Zwicker (1977), who has termed them Masking-Period patterns. A typical neural result is shown in Fig. 3. There are two inhibitory phases per cycle, with the maximum inhibition corresponding to BM displacement towards scala tympani. At high sound levels (of the HF tone), the response flattens out. This effect is partially due to the inner hair cell receptor potential and partially due to the nerve's higher average firing rate.
    Recording from inner hair cells (Fig. 4.), shows a similar pattern, but with the second inhibitory peak somewhat less, thus illustrating the enhancing effect of synaptic adaptation on transients. At high sound pressures, considerable flattening of the patterns is observed. In Fig. 4, the lowest curve is the extracellular 40 Hz CM and this gives an accurate picture of the relative phases of the modulation. A downward deflection of the CM corresponds to BM displacement towards scala tympani. Hence the phase of the modulation is a peak inhibition in synchrony with BM maximum displacement, with the greatest effect in the scala tympani direction and a smaller, but similar effect corresponding to scala vestibuli displacement.

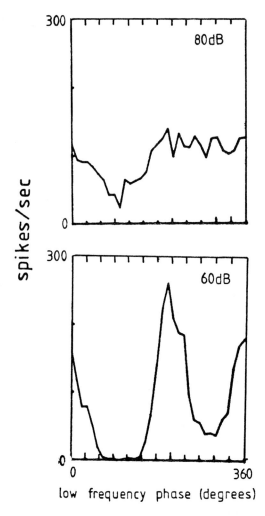

spikes/sec

low frequency phase (degrees)

*Fig. 3. Neural modulation patterns.
The 40 Hz tone was presented at 100
dB SPL, which was below neural threshold. The high frequency (Probe)
tone was at 17 kHz, the CF .of the
unit. The bottom scale is degrees
for one cycle of the 40 Hz tone and
zero phase is the same position as
Figs. 3 and 4. The suppression at
90–129 degrees is below spontaneous
activity*

Fig. 5 shows the modulation pattern
recorded on the BM. The pattern is
similar to the inner hair cell response, but lacks the compression or
flattening at high sound levels. An
apparent reduction in modulation of
the secondary dip at 83 dB may not be
real as it is not statistically significantly different from the dip of
the 73 dB curve. No enhancement is
seen at any phase. The extra flattening, most evident at the 180–360 degree phase recorded from inner hair
cells can be fully accounted for by
the high level non linear input/out-
put function of the hair cells. We
have followed modulation of CF responses on the BM for the low tones
varying from 40 Hz to 8 kHz. There is
only a little data at the moment for
frequencies above 1 kHz but those we
have show very similar behaviour to
the lower frequencies.

The modulation effect is maximal
for probe tones at CF and falls off
for lower frequencies. For probe
tones less than half an octave below
CF we have not been able to demonstrate modulation. The net result of
a low tone modulating a high is always inhibition. At modulating frequencies above a few hundred Hz, the
hair cell and neural synapse time constant will start smearing the pattern such
that above a few thousand Hz, only an average inhibition will remain in the neural response. These results strongly suggest that two tone inhibition is a function of BM mechanics.

It seems that BM mechanics can account for many of the parameters observed
in inner hair cell receptor potentials and neural responses and it is probable
that smaller Mössbauer sources placed nearer the spiral lamina would eliminate
the tuning curve discrepancies. More parameters must be tested, but the similarities are so strong that we question the need to hypothesize any further processing between BM response and inner hair cell stimulation.

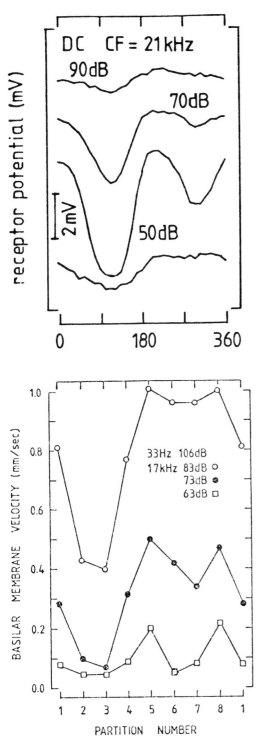

Fig. 4. Inner hair cell DC receptor potential modulation. The lowest curve is for the 40 Hz alone and represents the external CM

Fig. 5. Modulation pattern on the basilar membrane. The partition number refers to the division of the low frequency wave into eight segments. Note the two end points are repeated for clarity

Acknowledgement: *This work was supported by grants from the National Health and Medical Research Council and the Australian Research Grants Scheme (Australia).*

REFERENCES

Khanna, S.M. and Leonard, D.G.B. (1982). Basilar membrane tuning in the cat cochlea. *Science* 215, 305-306.

Patuzzi, R. and Sellick, P.M. (1983a). A comparison between basilar membrane and inner hair cell receptor potentials. *Submitted for publication.*

Patuzzi, R. and Sellick, P.M. (1983b). Modulation of the sensitivity of the mammalian cochlea. (to be published).

Sellick, P.M., Patuzzi, R. and Johnstone, B.M. (1982a). Measurements of basilar membrane motion in the guinea pig using the Mössbauer technique. *J. Acoust. Soc. Am.* 72, 131-141.

Sellick, P.M., Patuzzi, R. and Johnstone, B.M. (1982b). Modulation of responses of spiral ganglion cells in the guinea pig cochlea by low frequency sound. *Hearing Res.* 199-221.

Sellick, P.M., Yates, G.K. and Patuzzi, R. (1983). Influence of mass source size and position on phase and amplitude measurements of the guinea pig basilar membrane. *Hearing Res.* (in press)

Zwicker, E. (1977). Masking-period patterns. *J. Acoust. Soc. Am.* 61, 1031-1040.

GENERAL DISCUSSION

RUSSELL:

You observe sharper frequency selectivity in the basilar membrane mechanics when the Mössbauer source is located over the inner hair cells than when it is placed over the region of the outer hair cells. Have you considered the possibility that the source is somehow influencing the mechanical properties of the basilar membrane, and that this is position dependent?

JOHNSTONE:

We believe the source does influence the mechanics but only as a second order effect. However, more experiments are needed. Indeed it would be very interesting to record neurally after loading the membrane with various weights.

WILSON:

It seems to me to be a little unlikely that the hair cell excitation function should be exactly the same as basilar membrane tuning. Some slight longitudinal coupling in the tectorial membrane, for example, might account for the slight discrepancies that you observe.

JOHNSTONE:

Some slight coupling or disturbance by the tectorial membrane is certainly possible. Our results suggest this is a minor effect, at least in normal animals. It is not needed to account for any of the major properties of auditory neurons or hair cell responses that we have investigated to date.

KIM:

Regarding tuning characteristics of a cochlear neuron and of a point on BM, you and your associates (Sellick et al., JASA, 72, 131, 1982) have advocated that a 0.04 mm/sec iso-velocity curve of BM corresponds to the neural tuning curve. I wonder whether you have modified the notion that an iso-velocity curve provides a better match than an iso-displacement curve around the CF. I am asking this because we have found (Fig. 4 of Neely and Kim, Hear. Res. 9, 123, 1983) that replotting your BM data as a 10 Å iso-displacement curve provides a better match with the neural tuning curve than the 0.04 mm/sec iso-velocity curve or the 3 Å iso-displacement curve as originally plotted in Fig. 10 of Sellick et al. (1982).

JOHNSTONE:

We find a better fit to iso-velocity contours but it depends on what part of the curves is the fit to be emphasized. The tip to tail difference is better with iso-velocity, but the slope of the same intermediate frequencies may fit better to iso amplitude.

THERMAL NOISE AND ACTIVE PROCESSES IN THE INNER EAR:
RELATING THEORY TO EXPERIMENT

William Bialek

*Department of Biophysics and Medical Physics, and
Biology and Medicine Division, Lawrence Berkeley Laboratory
University of California, Berkeley
Berkeley, California 94720 U.S.A.*

1. INTRODUCTION

In 1948, Gold proposed that the filter characteristics of the auditory system may be influenced by active elements. In the same year, de Vries presented a preliminary analysis of thermal noise in the cochlea and its implications for the detection of the threshold auditory stimulus (cf. de Vries, 1956). With few exceptions, these papers were ignored until the 1970's, when a number of observations made the concept of active filtering an attractive hypothesis. At the same time, Flerov (1976) resurrected the issue of thermal noise, and we (Bialek and Schweitzer, 1980; 1983) began a more systematic investigation of this problem.

In this paper I discuss how the analysis of noise allows active filtering to be distinguished experimentally from passive filtering. For simplicity I use an elementary model of an inner ear filter, namely a mass-spring-damping system. Such a system could model an element of the basilar membrane, a bundle of stereocilia, or the dynamics of an otoconial mass (cf. Lewis, et al. (1983) for a review). The basic problem is to distinguish between a system in which the damping is intrinsically small, leading to a sharp passive resonance, and a system in which the damping is intrinsically large but is compensated by an active element, leading to a sharp active filter. Many observable properties of these two systems are identical for appropriate choices of the parameters; in particular, the frequency response of any stable active filter can be reproduced by some (perhaps quite complex) passive filter. Attempts to distinguish between active and passive filtering in the inner ear on the basis of frequency responses alone must therefore fail.

The central conclusions of this paper are that the characteristics of thermal noise in an active filter cannot be reproduced by any passive system, and that existing experiments point to the possibility of measuring these noise characteristics in the inner ear organs. These results are intended as a guide to the design of experiments which will finally decide the issue of active vs. passive filtering in the inner ear.

2. THERMAL NOISE IN ACTIVE AND PASSIVE SYSTEMS

The dynamics of the mass-spring-damping system are described by the differential equation

$$m\frac{d^2x(t)}{dt^2} + \gamma\frac{dx(t)}{dt} + \kappa x(t) = F(t), \qquad (1)$$

where x is the displacement, F is the applied force, and m, γ, and κ, are the mass, damping, and stiffness, respectively. This differential equation leads to the frequency response function,

$$\alpha(\omega) = \frac{x(\omega)}{F(\omega)} = [-m\omega^2 - i\gamma\omega + \kappa]^{-1}, \tag{2}$$

where $x(\omega)$ and $F(\omega)$ are, respectively, the Fourier transforms of $x(t)$ and $F(t)$:

$$x(\omega) = \frac{1}{(2\pi)^{\frac{1}{2}}}\int dt\ e^{i\omega t}x(t) \qquad\qquad F(\omega) = \frac{1}{(2\pi)^{\frac{1}{2}}}\int dt\ e^{i\omega t}F(t). \tag{3}$$

To describe thermal noise in the mass-spring system, we add to equation (1) a "Langevin force", $\delta F(t)$:

$$m\frac{d^2x(t)}{dt^2} + \gamma\frac{dx(t)}{dt} + \kappa x(t) = F(t) + \delta F(t). \tag{4}$$

Conceptually, the Langevin force arises from the random, incessant collisions between the mass and the molecules of the fluid which surrounds it (Einstein, 1956). The principles of statistical mechanics (Landau and Lifshitz, 1977) determine the properties of δF:

[1] δF is a stationary, Gaussian random variable with zero mean.
[2] δF has no "memory"; it has zero correlation time. That is, $<\delta F(t)\delta F(t')> = A\delta(t-t')$. Thus the probability of δF taking a particular value at one time is not influenced by its value at any previous time.
[3] The Fourier transform of $\delta F(t)$, $\delta F(\omega)$, forms a set of Gaussian variables, one at each frequency. To determine variances and co-variances, consider

$$<\delta F(\omega)\delta F*(\omega')> = \frac{1}{2\pi}\int dt_1\int dt_2 e^{i\omega t_1}e^{-i\omega t_2}<\delta F(t_1)\delta F(t_2)> = (A/2\pi)\delta(\omega-\omega'). \tag{5}$$

This shows that the Fourier components of δF fluctuate independently, and that each has the same variance per unit frequency interval, or spectral density, $S_F(\omega) = A/2\pi$.

[4] The spectral density of δF is given by $S_F(\omega) = A/2\pi = \gamma k_B T/\pi$, where $k_B = 1.36\times10^{-23}$ J/K is Boltzmann's constant and T (300 K) is the absolute temperature. It is important to note that the magnitude of the *random* Langevin force is completely determined by γ, which describes the response of the system to *deterministic* forces.

Using these properties of δF, together with equation (4), we can characterize the Brownian motion of the system, expressed as the fluctuation δx in the displacement. Like δF, δx is Gaussian. Further, its Fourier transform $\delta x(\omega)$ is given by $\delta x(\omega) = \alpha(\omega)\delta F(\omega)$, so the spectral density of δx is

$$S_x(\omega) = |\alpha(\omega)|^2 S_F(\omega) = \frac{\gamma k_B T/\pi}{(\kappa-m\omega^2)^2+(\gamma\omega)^2}. \tag{6}$$

Thus the fluctuations in x are filtered, and have the same dependence on frequency as does the tuning curve. The correlation function of δx, $<\delta x(t)\delta x(t')>$, is given by the Fourier transform of the spectral density function S_x (Rice, 1954):

$$<\delta x(t)\delta x(t')> = \frac{\gamma k_B T}{\pi}\int d\omega\frac{e^{-i\omega(t-t')}}{(\kappa-m\omega^2)^2+(\gamma\omega)^2}. \tag{7}$$

In particular, the total fluctuations in x,

$$<(\delta x)^2> = <\delta x(t)\delta x(t)> = \frac{\gamma k_B T}{\pi}\int\frac{d\omega}{(\kappa-m\omega^2)^2+(\gamma\omega)^2} = k_B T/\kappa, \tag{8}$$

are determined only by the stiffness κ.

How do these noise characteristics change when we introduce an active element? The molecules colliding with the mass, and giving rise to the Langevin force, do not "know" that the active element has been introduced, so that the statistics of δF do not change. To describe noise in the presence of feed-

back, we must therefore only add to equation (4) a term representing the feed-
back itself; for the case of a "negative damping" with magnitude η, we obtain

$$m\frac{d^2x(t)}{dt^2} + (\gamma-\eta)\frac{dx(t)}{dt} + \kappa x(t) = F(t) + \delta F(t). \tag{9}$$

From this equation we find the new frequency response function,

$$\alpha(\eta;\omega) = [-m\omega^2 - i(\gamma-\eta)\omega + \kappa]^{-1}; \tag{10}$$

the new spectral density of displacement fluctuations,

$$S_x(\eta;\omega) = \frac{\gamma k_B T/\pi}{(\kappa-m\omega^2)^2+(\gamma-\eta)^2\omega^2}; \tag{11}$$

and the new value of the total fluctuations in x,

$$<(\delta x)^2_\eta> = \frac{\gamma k_B T}{\pi}\int\frac{d\omega}{(\kappa-m\omega^2)^2+(\gamma-\eta)^2\omega^2} = (k_B T/\kappa)\frac{\gamma}{\gamma-\eta}. \tag{12}$$

The crucial point is that <u>the magnitude of the noise is no longer uniquely
related to the parameters of the response function</u>. Thus, if we measure the
ratio of force to displacement at low frequencies, which defines κ, and assume
the system is passive, we can use equation (8) to predict the magnitude of the
Brownian motion. If the system is in fact active, the observed Brownian
motion will be larger than predicted, and the magnitude of the discrepancy
measures the fraction of the damping which is compensated by the active element, as may be seen by comparing equations (8) and (12).

3. CAN WE SEE THERMAL NOISE IN THE HAIR CELL?

    In excised hair cells of the frog crista, Orman and Flock (1981) have
measured torsional stiffnesses for stereociliary bundles on the order of
5×10^{-11} Nt/rad, or $\kappa = 2\times10^{-6}$ Nt/m for bundles of length 25 μm. The assumption that these stereocilia are mechanically passive predicts the Brownian
motion amplitude $\delta x_{rms} = (k_B T/\kappa)^{\frac{1}{2}} = 0.05$ μm. If they are active, on the
other hand, the amplitude of Brownian motion may be significantly larger,
which will make it visible through a light microscope. In this case, then,
the mere visibility of the thermal noise would be strong evidence of an active
element in the mechanics of the stereocilium.
    An interesting, if indirect, method of observing thermal noise is through
its effect on the statistics of spontaneous activity at the afferent neurons.
To a first approximation the firing of the neuron is a Poisson process
(Siebert, 1965; Johnson, 1978) of rate λ which is modulated by motion of the
hair cell stereocilia. For small amplitude, low frequency motions, the modulation is linear, so that pure tones generate sinusoidal phase histograms with
modulation amplitude proportional to stimulus amplitude (Johnson, 1980):

$$\lambda(t) = \lambda_o + (\partial\lambda/\partial x)x(t). \tag{13}$$

If a spike occurs at time t=0, the probability that there are no spikes before
time t is given by

$$P_o(t) = <\exp [-\int_0^t d\tau\lambda(\tau)]>, \tag{14}$$

which, assuming Gaussian fluctuations in x, becomes

$$P_0(t) = e^{-\lambda_0 t} \exp \{ \tfrac{1}{2}(\partial\lambda/\partial x)^2 \int_0^t d\tau_1 \int_0^t d\tau_2 <\delta x(\tau_1)\delta x(\tau_2)> \}. \tag{15}$$

The conventional inter-spike-interval distribution is given by $P_{ISI}(t) = -dP_0(t)/dt$. Fourier transforming equation (12) allows us to find the correlation function,

$$<\delta x(\tau_1)\delta x(\tau_2)> = \frac{k_B T}{\kappa} \frac{\gamma}{\gamma-\eta} e^{-(\gamma-\eta)|\tau_1-\tau_2|/2m} \cos[\omega_0(\tau_1-\tau_2)], \tag{16}$$

where $\omega_0 = (\kappa/m)^{\frac{1}{2}}$ is the resonance frequency, and this can then be substituted into equation (15) to determine the interval distribution.

I shall consider the effects of thermal noise on the mean interval $<\tau>$ and on the behavior of the interval distribution for long times; these quantities are particularly interesting because it is possible to give analytic expressions for them by starting with equations (15) and (16). These expressions are (Bialek, unpublished):

$$\lim_{\tau \to \infty} P_{ISI}(\tau) = (\text{constant}) e^{-\lambda' \tau} \tag{17a}$$

$$<\tau> = \frac{2m}{\gamma-\eta} e^y \int_0^1 dz \exp[+(\ln z)\lambda' 2m/(\gamma-\eta)] I_0(zy), \tag{17b}$$

where I_0 is a modified Bessel function, and

$$\lambda' = \lambda_0 - \frac{\gamma-\eta}{2m} y, \tag{18a}$$

$$y = (\partial\lambda/\partial x)^2 (1/\omega_0)^2 (k_B T/\kappa) \frac{\gamma}{\gamma-\eta}. \tag{18b}$$

If there were no noise ($k_B T \to 0$), then we would have $P_{ISI}(\tau) = <\tau> e^{-\tau/<\tau>}$. Thus, in the absence of modulation by thermal noise, the interval distribution should decay with a time constant equal to the mean interval (Siebert, 1965; Johnson, 1978); if there is a significant refractory period τ_R, then the time constant will be reduced by this amount. A number of published experiments show clear deviations from this prediction. In particular, I have replotted in Fig. 1 the interval distribution for a vibratory receptor in the bullfrog saccule (Koyama, et al., 1982), illustrating a factor of two discrepancy between the "no noise" prediction and experiment.

If the discrepancy illustrated in Fig. 1 is indeed due to the effects of thermal noise, we can try to determine the magnitude of this noise, and hence decide whether active filtering occurs in this system. From equations (17) and (18), it is clear that the mean interval $<\tau>$ and the decay constant λ' allow us to determine λ_0 and y if we know $(\gamma-\eta)/2m$, and it is y which carries the information regarding the thermal noise. In fact, $(\gamma-\eta)/2\pi m$ is just the bandwidth of the frequency response, as may be shown from equation (10), which is 20 Hz for the saccular unit (the characteristic frequency is also 20 Hz). Using this estimate, together with the fit to the data shown in Fig. 1, I find y = 0.9+0.1 for this neuron. To convert this value of y into an estimate of $(\gamma-\eta)/\gamma$ through equation (18), we must determine $\partial\lambda/\partial x$.

The vibratory receptor provides an important advantage for the type of analysis presented here, since the stimulus is linear acceleration. In the mass-spring model, an acceleration a applies a force ma, and hence a displacement $\alpha(\eta;\omega)$ma. Therefore the measured quantity $\partial\lambda/\partial a$ is related (at the characteristic frequency) to $\partial\lambda/\partial x$ by $\partial\lambda/\partial a = [m/(\gamma-\eta)\omega_0](\partial\lambda/\partial x)$. Thus equation (18b) becomes

$$y = [\frac{\gamma-\eta}{m}]^2 (k_B T/\kappa) \frac{\gamma}{\gamma-\eta}(\partial\lambda/\partial a)^2$$

$$= [\frac{\gamma-\eta}{m\omega_0}]^2 (k_B T/m) \frac{\gamma}{\gamma-\eta}(\partial\lambda/\partial a)^2. \tag{19}$$

Experimentally, $\partial\lambda/\partial a = 3\times10^3$ spikes-sec-cm^{-1}, as estimated from the fact (Koyama, et al., 1982) that a 0.01 cm-sec^{-2} stimulus is sufficient to cause nearly complete phase-locking of a neuron with mean firing rate $(34.3 \text{ ms})^{-1}$. This value, together with our estimates of $(\gamma-\eta)/m$ and ω from the tuning curve and y from the interval distribution (and k_bT from above), allows an evaluation of $\gamma/(\gamma-\eta)$ in terms of m:

$$\frac{\gamma}{\gamma-\eta} = \frac{m}{1.16\times10^{-9} \text{ gm}}. \qquad (20)$$

Thus, if the mass-like element in the vibratory receptor of the saccule exceeds 10^{-9} gm, then a consistent interpretation of the tuning curves and spontaneous activity pattern requires $\gamma/(\gamma-\eta) > 1$: an active filter. In fact, from the dimensions of the individual otoconia in this organ, a single stone is likely to have a mass larger than this, and there are many stones per hair cell.

Detailed tests of this interpretation of neural statistics may be made by examining the joint probability distribution for successive intervals. As is well known, the simple Poisson model predicts that successive intervals are independent. In the presence of thermal noise, this is no longer true, and we must consider the generalization of equation (14),

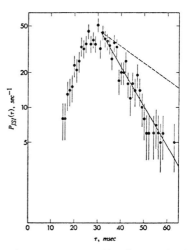

Fig. 1. Inter-spike-interval distribution $P_{ISI}(\tau)$ for a vibratory receptor in the bullfrog saccule (Koyama et al., 1982: unit 071581-3). Error bars are taken as the square root of the number of intervals observed in each bin; data rejected for fewer than 5 intervals. Mean interval $\langle\tau\rangle=34.3msec$, refractory period $\tau_R=5$ msec. Solid line: best fit to exponential at long intervals, Eq. (17) with $\lambda'=79$ s^{-1}. Dashed line: behavior expected form Poisson model with no thermal noise (see text)

$$P_o(t_1,t_2) = \langle\exp[-\int_0^{t_1}d\tau\lambda(\tau)]\lambda(t_1)\exp[-\int_{t_1}^{t_1+t_2}d\tau\lambda(\tau)]\rangle, \qquad (21)$$

where the conventional joint interval distribution (cf. Kiang, 1965) is given by $P_{JI}(t_1,t_2) = -dP_o(t_1,t_2)/dt_2$. As in the case of P_{ISI}, general results for the joint interval distribution are complicated, but they simplify in the limits of long and short intervals. In particular, it may be shown from equation (21) that the average interval $\langle t_2\rangle$ is a function of the length of the preceeding interval t_1. If the previous interval was very short, then $\langle t_2\rangle = \langle\tau\rangle$, while if the previous interval was long $\langle t_2\rangle = 1/\lambda'$. For the saccular neuron of Fig. 1, this means that the mean interval should vary by a factor of two, depending on the length of the previous interval. The direction of this variation is such that long intervals tend to be followed by abnormally short intervals – the spikes cluster. Observation of this effect would be strong evidence for the specific theory proposed here, and would support the general conclusion that the statistics of neural firing can be interpreted in terms of the magnitude and spectrum of thermal noise in the inner ear.

4. COMMENTS AND CONCLUSIONS

The next generation of optical instrumentation for inner ear studies should be capable of resolving nanometer motions of the stereocilia. The analysis presented here demonstrates that observation of both driven motions and Brownian motions on this scale will allow direct test of the hypothesis that the stereocilium is mechanically active. Further statistical analysis of spontaneous neural activity and hair cell voltage fluctuations will provide indirect probes of active elements in the inner ear. Both types of investigation should also allow the absolute magnitude of the thermal noise to be estimated and compared with the responses to behavioral threshold stimuli, and will therefore test the claim that the threshold of hearing is limited by thermal noise (de Vries, 1956; Flerov, 1976; Bialek and Schweitzer, 1980; 1983). The preliminary analysis presented here argues strongly in favor of active filtering and for the significance of Brownian motion as a source of noise in the inner ear.

Acknowledgements: These results developed out of work with Allan Schweitzer. I thank Professor E.R. Lewis for providing the data of Fig. 1. I am grateful to C. van Andel for preparing the figure, to R.F. Goldstein for comments on the manusciprt, to Professor G. Zweig for valuable discussions, and to Professor A. Bearden for providing both constructive criticism and a productive environment in which to carry out this research. This work was supported by the Office of Basic Energy Sciences, Office of Energy Research, U.S. Department of Energy, under contract No. DE-AC-03-76SF00098, and by the NAtional Science Foundation Biophysics (PCM 78-22245) and Pre-Doctoral Fellowship programs.

REFERENCES

Bialek, W., Schweitzer, A. (1980). Thermal fluctuation of stereocilia require active mechanical tuning. *J. Acoust. Soc. Am.* **68**, 42.

Bialek, W., Schweitzer, A. (1983). Thermal noise and the auditory receptor cell. In preparation.

de Vries, H. (1956). Physical aspects of the sense organs. *Prog. Biophys. Biophys. Chem.* **6**, 207 – 264.

Einstein, A. (1956). Investigations on the Theory of Brownian Movement. (R. Furth, ed.). New York, Dover.

Flerov, M.N. (1976). Thermal noise of the hair cells in the organ of Corti. *Biofizika* **6**, 1092 – 1096.

Gold, T. (1948). Hearing II. The physical basis of the action of the cochlea. *Proc. Roy. Soc. Edinb.* B135, 492 – 498.

Johnson, D.H. (1978). The relationship of post-stimulus time and interval histograms to the timing characteristics of spike trains. *Biophys. J.* **22**, 413 – 430.

Johnson, D.H. (1980). The relationship between spike rate and synchrony in responses of auditory nerve fibers to single tones. *J. Acoust. Soc. Am.* **68**, 1115 – 1122.

Kiang, N.Y.-S. (1965). Discharge Properties of Single Fibers in the Cat's Auditory Nerve. Cambridge, MIT Press.

Koyama, H., Lewis, E.R., Leverenz, E.L., Baird, R.A. (1982). Acute seismic sensitivity in the bullfrog ear. *Brain Res.* **250**, 168 – 171.

Landau, L., Lifshitz, E.M. (1977). *Statistical Physics* (2nd revised English edition). 343 – 400. Oxford, Pergamon.

Lewis, E.R., Leverenz, E.L., Bialek, W.S. (1983). The vertebrate inner ear. To appear in *C.R.C. Crit. Rev. Biomed. Eng.*

Orman, S., Flock, A. (1981). Stiffness measurements of stereociliary bundles in frog crista ampullaris. *Soc. Neurosci. Abs.* **7**, 536.

Rice, S.O. (1954). Mathematical analysis of random noise. In: *Selected Papers on Noise and Stochastic Processes.* (N. Wax, ed.). 133 – 294, New York, Dover.

Siebert, W.M. (1965). Some implications of the stochastic behaviour of primary auditory neurons. *Kybernetik* **2**, 206 – 215.

GENERAL DISCUSSION

EVANS:

Can you say why these characteristics should not be observed easily in <u>mammalian</u> (e.g. cochlear nerve fibre) preparations?

BIALEK:
The theory presented here is for linear modulation of firing probability by stereocilium (or basilar membrane) motion; this is realistic only for small amplitude, low frequency situations, and does not apply to most mammalian units with
CF $\geq$ 6 kHz. Also the effects are largest when the CF is not too much larger than
the mean firing rate, again not true in mammals. Published experiments on mammals
do, however, exhibit anomalous decay constants for the interval distribution, but
the effects are not as dramatic as in the frog sacculus.

WIT:
You said that there is no direct proof for the existence of active processes within the cochlea. What then is your opinion on spontaneous acoustic emissions from
the ear canal?

BIALEK:
I believe that the spontaneous acoustic emissions reflect the instabilities of
an active filter in the cochlea, but I do not think that this can be convincingly proven. At best we imagine that the emission occurs only in pathological situations, and it is difficult to argue from those observations to the "normal"
case. I would not want to base a theory of active processes on the emissions
alone, although obviously they provide support for such a theory; part of the
problem is that active filters do not necessarily produce emissions.

DE BOER:
According to your calculations, the magnitude of thermal noise will be (much)
larger in an active system. I fail to see the physical reason for it since the
resistance as well as the amplifier must interact energetically with their surroundings.

BIALEK:
Amplifiers and resistors interact with the environment very differently. The resistor represents a dissipation pathway for the system to come to thermal equilibrium, while the amplifier holds the system away from thermal equilibrium
(using the energy from its power supply). It is this difference which accounts
for the results I present. I emphasize that the calculation methods are completely rigorous in the case of a noiseless amplifier; real amplifiers, with non-zero
noise temperatures of their own, will increase the noise still further above the
passive case.

KEMP:
We can do something like the experiment you propose with the whole cochlea. In
spontaneous acoustic emissions I believe the cochlea acts as a delay line loop resonator with a level dependent loop gain (Kemp, in: Tinnitus, Evered and Lawrenson,
Eds., London, p. 54-81, 1981). We took observations of the level dependence of the
system and the bandwidth and intensity of the spontaneous tonal emissions at the
ear canal. At zero stimulation the system should have a very high Q, limited by
the level of noise in the system. We worked back from the spontaneous emissions
data to compute the background noise environment, needed to create the 'emissions'.
The result was a noise 10 dB above the computed thermal noise in the ear canal,
which was above the level of external acoustic noise. My question is: Does this
prove the cochlea has active amplification? Could not the cochlear just be a
noisy place? How would you discriminate against noisy and functionless active processes in your model?

BIALEK:
As you suggest, the cochlea could include a number of extraneous noise sources,
particularly in pathological situations such as emissions. Thus I agree with your
(implicit) suggestion that experiments at the ear canal could not be conclusive.
My argument that measurements of noise can discriminate active from passive
filters must be qualified: Experiments must be done on isolated systems, such as
the stereocilia of individual hair cells, which are shielded from 'trivial' noise
sources.

COCHLEAR POTENTIALS IN HOMOZYGOUS AND HETEROZYGOUS BRONX WALTZER MICE

Gregory R. Bock

MRC Institute of Hearing Research
University of Nottingham, Nottingham NG7 2RD, U.K.

1. THE BRONX WALTZER MUTATION

Deol and Gluecksohn-Waelsch (1979) reported the occurrence of a new mutation in a mouse colony at Albert Einstein College of Medicine in New York. This mutation, which was named "Bronx waltzer" (symbol *bv*), was autosomal recessive, with homozygotes (*bv/bv*) exhibiting two principal abnormalities:
1. A behavioural disorder, associated with many single-gene mutations causing deafness in mice, and characterized by shaking or waltzing (Steel *et al*, 1982).
2. An absence of inner hair cells in the cochlea.
Deol and Gluecksohn-Waelsch (1979) reported that mice homozygous for the Bronx waltzer gene responded to sound, if at all, only for a brief period following the normal time of onset of auditory function (around postnatal day 13 in mice). Deol (1981) subsequently reported that homozygous Bronx waltzers show severe and early degeneration of the maculae and cristae of the vestibular system.
Bronx waltzers from the original colony in New York were imported to the U.K. by M.S. Deol and were then outcrossed onto CBA animals in order to produce a more robust breeding stock. Data in the present paper were obtained from animals from this outcrossed stock.

2. HOMOZYGOUS ANIMALS

The general methods used in our laboratory for measuring cochlear potentials have been described in detail elsewhere (Bock and Steel, 1982; Steel and Bock, 1982) and will only be briefly described here. The auditory bulla was exposed in urethane-anaesthetized animals (2.0mg/g) and a recording electrode placed on the round window. Stimuli were delivered via a closed calibrated sound system and responses were amplified, digitized, and averaged on a microcomputer.
Responses to tone bursts in homozygous Bronx walzer mice (Bock *et al*, 1982) were compared with responses in CBA controls. The compound action potential (C.A.P.) in response to tone bursts was either very small or was completely absent. Microphonics were present but were of very small maximum amplitude (0.1µV at most frequencies). Summating potentials were present in the round window response, and the patterns of polarity reversal with changes in tone frequency and amplitude were similar to those in CBA controls.
It was not possible to construct audiograms for Bronx waltzer mice since the C.A.P. was not clearly recognisable. All animals examined in our laboratory showed a behavioural response to loud sound, although the response was clearly abnormal in magnitude in comparison with responses of C.B.A. animals.

3. HETEROZYGOUS ANIMALS

Animals heterozygous for the Bronx waltzer gene (+/bv) examined in our laboratory have no waltzing-type behavioural abnormality but their behavioural response to loud sound is poor. C.A.P. thresholds from a typical heterozygote are shown in Fig. 1, together with thresholds from a typical CBA mouse. Although thresholds in heterozygotes are relatively normal below 10 kHz, they deteriorate rapidly at higher frequencies. An example of the averaged round window response at 10 kHz in the heterozygous animal is shown in Fig. 1. The C.A.P. responses in heterozygotes, although showing poor thresholds, were relatively normal in form, with clear N_1 and N_2 peaks. Summating potentials were, however, very small.

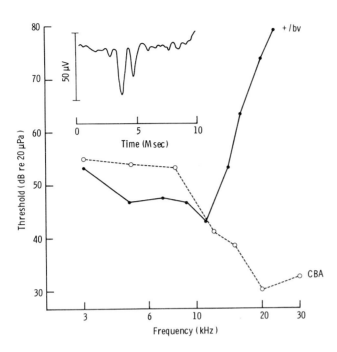

Fig. 1. Represent-ative C.A.P. audio-grams of one CBA and one +/bv mouse. The insert shows the averaged round window response to a 10 kHz tone burst (83dB re 20μPa) in the +/bv animal

Microphonic amplitudes at various frequencies are shown in Fig. 2 for a typical heterozygote and a typical C.B.A. control. Peak amplitudes in hetero-zygous animals were usually around 10 to 50μV which, although larger than peak amplitudes in homozygotes (usually <10μV), is well below peak amplitudes in C.B.A. controls (100-200μV).

4. DISCUSSION

The finding of severely diminished C.A.P. responses in homozygous Bronx waltzers is not surprising in view of the rapid and early degeneration observed in the spiral ganglion cell population (Deol and Gluecksohn-Waelsch, 1979). The poor C.A.P. thresholds and microphonics in heterozygous animals are, however, unexpected and suggests that the expression of the Bronx waltzer gene is rather more complicated than was at first thought.

When the Bronx waltzer mutation was first reported, it seemed likely that mutant animals would provide interesting data on cochlear physiology, since a uniform inner hair cell lesion is difficult to produce experimentally. Several considerations must now give rise to caution in interpreting data in homozygous animals. Although it was originally reported that inner hair cells in homozygotes are all either absent or structurally abnormal, more recent studies (Pujol, personal communication) suggest that some inner hair cells are present and of normal appearance. Furthermore, the finding of physiological abnormalities in heterozygotes in the present study suggests that corresponding anatomical abnor-malities may be present in these animals, in which case the Bronx waltzer gene would not be fully recessive in its effect on hearing. Careful anatomical study using scanning and transmission electronmicroscopy is clearly needed for both homozygous and heterozygous Bronx waltzers. It remains possible that such a study will provide useful information about the development and maintenance of cochlear innervation.

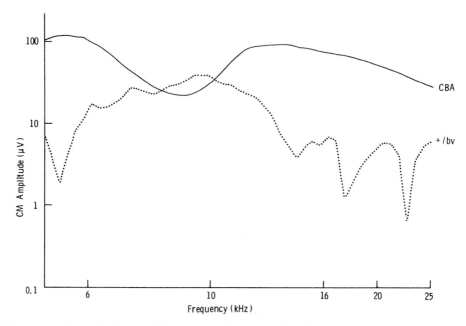

Fig. 2. *Curves showing cochlear microphonic amplitude as a function of frequency with a constant attenuation of 20 dB in the sound system for representative CBA and +/bv mice*

Acknowledgement: *I am grateful to M. Haggard, K. Steel and K. Horner for their comments on the manuscript.*

REFERENCES

Bock, G.R. and Steel, K.P. (1982). Inner ear pathology in the deafness mutant mouse. *Acta Otolaryngol.*, in press.

Bock, G.R., Yates, G.K. and Deol, M.S. (1982). Cochlear potentials in the Bronx waltzer mutant mouse. *Neuroscience Letters*, in press.

Deol, M.S. (1981). The inner ear in Bronx waltzer mice. *Acta Otolaryngol.*, 92, 331-336.

Deol, M.S. and Gluecksohn-Waelsch, S. (1979). The role of inner hair cells in hearing. *Nature*, 278, 250-252.

Steel, K.P. and Bock, G.R. (1982). Cochlear dysfunction in the jerker mouse. *Behav. Neuroscience*, in press.

Steel, K.P., Niaussat, M.M. and Bock, G.R. (1982). The genetics of hearing. In: *Auditory psychobiology of the mouse.* (J.F. Willott, ed.) Springfield, Ill. C.C. Thomas.

GENERAL DISCUSSION

STOPP:

It would be of interest to know what kind of innervation exists on the OHCs of both homozygous and heterozygous <u>bv</u> mice. Do you have any information on this?

BOCK:

Unfortunately there are no published data relevant to this problem. The original publication (Deol and Gluecksohn-Waelsch, cited above) presented data on light microscopy but no data on innervation. Recent unpublished studies by Pujol (pers. comm.) suggest that innervation of outer hair cells in cochleae of homozygous (bv/bv) mice is relatively normal, but we will have to wait for the completion of Pujol's study before we have an adequate answer to your question.

DUAL ACOUSTICAL SENSITIVITY IN FROGS

Edwin R. Lewis

Electronics Research Laboratory, University of California
Berkeley, California 94720, USA

While deriving new auditory structures that may be unique among terrestrial vertebrates, frogs and toads (anurans) apparently retained the auditory apparatus of fish, adapting it to seismic sensitivity (sensitivity to substrate-borne vibration). The present paper will compare and contrast the seismic and auditory senses in one species, the American bullfrog (*Rana catesbeiana*), presenting new observations from single-axon recording along with recent observations from intracellular dye-injection studies and morphological studies. The principal new conclusions are the following: a) Bullfrog seismic axons apparently reflect vibratory *acceleration* sensitivity, some exhibiting small-signal linear transfer ratios between acceleration amplitude and spike rate that are within ±2 dB of being constant over more than three octaves of stimulus frequency. b) Bullfrog seismic axons with substantial resting spike rates (approximately half of those observed) exhibit remarkably linear small-signal transfer ratios, some reflecting truly extraordinary sensitivity (as high as 2000 spikes/sec per cm/sec^2). c) Bullfrog seismic axons with very low resting spike rates (approximately half of those observed) typically exhibit quadratic relationships between acceleration amplitude and spike rate. d) While the tuning properties vary from axon to axon, at high frequencies (e.g., 100 to 200 Hz) all bullfrog seismic axons exhibit sensitivity declines that are much too steep (e.g., 40 dB or more per octave) to reflect the simple second-order dynamics of a conventional inertial accelerometer. e) Some bullfrog auditory axons exhibit tuning properties remarkably similar to those of mammalian cochlear fibers, with pronounced low-frequency tails and extraordinarily steep high-frequency slopes (e.g., 120 dB per octave). f) The small-signal transfer ratios of bullfrog auditory axons close to the resting (zero-input) state appear consistently to have dominant nonlinear (even-order) components, occasionally with large linear components superimposed (with maximum linear transfer ratios in the neighborhood of 5000 spikes/sec per dyne/cm^2). g) The auditory and seismic senses of the bullfrog inner ear are quite separate, with seismic axons exhibiting only very crude sensitivity to auditory stimuli and auditory axons exhibiting at best only crude sensitivity to vibratory stimuli.

1. PHYSIOLOGICAL PREPARATION AND SETUP

The bullfrog preparation was adapted from that of Capranica and his colleagues (Capranica and Moffat, 1975; Feng *et al.*, 1975). Animals were anesthetized with approximately 70 µg sodium pentobarbital per g body weight. Through a small hole in the roof of the mouth, the VIIIth nerve was exposed on its way from the intact otic capsule (with intact circulation) to the brain. The animal was mounted upside down on a rigid platform, with its head held firmly against the platform surface. Individual axons were penetrated with conventional glass microelectrodes, filled either with 0.5M KCl or with the ionic dye *Lucifer Yellow* (Stewart, 1978).

a) *Auditory Isolation and Stimulation*
Partial isolation from ambient auditory noise was achieved with a lab-built chamber providing at least 35 dB attenuation over the entire frequency range (50-3000 Hz) of bullfrog audition. Over the same range, the peak acoustical noise outside the chamber typically was 50-60 dB SPL. A closed-field auditory stimulus system, comprising a *KOSS* PRO-4X headphone and a calibrated *Bruel & Kjaer* 4186 condenser microphone mounted together in a brass housing, was placed next to the animal's tympanum and sealed with silicone grease around the entire perimeter of

that structure (see Capranica and Moffat, 1975). The housing provided further i-
solation of approximately 40 dB. However, since the experiments were conducted
with the animal's mouth wide open, exposing the large Eustachian tubes to ambient
sound pressure, this last stage of isolation served primarily to localize the applied auditory stimuli.

b) *Seismic Isolation and Stimulation*
    Partial isolation from ambient seismic noise was achieved by carrying out
the experiments on a lab-built vibration-isolation table comprising four second-
order mechanical filter stages, each slightly underdamped and with corner frequencies in the neighborhood of 1 Hz, topped by a fifth second-order stage in the
form of a commercial optical platform, also with corner frequencies in the neighborhood of 1 Hz. The entire structure was contained within the outer walls (reinforced concrete, 14 cm thick, with gasket-sealed double doors) of the acoustical
isolation chamber; the last two stages were contained within the inner walls
(plywood, 1.9 cm thick, with gasket-sealed doors) of the chamber. Thus vibrations induced in the table surface by air-borne sound were greatly reduced. With
this system, linear vibrations in the frequency range of interest (10-300 Hz)
were reduced to levels below the noise floor of our measuring system (approximately 0.0002 cm/sec^2).
    Dorsoventral sinusoidal vibrations were generated by a *Bruel & Kjaer* 4810 ex-
citer connected to the underside of the platform on which the frog was mounted.
The stimuli were monitored with a calibrated *Bruel & Kjaer* 4370 accelerometer.
The loaded platform was calibrated with respect to spatial variation of vibration
amplitude and found to be uniform to within ±1 dB over the frequency range of interest (10-300 Hz). When the peak acceleration of these vibratory sinusoids was
fixed at 7 cm/sec^2, the resulting open-field sound intensity measured at the level of the frog's tympanum was less than 50 dB SPL over almost the entire 10-300
Hz range, the only exception being between 140 and 160 Hz, where the intensity
reached 60 dB SPL. The amplitudes of all small-signal vibratory stimuli used in
the experiments were at least 40 dB below the 7 cm/sec^2 level, by linear extrapolation placing the concomitant airborne sound intensity well below the lowest
threshold levels reported for the bullfrog. Coupling from the closed-field auditory source to platform vibration was too weak to measure, presumably owing to
the isolation provided by the brass housing of the former. No attempts were made
to measure vibrations induced in the skeletal components of the otic capsule by
auditory stimuli.

2. EXPERIMENTAL PROCEDURES AND DATA PROCESSING

a) *Stimulus Protocols*
    Auditory and seismic axons were identified by their responses to sinusoidal
stimuli rapidly swept through the appropriate frequency ranges. Subsequent stimulus protocols for auditory fibers typically comprised tone bursts with 0.8-sec
periods, 50% duty cycles, and 50 ms rise and fall times. The tone-burst modulation usually was applied to a sinusoidal carrier whose frequency was swept logarithmically and sufficiently slowly that the frequency varied by less than 4%
(0.05 octave) during a single burst. Protocols for seismic fibers included continuous (logarithmic) frequency sweeps at 8 octaves/min, continuous single-
frequency stimuli, and (in cases where adaptation had been identified or suspected) series of widely separated tone bursts at a single carrier frequency.
The amplitudes of seismic stimuli were monitored continuously throughout each experiment; auditory stimulus amplitudes were calibrated at the beginning and the
end of each experiment.

b) *Data Processing*
    Stimulus waveforms and fiber responses were recorded on audio tape and sub-
sequently translated by comparator/Schmitt-trigger circuits to series of pulses,
one pulse for each spike and one for each positive-going zero crossing of the
stimulus sinusoid. The pulse series were converted by a digital computer with a
real-time clock to series of event times, reflecting the leading edges of the

pulses with 4 µsec accuracy except in cases where two pulses occurred within 33
µsec (i.e., the pulse representing a spike occurred within 33 µsec of that representing a zero crossing), in which case the inter-event interval was rounded to
33 µsec. Conventional signal-processing algorithms were applied to the event-
time series.

c) *Fiber-Marking*

Lucifer Yellow was selected as the intracellular dye because of its ability
to fill small-diameter fibers (e.g., the bullfrog auditory and seismic afferents,
which typically have diameters in the neighborhood of 2 µm, including myelin
sheath), an attribute not shared by Horseradish Peroxidase. Following physiological characterization, selected fibers were iontophoretically injected with the
dye, then processed and traced according to the published protocols (Lewis *et al.*,
1982a). The presence of a dye-filled cell body in one of the two VIIIth-nerve
ganglia served to identify a fiber as afferent. From the ganglion, each dye-
filled fiber was traced peripherally as far as possible, all the way to its termi-
nations in successful cases.

3. GENERAL RESULTS

a) *Auditory Tonotopy*

The dye tracing studies definitively confirmed the conclusions of earlier
investigators (Frishkopf and Goldstein, 1963; Feng *et al.*, 1975) that the sound
spectrum is divided between the two auditory papillae, with the amphibian papillar fibers exhibiting CFs from 100 Hz to 1000 Hz and the basilar papillar fibers
exhibiting CFs in the 1200 to 1600 Hz range. Within the two subdivisions of the
amphibian papilla, the studies revealed refined tonotopic organization (Lewis *et
al.*, 1982a; Lewis and Leverenz, 1983). The afferents from the triangle-shaped
anterior portion of the papilla exhibiting CFs ranging approximately from 100 to
300 Hz and gradually increasing as the location of fiber origin (peripheral termination) shifted from the posteromedial apex of the triangle to the antero-
lateral base. The afferents from the posterior, S-shaped stripe-like portion of
the papilla exhibited CFs ranging from less than 200 Hz to approximately 1000 Hz,
gradually increasing as the location of fiber origin shifted from the anterior
end to the posterior end.

b) *Seismic Endorgans*

The dye tracing studies revealed that seismic afferents originate either at
the center (striolar region) of the lagenar macula or at any location on the saccular macula, the most sensitive being saccular in origin (Koyama *et al.*, 1982;
Lewis *et al.*, 1982b). Purely-seismic lagenar afferents originated at the very
center of the striola; lagenar afferents exhibiting both seismic and gravity
sensitivities all terminated both at the center and the edge of the lagenar
striola, the latter also being the site of origin of purely gravity-sensitive fibers (Baird, 1982). No gravity-sensitive fibers were traced to the saccular macula, although many in the same major branch of the VIIIth nerve were traced past
the sacculus to the utriculus (Baird, 1982).

c) *Bulbed Kinocilia*

Hillman (1969) observed that most of the hair cells of the bullfrog sacculus
possess large bulbs at the distal ends of their kinocilia. The exceptions are a
few developing hair cells around the perimeter of the macula (Lewis and Li, 1973).
Similar bulbs are found in three other locations in the bullfrog inner ear (Lewis
and Li, 1975): all of the hair cells at the center of the lagenar striola possess bulbs; all but a few (lateral-most, developing) hair cells of the amphibian
papilla possess bulbs; and all of the hair cells of the medial-most four or five
rows of the basilar papilla possess bulbs. Interestingly, to date all of the
functionally-identified afferents traced to the basilar papilla have originated
from one or more of these rows. The only other kinociliary bulbs in the bullfrog
ear occur on a few scattered hair cells of unknown function along the center of
the utricular striola. Thus bulbed hair cells are strongly linked to both auditory and seismic sensitivity, providing a common denominator between the two.

4. SOME SPECIFIC PHYSIOLOGICAL OBSERVATIONS

a) *Saccular Afferents with Moderate to High Resting Discharge*

Qualitatively, the phase histograms of Figure 1 apparently are typical of all bullfrog seismic afferents that have moderate to high mean resting spike rates. At high stimulus intensities, response spike rates saturate at one per stimulus cycle for high frequencies (>40 Hz) and two or more per stimulus cycle for lower frequencies. When the stimulus intensity is reduced sufficiently, the histogram reflects a linear ac component at the frequency of the stimulus, super-imposed on the background discharge-- which in turn can be taken to comprise a dc (mean) component plus noise. From the ac component one can identify a small-signal, linear transfer ratio (defined to be the ratio of the peak amplitude of the ac response to the peak amplitude of the stimulus). The fiber of Figure 1 was especially sensitive, exhibiting a linear transfer ratio of approximately 1500 spikes/sec per cm/sec^2 at 60 Hz.

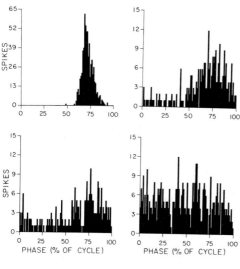

Fig. 2 (below). Small-signal linear transfer ratio (instantaneous spike rate/acceleration) plotted against stimulus frequency for a seismic afferent fiber from the bullfrog sacculus

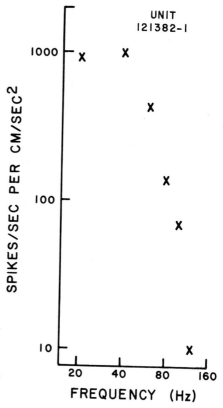

Fig. 1. Phase (cycle) histograms from a bullfrog saccular afferent fiber (unit 081282-4). Stimulus frequency = 60 Hz. Peak stimulus intensity (cm/sec^2)/response sampling time (sec) = 0.1/24 (upper left), 0.01/24 (upper right), 0.006/24 (lower left), 0/80 (lower right)

The transfer-ratio tuning curves of saccular afferents varied markedly from fiber to fiber, with 3-dB bandwidths ranging from less than 10 Hz to more than 80 Hz, typically centered about frequencies below 100 Hz. These tuning curves invariably exhibited extremely steep high-frequency rolloff, exemplified by that in Fig. 2, which approaches 40 dB/octave-- indicative of linear dynamics of order seven or more. Some fibers exhibited 3-dB bandwidths extending an octave or more beyond the approximately 50-Hz corner frequency of the unit of Fig. 2. For example, unit 121382-4 exhibited a bandwidth extending from less than 10 Hz to approximately 100 Hz, with small-signal, linear transfer ratios at 10, 20, 40, 60 and 80 Hz all lying between 170 and 240 spikes/sec per cm/sec^2. Low-frequency rolloff often began well above 20 Hz. Unit 121382-2, for example, exhibited a 3-dB bandwidth extending upward from approximately 35 Hz, the small-signal, linear transfer ratio at 20 Hz being down 12 dB from its midband value of approximately 1000 spikes/sec per cm/sec^2. Thus, the dynamics of saccular afferents seem not to be determined by a common mechanical filter.

b) *Seismic Afferents with Low Resting Spike Rates*
    In seismic afferents with low resting spike rates (i.e., much less than one spike per sec), every response of necessity included a dc component, which inherently is nonlinear (i.e., is generated by even-order distortion). Small signal responses exhibited strong phase preference with respect to the stimulus sinusoid at *all* stimulus intensities, but both peak and mean (ac and dc) response amplitudes (instantaneous spike rates) increased as the stimulus amplitude (peak acceleration) raised to the 2nd power, occasionally with conspicuous higher-power components as well. For example, at approximately the middle (50 Hz) of its sensitivity band, lagenar unit JH02-010 exhibited dc levels of 2.80 spikes/sec in response to 0.2 cm/sec^2 acceleration and 18.4 spikes/sec in response to 0.5 cm/sec^2. Saccular unit 072982-2 exhibited an extremely narrow sensitivity band (10-dB bandwidth less than 10 Hz) centered at approximately 90 Hz and a broader band (3-dB bandwidth approximately 20 Hz) centered at approximately 40 Hz. At 90 Hz, the unit exhibited dc levels of 1.32 spikes/sec in response to 0.2 cm/sec^2 and 15.6 spikes/sec in response to 0.7 cm/sec^2. Apparently consistent presence of higher-order terms (in addition to a quadratic term) is exemplified by the transfer ratio of lagenar unit JH02-004, whose sensitivity was greatest in the vicinity of 120 Hz. It exhibited the following dc responses at that frequency: 0.71 spikes/sec at 0.07 cm/sec^2, 6.8 spikes/sec at 0.2 cm/sec^2, and 55 spikes/sec at 0.5 cm/sec^2.

c) *Auditory Afferents*
    Amphibian papillar units typically exhibited very low resting spike rates (less than 1 spike/sec). Therefore, once again, every response included a nonlinear (dc) component. Auditory afferents with CFs below 500 Hz exhibited conspicuous linear ac responses superimposed on the dc responses, as exemplified by the phase histogram of Fig. 3, generated in response to 0.75-sec tone bursts, 10 dB above threshold (see next paragraph) at CF (440 Hz). The unit of Figs. 3 and 4 was the most sensitive amphibian-papillar fiber we have identified so far. Its small-signal linear transfer ratio (from Fig. 3) was approximately 5000 spikes/sec per $dyne/cm^2$. A unit with CF = 425 Hz, on the other hand, exhibited only marginally identifiable ac response (on a large dc component) when stimulated at CF, 10 dB above threshold. Thus the relative amplitude of the ac response was not simply related to frequency. This may be due to the fact that some amphibian-papillar afferents innervate hair cells of one polarity only, others innervate hair cells of opposite polarities (Lewis *et al.*, 1982a). The latter should exhibit partial cancellation of linear (and other odd-order) response components. Basilar-papillar fibers all innervate hair cells of one polarity only; yet to date we have found no evidence of a linear, small-signal response in any of them, even at relatively low stimulation frequencies (less than 500 Hz).
    For amphibian papillar units that were essentially silent at rest, the coordinates of a threshold point were taken to be the frequency and amplitude of the first 0.4-sec tone burst producing spikes during a descending or ascending frequency sweep. For frequencies above CF they were established on descending sweeps; for frequencies below CF they were established on ascending sweeps. The shapes of threshold tuning curves so derived varied markedly from afferent to afferent; that of Fig. 4 cannot be called typical. Indeed, it was extraordinary inasmuch as it was taken from the most sensitive amphibian papillar unit we have identified so far. Other amphibian papillar units with comparable sensitivities exhibited similarly steep rolloff at high frequencies and similar low-frequency tails. Units with considerably higher thresholds at CF typically exhibited more symmetric tuning curves, with more gentle rolloff at high frequencies. Using the Megela-Capranica (1982) protocol (tone bursts at CF, 10 dB above threshold, 10-ms

rise times), we found that almost all auditory afferents (including that of Figs. 3 and 4) exhibited a high probability of response within the first few cycles (long before the tone burst was fully on), indicating that the gradual accumulation of excitation typical of high-Q resonant systems was not present.

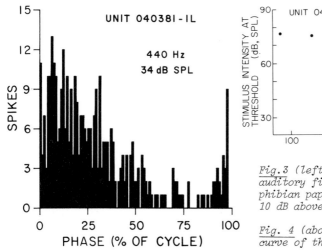

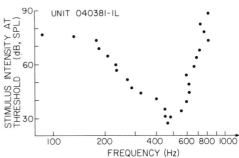

Fig.3 (left). Phase histogram of an auditory fiber from the bullfrog amphibian papilla, stimulated at CF, 10 dB above threshold

Fig. 4 (above). Threshold tuning curve of the unit of Fig. 3

REFERENCES

Baird, R.A. (1982). *Correspondences between Structure and Function in the Bullfrog Otoconial Organs*. Berkeley: University of California (dissertation).

Capranica, R.R., Moffat, A.J.M. (1975). Selectivity of the peripheral auditory system of spadefoot toads (*Scaphiopus couchi*) for sounds of biological significance. *J. Comp. Physiol.* 100, 231-249.

Feng, A.S., Narins, P.M., Capranica, R.R. (1975). Three populations of primary auditory fibers in the bullfrog (*Rana catesbeiana*): their peripheral origins and frequency sensitivities. *J. Comp. Physiol.* 100, 221-229.

Frishkopf, L.S., Goldstein, M.H. (1963). Responses to acoustic stimuli from single units in the eighth nerve of the bullfrog. *J. Acoust. Soc. Am.* 35, 1219-1228.

Hillman, D.E. (1969). New ultrastructural findings regarding a vestibular ciliary apparatus and its possible functional significance. *Brain Res.* 13, 407-412.

Koyama, H., Lewis, E.R., Leverenz, E.L., Baird, R.A. (1982). Acute seismic sensitivity in the bullfrog ear. *Brain Res.* 250, 168-172.

Lewis, E.R., Baird, R.A., Leverenz, E.L., Koyama, H. (1982b). Inner ear: dye-injection reveals peripheral origins of specific sensitivities. *Science* 215, 1641-1643.

Lewis, E.R., Leverenz, E.L. (1983). Morphological basis for tonotopy in the anuran amphibian papilla. *Scanning Electron Microscopy* (in press).

Lewis, E.R., Leverenz, E.L., Koyama, H. (1982a). The tonotopic organization of the bullfrog amphibian papilla, an auditory organ lacking a basilar membrane. *J. Comp. Physiol.* 145, 437-445.

Lewis, E.R., Li, C.W. (1973). Evidence concerning the morphogenesis of saccular receptors in the bullfrog. *J. Morph.* 139, 351-361.

Lewis, E.R., Li, C.W. (1975). Hair cell types and distributions in the otolithic and auditory organs of the bullfrog. *Brain Res.* 83, 35-50.

Megela, A.L., Capranica, R.R. (1982). Differential patterns of physiological masking in the anuran auditory nerve. *J. Acoust. Soc. Am.* 71, 641-645.

Stewart, W.W. (1978). Functional connections between cells as revealed by dye-coupling with a highly fluorescent naphthalimide tracer. *Cell* 14, 741-759.

Research supported by the National Science Foundation, Grant BNS-8005834 and by the National Institute of Neurological and Communicative Disorders and Stroke, Grant NS12359. I gratefully acknowledge the invaluable assistance of my colleagues.

GENERAL DISCUSSION

KIM:
Is there correlation among the sensitivity at CF, the sharpness of tuning and
the number of hair cells innervated by one neuron in the saccule?

E.R. LEWIS:
In order to collect data from many axons, we have carried out most of our quantitative studies of seismic sensitivity without dye (unambiguous dye-tracing is
limited to one fiber per animal). We soon will resume dye-tracing studies in the
sacculus, at which time one should be able to answer your fascinating question.

FETTIPLACE:
Could the square-law dependence on stimulus amplitude of the seismic afferent
discharge be due to the exponential transfer function of the afferent synapse?

E.R. LEWIS:
The stimulus-response relationships we find are very close to

$$R = S^2 \text{ for } S > 0; \quad R = 0 \text{ for } S \leq 0$$

where R is response amplitude and S is stimulus amplitude. Therefore a candidate
function should possess a Taylor's expansion (about some point) in which the zero-
degree and first-degree terms, $f(x_o)$ and $f'(x_o)(x-x_o)$, are negligible in comparison to the second-degree term $f''(x_o)(x-x_o)^2/2$. For the function

$$f(y) = e^{ay}-1 \; ; \; y = x-x_o$$

we have $f(y) \simeq ay + \dfrac{(ay)^2}{2} + \cdots\cdots\cdots$
in which case the second-degree term begins to dominate as ay becomes greater
than two. Unfortunately, as this takes place the third-degree term $(ay)^3/6$ also
becomes prominent. We see no evidence of cubic components in the observed stimulus-response relationship, leaving us with a puzzle indeed.

DE BOER:
Did you monitor the physiological condition of the animal? Do you encounter more
insensitive units near the end of the experiment?

E.R. LEWIS:
The one parameter we monitor is blood flow to the inner ear, and our resolution
of that is crude ("rapid flow of RBCs through arteries to the ear" vs "sluggish
flow" vs "no flow"). We typically record for 40 to 60 minutes from a single axon.
Over that period of time we have seen no obvious changes in either sensitivity
or tuning. Nor have we noted any obvious trends with respect to tuning or sensitivity as we have proceeded from unit to unit over our typical five to eight hour
experimental sessions with individual animals. In the series of four units
(032283-1 through 032283-4) presented in my talk, the peak sensitivity increased
by a factor of six from the first unit studied to the third then remained high
in the fourth. The units were studied for approx. one hour each. In other animals
the most sensitive units were found first rather than last. We have not looked
for subtle trends.

GUMMER:
1. How does the shape and, in particular, the CF of a tuning curve obtained from
the mean firing rate compare to that obtained from the relative modulation depth?
2. In this frequency range would you expect ongoing neural filtering to contribute significantly to the shape of your tuning curves and therefore complicate an
interpretation in terms of a cochlear tuning mechanism.

E.R. LEWIS:
1. So far I have taken small-signal, linear-transfer ratio tuning curves only for
seismic axons with substantial background discharge; and for those same units I
have not taken separate tuning curves in the nonlinear range (i.e., not for stimuli producing sufficient even-order distortion to cause clear shifts in mean

firing rate - even a few spikes per second). However, the small-signal linear
transfer ratio for linear seismic axons remains essentially constant for modulations of spike rate ranging from zero to nearly 100%. Thus, conspicuous effects
of nonlinearities (principally even-order harmonic distortion products) first
appear at response levels close to 100% modulation. From this I infer that tuning
curves based on criterion changes in mean firing rate would be qualitatively similar to those based on small-signal, linear responses. However, depending on
whether the stimulus frequency is greater or less than the mean resting spike
rate, the mean spike rate may shift up or down as 100% modulation is exceeded.
Thus the criterion changes must be double valued in order to yield reasonable
results.

2. Following a depolarizing event (e.g., a spike or a volley of EPSPs) one expects
an axon to undergo highly-damped oscillation of excitability. This expection arises from the observations of positive and negative afterpotentials in various neurons and from the theoretical consequences of the Hodgkin-Huxley model for the
stellate axons of Loligo. Whereas the first half cycle of oscillation (the period
of classical relative refractoriness) always becomes significant at high spike
rates, subsequent components usually seem to be very subtle. Spike interval histograms for the resting discharges of the auditory and seismic axons described in
my paper, for example, reflect an aperiodic spike-initiation process and exhibit
no conspicuous contributions (e.g., conspicuous multiple modes) from oscillating
axonal excitability. The mean and the single obvious mode of resting spike interval, on the other hand, presumably reflect the effects of relative refractoriness
(among other things). However, the peak modulations used by me to compute small-
signal linear gain seldom exceeded ten spikes per second, even at high stimulus
frequencies. Therefore, I expect the influence of relative refractoriness on
small-signal linear tuning curves to be subtle. Basically, I believe we are ex-
periencing simply stimulus-induced, weak periodic modulation of an essentially
aperiodic process. However, your question definitely will provoke a more careful
examination of spike-interval data by me.

R.S. LEWIS:
As you know, Jim Hudspeth and I have found that hair cells in the excised bullfrog
sacculus show spontaneous electrical oscillations, reaching 5 - 10 mV peak-to-
peak. Assuming that this behaviour extends to cells in the animal, can you suggest
how the frog detects threshold-level vibrations, which would add only a small
change in hair-cell membrane potential to this large spontaneous noise level?

E.R. LEWIS:
I am not sure what levels of seismic stimuli are detected by the bullfrog. However, in the few linearly-responding sacculus axons in which I have analyzed the
resting noise, I found that the rms deviations of instantaneous spike rates from
the mean resting spike rates were of the order of several tens of spikes per sec.
Peak linear transfer ratios of the same axons were of the order of several hundred spikes/sec per cm/sec^2. Thus the instantaneous-spike-rate representation of
the seismic stimulus is equal to the spike-rate noise amplitude when the stimulus
amplitude is of the order of tenths of cm/sec^2. If the noise is only weakly correlated from axon to axon, then signals and noise from approx. 100 fibers of this
type could be summed to yield a system in which signal and noise amplitudes were
equal for stimulus amplitudes of the order of hundreds of cm/sec^2 (e.g. tens of
Angstrom of peak vibrational amplitude). Pursuing the matter in a more rigorous
manner, we need to compare the values of the parameters of resting spike rate noise with those of typical hair-cell electrical noise. This would be most revealing
for dye-filled axons for which the numbers of innervated hair cells have been determined. We should look for relationships that might exist between the linear
transfer ratio of an axon and its resting noise level. We should try to determine
behaviourally the intensities and spectral qualities required for significant detectability of seismic signals by bullfrogs.

KLINKE:
How do you define the difference between seismic and acoustic sensitivity? In the
auditory nerve of caiman we also found fibres with CF of 30 Hz, possibly even
below, but these were the limitations of our acoustic system (Klinke and Pause,
Exp. Brain Res. 38, 137, 1980).

E.R. LEWIS:
We define seismic sensitivity as responsiveness to substrate-borne vibration,
auditory sensitivity as responsiveness to airborne sound. The problem, of course,
is stimulus-mode isolation; we must be sure that applied substrate vibrations are
not inducing airborne sound of sufficient intensity to elicit response, and
vice versa. We have done this by careful calibration of our stimulus apparatus.

LANGNER:
I like to add that the European water frog (Rana temporaria) is also highly sensitive to substrate vibrations. In the Torus semicircularis or at least nearby I
recorded units responding vividly, e.g. to tiny vibrations due to a drop of a small
piece of a paper towel from a hight of 5 cm onto the heavy recording table.

FREQUENCY CODING IN THE INNER EAR OF ANURAN AMPHIBIANS

P. M. Narins* and C. M. Hillery

*Department of Biology and Brain Research Institute**
University of California at Los Angeles
Los Angeles, CA 90024 USA

1. INTRODUCTION

The amphibian inner ear is unique among vertebrates in that it contains two separate auditory organs: the amphibian and basilar papillae. Each organ has its own complement of hair cells and overlying tectorial membrane. However, neither organ possesses a basilar membrane or two populations of sensory receptor cells corresponding to inner and outer hair cells. The polarization patterns of the hair cells of both the amphibian papilla (a.p.) and the basilar papilla (b.p.) are a complex function of sensory surface geometry and for the most part are family- if not species-specific (Lewis, 1978). Despite the distinctive inner ear morphology of amphibians, FTCs obtained from auditory nerve fibers in the frog have shapes similar to those of comparable CFs recorded from the eighth nerves of fish, reptiles, birds and mammals.

Selective lesioning and dye tracing experiments have demonstrated the existence of three populations of fibers originating in the inner ear of the American bullfrog, *Rana catesbeiana* (Feng *et al.*, 1975; Lewis *et al.*, 1982). The low- and mid-frequency populations have their CFs below 1100 Hz and derive from the a.p., whereas the high-frequency fibers innervate the b.p. and have their CFs above 1200 Hz. The ability of single auditory fibers to "follow" click trains presented at rates up to 150/s has been demonstrated in the bullfrog (Frishkopf *et al.*, 1968) and up to 250/s in the spadefoot toad (Capranica and Moffat, 1975). Although the suggestion has been made that amphibian auditory nerve fibers are capable of phase-locking to low-frequency sinusoidal stimuli (Feng, 1982), neither phase-locking *per se* nor its frequency dependence has been directly demonstrated.

We now report the results of a study of frequency selectivity and phase-locking by auditory fibers in the eighth nerve of the neotropical treefrog, *Eleutherodactylus coqui*. This species also possesses three auditory fiber populations (Narins and Capranica, 1976, 1980). Phase-locking is described for amphibian auditory nerve fibers which, like mammalian fibers, can occur in response to stimuli presented as much as 10-15 dB below their discharge rate threshold determined by their FTC. In addition, we show quantitatively that phase-locking in *E. coqui* falls off monotonically with stimulus frequency such that fibers innervating the both the a.p. and the b.p. are capable of reliable phase-locking to sinusoidal stimuli only up to 0.9 kHz.

2. METHODS

Adult *E. coqui* were placed ventral side up on a rigid platform, immobilized with d-tubocurarine chloride and topically anesthetized with Lidocaine prior to surgical exposure of the auditory nerve. Conventional glass micropipettes filled with 3M KCl were used to record from single auditory fibers. The preparation was placed inside a sound-proof chamber (Industrial Acoustics 1202A) which was maintained at a constant temperature of 23o-24oC.

A brass housing was specially constructed in order to accomodate a Beyer DT-48 earphone for sound presentation and a Bruel & Kjaer 4134 microphone used to monitor and calibrate the stimulus. The output port of the housing accepts a short length of rubber tubing which was sealed around the frog's eardrum with silicone grease, creating a closed-field acoustic delivery system. The system was calibrated before each experiment and its frequency response equalized such that it was flat (+ 2 dB) from 0.05-6.40 kHz.

When a single fiber was isolated, its FTC was obtained using an automated threshold-tracking paradigm (Liberman, 1978; Evans, 1979). FTCs were determined using frequency increments of 1/40 octave and intensity increments of 1 dB. The test stimulus was a low-distortion, 50 ms tone with 5 ms rise-fall times presented once per 160 ms. Two FTCs were obtained in succession by sweeping through a five octave frequency range approximately centered on the CF; first from high to low frequencies, and then in the reverse sweep direction. These two curves were then merged and smoothed using a Hamming window of about one-third octave. LF and HF cut-off slopes were estimated by the slope of the least-squares regression lines through the threshold points between 10 and 25 dB above the unit's best threshold. In addition, period (cycle) histograms were generated using the positive-going zero-crossing of the stimulus waveform to trigger a fast data acquisition unit (Cambridge Electronic Design, Ltd., model 502). Period histograms were obtained for CF stimuli at a series of intensities and at as many additional frequencies and intensities as time would allow. Vector strength (Goldberg and Brown, 1969; Woolf et al., 1981) was calculated for each period histogram. A conservative criterion for significant phase-locking of V.S. 0.4 for at least 20 spikes was adopted.

3. RESULTS AND DISCUSSION

a) Frequency Threshold Curves

We have determined FTCs with a high resolution technique to examine their shape, sensitivity and variability and to correlate these physiological measures with observed morphological and mechanical properties of the peripheral auditory system. Fig. 1 shows a family of typical FTCs obtained from several E. coqui.

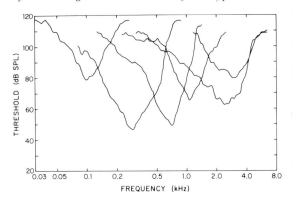

Low-frequency peripheral auditory fibers (CFs below 0.6 kHz) in the treefrog having best thresholds in the range of 30-90 dB SPL exhibit FTCs which are symmetrical when plotted on a logarithmic frequency scale. Mid- and high-frequency-sensitive fibers (CFs between 0.5 and 3.3 kHz) tend to be more asymmetrical, with high-frequency cut-off slopes of up to 80 dB/octave and more gradual low-frequency cut-off slopes typically about 25 dB/octave. This trend is confounded however, by the unit's absolute sensitivity since in general, the least sensitive cells tend to be highly symmetric regardless of their CF (see also Lewis, this volume). Fig. 2 illustrates the relationship between the a unit's

Fig. 1. Typical FTCs obtained from single eighth nerve fibers of adult male and female E. coqui

FTC cut-off slopes and its CF. Fibers which innervate the a.p. (CFs < 1.35kHz; N=32) show no significant difference (p>0.05) between their mean HF and LF cut-off slopes ($|\bar{S}_{HF}|$ =35.0 dB/octave; $|\bar{S}_{LF}|$ =29.5 dB/octave). In contrast, b.p. fibers (CFs > 1.7 kHz; N=35) have significantly greater (p<0.001) mean HF cut-off slopes than LF cut-off slopes ($|\bar{S}_{HF}|$ =45.7 dB/octave; $|\bar{S}_{LF}|$ = 23.4 dB/octave). Direct mechanical measurements of middle ear transmission in amphibians suggest that a portion (30 dB/octave) of the steep high-frequency roll-off may be explained by the low-pass characteristic of the anuran middle ear transfer function (Saunders and Johnstone, 1972; Moffat and Capranica, 1975). On the other hand, the greater relative skew (|HF cutoff slope/LF cutoff slope|) of high-frequency sensitive neurons may be indicative of different modes of stimulation or receptor/neural responsiveness of the a.p. and b.p. fibers in amphibians.

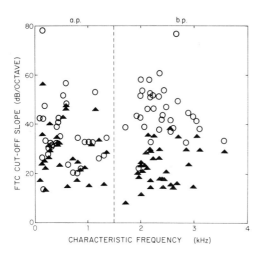

Fig. 2. Low-frequency cut-off slopes (▲)
and high-frequency cut-off slopes (○) of
FTCs of 67 eighth nerve fibers as a func-
tion of CF for the treefrog, E. coqui

b) *Phase-locking Characteristics*

Our motivation for investigating phase-locking by auditory fibers in frogs is the fact that most anuran communication signals have their principal frequency components < 6.0 kHz. In this range phase-locked responses could potentially (a) code information concerning the stimulus frequency (Fay, 1978a,b), (b) increase the dynamic range of a fiber (Evans, 1980), and/or (c) provide cues for localization of the stimulus in space (Barrett, 1981). Fig. 3 shows the ability of a single a.p. fiber to phase-lock to continuous tones at its CF (a-c) and 0.64 octave above its CF (d-f). This fiber was typical of a.p. fibers in that significant phase-locking occurred in response to CF tones presented at a level *below* its discharge rate threshold (Fig. 3C). Mammalian (Rose *et al.,* 1967; Evans, 1980) avian (Sachs *et al.,* 1980) and fish (Fay, 1978a) auditory nerve fibers are capable of phase-locking to low-frequency tones presented as much as 20 dB (mammalian) and 10-15 dB (birds and fish) below their

discharge rate threshold. Thus, altering the temporal pattern of firing in response to a low-level tone with no concomitant increase in discharge rate appears to be a characteristic common to at least four vertebrate classes.

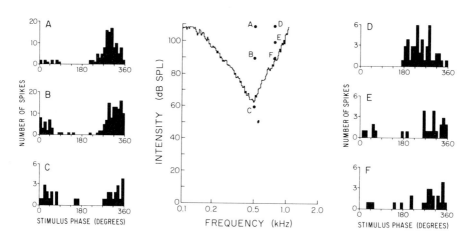

Fig. 3. Center, FTC for an a.p. fiber with a CF=0.49 kHz at 64 dB SPL. The
period histograms were recorded in response to 5-8 seconds of continuous tone at
0.50 kHz (a-c) or at 0.77 kHz (d-f). Spikes are accumulated over every second
cycle of the stimulus. Stimulus intensities in dB SPL and resulting vector
strengths (a) 109, 0.77, (b) 89, 0.74, (c) 59, 0.62, (d) 109, 0.72, (e) 89,
0.58, and (f) 79, 0.41. Histogram bin widths: 10°

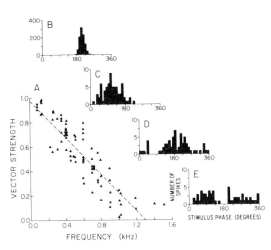

Fig. 4. Vector strength of phase-locking as a function of stimulus frequency for six a.p. fibers from a single male E. coqui. Vector strengths (N=81) were determined from period histograms collected at various frequencies; stimulus levels used were between 5 and 65 dB above rate threshold for each test frequency. Histograms (bin widths: 10°) were derived from either 2000 or 4000 cycles of the stimulus tone, in which spikes were accumulated during every second cycle. The test frequencies (kHz), stimulus levels (dB SPL), and the vector strengths for the resulting period histograms shown are (a) 0.13, 75, 0.97, (b) 0.41, 85, 0.72, (c) 0.70, 105, 0.42, and (d) 1.01, 105, 0.13

The frequency-dependence of phase-locking, however, appears to be a class-dependent or even a species-dependent phenomenon. The best-fit regression line ($r=0.89$) through the data in Fig. 4 illustrates that vector strength calculated for period histograms for a.p. units in the treefrog falls off monotonically with stimulus frequency. Significant phase-locking (V.S. $\geq$ 0.4) was never observed at any stimulus level at test frequencies greater than 0.9 kHz. For a constant stimulus level above threshold (15 dB), vector strength was greater at frequencies below CF than at frequencies at or above CF for all units encountered. Moreover, we found no systematic correlation of vector strength with stimulus intensity within a unit's response area. Preliminary observations of basilar papillar fibers suggest that if their frequency response range includes frequencies below 0.9 kHz, then phase-locking may also be observed in these fibers (Fig. 5). Thus, phase-locking does not appear to be an exclusive property of the a.p. but depends rather on the extent of a fiber's low-frequency sensitivity, irrespective of its peripheral origin.

The 0.9 kHz upper frequency limit for phase-locking in the treefrog is similar to that described for goldfish (1.0 kHz, Fay, 1978a,b) and the Tokay gecko (0.6-0.8 kHz, Eatock et al., 1981)[1], but significantly lower than the 6.0 kHz cut-off for birds (Sachs et al., 1980) or the 4.0-5.0 kHz upper limit in mammals

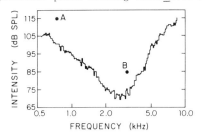

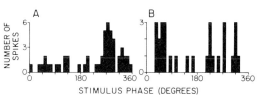

Fig. 5. FTC (unsmoothed) of a b.p. fiber with a CF of 2.6 kHz at 68 dB SPL. a) a tone presented at 15 dB above threshold at 0.74 kHz resulted in a period histogram with a vector strength of 0.40 whereas in b) a tone at 15 dB above threshold at 3.0 kHz resulted in a histogram with a vector strength of 0.17. Thus, b.p. fibers in the frog are capable of significant phase-locking at low frequencies (<0.9 kHz)

[1] In the caiman, phase-locking has been demonstrated up to 1.5 kHz (Klinke and Pause, 1980); its existence at higher frequencies is uncertain at this time.

(Kiang *et al.*, 1965). The close agreement of the upper frequency limits for
phase-locking in fish, amphibians and reptiles does not reflect the disparate
structural organizations of their inner ears (Fay and Popper, 1980; Wever, 1976;
Miller, 1973a,b). Thus, we doubt that specific structural limitations on the
auditory systems of fish, amphibia and reptiles are likely to account for the
similar low upper frequency limits for phase-locking in these groups. We propose
instead that the dichotomy in the frequency range of phase-locking between
birds/mammals and other vertebrates (fish, amphibians, reptiles) is a
manifestation of the evolutionary dichotomy between endothermy and ectothermy.
That is, we suggest that the evolution of endothermy was accompanied by
concomitant changes in the physiological or membrane properties of the receptors
which permitted the increase in the upper limit of phase-locking in these
vertebrates. A similar dichotomy between mammals and nonmammalian vertebrates
has been suggested by Eatock and Manley (1981) for temperature-dependent tuning
shifts of auditory nerve fibers. We believe that our phase-locking data may
reflect another indication of a basic difference in receptor function between
these two vertebrate groups.

REFERENCES

Barrett, A.N. (1981). A theoretical explanation of directional hearing
    characteristics in Amphibia. *J. Theor. Biol.* 93, 591-596.
Capranica, R.R., Moffat, A.J.M. (1975). Selectivity of the peripheral auditory
    system of Spadefoot toads *(Scaphiopus couchi)* for sounds of biological
    significance. *J. Comp. Physiol.* 100, 231-249.
Eatock, R.A., Manley, G.A. (1981). Auditory nerve fibre activity in the Tokay
    gecko. II. Temperature effect on tuning. *J. Comp. Physiol.* 142, 219-226.
Eatock, R.A., Manley, G.A., Pawson, L. (1981). Auditory nerve fibre activity in
    the Tokay gecko. I. Implications for cochlear processing.
    142, 203-218.
Evans, E.F. (1979). Single unit studies of mammalian cochlear nerve. In: *Auditory
    Investigation: The Scientific and Technological Basis.* (H.A. Beagley, ed.).
    pp 324-367. Oxford, Clarendon Press.
Evans, E.F. (1980). 'Phase-locking' of cochlear fibres and the problem of dynamic
    range. In: *Psychophysical Physiological and Behavioural Studies in Hearing.*
    (G. van den Brink, F.A. Bilsen, eds.). pp 300-309. Delft, Delft Univ. Press.
Fay, R.R. (1978a). Coding of information in single auditory-nerve fibers of the
    goldfish. *J. Acoust. Soc. Am.* 63, 136-146.
Fay, R.R. (1978b). Phase-locking in goldfish saccular nerve fibres accounts for
    frequency discrimination capacities. *Nature* 275, 320-322.
Fay, R.R., Popper, A.N. (1980). Structure and function in teleost auditory
    systems. In: *Comparative Studies of Hearing in Vertebrates* (A.N. Popper,
    R.R. Fay, eds.). pp 3-42. New York, Springer-Verlag.
Feng, A.S. (1982). Quantitative analysis of intensity-rate and intensity-latency
    functions in peripheral auditory nerve fibers of northern leopard frogs.
    Hearing Res. 6, 241-246.
Feng, A.S., Narins, P.M., Capranica, R.R. (1975). Three populations of primary
    auditory fibers in the bullfrog *(Rana catesbeiana)*: their peripheral origins
    and frequency sensitivities. *J. Comp. Physiol.* 100, 221-229.
Frishkopf, L.S., Capranica, R.R., Goldstein, M.H., Jr. (1968). Neural coding in
    the bullfrog's auditory system-a teleological approach. *Proc. IEEE* 56, 969-
    980.
Goldberg, J.M., Brown, P.B. (1969). Response of binaural neurons of dog superior
    olivary complex to dichotic tonal stimuli: some physiological mechanisms of
    sound localization. *J. Neurophysiol.* 32, 613-636.

Kiang, N.Y.-S., Watanabe, T., Thomas, E.C., Clark, L.F. (1965). *Discharge Patterns of Single Fibers in the Cat's Auditory Nerve.* Res. Monograph No. 35, Cambridge, Mass., M.I.T. Press

Klinke, R., Pause, M. (1980). Discharge properties of primary auditory fibres in *Caiman crocodilus*: Comparisons and contrasts to the mammalian auditory nerve. *Exp. Brain Res.* 38, 137-150.

Lewis, E.R. (1978). Comparative studies of the anuran auditory papillae. In: *Scanning Electron Microscopy/1978*, Vol. 2. (O. Johari, I. Corvin, eds). pp 633-642. O'Hare, Ill., SEM Inc.

Lewis, E.R., Leverenz, E.L., Koyama, H. (1982). The tonotopic organization of the bullfrog amphibian papilla, an auditory organ lacking a basilar membrane. *J. Comp. Physiol.* 145, 437-445.

Liberman, M.C. (1978). Auditory nerve response from cats raised in a low-noise chamber. *J. Acoust. Soc. Am.* 63, 442-455.

Miller, M.R. (1973a). A scanning electron microscope study of the papilla basilaris of *Gecko gecko*. *Z. Zellforsch.* 136, 307-328.

Miller, M.R. (1973b). Scanning electron microscope studies of some lizard basilar papillae. *Am. J. Anat.* 138, 301-330.

Moffat, A.J.M., Capranica, R.R. (1978). Middle ear sensitivity in anurans and reptiles measured by light scattering spectroscopy. *J. Comp. Physiol.* 127, 97-107.

Narins, P.M., Capranica, R.R. (1976). Sexual differences in the auditory system of the treefrog, *Eleutherodactylus coqui. Science* 192, 378-380.

Narins, P.M., Capranica, R.R. (1980). Neural adaptations for processing the two-note call of the Puerto Rican treefrog, *Eleutherodactylus coqui. Brain, Behav. Evol.* 17, 48-66.

Rose, J.E., Brugge, J.F., Anderson, D.J., Hind, J.E. (1967). Phase-locked response to low-frequency tones in single auditory nerve fibres of the squirrel monkey. *J. Neurophysiol.* 30, 769-793.

Sachs, M.B., Woolf, N.K., Sinnott, J.M. (1980). Response properties of neurons in the avian auditory system: Comparisons with mammalian homologues and consideration of the neural encoding of complex stimuli. In: *Comparative Studies of Hearing in Vertebrates* (A.N. Popper, R.R. Fay, eds.). pp 323-353. New York, Springer-Verlag.

Saunders, J.C., Johnstone, B.M. (1972). A comparative analysis of middle-ear function in non-mammalian vertebrates. *Acta Otolaryng.* 73, 353-361.

Wever, E.G. (1976). Origin and evolution of the ear in vertebrates. In: *Evolution of Brain and Behavior in Vertebrates* (R.B. Masterton, M.E. Bitterman, C.B.G. Campbell, N. Hotten, eds.). pp 89-105. New York, John Wiley & Sons.

Woolf, N.K., Ryan, A.F., Bone, R.C. (1981). Neural phase-locking properties in the absence of cochlear outer hair cells. *Hearing Res.* 4, 335-346.

GENERAL DISCUSSION

EGGERMONT:
I wonder if the 900 Hz boundary of phase locking in your experimental animal (studied at 22 - 24°C) together with data from Klinke and Pause (Exp. Brain Res. 38, 137, 1980) in caiman (upper limit 1500 Hz at 28°C) and our own results in *Rana temporaria* (upper limit 350 Hz at 15°C) point to a main effect of temperature. Including the 4 - 5 kHz upper boundary in mammals (38°C) one tentatively arrives at a temperature coefficient (Q_{10}) of about 3. This could point to synaptic mechanisms as the limiting factor, e.g. as found in the time jitter of the transmitter release.

TEN KATE:
Have you used any statistical measure like $L = 2nR^2$ (n = number of spikes; R = vector of synchronization) in order to know, whether the phase-locking of the neurones were statistically significant or not ?

NARINS:

Our criteria for significant phase-locking was based on obtaining a vector strength of greater or equal to 0.4 for a minimum of 20 spikes. In most cases, however, these criteria were far exceeded.

KIM:

Is the phase locking behaviour for various frequencies similar between neurons in the basilar papilla and in the amphibian papilla?

NARINS:

To date, we have not collected enough data on phase-locking of basilar papillar fibers to make such a comparison, but this is planned.

KLINKE:

Let me extend your reference to temperature studies. We have further studied this phenomenon in caiman, pigeon and guinea pig, using temperature changes over more than 20°C. There is a significant change of CF (eventually more than 2 octaves) to lower values with lower temperature in caiman and pigeon without significant elevation of threshold except for extreme temperatures (Smolders and Klinke, Arch. Otolaryngol. 234, 187, 1982; Schermuly and Klinke, Pflügers Arch. Suppl. 394, R 63, 1982). In the guinea pig the main effect of a temperature decrease is an elevation of threshold and only a small CF shift to lower values (Gummer and Klinke, in prep.). These studies were all done with fibres below 1 kHz CF and are thus comparable. So the dichotomy in cochlear mechanisms I was mentioning yesterday in relation to Furosemide appears to be between mammals and submammalian vertebrates.

ON THE FREQUENCY-DISTRIBUTION OF SPONTANEOUS COCHLEAR EMISSIONS

W. Fritze

2nd Department of ENT, University of Vienna, Medical School
Head: Prof. Dr. K. Burian
A-1090 Vienna, Garnisongasse 13

The method used by the author is distinct from the usually employed procedures: In a camera silens the subject lies comfortably and relaxed on a bed.
The microphone (B & K 4145) is freely suspended at the entry to the external
auditory canal (Fig. 1). While the system should be very sensitive, the entire
acoustic output from the auditory canal should be captured rather than a limited
section of it. Although the sound-flow from the auditory canal is widened to the
membrane, little energy is lost.

After the signal has passed a pre-amplifier (B & K 2619), it is subjected
to Fourier transformation outside the camera silens (B & K 2033). The averaged
spectra are then transferred to a computer for
storage and plotting. For the sound exposure experiments a Synthesizer Exact 605 with a loudspeaker
Peerless KO4OMRF, which is coupled to the ear, is
used.

The camera silens is suited for frequencies
from about 1 kHz upwards. For 400 lines, the
background noise in the frequency range of interest
is -13 dB. When 4.000 lines are computed, the noise
level is about 10 dB lower. This difference is due
to the fact that the machine computes a power
spectrum: When changing from a 400 to a 4.000 line
spectrum, the energy of 1 line is alloted to
10 lines.

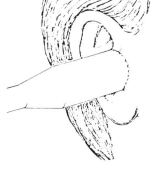

SPONTANEOUS COCHLEAR EMISSIONS

The frequency spectrum of spontaneous
cochlear emissions was described by several

Fig. 1.
Position of the microphone

researchers (among them Zurek, 1981, Wit et al.,
1981, Grandori, 1983, Fritze, 1983).

The author had an opportunity to examine the
right ear of subject K.B. (negative history, normal audiogram, 20 years old),
68 times within a period of 13 months. On 55 of the 68 examination-days spontaneous emissions were recorded. Their intensity varied from just above the
system noise level to 11 dB rel. On 13 days emissions were absent. The frequencies of these emissions varied between 1633 and 1650 Hz. However, the variations
failed to show any specific pattern, in particular, there was no trend towards
one of the two frequencies. While the subject had spontaneous emissions from the
right ear, an acoustic output from the left ear was not demonstrable.

Fig. 2 shows the audiogram of another subject (M.V.) aged 48 years who repeatedly suffered from episodes of hypotension (venticular septum defect). From
the right ear spontaneous emissions were recorded at about 1.780 Hz on 12 different days. As in the previous case frequency shifts were observed. The frequency-centered and averaged spectrum is shown in Fig. 3. It is characterized
by a narrow frequency profile, while the base is somewhat wider. Apparently,
there is poor synchronization at the margins of a more extended area, which explains the wider base: at the margins of this area frequencies are some Hz lower
or higher. Another conspicuous feature is that the base of the emission imper-
ceptibly fades into the base line. This base line is tantamount to the noise

level of the system and is generated by the microphone, as can easily be demon - strated by zero testing. If the cochlea has any basal activity of its own, this would not seem to be appreciably below the resolution of the microphone used, at least not in the vicinity of the emission.

INVESTIGATION OF PATIENTS

Three groups were investigated:
1. Normal subjects with normal audiograms and a negative history:
    In 21 subjects 37 ears were examined. Of these 37 ears, 7 had spontaneous emissions. From 1 ear two emissions were recorded.
2. In 12 patients with minor inner ear deafness the right ears were examined. Seven of these 12 ears showed cochlear emissions. In 5 several emissions were demonstrable.
    It seems to be noteworthy that in this group of persons spontaneous emissions are to be seen much more frequently than in the group of the "normals".
3. In 12 patients with severe inner ear deafness (30 dB and more) no emissions were found to be present.

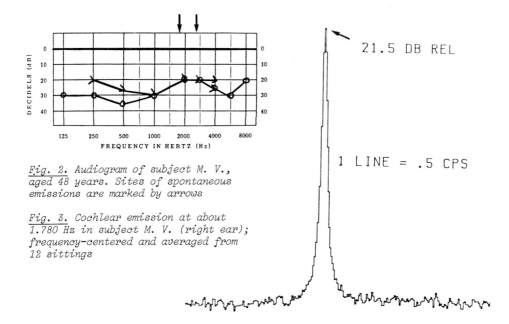

Fig. 2. Audiogram of subject M. V., aged 48 years. Sites of spontaneous emissions are marked by arrows

Fig. 3. Cochlear emission at about 1.780 Hz in subject M. V. (right ear); frequency-centered and averaged from 12 sittings

This implies that the critical level for cochlear emissions is about 25 dB. On the other hand it seems logical to assume that normal subjects with cochlear emissions have some minor cochlear lesion. Histological studies have shown (see Schuknecht, 1974) that even a substantial loss of hair cells, particularly of the outer hair cells, need not be associated with an appreciable reduction of the auditory perception threshold in the audiogram. This and the above critical level for the occurrence of emissions suggest that areas of damaged outer hair cells are prominently involved in this mechanism.

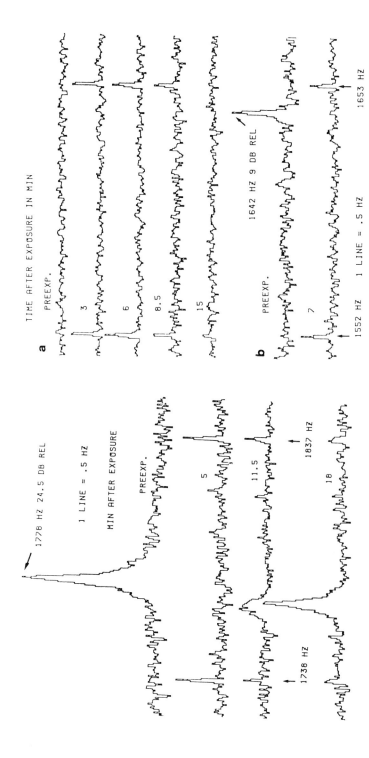

Fig. 5. Two exposure-experiments (900 Hz Sinus, 100 dB SPL, 3 min.) with subject K. B. (normal). In a) there was no spontaneous emission but the "secondary emission" were located at the site at which they normally occurred (b)

Fig. 4. Same subject as in Fig. 3 before and after exposure to a sinus tone of 1000 Hz, 100 dB SPL, 5 minutes

COCHLEAR EMISSIONS AFTER SOUND EXPOSURE

Assuming that the cochlear emitting sites are damaged rather than destroyed, acoustic stimulation can be expected to produce some effects. Figs. 4 and 5 show 2 pertinent experiments.

As can be seen, the emissions tend to become less prominent or disappear altogether depending on the (interindividually quite variable) sound energy applied. They recur after a variable recovery phase; however, their frequency is somewhat shifted downward and their shape is different, as if "deformed". In one instance a double-peaked emission was recorded. (It may be of interest to note that the distance between the two peaks - in anatomical dimensions - corresponded to the distance between two hair cells.) In addition to the disappearance and recurrence of the original emission 1 to 2 other emissions were usually found to occur in the adjacent frequency range. These tended to disappear again as the original emission returned. On repeated sound exposure these "secondary emissions" recurred at the same site.

Sound exposure apparently interferes with the capability of synchronisation within the cochlea: From a cochlear area from which signals are normally syn - chronized to give one emission, two emissions are produced at sites which are particularly active.

DISCUSSION

Spontaneous cochlear emissions apparently reflect cochlear dysfunction due to cochlear lesions, with presumably physiologic synchronization occurring spontaneously, i. e. without acoustic stimulation.

A closer analysis of the evoked cochlear emissions, which have been studied in many centers, will show that these, just like the spontaneous emissions, are excellently reproducible. This prompted some authors (Johnsen & Elberling, 1982, Wit et al., 1981, Grandori, 1983) to regard them as "finger print like" features. But unlike finger prints, the emissions only relate to one ear and are not symmetrical on both sides. In 1981 Wit and associates reported on the frequency relations between spontaneous and evoked emissions. They found evoked emissions to be by far more common than spontaneous emissions. However, the cochlear sites from which spontaneous emissions originated were the same as those for evoked events. As evoked emissions are not consistently recordable in normal subjects (Johnsen & Elberling, 1982; Rutten, 1980; Grandori, 1983), it may well be that those known evoked emissions so far originated from sites of cochlear damage. This assumption is not necessarily refuted by the consistently recordable evoked acoustic output in newborns found by Johnsen et al., 1983. In fact, what may be attributable to cochlear lesions in adults may well be referable to the maturation process in newborns.

If this assumption were right, it would by no means rule out emissions from a normal cochlear area in the course of physiologic hearing. These could well be related to the second filter. In the author's view the search for such emissions would, however, need more sensitive microphones.

Acknowledgement: I gratefully acknowledge the valuable suggestions by Dr. L.U. Kohllöffel.

REFERENCES

Fritze, W., Registration of Spontaneous Cochlear Emissions by Means of Fourier-Transformation, *Arch. Otolaryngol.*, in press.

Grandori, F. (1983). Otoacoustic Emission and nonlinear cochlear filtering, submitted to *Hearing Research*, in press.

Johnsen, N. J., Elberling, C. (1982). Evoked acoustic emissions from the human ear. II normative data in young adults and influence of posture; *Scand. Audiol.* 11/69

Johnsen, N. J., Bagi, P., Elberling, C. Evoked acoustic emissions from the human ear. *Scand. Audiol.*, in press.

Kemp, D. T. (1979). The evoked cochlear mechanical response and the auditory
     microstructure - evidence for a new element in cochlear mechanics.
     Scand. Audiol. Suppl. 9.
Rutten, W.L.C. (1980). Evoked acoustic emissions from within normal and abnormal
     human ears: Comparison with audiometric and electrocochleographic findings;
     Hearing res. 2, 68.
Schuknecht, H.F. (1974). Pathology of the Ear, Harvard Univ. Press, Cambridge,
     Massachusetts.
Wit, H.P., Langevoort, J.C., Ritsma, R.J. (1981). Frequency spectra of cochlear
     acoustic emissions ("Kemp-echoes"). *J. Acoust. Soc. Am.* 70, 437 - 445.
Zurek, P.M. (1981). Spontaneous narrowband acoustic signals emitted by human ears.
     J. Acoust. Soc. Am. 69, 514 - 523.

GENERAL DISCUSSION

TYLER:
We (Tyler and Conrad-Armes, Brit. J. Audiol. 16, 193, 1982) were unable to find
any correspondence between pathological sensorineural tinnitus and spontaneous
acoustic emissions. Do any of your hearing-impaired subjects have tinnitus, and
if so, can this be related to the emissions?

FRITZE:
In common there seems to be no correlation between subjective tinnitus and spontaneous cochlear emissions.

WIT:
After noise exposure secondary emissions appear. In both cases that you showed,
these emissions were almost exactly 100 Hz apart. Does this in your opinion have
any meaning ?

FRITZE:
Indeed, the difference is very similar (99 resp. 101 Hz). I don't see any systematic effect in it as it was not reproducible in other subjects.

KEMP:
Concerning the day-to-day changes you showed in the emission frequency I believe
this could be due to mechanical changes in the middle ear rest position - caused
for instance by pressure.
The impedance of the cochlear windows play a major role in determining the frequency at which spontaneous oscillation can occur, but the existence of a good
'echo'response at that frequency is essential to provide the energy. I agree
with you that frequencies which give especially good echo responses are probably
related to an untypical area of the organ of Corti. The widespread existence of
echo responses leads me to suspect that a background level of response will be
found at all frequencies in healthy ears.

FRITZE:
I didn't check a possible influence of the middle ear, but increasing the re-
sonance-volume far above 15 cm^3 did not show any alteration of the frequency
(the resolution was 0.25 %).

A COMPARISON OF MECHANICAL NONLINEARITIES IN THE COCHLEAE OF MAN AND GERBIL FROM EAR CANAL MEASUREMENTS

D.T. Kemp and A.M. Brown

Institute of Laryngology and Otology, Gray's Inn Road, London WC1X 8DA

With the increasing certainty that cochlear mechanics is the determining factor in auditory sensitivity and frequency selectivity, we need to develop our understanding of the evoked biomechanical responses of the cochlea just as we have come to understand and use its electrophysiological responses. Here we compare and contrast ear canal manifestations of cochlear biomechanics in human and gerbil, and consider some parallels with the round window potential.

1. OTOACOUSTIC PHENOMENA AND COCHLEAR MECHANICS

The acoustic response of the external ear canal to sound is influenced by mechanical events inside the cochlea. The bio-hydrodynamic reaction to cochlear excitation at the oval window contributes two factors to middle ear dynamics - a passive mechanical loading, and a complex nonlinear physiologically dependent element.

The physiological element gives rise to otoacoustic phenomena, the most striking of which in primates is the 'cochlear echo' response to transient stimulation (Anderson and Kemp 1979, Kemp 1982), and its continuous stimulation equivalent (Kemp and Chum 1980). Intermodulation distortion, results in another otoacoustic phenomenon - ear canal combination tones. This effect is present weakly in man (Kemp 1979, Wilson 1980) but strongly in chinchilla, guinea pig and gerbil, in contrast to a weak or undetectable stimulus echo effect in these animals (Kim 1980, Schmiedt and Adams 1981, Zwicker and Manley 1981).

Do the apparently differing relative magnitudes of these two nonlinear phenomena in different animals indicate independent origins? Are there real differences in the detailed auditory bio-micromechanics or are the levels obtained externally, spuriously determined? What are the best otoacoustic emission parameters with which to investigate and monitor cochlear biomechanical activity?

As a first step towards answering these questions we set out to make exactly parallel measurements of ear canal acoustic nonlinearities in human and gerbil ears.

2. MEASUREMENTS AND TECHNIQUES

The sound field in the closed external meatus was recorded via a Knowles microphone and analysed by a narrow band (5 - 0.5 Hz) hetrodyne analyser, tunable and phase lockable to the stimuli or any combination tone. The amplitude and phase of the selected component was recorded. Stimulation was tonal and continuous. For human ears it was applied via two transducers incorporated in the meatal probe. For gerbil (*Meriones unguiculatus*) the transducers fed sound into the closed bulla. To minimise artefactual distortion product generation, each source transducer was screened from its partner's output via a high acoustic resistance element in the 10 mm feed tubes.

Two response components were examined. A nonlinear stimulus-frequency (NS) response component was extracted from the ear canal sound pressure. This was obtained by vector subtraction of the stimulus sound pressure in the presence of a non-synchronous suppressor tone, of 10 dB greater intensity and 100 Hz greater frequency, from the sound pressure measured during single tone stimulation. The residual comprises any level dependent stimulus frequency component in the sound field. The technique is a variation of that used by Kemp and Chum 1980 to isolate the continuous equivalent of the cochlear echo. In the present system the artefact level for this measurement was 55 dB below the stimulus.

The second component studied was the acoustic distortion product 2f1-f2 (DP). This was recorded in amplitude and phase, for two equal intensity stimuli, f1 and f2. The artefact level was 75 dB below stimulus level. For both NS and DP measurements the noise floor was -10 dB SPL. Responses were digitally divided by the measured ear canal stimulus vector sound pressure, in order to minimise the effects of transducer responses.

Response latency was determined from the rate of change in phase with response frequency observed during a stimulus frequency sweep typically of half an octave. For DP measurements, f1 or f2 was swept to give an f2/f1 ratio change from 1.4 to 1.05. Figure 1 a-c shows raw frequency sweep data for DP.(See Kemp and Chum 1980 for NST sweep data).

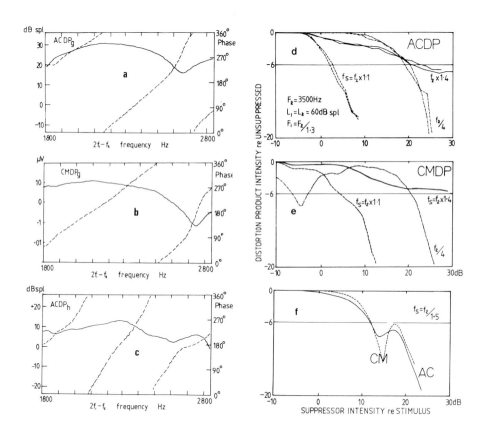

Fig. 1. Left. Raw data DP from frequency-sweep measurements showing gerbil acoustic (a), cochlear microphonic (b), and human acoustic (c), intensity data (solid line) and phase changes (broken line) with frequency, all under the same conditions. Stimuli were - f1, 2330 to 2842 Hz at 70 dB SPL and f2 fixed at 3500 Hz 70 dB SPL. Latency (the rate of change of phase with output frequency) is 1.4, 1.3, and 2.2 ms respectively. On the right are examples of gerbil DP in the range shown left, under suppression by various tones at frequencies stated. Reproducibility is good, (d) and both the CM and acoustic DP's behave similarly (e & f)

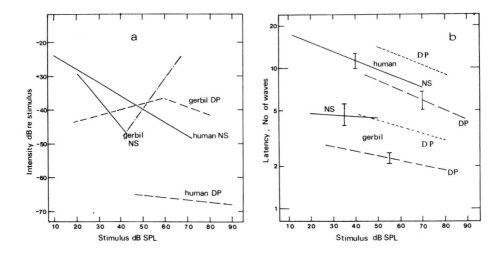

Fig. 2.a) Mean NS and DP intensity data as a function of stimulus intensity for man (5 ears) and gerbil (DP 6 ears, NS 2 ears). The gerbil NS has a latent (solid line) and a non-latent (dash-dot line) region. Individual ear's responses were in the range ± 6 dB of the means shown. Stimuli frequencies were as in Fig. 1 for gerbil, but one octave lower for human data as this offered a greater dynamic range for comparison. 2b) latencies measured under the same conditions are shown. The use of 'waves delay' rather than ms, removes features due solely to the frequency band. The high level gerbil NS is not shown. Its latency was 0.3 waves. The short dashed lines show DP latency for f2 changes, (one ear each). The ratio of about 2 is not trivially due to the '2 f1' factor as we take the ratio — 'change in DP phase/change in DP frequency'

Inherent tuning of the mechanism responsible for the DP and NS responses was determined by constructing a −6 dB isosuppression tuning curve with the aid of a computer-controlled suppressor tone of variable intensity and frequency.

A round window CM signal was recorded from the gerbil and was subjected to the same analysis as the ear canal acoustic signal to give a CMDP and a CMNS.

This study is ongoing. The data presented here is restricted in the frequency ranges for which data is available for comparison.

3. RESULTS

The intensities of nonlinear acoustic ear canal components in the two ear types are shown in figure 2a. The gerbil DP is 40 dB below the stimulus levels with some evidence of a relative maximum at 60 dB SPL stim. In the human ear the DP level is more than 20 dB lower, being 65 dB below the stimulus level.

The NS appears to be of comparable size in man and gerbil, but there are two very different NS components in gerbil. In man the relative NS level drops consistently below the stimulus level by an additional 4 dB/10 dB stimulus increase. In gerbil it drops 8 dB/10 dB stimulus increase (i.e. almost saturated) up to a stimulus level of 40 dB SPL, then it increases rapidly by 10 dB/10 dB (i.e. an absolute slope of 2). This accelerating gerbil NS component had almost zero latency unlike the low level gerbil NS and the entire human NS.

Figure 2b shows the latency of NS and DP for gerbil and man. Gerbil response latency is on average a factor of 3 less than that for human ears. The DP latency for f1 and f2 sweep data differ but the means are compatible with the NS latency for each animal.

In the gerbil CM response the DP component was present at a 20 dB greater

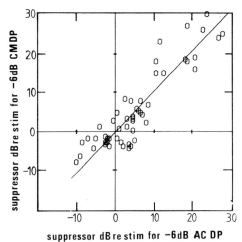

suppressor dB re stim for −6dB AC DP

Fig. 3. Suppressor levels compared for 6 dB suppression of CMDP and ACDP from all gerbils between 1 kHz and 10 kHz. A good overall correlation between the simultaneously measured acoustic and CM DP signals is demonstrated. CM DP tuning curves match acoustic DP curves

intensity relative to the linear stimulus component. The CMDP latency was found to be equal to or slightly below the acoustic DP latency. The CMNS intensity was only 12 dB below stimulation at 60 dB SPL and it remained at a similar ratio for 40 dB stimulation. No latent component was identified.

Figure 1d-e shows the progressive suppression of the gerbil DP for increasing suppressor intensities at various frequencies. Also shown is the suppression behaviour of the CMDP. Note the similarity between the mechanical and electrical DP properties (d & e). Often the CM alone showed a hyper-suppressibility as in 1e. Sometimes interference effects showed on both CM and AC DP suppression curves (1f). Figure 3 summarises the close correspondence between ACDP and CMDP suppression characteristics. Both are sharply tuned for suppression.

Figure 4 gives examples of acoustic DP 6 dB iso-suppression tuning curves for man and gerbil. The DP is most susceptible to suppressors around f2. spreading to f1, but not especially to suppressors at the DP frequency itself. Note the high inter-animal consistency (4a). We find gerbil Q10 dB to be lower than for man (1.1:1.6) and the human curves to have steeper slopes. Human NST suppression curves have previously been reported (Kemp and Chum 1980) for 40 dB SPL stimulation. They exhibited maximum suppressibility 100 Hz above the stimulus frequency and are sharper than the human DP curves obtained at 60-70 dB SPL, with a mean NS Q10 dB of 5. The Q10 dB difference may be due in part to the stimulation level difference and in part to the DP tuning curve being broadened by its two-tone origin. The dependence of DP Q10 dB on primary spacing will be reported elsewhere. We have insufficient data as yet on gerbil NS tuning, but it appears the low level component is tuned, the high level one is not.

The gerbil acoustic DP, NS and CMDP responses fell by more than 20 dB within three minutes of death as did the general stimulus CM potential.

4. DISCUSSION AND CONCLUSIONS

With the exceptions of the non-delayed gerbil high level NS component we have been able to directly compare nonlinear acoustic behaviour in human and gerbil ears in the frequency range 1 kHz to 4 kHz. It should be noted that this range is the most sensitive for human hearing but not for gerbil.

Gerbil ear canal nonlinear mechanical activity is less sharply tuned and exhibits less latency than man's. Such a latency-sharpness association is to be expected from filter theory. The DP Q10 dB ratio, about 1:1.5 is less than the 1:3 latency ratio, but the Q10 does not fully incorporate the slope differences important in determining latency. The shorter latency and smaller saturated intensity of the gerbil NS perhaps explains the non-appearance of a cochlear echo in this animal (Schmiedt and Adams 1981).

The NS/DP intensity ratios are very different in the two ear types. In gerbil the low level DP and NST are roughly equal but in man the DP is 20 to 30 dB less than the NS. It is unlikely that this is due to frequency selective middle ear transmission effects, as the frequencies involved are within 1 octave

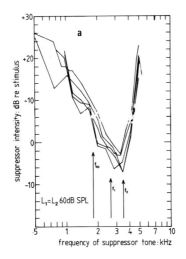

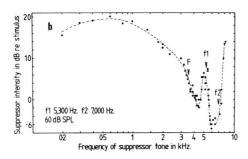

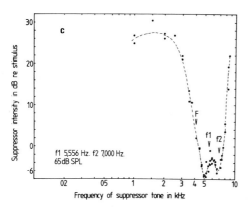

of each other. We must conclude that the two components are produced in different proportions in the two ears. The very different growth rates, i.e. saturating NS versus linear DP, point to separate generating mechanisms. However, a total dissociation of origin is unlikely in view of the broad agreement in NS and DP latencies, tuning, and physiological vulnerabilities.

The CM study has revealed that the DP component of the CM is closely associated with its acoustic counterpart, having similar tuning latency and vulnerability. As would be expected from the middle ear mechanics, the DP component in the meatus is a smaller proportion of the stimulus component than at the cochlea itself. Their origin must be highly localised on the basilar membrane, and from the suppression data it seems they strongly involve the f2 (higher frequency) site. We do not find evidence in the suppression behaviour that the echo (NS) process is an intermediate stage in DP acoustic output in man as suggested by Wilson (1980). We do find that the latency of DP is unequally contributed to by the two primaries in keeping with generation at the f2 site.

An unexpected outcome of this study has been the identification of a rapidly growing stimulus-frequency nonlinearity in gerbil with very little delay (less than 1/3 cycle). This obscures the weak delayed NS above 40 dB stimulation. We have not found this effect in man, but have in each of the 4 gerbils used in NS experiments. The component could not be induced in a model gerbil ear using the same transducers and instrumentation and the response was present at the same level in a gerbil with both tensor tympani and stapedius muscles sectioned. The response was abolished by death. We are forced to conclude that this is a physiological cochlear mechanical effect.

Fig. 4. Acoustic distortion product iso-suppression tuning curve examples for gerbil (a & b) and man (c). In a) the stimuli were f1, 2 650 Hz, f2, 3 500 Hz at 60 dB SPL. Results from 5 different animals are shown. F is the 2f1-f2 distortion product frequency 1 800 Hz. In b) a higher frequency stimulus pair is used. The greater resolution in this plot reveals a bimodal tuning curve as can be obtained for man (c). Note the sharper slopes in the human ear

It may be that just as the round window potential NS obtained demonstrates the well known fact that the mechanical-to-electrical conversion factor of the cochlea is level dependent; so the acoustic NS demonstrates that the mechanical input impedance of the cochlea is also level dependent. This is in keeping with the idea of physiologically-maintained cochlear dynamics. The effect may be present in man, but if it is of the same order of intensity as the DP, it would be below current noise levels and masked by the stronger delayed NS., or cochlear echo.

Although substantial qualitative similarities have been found between human and gerbil otoacoustic nonlinear behaviour, major quantitative differences do exist. We suggest that the nature and intensity of biomechanical energy release from the cochlea is critically dependent on as yet unknown factors involved in the mechanical amplification process (Kemp 1979). It seems that stimulus frequency and distortion product frequency escape depend on different parameters of a common mechanism, which could be determined by species and/or best-frequency.

Acknowledgements: This work is supported by the Medical Research Council and the Iron Trades Insurance Group.

REFERENCES

Anderson, S.D. and Kemp, D.T. (1979) The evoked cochlear mechanical response in laboratory primates. *Arch. Otorhinolaryngol.* 224, 47-54.
Kemp, D.T. (1979). Evidence of mechanical nonlinearity and frequency selective wave amplification in the cochlea. *Arch. Oto-Rhino-Laryngol.* 224, 37-45.
Kemp, D.T. (1982) Cochlear echoes-implications for noise-induced hearing loss. In: *New perspectives in noise-induced hearing loss.* (D. Henderson *et al.*, eds). pp 189-207. Raven Press, New York.
Kemp, D.T. and Chum, R. (1980) Observations on the generator mechanism of stimulus frequency acoustic emissions-two-tone suppression. In: *Psychophysical, physiological and behavioural studies in hearing.* (van den Brink G., Bilsen, F.A. eds). pp 34-41. Delft University Press.
Kim, D.O. (1980) Cochlear mechanics: implications of electrophysiological and acoustical observations. *Hearing Res.* 2, 297-317.
Wilson, J.P. (1980) The combination tone, 2f1-f2, in psychophysics and ear canal recording. In: *Psychophysical, physiological and behavioural studies in hearing.* (G. van den Brink & F.A. Bilsen, eds). pp 43-73. Delft University Press.
Schmiedt, R.D. and Adams, C.D. (1981) Stimulated acoustic emissions in the ear canal of gerbil. *Hearing Res.* 5, 295-305.
Zwicker, E. and Manley, G. (1981) Acoustical responses and suppression-period patterns in guinea pigs. *Hearing Res.* 4, 43-52.

GENERAL DISCUSSION

KIM:
Regarding the non-delayed emission in gerbil at high stimulus level, have you examined the delay as a function of stimulus level? Does it abruptly change from delayed to non-delayed? Is the behaviour different for different frequencies?

KEMP:
The delayed and nondelayed stimulus frequency component in gerbil seem to be separate signals. In figure 2 we plotted a V-shape intensity function. We see a mixture of the two responses at the transition region, with the delayed component diminishing with level and the non-delayed increasing. There is no discontinuity.

DE BOER:
Is it possible that the no-delay component is due to middle-ear distortion?

KEMP:

The response was unaffected by sectioning both direct muscular attachments to
the middle ear in gerbil – so we have only to consider mechanical nonlinearity
in the non-muscle tissue comprising the middle ear system. It would not be surprising if any such nonlinearity changed at death – but we found it went rapidly
to zero. To summarize, we cannot yet rule out the possibility that the gerbil
middle ear has or couples to sensitive level dependent components other than
muscles, which are physiologically vulnerable. Hopefully suppression tuning
studies will establish if the cochlea is this component or not.

EVANS:

Were the gerbils anaesthetized? Could this account for differences observed
between gerbil and human responses?

KEMP:

Gerbils were first anaesthetized with Nembutal, Phenoperidine and Droperidol:
Anaesthesia was maintained with just the first two. We saw no change in the response components with varying depth of anaesthesia in gerbil. We have not performed measurement on an anaesthetized human, so we cannot say that anaesthesia
has no effect on the response pattern, only that we have no reason to suspect
that as yet.

PSYCHOPHYSICAL ASPECTS OF COCHLEAR ACOUSTIC EMISSIONS ("KEMP-TONES")

J.W.Horst, H.P.Wit and R.J.Ritsma

Institute of Audiology, University Hospital,
Groningen, The Netherlands.

1. INTRODUCTION

In 1958 Elliott reported that the normal audiogram may fluctuate strongly over a few tens of Hz. This phenomenon was a.o. confirmed by V.d.Brink (1970), Thomas (1975) and Kemp & Martin (1976). The last authors, intrigued by the high Q-factors of the ripples in the audiogram, predicted active mechanisms as the cause of the ripple structure. Indeed Kemp (1978) was able to show emissions from human ears. Kemp (1979b) also investigated several subjective phenomena near absolute thres- hold. In particular he found strong loudness variations of low-level stimuli as a function of frequency. He found the distance Δf between consecutive maxima to be smaller than the critical bandwidth: For frequencies above 1 kHz Δf equals on the average about 7% of the test-tone frequency. Schloth (1982) found from audiogram measurements in the range 0.8 to 3 kHz that the mean distance between consecutive sensitivity maxima is 90 Hz if only distances smaller than 200 Hz are taken into account. Both Kemp and Schloth suggested regularity to be present in the fine structure of the audiogram. Cohen (1982) investigated audiogram structure in re- stricted frequency intervals. But, although she found strong variations in the audiogram, she did not find any regular structure. The main aim of this paper is to show that for subjects with pronounced emission peaks in the frequency spectra for both ears no strong regularity can be found in the fine structure of the audiogram.

2. METHODS

Click-evoked cochlear acoustic emissions were measured using the method described in detail by Kemp (1979a). From the time averaged responses (1024 averages) frequency spectra were calculated using an FFT-algorithm (Wit,Langevoort, and Ritsma, 1981).
Audiograms were measured with a computer-controlled Békésy-tracking procedure. The subject was seated in a sound-insulated booth, wearing TDH-49 headphones mounted in GS001A circumaural cushions. The signals were presented in a 400 ms period with 255 ms on-time. During the measurement of one track the signal frequen- cy was changed in steps δf, every time when the response button was pressed or re- leased by the subject. Reversal points in the Békésy audiogram were connected by straight lines. Typical values for δf were 3 and 10 Hz. Typical values for the number of frequency steps in a run were 50 or 75. Eight subjects participated in the experiments. All had normal hearing below 4 kHz. From the subjects we did not require any experience in psycho-acoustical tasks in general or training in this task in particular.

3. RESULTS

a. Acoustic emissions

Of all subjects six showed pronounced emission peaks in tne frequency spectra for both ears. The other two subjects had no or only very weak emissions in either ear. (Since we were especially interested in subjects with strong emissions, this ratio of 75% of the ears having emissions is not regarded as representative; see e.g. Zurek (1981), Schloth (1982)). In fig.1 evoked emission spectra of both ears of subject PK are shown. Strong emissions are found at a few frequencies which are

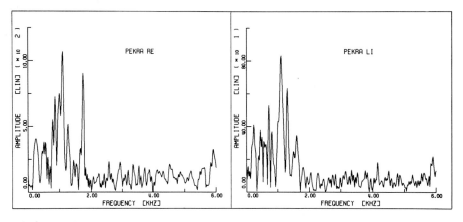

Fig.1. *Amplitude spectra of acoustic emissions from both ears of subject PK. The amplitude is plotted on a linear scale in arbitrary units*

specific for each ear. This is representative for all the subjects participating in the experiments and in agreement with other data (Zurek, 1981; Wit, et al.,1981; Schloth, 1982).

b. Absolute threshold

Fig.2 gives Békésy tracks for subject PK's right ear. One track was measured with 10 Hz frequency steps. A sharp sensitivity maximum is found near 1.74 kHz. The width of this peak is rather small compared to δf. Sharp maxima were found in audiograms from other ears too. In order to investigate whether 10 Hz is an appropriate step size for finding microstructure in the audiogram, several tracks were measured with smaller step size. The other track in fig.2 is an example of a measurement with $\delta f=3$ Hz. It can be seen that the smaller step size does not give extra information. Therefore, we feel that a step size of 10 Hz is a good compromise to investigate microstructure in the audiogram.

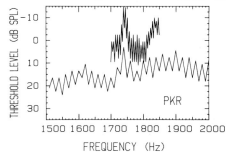

Fig.2. Békésy audiogram tracks of subject PK (right ear) with frequency steps of 10 Hz and 3 Hz respectively. The 3-Hz track was shifted by -15 dB for clarity

In order to estimate the shape of the audiogram, the Békésy tracks were smoothed. This was simply done by determining level and frequency midway between consecutive reversals. These points were interconnected for clarity. Examples of smoothed Békésy tracks are shown in fig.3 for subject PK. These data were collected during two sessions. In each session the frequency range from 1000 Hz to 4000 Hz was covered by 6 subsequent runs. Although there are small differences in absolute threshold, the overall structure of the audiogram, including the frequency position of the sensitivity maxima, is retained. The two sessions of fig.3 took place on the same day. Fig.2 on the other hand shows similar data from sessions about two months apart, indicating that for an isolated maximum the frequency remains constant for several months. We found the same stability for the microstructure in the audiograms of the other investigated ears.

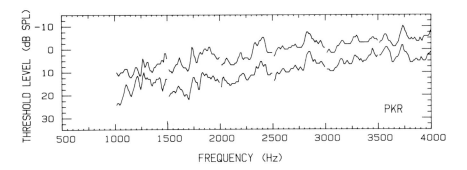

Fig.3. Smoothed Békésy audiograms for subject PK's right ear. Results of 2 sessions consisting of 6 runs each. The data of one session are shifted by -10 dB

c. On the relation between Kemp-tone frequency and microstructure of the audiogram.

Six out of our eight subjects exhibited fine-structure in the audiograms from both their ears. These were the subjects with acoustic emissions from both ears. The two subjects with no or only weak emissions turned out to have smooth audiograms. So, audiogram fine structure and cochlear emission seem to be interrelated phenomena. The data in fig.4 show that a maximum in the audiogram is generally at or close to an emission frequency. This is in agreement with data given by Wilson (1980) and Schloth (1982). As we can see in the upper panel of this figure, subject LE shows strong fluctuations in her right-ear audiogram. However, the maxima near the emission frequencies are not very pronounced. Yet the levels of her emissions are rather high (e.g. 12 dB SPL at 1.61 kHz (Wit et al., 1981)). No clear relation could be found between emission level and maximum/minimum level ratio in the fine structure of the audiogram for frequencies around the emission frequency.

d. Maxima spacing in the audiogram.

The above data show that the number of maxima in the audiogram clearly exceeds the number of frequencies at which strong emissions occur in the same ear. Kemp (1979b) gives a theory for the mechanism responsible for these sensitivity maxima. This theory requires the existence of standing waves in the cochlea. The theory predicts maxima in the audiogram at regular intervals and is in accordance with Kemp's own findings concerning loudness maxima near the absolute threshold. The average spacing of these loudness maxima is a constant fraction of the signal frequency f, if f is between 1 and 4 kHz. Thomas (1975) found the distance Δf between consecutive maxima to correspond closely to the critical bandwidth. The data in fig.4 show in the regions with a strong ripple structure that several maxima are present within a critical band.

We analysed our data in order to investigate if there was any regularity in the frequency of the sensitivity maxima. Only sensitivity maxima that were at least 3 dB above the contiguous minima were considered. In fig.5 we plotted the distance Δf between consecutive maxima as a function of frequency for four subjects. No regularity can be seen. Our data are in agreement with other data (Elliott, 1958; Cohen, 1982; Schloth, 1982) with respect to the fact that fine-structure audiograms do not show inter- and intrapersonal correlations. Our data also show a dependence of Δf on f which is specific for each ear.

For two ears we investigated the fine structure of the audiogram with Fourier analysis. The finite Fourier transform (FFT) was calculated for 600-Hz-long subsequent intervals of the audiogram. This analysis did not give information about the regularity in maxima spacing, that had not already been obtained from the frequency difference method (fig.5).

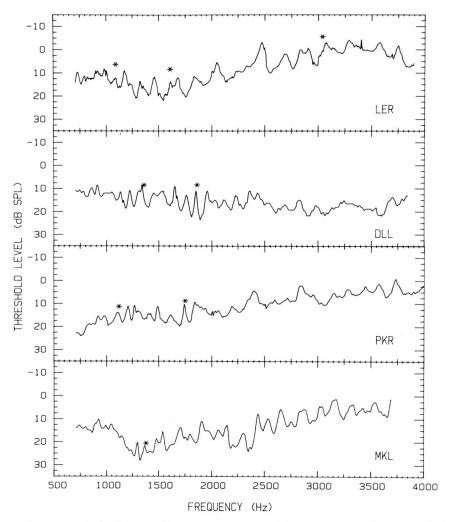

Fig. 4. Smoothed Békésy audiograms for four subjects. Frequencies of evoked emissions of each subject are indicated with * (arbitrary level)

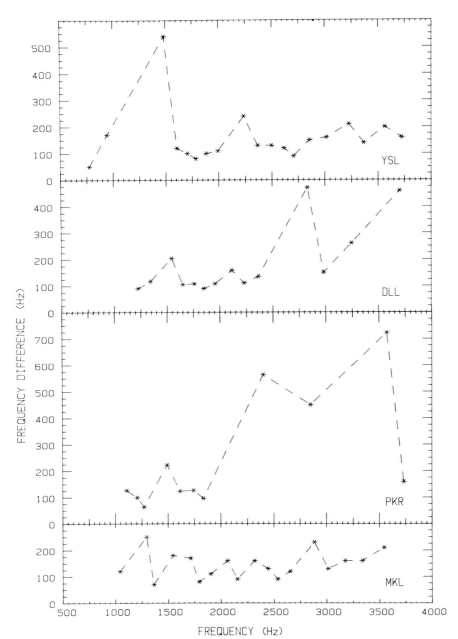

Fig.5. Frequency difference $\Delta f = f_h - f_l$ between neighbouring sensitivity maxima as a function of f_h

Acknowledgement: The authors wish to thank Arend Smit for giving programming assistance.

REFERENCES

Brink, G.v.d. (1970). Experiments on binaural diplacusis and tone perception. In: *Frequency analysis and periodicity detection in hearing,* (R.Plomp, G.F. Smoorenburg, eds.).pp.362-374, Leiden, A.W.Sijthoff.

Cohen, M.F. (1982). Detection threshold microstructure and its effects on temporal integration data. *J.Acoust.Soc.Am.*71, 405-409.

Elliott, E. (1958). A ripple effect in the audiogram. *Nature* 181, 1076.

Kemp, D.T., Martin, J.A. (1976). Active resonant systems in audition. 13th. International Congress of Audiology, Florence, *Abstracts*, 64-65.

Kemp, D.T. (1978). Stimulated acoustic emissions from within the human auditory system. *J.Acoust.Soc.Am.*, 64, 1386-1391.

Kemp, D.T. (1979a). Evidence of mechanical nonlinearity and frequency selective wave amplification in the cochlea. *Arch.Otorhinolaryngol.* 224, 37-45.

Kemp, D.T. (1979b). The evoked cochlear mechanical response and auditory micro- structure – Evidence for a new element in cochlear mechanics. In: Models of the auditory system and related signal processing techniques, (M.Hoke and E.de Boer, eds.). *Scand.Audiol.Suppl.*9, 35-47.

Schloth, E.(1982). Akustische Aussendungen des menschlichen Ohres (oto-akustische Emissionen). *Doctoral dissertation,* Technical University of München.

Thomas, I.B. (1975). Microstructure of the pure-tone threshold. *J.Acoust.Soc.Am.* 57, Suppl.1, S26-S27.

Wilson, J.P. (1980). Evidence for a cochlear origin for acoustic re-emissions, threshold fine-structure and tonal tinnitus. *Hear.Res.* 2, 233-252.

Wit, H.P., Langevoort, J.C. and Ritsma, R.J. (1981). Frequency spectra of cochlear acoustic emissions ("Kemp-echoes"). *J.Acoust.Soc.Am.*70, 437-445.

Zurek, P.M. (1981). Spontaneous narrowband acoustic signals emitted by human ears. *J.Acoust.Soc.Am.* 69, 514-523.

ADDENDUM by HORST, WIT and RITSMA:

In order to remove all doubts about the influence of day to day variations and body posture on the relation between emission frequency and audiogram fine

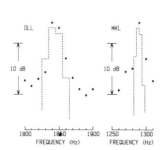

structure, we have performed an experiment in which emission spectrum and absolute threshold were measured simultaneously. Békésy tracking was performed at distinct frequencies around a strong emission peak. In the 300 ms long si- lent intervals between the stimuli the micro- phone signal was sampled and the spectrum of it was calculated with a real-time FFT spectrum analyser. Successive spectra were averaged (128 averages for one stimulus frequency value). The figure shows the shape of a pronounced ma- ximum in the acoustical emission frequency spec- trum, together with the absolute thresholds (stars) on a dB-scale (arbitrary reference va- lues; the emission level increases in upward direction, whereas the threshold level decreases in this direction). The close correspondence of the emission peak and the peak in hearing sensitivity is striking. (Both in center frequency and in width). It looks as if a very frequency selective region of the cochlea where the emission is generated has an increased sensitivity for tones with a frequency equal to the emission frequency.

GENERAL DISCUSSION

DE BOER:
Can there be a peak of auditory sensitivity at a location where, because of
day-to-day variations, a normally present spontaneous emission is absent?

HORST:
An indication may be that we find sharp sensitivity peaks at frequencies where
evoked emissions are either absent or relatively weak.

WILSON:
I (Wilson, Hear. Res. 2, 233, 1980; fig. 10) looked at a very similar problem:
the relationship between sound pressure maxima in the sealed ear canal for continuous tonal stimulation and threshold minima. (The latter was performed with
a free-field earphone to avoid ear canal pressure irregularities). Of the three
subjects used, one had threshold minima at the SPL peaks, another had maxima and
the third was intermediate. It is my view that these and your results with click
stimulation are consistent because the objective measurements are being made at
a different level of the system from that involved in psychophysical measurements.
With phase shift between these locations interference minima will occur at slightly different frequencies. Exact correspondance should not therefore, be expected
in all subjects even with the same acoustical system. With spontaneous emissions
I also observed (same fig.) a correspondence between emission frequencies and
threshold minimum. This may simply be due to the detection of beats as found in
tone-to-tone masking curves !

JOHNSTONE:
Were the threshold curves corrected for sound pressure in the ear canal? If not
then any emission would add to the sound field and thus give an apparent change
in sensitivity of the audiogram at the emission frequency. Hence all emissions
would coincide with a peak in the audiogram, some or all of which could be an
artefact.

HORST:
The results we present here, were obtained during the last week. We have not measured sound pressure levels yet. But as far as I remember from the oscilloscope
screen, the stimulus level was much higher than the level of the emission signal
during the silent periods. Besides from this, I think that your view is too
simple. If the emission would not be generated within the cochlea, we could simply add its level to that of the stimulus (at the emission frequency) if both signals are in phase all the time; which is unlikely to be the case. But as we think
that the emission is generated within the cochlea, the situation is even more
complicated: The site where the emission is generated may be the same site as
where the stimulus is detected. As we have no idea how this detection mechanism
works, we cannot say anything with certainty about the interaction of the stimulus and the emission signal.

KIM:
Is your data plot of hearing threshold actually the electric voltage level applied
to the earphone, or the genuine SPL directly measured in the ear canal? This subtle difference is important to distinguish because the total acoustical signal in
the ear canal in general can include three components: 1) the spontaneous emission component; 2) the stimulus-frequency evoked emission component; and 3) the
"applied stimulus" component. The first two components originate from inside the
ear, whereas the third originates from the earphone.

HORST:
It is the voltage level.

LONG:
Kim's comment suggests that the threshold microstructure may depend on the sound
pressure in the ear canal. I measured the sound pressure in the ear canal while
tracking threshold in an ear with marked microstructure and a clear microstructure could still be seen. Changes in threshold for tones in an area at micro –
structure are probably not simply dependent on changes in acoustical input.

KEMP:
If the sensitivity maxima in the audiograms are the result of constructive interference between the stimulus and its reverberating echo then we would expect the
sharpest and greatest maxima at frequencies where the most emission could be elicited. Have you examined the Q-factor of the sensitivity maxima in relation to
the intensity of evoked emissions, or the existence of spontaneous emission at
that frequency. Of course, for evoked emission measurements the sample time must
be short enough to exclude the interference effect.

HORST:
This is an interesting point, we have not checked that yet.

"A FAMILY WITH HIGH-TONAL OBJECTIVE TINNITUS" - AN UPDATE

J.P. Wilson & G.J. Sutton

Department of Communication & Neuroscience,
University of Keele, Keele, Staffordshire, ST5 5BG, U.K.

1. INTRODUCTION

In 1971 Glanville, Coles & Sullivan reported on three members of a family whose ears produced externally-audible high-pitched whistles. Although Gold (1948) had proposed an active mechanical feedback mechanism which he postulated might oscillate and cause tinnitus, this possibility did not receive serious attention until Kemp described the cochlear echo phenomenon in 1978. At the time, a vascular hypothesis for the whistles appeared most plausible and appeared to be supported by some of their evidence. The whistle components found, ranged from 5.6-14 kHz with a maximum reported level of 60 dB SPL. Most recent investigations of stimulated and spontaneous oto-acoustic emissions, on the other hand, have found them occurring most strongly in the 1-3 kHz range and saturating at, or limited to, a maximum of about 20 dB SPL in the sealed ear canal (Kemp, 1979b, 1981; Wilson, 1980a,b,c; Wilson & Sutton, 1981; Zurek, 1981). This low saturating level and the restriction of emissions to certain frequency regions, specific to each ear, led to the suggestion of a model (Wilson, 1980cd) based on two hypotheses: firstly, that the signal represents summed activity from the cochlea, and secondly, that the activity might represent signal-synchronous swelling and shrinking of hair cells. For a uniformly-graded cochlea the summed activity would be very small, but with an irregularity in the place/frequency map a large local component would appear in the summed response. Clearly, the existence of emission levels of 60 dB SPL would render the second hypothesis implausible. It was therefore desirable to reinvestigate the original subjects to determine whether their whistles have a similar oto-acoustic origin and, if so, to obtain further clues to the underlying mechanisms.

The various criteria that have been used to link spontaneous emissions with cochlear transduction mechanisms have been discussed previously (Kemp, 1979ab; Wilson, 1980b) and include: relationship with audiogram fine-structure, appropriately-tuned suppression and synchronisation functions, and an envelope periodicity of 10-20 waves. One unexplained feature of previous measurements which might be looked for was a small but consistent shift of emission frequency in the presence of an external tone (Wilson & Sutton, 1981). Middle-ear pressure has also been reported to influence emissions (Kemp, 1979a; Wilson, 1980b; Wilson & Sutton, 1981) but this is less likely to be observable at very high frequencies.

2. METHODS

The boy, SF, was first investigated at $2\frac{1}{2}$ yrs., and more thoroughly at 4 yrs. (1969), and was 17 yrs. old during the present study. The girl, CF, was first investigated at 4 months and was 13 yrs. old for the present investigation.

The instrumentation and methodology were as described previously (Wilson, 1980b). Another microphone (B & K 4155) with miniature low-noise (15 dBA with 4155) head amplifier was also used because of its better high frequency response. Spectral components were analysed with a quadrature, ganged pair of Brookdeal 401 lock-in amplifiers and with a B & K 2020 slave filter set to 10 Hz bandwidth, and plotted on a B & K 2305. Clinical audiograms were obtained on a Rion Békésy audiometer, and expanded audiograms obtained using a B & K 1024 oscillator driven by a 2305 recorder, with a reversible motor-driven log attenuator. The signal was chopped by a diode gate at 1.5 Hz and filtered by a B & K 2020 slave filter set at 3.16 Hz, and presented by a free-field electrostatic earphone (Wilson, 1968).

3.   RESULTS

a) *Spectral components.* These are shown in Fig. 1 for the four ears tested.
Each ear shows many components covering a wide frequency range (from 1.4-17 kHz
to 2.8-12 kHz), although some regions show stronger and more closely-grouped components.   In each case the lower components fall within the frequency and level
ranges found for many normal hearing subjects (Kemp, 1979b, 1981; Wilson, 1980a,b,
c; Wilson & Sutton, 1981; Zurek, 1981).   In each ear, however, the strongest component is about 40 dB SPL and lies in the range 5.2-8.5 kHz.   These are
higher in frequency and level than found for other subjects, although the maximum levels are lower than the highest levels (55 and 60 dB SPL using a $\frac{1}{4}$" microphone in the ear canal) measured in SF in 1968, although quite comparable to
the more extensive 1969 measurements (Glanville *et al.*, 1971, table I, using a
$\frac{1}{2}$" microphone at the ear canal entrance) which are shown for comparison below the
present measurements.   There is remarkable correspondence in the frequencies of
major components in view of the long interval between measurements.   The absence
of lower components in the 1969 measurements is explicable because the microphone
was positioned at the entrance of the ear canal but not sealed to it.   The
components which seem to correspond, appear to have shifted downward in frequency
slightly (-4%).   This continues a trend observable in the data of Glanville *et al.*,
(1971).

*Fig. 1. Spectra of oto-
acoustic emissions found
in the ears of subjects CF
and SF in the present
study (1982) and by
Glanville et al. (1971,
table 1) in 1969. Also
shown for each ear is a
4 ms sample of the
acoustic waveform.
Measured with B & K 4155
microphone (pressure
calibration) sealed into
ear canal with 2 cm of
4 mm i.d. tube*

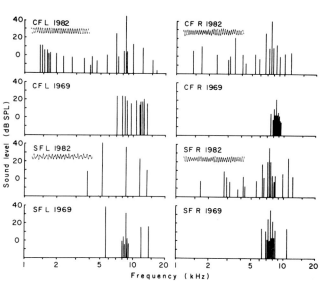

The above measurements were made "live" using the lock-in amplifier and
afterwards from tape loops made from continuous recordings using the slave
filter.   It was apparent from these measurements, and from listening to the emissions, that they were stable sometimes but fluctuated or took up other stable
states at other times.   Sonagram analyses were therefore made from the tape
recordings during periods of fluctuation.   Examples from three ears are shown in
Fig. 2: some components are steady throughout or undergo irregular periodic
fluctuations of frequency; other components come and go or switch frequency by a
fixed amount.   The time markers indicate some positions at which a number of
correlated changes can be observed.   The sudden change to a much more complex
spectrum is also indicated in Fig. 4 by the broken vertical lines from a slave-
filter analysis.   In view of these short-term changes, some of the apparent
differences from the earlier measurements may not be significant.

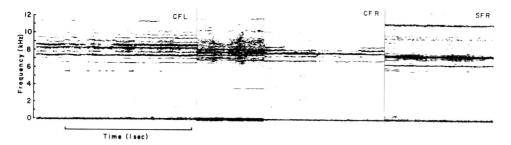

Fig. 2. Sonagram analyses from three ears during periods of spectral instability.
The two sections for CFR were recorded at different times

b) *Audiograms.* Although frequency regions of emissions are often associated
with audiogram fine-structure (Kemp, 1979a; Wilson, 1980b) they do not usually
occur in regions of grossly elevated threshold. This is assumed to be because
cochlear pathology may reflect damage to the same active process that is involved
in acoustic emissions and in determining low threshold and sharp tuning properties. The 1969 audiograms of SF, however, showed losses of 50 and 60 dB at the
major emission frequencies. Recent audiograms are shown in Fig. 3 and show
remarkable agreement with the previous measurements (squares and dots). The
question arises therefore, whether this loss represents some kind of pathology
or simply represents masking of the external signal by the internal one. Somewhat fortuitously, the sensation levels for emissions in the 1-3 kHz range have
been found to be comparable to the SPL's measured in the sealed ear canal (Kemp,
1979b, 1981; Wilson, 1980ab; Wilson & Sutton, 1981; Zurek, 1981). As a masker
has to be 10-20 dB above the maskee, this explanation would appear not to suffice in the present case. At these high frequencies, however, the middle ear is
likely to be less efficient so that the internal (masking) level would exceed
the external level by a corresponding amount. To investigate this further, an expanded audiogram was taken (Fig. 4) and compared with the emission spectrum. Idealised critical band masking curves are indicated by the dashed lines. For SFL
there is clearly some disagreement in that the maximum expected elevation occurs
at too low a frequency. A similar but less marked discrepancy occurs also for
CFL. It should also be noted that the high frequency deficit for CFR (Fig. 2)
is appreciably less than for the other three ears even though the emission
level is comparable. The audiogram curve may therefore represent a mixture of
masking and pathological influences. The fine-structure observed in Fig. 4
occurs in many regions associated with objective components but also in other

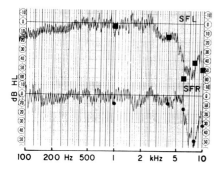
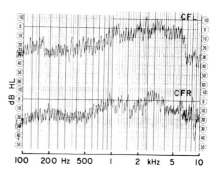

Fig. 3. Clinical Békésy audiograms showing considerable hearing loss in the
region above 5 kHz for three of the four ears. The fourth ear (CFR) was measured
twice in this region. Squares and dots show the 1969 measurements (Glanville
et al., 1971)

regions. It is apparent that CF in particular had difficulty in determining
threshold in the region of the strongest components. Both subjects reported
difficulties because of beats in certain frequency regions.

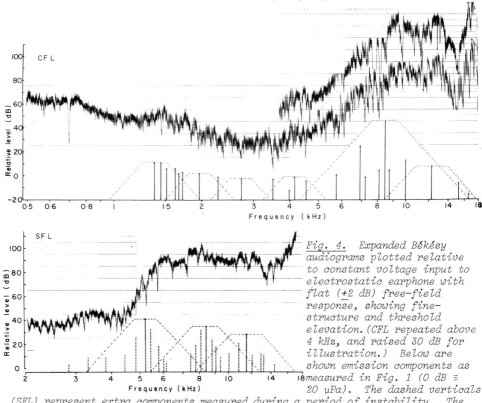

*Fig. 4. Expanded Békésy
audiograms plotted relative
to constant voltage input to
electrostatic earphone with
flat (+2 dB) free-field
response, showing fine-
structure and threshold
elevation.(CFL repeated above
4 kHz, and raised 30 dB for
illustration.) Below are
shown emission components as
measured in Fig. 1 (0 dB ≡
20 μPa). The dashed verticals
(SFL) represent extra components measured during a period of instability. The
dashed outlines represent idealised critical band masking functions*

c) *Interactions with an external signal*. Attempts to synchronise the strongest
component to an external click were unsuccessful for SFR although it should be
pointed out that for various reasons the dynamic range of the equipment was quite
limited. Even so, this was unexpected in view of the low levels required
for synchronisation in other subjects (Wilson, 1980b; Wilson & Sutton, 1981). A
continuous tone, close in frequency to the emission, however, did synchronise
(and pull-in) the emission frequency but there was too little dynamic range
to obtain a synchronisation curve.

As reported earlier (Wilson & Sutton, 1981) care must be taken to separate
the influence of change of emission frequency from true suppression, the procedure being to retune the slave filter to centre it on the emission while suppression is adjusted to 3 dB. The resulting emission frequencies and suppressor
levels are shown in Fig. 5. The suppressor level curve is a less convincing
critical band curve than previous measurements and also shows two higher-frequen-
cy suppression lobes (see Evans *et al.*, 1981; Wilson & Sutton, 1981; Zurek, 1981)..
The shift-of-emission-frequency curve, however, is quite similar to that shown
in Wilson & Sutton (1981) and to other unpublished curves. This is strong
evidence linking these high-level high-frequency emissions with previously reported ones. With subject CF, tonal suppression was confirmed, but the less stable
level, and emission frequency, made the determination of a complete curve
impracticable.

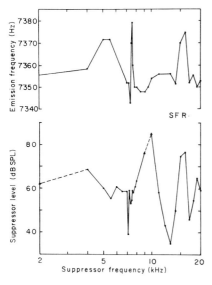

Fig. 5. *Shows (upper) the frequency of the*
major emission component as a function of
suppressor frequency at 3 dB suppression,
and (lower) the level of suppressor, as a
function of frequency, required for 3 dB
suppression. (The dashed lines represent
levels producing some instrumental
overload.)

d) *Tinnitus.* Both subjects, when asked initially, denied awareness of their
signals as tinnitus. However, they both later volunteered that after sitting in
the sound-proofed room for recording and audiogram determinations, they could
indeed hear them. Clearly, however, they cannot be considered as tinnitus
sufferers. This comparative lack of awareness is not consistent with masking as
an interpretation of threshold elevation. Conversely, however, the elevated
thresholds at these frequencies are consistent with their low sensation levels.

4. CONCLUSIONS

In view of the above findings it appears reasonable to suppose a common
underlying mechanism for these and the previously reported spontaneous emissions
and the stimulated emission phenomenon. There are, however, certain aspects
such as the high level required for synchronisation, the poor suppression curve
shape and the high degree of threshold elevation, and perhaps also the apparent
heredity element (Glanville *et al.*, 1971) which suggest a greater possible
involvement of pathology in these cases. Clearly, however, the latter is not
progressive over a period of 13 yrs. The high sound levels appear to rule out
the suggestion (Wilson, 1980cd) that the source of sound pressure variation
could be the periodic swelling and shrinking of hair cells. This suggestion was
in any case intended to satisfy a condition that comparatively little influence
of such processes should be seen in basilar membrane motion as indicated by
early measurements. Recent measurements in the cat (Khanna & Leonard, 1982) and
guinea pig (Sellick *et al.*, 1982) have found sharp basilar membrane tuning and
large displacements for small input signals indicative of a mechanical positive
feedback mechanism (Gold, 1948; Kemp, 1978; Kim *et al.*, 1980). The other part
of the model proposed by Wilson (1980cd) however, appears to remain plausible:
i.e. that acoustic emissions represent summed activity over the whole cochlea,
and that for a uniformly graded cochlea, this must be small, whereas for regions
of irregular mapping or sensitivity the summed activity shows a large local
component. This summed activity would now appear to represent simply net
basilar membrane displacement.

The authors thank Mr. J.D. Glanville and Dr. R.R.A. Coles for permission and
initial arrangements to see SF and CF, the Medical Research Council for Grant
G80/0495/0/N, the Science Research Council for a Studentship for G.J.S., Prof.
E.F. Evans and Dr. S.R. Pratt for comments on manuscript, Mr. J.B. Ruscoe for
technical assistance and Ms. M. Hodgson for typing.

REFERENCES

Evans, E.F., Wilson, J.P., Borerwe, T.A. (1981). Animal models of tinnitus. In:
    Tinnitus. Ciba Found. Symp. 85. (D. Evered and G. Lawrenson, eds.).
    pp 108-138. London, Pitman Medical.
Glanville, J.D., Coles, R.R.A., Sullivan, B.M. (1971). A family with high-tonal
    objective tinnitus. J. Laryngol. Otol. 85, 1-10.
Gold, T. (1948). Hearing II: The physical basis of the action of the cochlea.
    Proc. R. Soc. Lond. B. Biol. Sci. 135, 492-498.
Kemp, D.T. (1978). Stimulated acoustic emissions from within the human auditory
    system. J. Acoust. Soc. Am. 64, 1386-1391.
Kemp, D.T. (1979a). The evoked cochlear mechanical response and the auditory
    microstructure - evidence for a new element in cochlear mechanics.
    Scand. Audiol. Suppl. 9, 35-47.
Kemp, D.T. (1979b). Evidence of mechanical nonlinearity and frequency selective
    wave amplification in the cochlea. Arch. Oto-Rhino-Laryngol. 224, 37-45.
Kemp, D.T. (1981). Physiologically active cochlear micromechanics - one source
    of tinnitus. In: Tinnitus. Ciba Found. Symp. 85. (D. Evered and G.
    Lawrenson, eds.). pp 54-81. London, Pitman Medical.
Khanna, S.M. and Leonard, D.G.B. (1982). Basilar membrane tuning in the cat
    cochlea. Science 215, 305-306.
Kim, D.O., Neely, S.T., Molnar, C.E., and Matthews, J.W. (1980). An active
    cochlear model with negative damping in the partition. In: Psychophysical,
    Physiological & Behavioural Studies in Hearing. (G. van den Brink & F.A.
    Bilsen, eds.). pp 7-14. Delft University Press.
Sellick, P.M., Patuzzi, R. and Johnstone, B.M. (1982). Measurement of basilar
    membrane motion in guinea pig using the Mössbauer technique. J. Acoust.
    Soc. Am. 72, 131-141.
Wilson, J.P. (1968). High quality electrostatic headphones. Wireless World
    74, 440-443.
Wilson, J.P. (1980a). Recording of the Kemp echo and tinnitus from the ear
    canal without averaging. J. Physiol. 298, 8-9P.
Wilson, J.P. (1980b). Evidence for a cochlear origin for acoustic re-emissions,
    threshold fine-structure and tinnitus. Hearing Research 2, 233-252.
Wilson, J.P. (1980c). Model for cochlear echoes and tinnitus based on an
    observed electrical correlate. Hearing Research 2, 527-532.
Wilson, J.P. (1980d). Model of cochlear function and acoustic re-emission. In:
    Psychophysical, Physiological & Behavioural Studies in Hearing. (G. van
    den Brink & F.A. Bilsen, eds.). pp 72-73. Delft University Press.
Wilson, J.P. and Sutton, G.J. (1981). Acoustic correlates of tonal tinnitus.
    In: Tinnitus. Ciba Found. Symp. 85. (D. Evered and G. Lawrenson, eds.).
    pp 82-107. London, Pitman Medical.
Zurek, P.M. (1981). Spontaneous narrowband acoustic signals emitted by human
    ears. J. Acoust. Soc. Am. 69, 514-523.

GENERAL DISCUSSION

SCHARF:
Do you have evidence of loudness recruitment in the frequency region where
the emissions occur and where the thresholds are elevated ?

WILSON:
Unfortunately we did not have time to test this. I think that it might have been
found either if the region is pathological or if it represents masking by the
internal signal.

TYLER:
Once the subjects were in the sound-proof room and able to hear a tinnitus,
where did they localize the perception?

WILSON:
We asked about tinnitus before the experiments and got negative replies (apart
from S.F. having heard his signals via a tube between the ears). They did not
report having observed tinnitus until the end of the experiments when it was too
late to investigate further. We did, however, have an unexpected "localisation"
observation in another subject who will be discussed after the paper of Long and
Cullen. She localised her tinnitus centrally even though the emission frequencies
in the two ears were slightly different. The same tone frequencies given to normal subjects however, also fused to give a central image.

JOHNSTONE:
Is it possible that the cochlear emission has caused adaptation and this is one
reason for the elevated threshold.

WILSON:
I do not know very much about this type of adaptation. I rather thought that
even though loudness may decrease, threshold does not change very much. Otherwise, I think that this is a possibility.

BROWNELL:
The subjects showing changes in the frequency of their cochlear acoustic emissions
in both Fritze's and your presentation were female. Did you monitor androgen levels in your subjects? Meyer and Zakon (Science 217, 635, 1982) have recently reported androgen modulation of the frequency of lateral line electroreceptor oscillations in a weakly electrical fish. The possible influence of androgen on cochlear
acoustic emissions might be assessed by monitoring androgen levels in humans or ad-
ministering the hormone to experimental animals.

WILSON:
No, we have not done this yet, but we hope to do so.

ON PERIPHERAL PROCESSING IN HUMAN HEARING

E. Zwicker

*Institute of Electroacoustics, Technical University München, D-8000 München 2
F.R. Germany*

INTRODUCTION

It was confirmed, through the discovery of traveling waves along the basilar membrane, that most of the ear's frequency selectivity is established peripherally, i.e. within the cochlea and without neural lateral inhibition. some very carefully collected physiological data (e.g. Sellick et al., 1982a) have recently revealed that the frequency selectivity of the basilar membrane is sharper than was previously assumed. These results also agree quite well with data based on psychoacoustical and neurophysiological measurements. The latter data, however, are more level dependent. As summarized earlier (Zwicker, 1979) significant non-linearities are found in many psychoacoustical measurements, not only in ordinary masking. Examples include difference tone production, two-tone interaction, specific loudness, post-masking (Zwicker and Fastl, 1972) and overload protection (Zwicker and Hesse, 1983). Some of these nonlinearities have already been shown to be related (Zwicker, 1979) but the combination with frequency selectivity complicates the discussion, since the efficiency of networks composed of linear (frequency selective) and nonlinear parts depends strongly on the sequence of these parts. In order to understand and to model the auditory system it is therefore necessary to find out which of the nonlinearities are located peripherally and which after neural transduction. It has been shown (Zwicker, 1983a), that masking – at least for lower SPLs – is performed peripherally. The location of two other nonlinear effects, overload protection and post-masking, has not yet been determined. The two experiments described below are designed to investigate this question.

EXPERIMENT I

A temporary threshold shift of 10 to 15 minutes duration occurs after a 112-dB/40-Hz tone of 20 minutes duration is switched off. This masker tone does not release the stapedius reflex as was monitored using an impedance bridge in the contralateral ear. Such sounds are by no means unbearably loud if switched on gradually without a click. (Driving an automobile at high speed with the windows open produces much higher SPLs than this at the ears of the passengers.)

The level L_T^* of 2-ms/1350-Hz tone impulses (repetition rate 46 Hz) at threshold was measured after offset of the 112-dB/40-Hz masker (indicated in Fig. 1a by the shaded area at the left side) as a function of time t. The first minute after offset, L_T^* remains at normal threshold in quiet, but rises afterwards by as much as 15 dB. It reaches a maximum near t = 2.5 min and decreases more slowly and with one or two slightly pronounced "bumps" to normal threshold in quiet, which is reached after about 10 min. Several examples of such temporal threshold shifts are described elsewhere as functions of different masker parameters (Zwicker and Hesse, 1983).

Subject "E.Z.r." shows a delayed evoked oto-acoustic emission at 1350 Hz. Such emissions originate within the cochlea and are therefore excellent indicators of peripherally located effects. In order to evoke the emissions 2-ms/1350-Hz tone impulses with a repetition rate of 46 Hz and a SL of 15 dB (corresponding to the maximal threshold shift in Fig. 1a) were used. Their sound pressure p_{OAE} was measured once a minute after the offset of the 40-Hz masker. These time functions are plotted in Fig. 1b. On average, about 22 seconds were needed for 1000 runs. The uncertainty in temporal position was therefore ± 11 sec. Despite this relatively wide margin, the emissions reflect very clearly the temporal behaviour

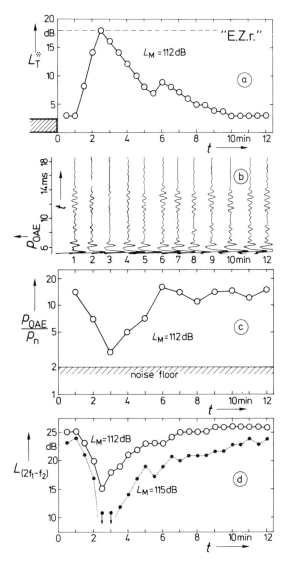

Fig. 1. (a): Temporary threshold shift of 1350-Hz tone bursts after the 40 Hz/112 dB masker's offset. (b) Time functions of delayed oto-acoustic emissions (p_{OAE}) evoked by the same 1350-Hz tone bursts at a sensation level of 15 dB. (c) Normalized amplitude of p_{OAE} on a logarithmic scale as a function of time t after masker's offset. (d) Level of CDT necessary to produce cancellation after offset of the masker. In addition to the data produced by the 40 Hz/112 dB masker, the data produced by a 115-dB masker are included (as dots)

of the threshold: the emission is strong if measured 1 minute after offset of the 40-Hz masker, but diminishes strongly afterwards, disappears almost completely for t = 3 min, and finally appears again exhibiting some "bumping" behaviour. The emission's sound pressure registered within the time window between 10.5 and 14.5 ms was calculated. It is graphed in Fig. 1c on a logarithmic scale (related to an arbitrary pressure p_n) again as a function of time t after offset of the 40-Hz masker. The result is a mirror image of Fig. 1a. This strongly suggests that this kind of temporary threshold shift originates within the cochlea. It also strengthens the assumption (Zwicker and Hesse, 1983) that a change of metabolic requirements in the scala media may cause this temporary threshold shift.

In order to find out whether this temporal effect also relates to the production of distortions, the variation of the level of the $(2f_1-f_2)$-difference tone was measured after the 40-Hz masker's offset using the method of cancellation. The frequencies and levels of the primaries were chosen to be: f_2 = 1920 Hz, L_2 = 43 dB, f_1 = 1680 Hz, L_1 = 48 dB. Consequently, $(2f_1-f_2)$ corresponds to a frequency of 1440 Hz. The cancellation level $L_{(2f_1-f_2)}$ adjusted under the normal condition, i.e. without previous masker, was set to 26 dB. In order to investigate also the amount of simultaneous masking produced by the 40-Hz/112-dB tone, masked thresholds were determined for the three above-mentioned frequencies of 1920, 1680, and 1440 Hz at sound pressure levels of 38, 39, and 40 dB, respectively (masker on for more than 5 min).

In Fig. 1d, cancellation level $L_{(2f1-f2)}$ is plotted as a function of time after offset of the masker. The open circles belong to a 112-dB masker, as used above, the filled circles to one of 115 dB. While for the former masker cancellation could be maintained throughout the prescribed time, this was not possible for the latter at t = 2.5 and 3.0 min. The cancellation level's time behaviour shows a very close relation to the results plotted in Fig. 1a and 1c for both conditions indicating

that the production of the cubic difference tone $(2f_1-f_2)$ occurs not only within
the cochlea but may also be influenced by the metabolic balance in the scala
media.

It should be mentioned that the described effect is actually twofold. The audible $(2f_1-f_2)$-tone gets fainter during the minimum *and* cancellation level decreases for subject "E.Z.r". For other subjects, conditions have been found for which
only the audible difference tone became fainter but cancellation level remained
almost constant. Other methods are necessary to separate these two effects, which
are closely related but seem to depend on the individual amount of masking (or
better, excitation) produced by the low-frequency tone on the one hand and the
possible change of the individual distribution of the metabolism along the scala
media on the other.

EXPERIMENT II

Post-masking (forward masking) is a significant effect, whose duration dependence, i.e. nonlinearity is only rarely discussed (see Zwicker and Fastl, 1972;
Zwicker, 1983b). An example of post-masking is given in Fig. 2a. A bandpass noise
(700 Hz to 2 kHz) with a level L_M = 48 dB is cut into bursts of 20 ms duration with
a repetition rate of 10 Hz, so that post-masking can be measured for at least 60 ms
within the pauses of 80 ms. The test-tone burst is composed of 1.5-kHz impulses of
2 ms duration with rise and fall times of 0.5 ms. Its masked threshold due to the
noise burst is measured as a function of the delay time t_v between the end of the
masker and the end of the test-tone impulse, as indicated in the insert of Fig. 2a.
The open circles indicate the sensation level SL_T^* of the test tone burst for different delay times t_v on a logarithmic scale. Note that the data for -3 and 0 ms do
not belong to that scale, because they involve simultaneous masking. SL_T^* decreases
more and more with increasing t_v, starting at t_v = 2 ms. At t_v = 20 ms, the half-
way mark for simultaneous masking is reached, and at t_v = 40 ms only 10 dB threshold shift remains. Threshold in quiet (marked with a filled circle at "L_M = 0") is
not reached within the 80-ms pause between two consecutive noise impulses.

The set up as well as the paradigm with the masker remained unchanged for the
measurement of delayed evoked oto-acoustic emissions, which for "A.S.1" are prominent near 1.5 kHz. Two sensation levels, SL_T^* = 20 dB and SL_T^* = 10 dB, were chosen.
These levels are marked in Fig. 2a by open square and open diamond; the connected
horizontal arrows point to the corresponding sensation levels. The sound pressures
p_{OAE} of the oto-acoustic emissions are plotted in Fig. 2b and 2c as a function of
the time t, with the corresponding delay time t_v as parameter, for SL_T^* = 20 dB and
SL_T^* = 10 dB respectively. The emissions marked with "L_M = 0" are produced in quiet,
i.e. with the masker switched off, and indicate the unmasked or unsuppressed condition. At t_v = 60 ms, the emission remains very similar to that produced for "L_M
= 0". The emissions remain unchanged as t_v decreases from 60 to 30 to 16 ms for
both conditions: SL_T^* = 20 dB in Fig. 2b as well as SL_T^* = 10 dB in Fig. 2c. For t_v
= 2 ms, the emissions decrease significantly and are hardly measurable for t_v = 0,
indicating that simultaneous masking coincides with suppression of the emissions.
The emissions' time functions are evaluated quantitatively by calculating the sound
pressure produced within the time window between 9 and 14.5 ms after onset as indicated by the dashed lines. This pressure p_{OAE} is plotted in Fig. 2d (relative to
an arbitrary pressure p_n) as a function of the delay time t_v. Squares belong to
SL_T^* = 20 dB and diamonds to SL_T^* = 10 dB, as in Fig. 2a. Closed symbols indicate
values for switched-off masker (L_M = 0). While discussing these results, it should
be remembered that the test tone bursts are audible for levels SL_T^* and delay times
t_v above and to the right of the solid-line curve of Fig. 2a connecting the open
circles. In all experiments with simultaneous masking (Zwicker 1981; Zwicker 1983b)
it was found that delayed evoked emissions are very strongly reduced if conditions
are reached at which the test sound evoking the emission is masked and becomes in-

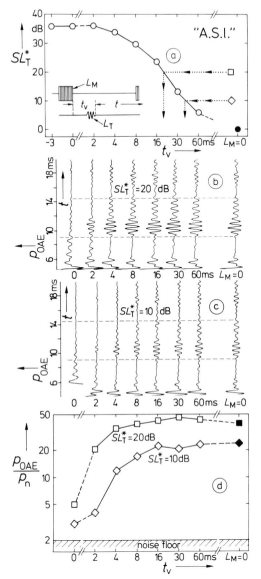

Fig. 2. (a) Post-masking (SL*_T) of a 1.5-kHz/
2-ms sequence of tone bursts masked by bursts
of bandpass noise (0.7 to 2 kHz) with an SPL
of 48 dB, as a function of the delay time t_v.
"L_M = 0" indicates data without masker.
(b) Delayed oto-acoustic emissions (p_OAE) e-
voked by the same test tone bursts with SL*_T
= 20 dB, for different delay times as marked.
(c) Same as (b) but with SL*_T = 10 dB.
(d) Normalized amplitude of p_OAE on a logarithmic scale as a function of the delay
time t_v, for the cases SL*_T = 10 dB and 20 dB.

audible. In the case displayed in
Fig. 2, this would be expected at
delay times t_v of 20 ms and 40 ms
for SL^*_T = 20 dB and 10 dB, respectively, as indicated by the downward pointing arrows in Fig. 2a.
For these delay times, however, no
change of the amplitude of the
emissions can be observed, indicating strongly that post-masking is
not a peripheral effect but is
established more centrally within
the neural pathway. The decrease
in the size of the emissions at t_v
= 2 ms is presumably the result of
simultaneous masking produced by
the decaying tail of the masker
burst, and is therefore a consequence of the ear's frequency
selectivity.

It is a remarkable fact - for
both the subject and the experimen-
ter - that a totally inaudible test
sound can produce strong emissions
of this kind. This simple observation has the important consequence that the information in the test
sound is available, i.e. not masked,
at the peripheral level within the
cochlea. Otherwise it could not
have produced the emission. In
other words, the peripheral information processing system acts very
quickly - in fact, as quickly as
its frequency selectivity allows.

DISCUSSION AND CONCLUSIONS

The use of delayed evoked oto-
acoustic emissions to establish
whether nonlinear effects are peripheral or nonperipheral was found
to be very effective. It should be
mentioned, however, that for extraction of quantitative relations
subjects are needed who show no
spontaneous emission of significant value (see Zwicker, 1983a)
apart from the evoked emission in
question in the frequency range
of interest. The level range within which the evoked sound pressure
of delayed emissions grows in proportion to the evoking stimulus is
limited to the region below about
20 dB above the stimulus' threshold in quiet. The discussion is
therefore limited to lower sound
levels.

The effect of temporary threshold shift produced after offset of low frequency maskers has a typical duration of some minutes. Similar periods and time constants have been found for the dependence of delayed oto-acoustic emissions on hypoxia in guinea pigs (Zwicker and Manley, 1981). Hypoxia strongly influences the metabolism within the scala media. It may therefore be concluded that low frequency sounds of high level bear upon this metabolism, even though these sounds are not very loud. Taking these assumptions for granted, the data elaborated in Fig. 1 can be understood as indications of the metabolism change. The following consequences ensue: the change reduces the sensitivity (raises threshold in quiet), it suppresses the evoked emissions, and it reduces the $(2f_1-f_2)$-difference tone, i.e. it decreases the nonlinearity. The very close relation between the temporal behaviour of these three effects implies that all three stem from the same source, which in turn is strongly dependent on the metabolic status. The feedback-saturation model discussed earlier (Zwicker, 1979, Fig. 6) may at least qualitatively describe these effects if the metabolic status is assumed to influence the gain of the amplifier (correlated to the OHC).

At low levels, the nonlinear saturation curve can be better approximated by a symmetrical power function with an exponent less than unity (for example square-root) instead of a straight line-break point curve, as drawn in Fig. 6 of the mentioned paper. This additionally suggests the possibility of spontaneous emissions (oscillations) which stabilize in amplitude at very low levels as a result of this nonlinearity. The input-output function of the corresponding amplifier (Zwicker, 1979, Fig. 6) is assumed to depend on the local change of metabolic requirements, as indicated in Fig. 3. From this point of view, CDT production,

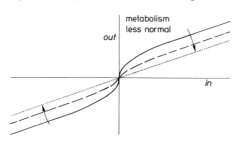

Fig. 3. Metabolism-controlled input-output function at low levels

(Zwicker, 1981b) two-tone suppression (Sachs and Kiang, 1968; Sellick et al., 1982b), and nonlinear growth of masked threshold (Schöne, 1979) all have the same source: the nonlinear metabolism-controlled gain function acting in the feedback loop. This means that the model proposed earlier (Zwicker, 1979) can be used to explain the facts described in Fig. 1, and leads to two interesting, almost exclusive combinations: the peripheral hearing system can act very sensitively but behaves highly nonlinearly or it can act linearly but then its sensitivity is strongly reduced. The actual condition depends not only on the present stimulus level, but also on the metabolism, which may as well be influenced by former stimuli.

The data elaborated in Fig. 2 indicate that post-masking is not produced peripherally, but rather more centrally in the neural pathway. They strongly confirm a result which was expected, but not previously well established. Since loudness depends on post-masking (Zwicker, 1977) it can be assumed that loudness – at least for lower levels – is also processed more centrally. The data also show that not all of the information available peripherally is transferred to higher centers. Post-masking therefore involves a reduction of information, an important aspect of the understanding of speech processing in humans.

AKNOWLEDGEMENT. This study was carried out within the Sonderforschungsbereich 204, "Gehör", supported by the Deutsche Forschungsgemeinschaft.

REFERENCES

Sachs, M.B. and Kiang, N.Y. (1968). Two-tone inhibition in auditory-nerve fibres. *J. Acoust. Soc. Am.* **43**, 1120-1128.
Sellick, P.M., Patuzzi, R. and Johnstone, B.M. (1982a). Measurement of basilar membrane motion in guinea pig using the Mössbauer technique. *J. Acoust. Soc. Am.* **72**, 131-141.

Sellick, P.M., Patuzzi, R. and Johnstone, B.M. (1982b). Modulation of responses
of spiral ganglion cells in the guinea pig cochlea by low frequency sound.
Hearing Res. 7, 199-221.
Schöne, P. (1979). Mithörschwellen-Tonheitsmuster maskierender Sinustöne. *Acou-
stica* 43, 197-204.
Zwicker, E. (1977). Procedure for calculating loudness of temporally variable
sounds. *J. Acoust. Soc. Am.* 62, 675-682.
Zwicker, E. (1979). A model describing nonlinearities in hearing by active pro-
cesses with saturation at 40 dB. *Biol. Cybernetics* 35, 243-250.
Zwicker, E. (1981a). Masking-period patterns and cochlear acoustical responses.
Hearing Res. 4, 195-202.
Zwicker, E. (1981b). Dependence of level and phase of the $(2f_1-f_2)$-cancellation
tone on frequency range, frequency difference, level of primaries, and sub-
ject. *J. Acoust. Soc. Am.* 70, 1277-1288.
Zwicker, E. (1983a). Delay evoked oto-acoustic emissions and their suppression
by Gaussian-shaped DC-impulses. *Hearing Res.* (submitted).
Zwicker, E. (1983b). Dependence of post-masking on masker duration and its rela-
tion to temporal effects in loudness. *J. Acoust. Soc. Am.* (submitted).
Zwicker, E. and Fastl, H. (1972). Zur Abhängigkeit der Nachverdeckung von der
Störimpulsdauer. *Acoustica* 26, 78-82.
Zwicker, E. and Hesse, A. (1983). Temporary threshold shifts after onset and off-
set of moderately loud low-frequency maskers. *J. Acoust. Soc. Am.* (submitted).
Zwicker, E. and Manley, G. (1981). Acoustical responses and suppression-period
patterns in guinea pigs. *Hearing Res.* 4, 43-52.

GENERAL DISCUSSION

EGGERMONT:
You are suggesting that forward masking is "not produced peripherally, but rather
more centrally in the neural pathway" because its effect is not seen in the oto-
acoustic emission. From results of Smith and Zwislocki (Biol. Cybernetics 17, 169
1975), Harris and Dallos (J. Neurophysiol. 42, 1083, 1979) and modelling by Eggermont (Biol.Cybernetics 19, 181, 1975) and Duifhuis and Bezemer (this volume) one
may conclude that forward masking is due to synaptic mechanisms to a large extend. It is also suggested that hair cells are involved in the oto-acoustic emission. Is therefore the division between peripheral and more central somewhere in
the middle of the hair cell ?

ZWICKER:
"Peripherally" to me means before the information is transferred neurally, i.e.
before it exists in action-potentials. The border may be regarded as at the synapses of the hair cells. Masking-period patterns produced by simultaneously-
presented low-frequency maskers have their correlates in suppression-period patterns produced with delayed oto-acoustic emissions. Post-masking decay, however,
does not produce a corresponding post-suppression time function.

EVANS:
I wanted to make the same point, namely that post-masking seems likely to correlate with the post-stimulation suppression effects seen at the cochlear nerve
level and more strongly still at the cochlear nucleus level. In the case of your
Fig. 1, the time-course of the threshold recovery does not match that of the
emission. Are other processes involved here too ?

ZWICKER:
Individual differences in the decay of the temporary threshold shift (Fig. 1) are
relatively large. Even changes from one measurement to the next with the same
subject are too large to discuss details of the "bouncing" (see Zwicker and Hesse,
(J.A.S.A., submitted).

WIT:
It is common finding that in the time-averaging procedure emissions can be evoked with stimuli far below auditory threshold (inaudible stimuli).

ZWICKER:
Subjects are chosen very carefully so that no spontaneous emission occurs within the frequency range in question. In the selected case the level of the delayed emission decreases in the same way as the stimulus level decreases and becomes very small for stimuli below threshold (Zwicker, Hear. Res., submitted)

MERZENICH:
Dr. Robert Shannon in our group has recently shown that there is strong forward masking seen with direct electrical stimulation of the auditory nerve array in cochlear implant patients. This recorded forward masking certainly arises from a location central to the hair cell / ganglion cell synapse.

ZWICKER:
Very fine, congratulations!

Section II
Auditory Nerve and Cochlear Nucleus,
Central and Centrifugal Auditory Systems

INTENSITY FUNCTIONS AND DYNAMIC RESPONSES
FROM THE COCHLEA TO THE COCHLEAR NUCLEUS

R. L. Smith, R. D. Frisina, and D. A. Goodman

Institute for Sensory Research, Syracuse University, Syracuse, N. Y. 13210, U. S. A.

Intensity functions, relating neural response to sound intensity level, are among the most commonly measured characteristics of auditory neurons. Nevertheless, questions remain unanswered concerning the detailed features of the functions. This paper describes intensity functions for the first three stages of the auditory system and presents some speculations about the significance of their shapes and the relationships between static and dynamic response components. All of the data come from single auditory neurons of anesthetized Mongolian gerbils, and the experimental techniques have been described in detail elsewhere (Frisina *et al.*, 1982; Goodman *et al.*, 1982; Smith, 1979).

1. INNER HAIR CELLS

In studies of inner hair cells (IHCs) of the guinea pig, Russell and Sellick (1978) showed that intracellular potentials in response to sound consist of two components: a dc response that follows the envelope of a tone burst and an ac response at the frequency of the tone burst. The response amplitudes increase monotonically with intensity and the responses do not appear to adapt in time. Intensity functions of gerbil IHCs are similar to those of the guinea pig (Goodman *et al.*, 1982) and some typical examples are shown in Fig. 1.

Figure 1 contains data from two IHCs where the filled circles show dc responses and the unfilled circles, ac responses. The ac functions have been normalized to coincide with the dc functions at the lowest intensity for which both responses were obtained. For each unit this point of commonality is indicated by a vertical cross which thus represents two data points. The tone-burst frequency is 2 kHz, well below the characteristic frequencies (CFs) of the units which are between 15 and 20 kHz. The dc functions are examples of the general observation that the dc receptor potential is proportional to sound intensity at low sound intensities and at frequencies less than or equal to the CF (Goodman *et al.*, 1982). This can be seen by comparing the slopes of the dc functions to the steeper dot-dash line which represents proportionality between the response and intensity or energy.

As previously noted (Goodman *et al.*, 1982), energy proportionality is in seeming conflict with cochlear microphonic (CM) measurements since the CM is proportional to sound

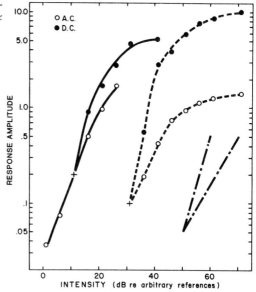

Fig. 1. Intracellular potentials of two IHCs plotted versus intensity level. The dc response is in millivolts and the ac response is normalized as described in the text. The dash-dot lines are proportional to stimulus amplitude and intensity. Solid curves: Unit AN-74.2; dashed curves: Unit AN-48

Fig. 2. Rate-intensity functions for an auditory-nerve fiber in response to a CF tone burst with a 1-msec rise-fall time. The unfilled circles are average firing rates computed over the first 40 msec of the response. The filled circles and crosses are maximum responses at onset, measured using 1-msec and 55-μsec time intervals, respectively. Note the different ordinates. The arrows indicate the intensity levels corresponding to the histograms in Fig. 3. Unit N7-11. CF: 16.1 kHz. Threshold: 33 dB SPL

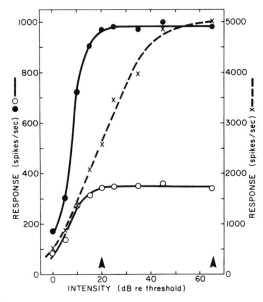

pressure level at low levels. The ac functions in Fig. 1 illustrate a similar dichotomy. At the lowest measured intensities they are less steep than the dc functions. However, the ac functions are somewhat steeper than amplitude proportionality as shown by the shallower dash-dot line. The slope difference between ac and dc functions is consistent with the speculation that the former may emphasize more linear aspects of transduction than does the latter (Goodman *et al.*, 1982). It should also be noted that the extracellular ac response measured in the basal turn of the gerbil cochlea sometimes exceeds the intracellular ac response. Hence a significant component of the ac response may be generated by sources other than the impaled IHC.

2. AUDITORY NERVE FIBERS

At high intensities the dc receptor potential of an IHC is a negatively accelerated function of intensity level, as illustrated in Fig. 1. Average and steady-state firing rates of gerbil auditory-nerve fibers are also negatively accelerated functions and typically reach saturation within 20-30 dB of threshold. An example is shown in Fig. 2 where average rates are given by unfilled circles. The rate-intensity function shows greater effects of saturation than does the dc intensity function, and the difference is even more apparent when the receptor potential is plotted using a linear ordinate (Goodman *et al.*, 1982). In comparison, the onset or unadapted rate-intensity function for a nerve fiber shows less effects of saturation and a greater operating range than does the steady-state function (Brachman, 1980; Smith and Brachman, 1980a,b). Hence the onset function may be a more direct reflection of the IHC intensity function than is the steady-state function, with the latter showing additional effects of synaptic transmission (Brachman, 1980; Smith and Brachman, 1982). Neural refractoriness can confound the situation by limiting the firing rate. The results that follow demonstrate that once the refractory limit is reached, the onset response of a fiber can still be influenced by intensity.

Many of the effects of time and intensity on auditory-nerve responses can be observed in Fig. 3. The histograms show responses of the fiber of Fig. 2 for a CF stimulus with a 1-msec rise-fall time and a duration of 50 msec. The short rise-fall time was chosen to maximize onset responses and yet still avoid significant frequency splatter (e.g. Özdamar and Dallos, 1978). The left-hand column contains various measures of the response to a tone 20 dB above threshold, and the right-hand column, a tone 65 dB above threshold. The upper row contains two peristimulus time histograms (PSTHs) generated using a 1-msec binwidth and 105 stimulus repetitions. Comparing the quasi steady-state responses reached at the end of each of the histograms, it can be seen that the 45 dB increase in intensity did not increase the steady-state response, i.e. the rate had reached

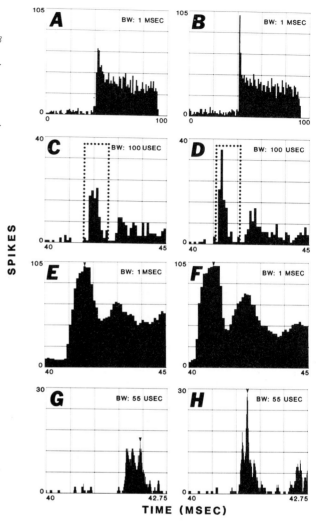

Fig. 3. Histograms of the responses of the unit of Fig. 2 for tone bursts 20 dB (left column) and 65 dB (right column) above threshold. A,B: PSTHs showing the full response to the stimulus. C,D: PSTHs showing the first few msecs of the response. The dots outline the 1-msec interval at onset that contains the maximum response. E,F: Smoothed PSTHs for the data in C and D. Successive bins are spaced 100 μsec apart. The arrows indicate the bins corresponding to the dotted intervals in C and D. G,H: Smoothed PSTHs with arrows indicating the maximum responses for an interval of 55 μsec. Bins are spaced 11 μsec apart

saturation, as had the average rate in Fig. 2.

The upper two histograms in Fig. 3 also appear to show that the onset response increases from 20 to 65 dB above threshold, as reported previously (Brachman, 1980; Smith and Brachman, 1980a, b). The maximum bin at the lower intensity contains 67 spikes and at the higher intensity, 102 spikes. The latter corresponds to almost one spike per presentation in a 1-msec bin, the maximum number of spikes possible for the refractory period of 1 msec (e.g., Gaumond *et al.*, 1982). However, comparing the maximum bins of Figs. 3A and 3B is somewhat misleading. The maximum response is changing, as described below, but it cannot be accurately measured with 1-msec bins. This is because the contents of the maximum bin depend upon its exact location and thus on the starting .point of the PSTH.

In order to improve resolution of the onset response, PSTHs were generated using a binwidth of 100 μsec and two of them are shown in Figs. 3C and 3D for the same data as Figs. 3A and 3B. Both histograms contain an initial mode less than 1 msec wide (Smith, 1973; Özdamar and Dallos, 1978). As intensity increases, the width of the mode and the latency to the maximum decrease. However, the maximum number of spikes in a 1-msec interval remains about the same, 101 for Fig. 3C and 102 for Fig. 3D. This is shown in the corresponding smoothed PSTHs (Smith and Brachman, 1980b) in Figs. 3E and 3F. The smoothed histograms consist of overlapping 1-msec bins located 100 μsec apart so that the intervals containing maxima can be located to within 100 μsec. In Fig. 2 the maximum onset responses, given by filled circles, are plotted versus intensity level. Consistent with the smoothed PSTHs, for intensities above 20 dB the onset firing rate has saturated at almost 1000 spikes/sec, i.e. the refractory limit of one spike per stimulus

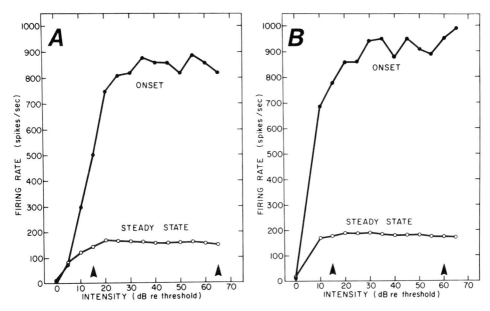

Fig. 4. Rate-intensity functions for two cochlear-nucleus units in response to CF tone bursts. The filled circles are maximum responses at onset measured using a 1-msec time interval. The unfilled circles are quasi steady-state rates measured during a 20-msec interval starting 25 msec after onset. The arrows indicate the intensity levels corresponding to the PSTHs in Fig. 5. A: Unit 74, CF: 6.3 kHz, Threshold: 20 dB SPL. B: Unit 80, CF: 5.5 kHz, Threshold: 18 dB SPL

presentation for a 1-msec interval.

The difference in width of the first mode in Figs. 3C and 3D indicates that, as intensity increases, the variability in the location of the first spike decreases and more spikes fall in a smaller time interval. This can be observed in more detail by using a still finer time resolution. Examples are shown in Figs. 3G and 3H which are smoothed PSTHs using overlapping 55-μsec bins located 11 μsec apart. The maximum number of spikes falling in a 55-μsec interval can be seen to increase substantially in going from 20 to 65 dB. The increase is also displayed by the dashed rate-intensity function in Fig. 2 where the crosses are the maximum onset responses obtained with this interval. It can be seen that this measure of the onset response increases with intensity in spite of the saturation of both the average response and the onset response for the 1-msec interval. Although the latter two rates saturate at about the same intensity in this example, this is not necessarily the case, and the two saturations presumably reflect different underlying mechanisms: neural refractoriness at onset and synaptic transmission in the steady-state.

3. COCHLEAR NUCLEUS

Rate-intensity functions of many cochlear nucleus units resemble those of auditory-nerve fibers. Two examples are shown in Fig. 4 for a CF stimulus with a rise-fall time of 2.5 msec. The onset responses, measured with a 1-msec interval, and the steady-state responses all increase monotonically with intensity. In addition, the onset function shows less pronounced saturation than does the steady-state function, as was previously observed in auditory-nerve responses (Brachman, 1980; Smith and Brachman, 1980a,b). The onset rates also appear to be somewhat higher than those observed in the auditory nerve with a 2.5-msec rise-fall time, although not as high as those produced in the experiment of Fig. 2 with a 1-msec rise-fall time.

Fig. 5. PSTHs of the responses of the units of Fig. 4 to stimuli containing a constant-intensity followed by an amplitude-modulated portion as shown schematically in the bottom row. The dotted rectangles outline the modulated intervals. Modulation was produced by multiplying the CF carrier by [2-cos(300πt)]. Intensity re threshold is 15 dB and 65 dB for the middle and upper rows, respectively. Number of repetitions: 98. Binwidth 640 μsec. A: Unit 74. B: Unit 80

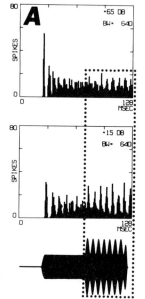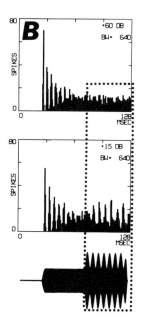

In order to investigate their dynamic response properties, the units of Fig. 4 were stimulated with amplitude modulated tones. The stimulus envelope is shown in Fig. 5, along with the PSTHs produced at two intensity levels. At the lower intensity, both units produce substantial response modulation in spite of the steady-state saturation, shown by the arrows in Fig. 4. The continued growth of the onset function may partially account for the response modulation, as was previously described for auditory-nerve responses (Brachman, 1980; Smith and Brachman, 1980b). However, in contrast to the auditory-nerve results and to the unit of Fig. 5B, the unit of Fig. 5A shows substantial response modulation even at high intensities where the onset rate has saturated. These results are typical of some units in the posteroventral cochlear nucleus of the gerbil (Frisina *et al.*, 1982) which provide enhanced responses to amplitude modulation (AM) with respect to both the predictions from their rate-intensity functions and to the responses of auditory-nerve fibers. These units may be similar to those described by Møller (1974) in the rat cochlear nucleus, and studies are underway to determine their properties in more detail.

4. DISCUSSION AND CONCLUSIONS

In each of the cases described above, a single intensity function was not sufficient to describe the effects of intensity on neural response. For the IHC, differences in the shapes of the ac and dc functions should provide insights into the transduction mechanism. The continued monotonic increase of the dc potential at high intensities may account for the increasing onset firing rate and decreasing latency to the maximum observed in auditory-nerve fiber responses. It may also allow for the large spread of thresholds reported for nerve fibers innervating the same IHC (Liberman, 1982). Some cells in the cochlear nucleus continue to respond to AM at high average intensities, in spite of the apparent saturation of both onset and steady-state firing rates. Both the decreasing jitter at stimulus onset and the responses to AM suggest the existence of an intensity-dependent synchronization of spikes, among units, that persists at high intensities and in the presence of various saturating nonlinearities. It remains to be seen whether the central nervous system can utilize such synchrony to further emphasize and analyze particular dynamic stimulus features.

Acknowledgements. We thank Drs. S. C. Chamberlain and J. J. Zwislocki for their valuable advice, and the former for guiding the histology accompanying these experiments. This research was supported by NSF grant BNS 82-42176, NIH grant NS 03950, and an NIH Research Career Development Award to R. L. Smith.

REFERENCES

Brachman, M.L. (1980). Dynamic response characteristic of single auditory-nerve
    fibers. Ph.D. Dissertation and Special Report ISR-S-19, Inst. for Sensory
    Res., Syracuse University, Syracuse, New York.
Frisina, R.D., Smith, R.L., Chamberlain, S. C. (1982). Specialized responses to
    amplitude modulation in the posteroventral cochlear nucleus: Single unit re-
    cordings with HRP-filled micropipettes. Soc. for Neurosci. Abstr. 8, 347.
Frisina, R.D., Chamberlain, S.C., Brachman, M.L., Smith, R.L. (1982). Anatomy and
    physiology of the gerbil cochlear nucleus: An improved surgical approach for
    microelectrode studies. Hearing Res. 6, 259-275.
Gaumond, R.P., Molnar, C.E., Kim, D.O. (1982). Stimulus and recovery dependence of
    cat cochlear nerve fiber spike discharge probability. J. Neurophysiol. 48,
    856-873.
Goodman, D.A., Smith, R.L., Chamberlain, S.C. (1982). Intracellular and extra-
    cellular responses in the organ of Corti of the gerbil. Hearing Res. 7,
    161-179.
Møller, A.R. (1974). Response of units in the cochlear nucleus to sinusoidally
    amplitude-modulated tones. Exp. Neurol. 45, 104-117.
Liberman, M.C. (1982). Single neuron labeling in the cat auditory nerve. Science
    216, 1239-1241.
Özdamar, Ö., Dallos, P. (1978). Synchronous responses of the primary auditory
    fibers to the onset of tone burst and their relation to compound action po-
    tentials. Brain Res. 155, 169-175.
Russell, I.J., Sellick, P.J. (1978). Intracellular studies of hair cells in the
    mammalian cochlea. J. Physiol. 284, 261-290.
Smith, R.L. (1979). Adaptation, saturation, and physiological masking in single
    auditory nerve fibers. J. Acoust. Soc. Am. 65, 166-178.
Smith, R.L. (1973). Short-term adaptation and incremental responses in single
    auditory-nerve fibers. Ph.D. Dissertation and Special Report LSC-S-11,
    Inst. for Sensory Res., Syracuse University, Syracuse, New York.
Smith, R.L., Brachman, M.L. (1982). Adaptation in auditory-nerve fibers: A revised
    model. Biol. Cyber. 42, 107-120.
Smith, R.L., Brachman, M.L. (1980a). Operating range and maximum response of
    single auditory-nerve fibers. Brain Res. 184, 499-505.
Smith, R.L., Brachman, M.L. (1980b). Dynamic response of single auditory-nerve
    fibers: Some effects of intensity and time. In: Psychophysical, Physiolog-
    ical and Behavioural Studies in Hearing. Eds. G. van den Brink and F.A.
    Bilsen, pp. 312-319, Delft, Delft University Press.

GENERAL DISCUSSION

SCHARF:
Does dynamic range of hair-cell DC response depend on stimulus rise time (for
longer duration sounds than you used here) ?

SMITH:
We have not studied the effects of rise time on the IHC response. However, the
response does not appear to adapt and rise time would not be expected to influence
operating range. In contrast, rise time does influence the operating range of
auditory nerve fibres (e.g. Smith and Brachmann, Brain Res. 184, 499, 1980;
Psychophysical, Physiological and Behavioural Studies in Hearing, van den Brink
and Bilsen, Eds, Delft, 1980, pp. 312 - 319).

LANGNER:
What were the periods of the chopper responses and how did these periods vary
with intensity?

SMITH:
The PSTs in fig. 5 are typical of the chopper units we have recorded from. The
period of chopping is several msecs and decreases as intensity increases. We are
presently preparing a quantitative description of the results. We are also investigating possible relationships between chopping frequency and best modulation
frequency and, more generally, between the response to AM and cell PST type.

EVANS:
Firstly, did you try frequencies of amplitude modulation substantially different
from the 'chopper' frequency?
Secondly, both you and I (Fig. 1, Evans. Psychophysical, Physiological and
Behavioural Studies in Hearing. van den Brink and Bilsen, Eds, Delft, 1980, pp.
300 - 309) have shown similar extensions of cochlear fibre dynamic range comparing shorter against longer duration ('steady-state') stimuli, but on a much
longer time-scale, where 'short' is tens of msec and 'steady-state' is of the
order of seconds. Should these be regarded as aspects of the same (e.g. adapta -
tion) process, and which is likely to be most relevant for accounting for psychoacoustic performance?

SMITH:
Preliminary results suggest that "chopping frequency" is not a good predictor of
best modulation frequency and that most chopper units will respond to AM, at high
intensities, give an appropriate modulation frequency (Frisina, Smith and Chamberlain, J.A.S.A. Abstr., 1983). I agree that there appear to be an hierarchy of
"adaptation" processes, often producing analogous results, but for different time scales (e.g. Smith and Brachmann, as above). Each may operationally produce
enhanced responses for the appropriate dynamic stimulus but I doubt if they all
reflect the same physiological process. Intensity also appears to differentially
affect the different processes (e.g. Westerman and Smith, Soc. for Neuroscience
Abstr., 1983). Relevance to psychoacoustics will depend on the dynamic aspects of
the stimulus paradigm as well as the interests of the central auditory nervous
system, and will undoubtedly differ for different kinds of stimulation.

PALMER:
We have also found a small number of cells in DCN which responded to CF tone intensity increments at sound levels well above those at which complete saturation
of onset and steady-state firing rates occurred (Palmer and Evans, unpublished).
Have you ever measured responses to tone intensity increments and/or amplitude
modulation, in cochlear nerve fibres, which persisted beyond complete saturation
of onset and steady-state firing rates?

SMITH:
The modulation of the stimulus shown in Fig. 5 consists of both a sinusoid and an
increment. At high intensities the most prominent response appears to be the periodic fluctuation in firing rate without an accompanying incremental response.
Other cells in the gerbil cochlear nucleus do exhibit incremental responses (e.g.
Smith, Dissertation, Syracuse University, 1973) in the presence of both onset
and steady-state saturation and may be similar to the units you are describing.
Individual auditory-nerve fibers do not appear to produce such large dynamic responses for comparable conditions.

REPRESENTATION OF ACOUSTIC STIMULI IN THE PRESENCE OF BACKGROUND SOUNDS:
ADAPTATION IN THE AUDITORY NERVE AND COCHLEAR NUCLEUS

Eric D. Young, John A. Costalupes and Daniel J. Gibson

*Department of Biomedical Engineering, The Johns Hopkins University
Baltimore, Maryland 21205 USA*

1. INTRODUCTION

    The difficulties involved in reconciling the wide intensity range over which
the auditory system operates with the limited dynamic range of auditory-nerve
fibers are well known (Evans, 1980). An interesting aspect of this problem is
the neural representation of narrowband stimuli presented with broadband masking
noise. High levels of background noise produce uniform excitation of auditory-
nerve fibers of all best frequencies; as the discharge rate produced approaches
saturation, rate changes in response to narrowband stimuli are reduced or eliminated (Rhode and Geisler, 1978; Geisler and Sinex, 1980; Sachs *et al.*, 1983).
Yet many measures of auditory performance such as speech discrimination (Borg and
Zakrisson, 1973) and intensity discrimination (Viemeister, 1974; Moore and Raab,
1975) do not show marked degradation in the presence of background noise at intensity levels up to 80-100 dB SPL.

    There are a number of aspects of the effects of background sounds on rate re-
sponses of auditory-nerve fibers which have not been worked out. Particular questions which have not been completely explored include the difference between the
effects of gated and continuous maskers, the effects of lateral suppression on
masked rate responses, and differences between the responses of auditory-nerve
fibers and cells in the cochlear nucleus. The latter question is particularly interesting in light of studies suggesting that cochlear nucleus cells' dynamic
ranges can shift to compensate for background stimuli, whereas those of auditory-
nerve fibers are fixed (Smith, 1973, 1977; Møller, 1976; Palmer and Evans, 1982).

    In this paper, we will report on the effects of a continuous background
sound on the rate response of auditory-nerve fibers and cochlear nucleus neurons.
In order that the neuron be in a near-steady state with respect to the effects
of the background, the background stimuli were on for at least 15-30 seconds
prior to presentation of test stimuli and remained on (except as noted below)
during the entire test period. Auditory-nerve fibers were recorded in anesthetized and decerebrate cats and cochlear nucleus neurons were recorded in decerebrate cats.

    Both simultaneous and non-simultaneous effects of the background must be
considered. By simultaneous effects, we mean processes such as two-tone or
lateral suppression (Sachs and Kiang, 1968) which are active when test and background stimuli are on at the same time. Non-simultaneous effects include all
influences on a unit's responses due to previously-presented stimuli; they are
usually referred to as adaptation. To study non-simultaneous effects, we use a
background stimulus which is on continuously except during 200 millisecond test
intervals (called negative gating, see the inset at the top of Fig. 1).

2. NON-SIMULTANEOUS EFFECTS OF EXPOSURE TO BF TONE BACKGROUNDS

    Figure 1 shows an example of the changes in an auditory-nerve fiber's rate
response which occur when a negatively-gated background (inset) is used. The
curves show the average discharge rate of the fiber during 200 ms BF tone bursts
as a function of the sound pressure level of the tone bursts (*rate-level functions*). Part A shows the rate-level function in quiet (Q) and in the presence

of negatively-gated BF tone backgrounds presented at three sound levels. Two
effects of the backgrounds can be observed. First, there is a reduction in the
driven discharge rate of the unit which becomes more severe as the level of the
background increases. It is most easily seen by the reduction of the fiber's
saturation rate to test tones. Second, there is a horizontal shift of the fiber's
dynamic range. That is, in the presence of the background, the range of sound
levels over which the unit's response rate goes from threshold to saturation moves
to the right along the abscissa, toward higher sound levels.

The horizontal shift in dynamic range shown in Fig. 1A is illustrated more
clearly in Fig. 1B which shows the rate-level functions of Fig. 1A after normalization. When rate functions are normalized, it is clear that negatively-gated
backgrounds cause a shift in the fiber's dynamic range to the right without
changing the width of the dynamic range. That is, the number of dB increase in
test level required to go from threshold to saturation is about the same with or
without background, and therefore the normalized rate functions are parallel-
shifted versions of one another. This behavior can be described by the following
equation relating the rate-level function in quiet $R_q(i)$ to the rate-level function in the presence of a background of level I, $R_I(i)$. i is the level of
the test tone.

$$R_I(i) = S \left[R_q(i-i_H) - R_{sp} \right] + R_{\ell o} \qquad (1)$$

R_{sp} is the spontaneous rate in quiet; $R_{\ell o}$ is the low-test-level discharge rate in
the presence of the background; i_H is the horizontal shift of the rate-level
function; and S is a scale factor expressing the reduction in driven discharge
rate produced by the background. We use the transformation of Eqn. 1 to determine values of horizontal shift i_H and scale factor S needed to superimpose a
unit's quiet rate-level function on its rate functions in the presence of backgrounds. The two parameters i_H and S provide a quantitative description of the
effects of background sounds on units' rate responses.

Figure 2 shows the dependence of scale factor (Fig. 2A) and horizontal shift
(Fig. 2B) on the level of the negatively-gated BF tone background. Figure 2A
shows that the scale factor decreases monotonically (note that the ordinate scale
of Fig. 2A is upside down) as background level increases, which is consistent with
the observation made in Fig. 1A that the reduction in driven discharge rate becomes more severe as background level in-
creases. The rate reduction in low and
medium spontaneous rate units (solid
lines) tends to be larger than that observed
in high spontaneous rate units (dashed lines
and unfilled circles). This is generally observed. At background levels of 40-50 dB
above threshold, scale factors average around
0.6 for high spontaneous rate units and around
0.4 for low and medium spontaneous rate units.

Figure 2B shows that the horizontal
shift of dynamic range increases monotonically

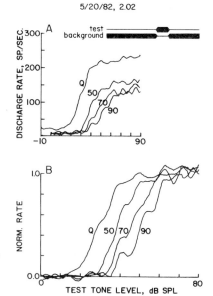

*Fig. 1. A. Rate-level functions for an auditory
nerve fiber in quiet (Q) and with three levels
of negatively-gated (see inset) BF tone background. Background levels next to curves.
Rates computed from presentations of 200 ms BF
tone bursts at 100 sound levels. BF = 2.9 kHz.
  B. Data of part A normalized as*

$$r(i) = (R(i) - R_{\ell o}) / (R_{sat} - R_{\ell o})$$

*R(i) is discharge rate, r(i) is normalized rate,
$R_{\ell o}$ is discharge rate at low test levels (spontaneous rate for Q), and R_{sat} is saturation
rate. Abscissa scale expanded for clarity*

and roughly linearly, with background level. An important aspect of this horizontal shift is the slope with which it occurs, i.e., how many dB of horizontal
shift are produced per dB increment in background level. Its importance lies in
the functional significance of the horizontal shift.

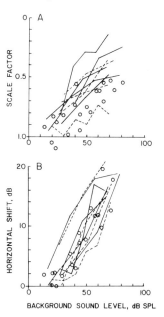

If the slopes were near 1, then the horizontal shift
would move units' dynamic ranges to the right exactly
far enough to compensate for changes in background
level. Such shifts would prevent saturation of rate
responses. The slope will be called *adaptation slope*
in this paper. For negatively-gated backgrounds, adaptation slope is significantly less than 1, and is
negatively-correlated with BF. Near 1 kHz, adaptation
slopes range from 0.2 to 0.5 and above 10 kHz, they are
smaller than 0.3. These shifts are relatively small
and they produce little or no expansion of units' overall dynamic ranges. The data of Fig. 2B are typical in
that differences are not observed between low, medium
and high spontaneous rate fibers either in the amount
of horizontal shift or the adaptation slope.

*Fig. 2. Dependence of scale factor S (A) and horizon-
tal shift i_H (B) on level of negatively-gated BF tone
background. 13 units from one cat with BFs ranging
from 0.7 to 4.7 kHz. Solid lines are low and medium
spont. units ($\leq$19/s), dashed lines and unfilled
circles are high spont. units*

3. SIMULTANEOUS AND NON-SIMULTANEOUS EFFECTS OF
    EXPOSURE TO NOISE BACKGROUNDS

      The effects of continuous broadband noise backgrounds are illustrated in Fig.
3A. The inset shows the test stimulus and background. The changes in the fiber's
rate-level function produced by the background are similar to the effects of negatively-gated backgrounds described above except that the discharge rate at the
lowest test levels increases monotonically with noise level. This is a response
to the noise background itself. Figure 3B shows the rate functions of Fig. 3A
after normalization. Significant horizontal shift is observed and it can be
measured by the same method as was used for negatively-gated backgrounds. The
horizontal shift and adaptation slopes produced by continuous noise backgrounds
are larger than those which result from negatively-gated tone or noise backgrounds. Adaptation slopes range from about 0.5 to 0.8 dB/dB. Adaptation slopes
with negatively-gated noise backgrounds are roughly equal to those obtained with
negatively-gated BF tone backgrounds (0.2-0.5 dB/dB).
      It is not surprising that horizontal shifts and adaptation slopes should be
larger with continuous than with negatively-gated noise backgrounds. With continuous backgrounds, both simultaneous and non-simultaneous effects operate. An
interesting question is the extent to which the horizontal shifts produced by
the two kinds of effects might summate. Comparison of the rate-level functions
in the top two panels of Fig. 3 with those in the bottom two panels demonstrates
the surprising finding that the horizontal shift due to non-simultaneous effects
is occluded by the larger horizontal shift due to simultaneous effects. Figure
3C shows rate-level functions obtained with simultaneously-gated noise (i.e.,
noise turned on only during test tones, as shown in the inset to Fig. 3C). In
this case, non-simultaneous effects are minimized and only simultaneous effects
are observed. There is little or no depression of driven discharge rate in this
case, so that saturation rate is approximately the same at all noise levels.
Nevertheless, horizontal shifts are observed, as can be seen in the normalized
rate functions of Fig. 3D.
      The important point to be made in comparing Figs. 3A and 3C is that the size
of the horizontal shifts are approximately the same for the continuous and

simultaneously-gated noise backgrounds. The shifts are 7 dB for both continuous and simultaneous noise at -45 dB and are 21 dB for simultaneous and 24 dB for continuous noise at -25 dB. This is consistently observed. In a population of 27 units from one cat, the slope of a linear regression equation fit to horizontal shifts from simultaneous noise plotted as a function of horizontal shifts from continuous noise is 0.94 (correlation coefficient of 0.96). Thus, the horizontal shift observed with continuous noise backgrounds is produced mainly by simultaneous effects. The non-simultaneous part of the noise, although capable of producing horizontal shift, does not contribute significantly to the shift observed with continuous noise.

The non-simultaneous part of a continuous background affects rate-level functions mainly by reducing the driven rate response to test stimuli. For example, saturation rate is significantly reduced in the presence of continuous noise (Fig. 3A), whereas saturation rate is changed only slightly by simultaneous noise (Fig. 3C). In most units, saturation rate is not changed at all by simultaneous noise. The non-simultaneous part of the noise produces a constant rate decrement, similar to the effects of short-term adaptation reported by Smith (1977). That is, the arithmetic difference between a rate function in simultaneously-gated noise and a rate function in continuous noise is a constant, independent of test level.

The horizontal shift of a fiber's dynamic range in the presence of a continuous noise background helps to prevent loss of rate response due to saturation by moving the sound level at which saturation occurs to higher levels. However, a continuous noise background also produces a net reduction in the range over which a fiber's discharge rate can increase (i.e., a reduction in $R_{sat}-R_{lo}$). This reduction is caused by the fiber's response to the background noise at low test levels. When R_{lo} reaches R_{sat}, the fiber's rate change to test stimuli disappears, regardless of the amount of horizontal shift of its dynamic range. This effect turns out to be the factor which ultimately limits rate responses to tones in the presence of continuous noise. Low and medium spontaneous rate fibers retain their rate response range to much higher noise levels than do high spontaneous rate fibers. In one experiment the scale factors (S, see Eqn. 1) of high spontaneous fibers were all below 0.2 in the presence of continuous noise at -30 dB, whereas the scale factors of medium and low spontaneous fibers ranged from 0.25 to 0.75 with the same noise background. This behavior reflects the fact that the response rate of low and medium spontaneous fibers grows more slowly with noise level than does the rate of high spontaneous fibers (Schalk and Sachs, 1980) and that their thresholds are higher (Liberman, 1978).

Fig. 3. A. Rate-level functions for BF tones with continuous noise backgrounds. Inset shows stimuli. Q is rate function in quiet, numbers are noise attenuations. Noise power at 0 dB is 35 dB re 20 µPa/√Hz. BF = 4.3 kHz.
B. Normalized rate functions for data in A.
C. Rate-level functions for BF tones with simultaneously gated noise. Inset shows stimuli.
D. Normalized rate functions for data in C

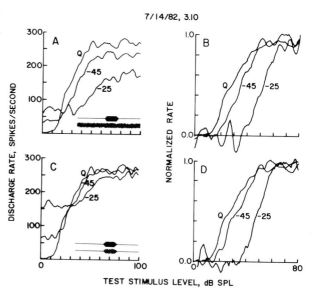

4. EFFECTS OF BACKGROUNDS ON COCHLEAR NUCLEUS CELLS

Unlike the auditory nerve, the cochlear nucleus (CN) contains a heterogeneous population of neurons. Single units in the CN display a variety of different response patterns, corresponding to the morphological diversity of the cell groups of which it is composed. For the purposes of this study, units in the CN were classified according to the location at which they were recorded and their response type. Units were ultimately lumped into two groups according to location, those in the dorsal cochlear nucleus (DCN) and those in the ventral cochlear nucleus (VCN). Response types were classified by the scheme introduced by Evans and Nelson (1973), as modified by Young and Voigt (1982). This scheme distinguishes four types of response, types I through IV, which differ in the amount of inhibitory response exhibited by the units.

Figure 4 shows three examples of the effects of continuous noise backgrounds on rate responses of CN neurons. The effects of negatively-gated and continuous backgrounds on CN cells are generally similar to those seen in auditory-nerve fibers. Horizontal shifts are always observed, but the behavior of the scale factor S is variable. Most units show rate reductions in the presence of backgrounds, but occasional units show rate increases at certain background levels.

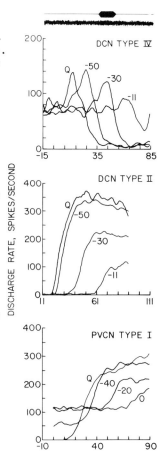

The example in the bottom panel of Fig. 4 is typical of many type I and type III units, which are the predominant response types in the VCN.

The behavior of the two response types found predominantly in the DCN, types II and IV, merits comment. Type II units are characterized by having little or no spontaneous activity and are the only units in the CN which do not respond to broadband noise. As is shown in the middle panel of Fig. 4, type II units show horizontal shift and rate reduction in the presence of continuous background noise. Since there is no response to the noise itself, these units retain excellent responsiveness to tones, even at the highest noise level. Type IV units give predominantly inhibitory responses to tones. They have characteristically nonmonotonic rate-level functions for BF tones, of which the curve marked Q in the top panel of Fig. 4 is a good example. Type IV units retain their sharp rate decrease at high levels in the presence of noise backgrounds; their whole BF response characteristic moves to higher sound levels, generally with some loss of prominence of the rate maximum.

Horizontal shifts are more difficult to quantify for CN cells because the shapes of rate functions sometimes change enough to prevent strict application of Eqn. 1. Horizontal shifts were still measured by shifting normalized rate functions into alignment, but maximum weight was given to the region near the point at which the slope of the rising portion of the rate function decreased sharply (i.e., the point of saturation or the point of maximum rate response). Table 1 summarizes the adaptation slopes of CN units and auditory-nerve fibers from decerebrate cats. Larger adaptation slopes are observed in the CN than in the auditory nerve and the largest slopes are found in

Fig. 4. Examples of the effects of continuous noise on the BF tone rate-level functions of cochlear nucleus cells. Stimulus shown at top of figure. Q is rate function in quiet, numbers give level of background noise in dB attenuation

the DCN. The in-
crease is small,
however, and the
distributions for
different regions
overlap consider-
ably. Apparently,
most of the dynamic
range adjustment
(horizontal shift)
of the rate re-
sponse of cells in
the CN actually
occurs in the
cochlea.

TABLE 1

Mean values of adaptation slope for various groups of units $\pm$ standard deviations. Numbers of units given in parentheses.

	negatively-gated BF tone backgrounds		continuous noise backgrounds
	BF$\leq$10 kHz	BF$\geq$10 kHz	
Auditory nerve fibers	0.33 $\pm$ 0.12 (14)	0.16 $\pm$ 0.07 (15)	0.79 $\pm$ 0.12 (15)
VCN units (types I and III)	0.38 $\pm$ 0.12 (15)	0.30 $\pm$ 0.08 (21)	0.86 $\pm$ 0.21 (30)
DCN units (types II,III and IV)	0.47 $\pm$ 0.17 (24)	no data	0.95 $\pm$ 0.20 (26)

Acknowledgement. This work was supported by NIH grants NS-12112 and NS-12524.

REFERENCES

Borg, E. and Zakrisson, J. (1973). Stapedius reflex and speech features. *J. Acoust. Soc. Am.* 54: 525–527.
Evans, E. F. (1980). "Phase–Locking" of cochlear fibres and the problem of dynamic range. In: *Psychophysical, Physiological and Behavioural Studies in Hearing.* (G. van den Brink and F. A. Bilsen, eds), pp. 300–307, Delft Univ. Press.
Evans, E. F. and Nelson, P. G. (1973). The responses of single neurones in the cochlear nucleus of the cat as a function of their location and the anaesthetic state. *Exptl. Brain Res.* 17, 402–427.
Geisler, C. D. and Sinex, D. G. (1980). Responses of primary auditory fibers to combined noise and tonal stimuli. *Hearing Res.* 3, 317–334.
Liberman, M. C. (1978). Auditory-nerve response from cats raised in a low-noise chamber. *J. Acoust. Soc. Am.* 63, 442–455.
Møller, A. R. (1976). Dynamic properties of primary auditory fibers compared with cells in the cochlear nucleus. *Acta physiol. scand.* 98, 157–167.
Moore, B. C. J. and Raab, D. H. (1975). Intensity discrimination for noise bursts in the presence of a continuous, bandstop background. *J. Acoust. Soc. Am.* 57, 400–405.
Palmer, A. R. and Evans, E. F. (1982). Intensity coding in the auditory periphery of the cat: Responses of cochlear nerve and cochlear nucleus neurons to signals in the presence of bandstop masking noise. *Hearing Res.* 7, 305–323.
Rhode, W. S., Geisler, C. D. and Kennedy, D. T. (1978). Auditory nerve fiber responses to wide-band noise and tone combinations. *J. Neurophysiol.* 41, 692–704.
Sachs, M. B. and Kiang, N. Y. S. (1968). Two-tone inhibition in auditory-nerve fibers. *J. Acoust. Soc. Am.* 43, 1120–1128.
Sachs, M. B., Voigt, H. F. and Young, E. D. (1983). Auditory-nerve representation of vowels in background noise. *J. Neurophysiol.* (in press).
Schalk, T. B. and Sachs, M. B. (1980). Nonlinearities in auditory-nerve fiber responses to bandlimited noise. *J. Acoust. Soc. Am.* 67, 903–913.
Smith, R. L. (1973). Short-term Adaptation and Incremental Responses of Single Auditory-nerve Fibers, Thesis, Syracuse Univ.
Smith, R. L. (1977). Short-term adaptation in single auditory nerve fibers: some poststimulatory effects. *J. Neurophysiol.* 40, 1098–1112.
Viemeister, N. F. (1974). Intensity discrimination in the presence of band-reject noise. *J. Acoust. Soc. Am.* 56, 1594–1600.
Young, E. D. and Voigt, H. F. (1982). Response properties of type II and type III units in dorsal cochlear nucleus. *Hearing Res.* 6, 153–169.

GENERAL DISCUSSION

EVANS:
At the Tutzing meeting I demonstrated the same effect of continuous noise on cochlear nerve fibre rate-level functions, shifting them along the level axis and reducing their dynamic range (Evans, in: Facts and Models in Hearing. Zwicker and Terhardt, Eds., Heidelberg 1974, pp. 118 - 129). Bandstop noise has analogous effects to continuous noise, but produces very strong effects on a high proportion of cells in the dorsal division of the cochlear nucleus (DCN), in terms of extension of the intensity dynamic range and in terms of the response 'dynamic range', i.e. the significance of the response relative to the background discharge. This results from the bandstop masker activating neural lateral inhibition (Evans and Palmer. J. Physiol. 252, 60 - 62P, 1975; Palmer and Evans, Hear. Res. 7, 305, 1982). Smaller effects are seen in a small proportion of cochlear nerve fibres having low spontaneous rates. Is there a danger that, by averaging data across populations, one disguises substantial differences in behaviour between subpopulations within the cochlear nerve and nucleus? We have even suggested that the DCN cells may receive their major input from the small subgroup of cochlear fibres with low spontaneous rates having larger dynamic ranges (Evans and Palmer, Exp. Brain Res. 40, 115, 1980) and stronger lateral suppression effects.

YOUNG:
I think the differences between our results and those presented in Palmer and Evans (1982) are mainly due to differences in the background stimulus. The notch-filtered noise backgrounds used by Palmer and Evans have significantly reduced power in the vicinity of the BF of the neuron under study. The strongest two tone suppression is known to be produced by frequencies near BF (Javel, J.A.S.A. 69, 1735, 1981). Therefore a notch-filtered noise should produce less suppression of a BF tone, and less horizontal shift of dynamic range, than a broad band noise. It is difficult to judge whether our results are inconsistent with those of Palmer and Evans concerning differences between cochlear nerve and nuclei. We are only claiming that the amounts of horizontal shift of dynamic range are approximately equal in the two loci. Palmer and Evans did not directly measure dynamic range shift. It is difficult to estimate dynamic range shift from their data using our technique since they generally did not determine the entire dynamic range. This does not mean that there are not differences in the effects of backgrounds on neurons in cochlear nerve and cochlear nuclei. Palmer and Evans have demonstrated one which probably has to do with the strong inhibitory effects which operate in dorsal cochlear nucleus. We have shown another in Fig. 4 of our paper from which it is clear that DCN units have significantly greater ability to resist saturation by rate response to the noise alone.
As to the question of averaging together the results from populations of neurones as we have done in Table I, we did not observe differences in the rate of horizontal shift of dynamic range between subpopulations of auditory nerve fibers or between response types in DCN. Thus I do not think we have covered up any correlations by averaging them together. We also suggested that low spontaneous rate units are specifically associated with one response type in DCN (Young and Voigt, Hear. Res. 6, 153, 1982). The response properties of type II units in DCN bear many similarities to those of low spontaneous rate auditory nerve fibers.

HARRISON:
The introduction of background noise may shift a fibre's characteristic frequency (CF). If so, and if the test stimulus is of fixed frequency, the rate versus intensity functions measured are progressively off CF. Your rate functions under masked conditions are very similar to above CF rate functions i.e. high threshold, low steepness of slope, not reaching saturation. In your experiments, did you have (downward) CF shifts with increasing background noise? If so, do you think that experiments involving a readjustment of the test tone to be always at CF would yield similar changes in rate-intensity functions?

YOUNG:
There are a number of similarities between our results and the effects expected
due to a shift in CF. It is my feeling that the effects of a shift in CF are not
large enough to explain our results. We are currently investigating this question
using the population approach.

NARINS:
For the past year, experiments have been carried out in our laboratory to determine the effects of noise on the coding of sounds of biological significance in
the frog. In one set of experiments we examined changes in the pure-tone rate-
level (R-L) functions produced by continuous or pulsed broadband noise (BBN). Recordings from single axons in the auditory nerve of treefrogs (eleutherodactylus
coqui) were made following the procedure described by Narins and Hillery (this
volume). Once a fiber was isolated and its FTC determined, a R-L function was obtained using 50 ms CF tones presented once per 130 ms. A digital attenuator under
program control allowed tone levels to be varied pseudorandomly in increments
equal to multiples of 2 dB (Palmer, Dissertation, Keele University, 1977). Five
consecutive R-L functions were averaged and smoothed with a Hamming window of
10 dB. BBN 0.05 - 6.4 kHz) was presented either (a) continuously or (b) in bursts
with identical characteristics as the tone bursts and coincident with them. Noise
level was controlled manually; its RMS level at 0 dB attenuation was 84 dB SPL
(BW: 100 Hz), corresponding to a total noise power over the system BW of -10 dB
re tone power.
R-L functions for frog auditory nerve fibers in the presence of BBN are more variable than those obtained with NB noise maskers, as in the cat (Geisler and Sinex,
Hear. Res. 3, 317, 1980). The fig. shows the results of continuous (A) and burst

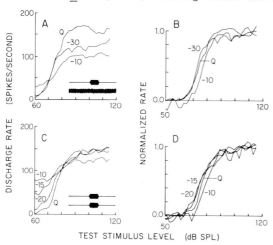

(C) BBN on the R-L functions for
the tone alone (Q) and for three
different BBN levels. Note the
lack of horizontal shift in the
normalized functions. This result
is typical of our observations to
date; no systematic shifts of the
R-L functions were observed with
increasing BBN level. Occasionally
small horizontal shifts are observed, but only by using the maximum noise levels our system is
capable of producing.
Unlike mammalian auditory nerve
fibers, eighth nerve fibers in amphibians exhibit two-tone suppression only for suppressing tones
above the fiber's CF. In other
words, inhibitory areas below the
unit's CF have not yet been reported in amphibians. Perhaps the ability of single auditory nerve fibers
to shift their operating range in
the face of broadband masking noise
is restricted to those vertebrates
which have suppressive areas below
their excitatory FTCs.

Fig. 1. R-L functions for BF tones in A)
continuous and C) simultaneous gated noise.
Insets show stimuli. B) and D) are normal-
ized according to Young et al. (this vol.).
R-L functions for 2 kHz tones in A)
continuous and C) simultaneous gated noise.
Insets show stimuli. B) and D) are normal-
ized according to Young et al. (this vol.)

COSTALUPES:
In related behavioural experiments, we have assessed the ability of cats to detect
pure tones at various frequencies in the presence of continuous noise backgrounds
over a wide range of intensities. We are interested in seeing whether behavioural
thresholds can be compared with the responses of auditory-nerve fibers to tones
in noise.

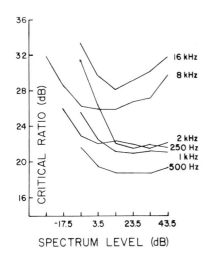

Fig. 2.
Mean critical ratios for three cats as a function
of noise spectrum level at the frequencies indi-
cated to the right of each contour

Results for three cats are shown in the figure.
Critical ratio - defined as the ratio of the power
of the tone at masked threshold to power of the
broadband noise background - is indicated along
the ordinate and spectrum level of the noise is
indicated along the abscissa. The absolute values
of the critical ratios obtained here and the behaviour of the critical ratios at low noise levels
are in accord with previous results from other
labs. What we wish to point out here is that for
frequencies up to 2 kHz, critical ratios tend to
remain constant over a wide range of noise levels
from moderate to high intensities. For frequencies
of 8 and 16 kHz, on the other hand, critical ratios
increase as noise level is raised from moderate to
high intensities.

One explanation of this difference is that detection of low frequency tones in noise is based on
timing information present in the discharge pattern of auditory-nerve fibres. Studies by Rhode et al. (J. Neurophys. 41, 692, 1978), Abbas (Hear. Res. 5, 69, 1981)
and others have shown that the dynamic range of phase-locking (as measured by synchronization) is shifted by noise at a rate equal to the rate of increase of the
noise background. For high frequencies, where timing information is not available,
detection must be based on rate changes and the dynamic range adjustments lag behind noise level increases about 65%, as we have just shown. Hence, masked thresholds might be expected to increase, as noise level is raised. At present, we are
extending these results to populations of fibres and to more precise predictions
of behavioural thresholds from the response of auditory-nerve fibres in the cat.

QUERFURTH:
I wonder whether the horizontal shift of the dynamic curves obtained during continuous noise stimulation is due to the inhibitory action of the Na-K ATPase,
which hyperpolarizes the encoding site during/after high frequency discharges.

YOUNG:
A contribution by metabolic effects cannot be entirely ruled out. However we
think it is unlikely for the following reasons. Since we observe the same horizontal shifts with brief, simultaneously gated backgrounds as with continuous
noise, it seems unlikely that horizontal shift is produced by metabolic effects.
Similarly, rate reduction can be observed following short exposures to tones and
noise (Smith, J. Neurophysiol. 40, 1098, 1977) and these reductions are proportional to the nerve fibre's discharge rate during the adaptation stimulus, suggesting that the rate reduction reflects processes in the hair cell/nerve fibre
synapse or in the fibre itself.

NONLINEAR BEHAVIOR AT THRESHOLD DETERMINED IN THE AUDITORY CANAL AND ON THE AUDITORY NERVE

J. B. Allen and *P. F. Fahey

*Bell Laboratories, Murray Hill, NJ and *University of Scranton, Scranton, PA*

In order to study mechanical nonlinearities in the mammalian hearing organ over a broad range of frequencies, we have both used and adapted the Kiang-Moxon threshold tuning curve paradigm (Liberman, 1978) to measure distortion products $2f_1-f_2$ (the CDT) and f_2-f_1 (the DT) and to measure two manifestations of two tone suppression.

The data presented here was primarily recorded from the auditory nerves of over twenty cats. Both the physiological techniques and the computer controlled audio and electrical instrumentation are discussed fully in Allen (1983). Most of the data presented here will be threshold curves defined such that the curve is the locus of points in frequency-amplitude space where the amplitude was adjusted until the neural unit under study generated one action potential more during a 50 ms interval with the signal on than the spontaneous rate during the immediately preceding 50 ms interval.

DISTORTION PRODUCTS

Using the Kiang-Moxon paradigm we measured the frequency threshold curve (FTC) for the neural units that we encountered on the auditory nerve. Given the FTC and, hence, the CF, we then input a tone pip comprised of two frequencies, f_1 and f_2, such that either $2f_1-f_2$ or, alternatively, f_2-f_1 was equal to the CF. Again we used the Kiang-Moxon paradigm to find the locus of points in the frequency amplitude (f_1,A_1) plane such that the unit responded with one more spike during the driven interval than during the silent interval. This locus of points defines a distortion threshold curve (DTC). For all of the data curves presented here the amplitudes of f_1 and f_2 are equal ($A_1=A_2=A$).

Effectively our procedure is to calibrate an auditory neuron (by measuring its FTC) and then to use this "calibrated" neuron to control the level of the primary frequencies. In Fig. 1 we show four FTC's superimposed on the units' $2f_1-f_2$ DTC's. The amplitude of the distortion product is equal to the FTC threshold at CF. Note that for frequencies less than the point of intersection of the DTC with the FTC both the distortion product and f_1 drive the unit. Hence this point of intersection (marked with a triangle in Fig. 1) is the last point in the DTC's in Figs. 2 and 3. Since the unit's threshold at CF is the amplitude of the distortion product (and the sensitivity of the detector) in the Figs. 2 and 3, the DTC will be normalized to the threshold at CF.

Fig. 2(a) shows cubic spline fits to all of the $2f_1-f_2$ DTC's for one cat. Although the individual curves in this figure can not be resolved, it is apparent that the non-monotonic behavior as seen in Fig. 1 is commonplace. It is further evident that at high CF's, the detectable distortion products can be generated at lower amplitude of the primaries.

As is seen in Fig. 2(b), if the DTC's are replotted versus log f_2/f_1, the slopes are found (non-monotonicities aside) to range from 50-70 dB/octave (of f_2/f_1), with a mean across animals of about 55 dB/octave (of f_2/f_1). For the CDT, the data spread is least using log (f_2/f_1) as the dependent variable. For the DT (f_2-f_1) f_1 seems to be an appropriate variable (Fig. 3).

In Fig. 3 we show a plot of the dependence of several f_2-f_1 DTC's upon frequency for one animal. As before the frequency of the distortion product equals the CF of the neural unit and the amplitude of the DT is equal to the threshold of the unit at CF. In this figure all responses have been normalized by the CF threshold. It is clear from Figs. 3 and 2(a) that the f_2-f_1 DTC is much less frequency dependent than the $2f_1-f_2$ DTC. Also we found a much larger variability

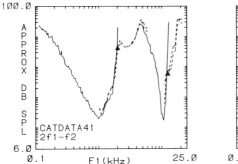
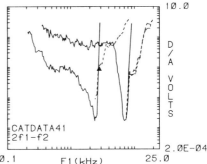

Fig. 1. *This figure shows some FTC's (solid lines) for Cat 41 with raw distortion product data (the DTC's, the dashed lines) for the respective units. With two units two passes at the DTC are shown. Also on some of the DTC's there is a triangle at the DTC-FTC intersection. Points on the DTC of lower frequency than the intersection point are not considered part of the DTC because the f_1 primary rather than the distortion product is driving the unit (10.0 volts to our driver results in an SPL of about 100 dB re 20 μPa at the tympanic membrane)*

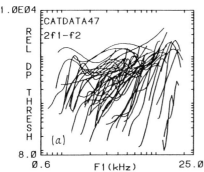
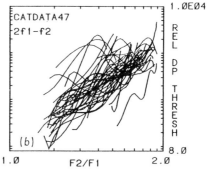

Fig. 2. *In (a) we show a collection of the cubic spline fits to the $2f_1-f_2$ DTC's of Cat 47. Cubic spline fits were used to average multiple passes at the DTC. The density of curves is too great to resolve the individual curves in most cases, but the trends in the DTC's with frequency are apparent. In (b) the same data as in (a) is replotted using log (f_2/f_1) as the independent variable (note the log scale). Disregarding non-monotonicities, generally the DTC's approximate straight lines of the same slope independent of the CF of the unit*

Fig. 3. *In this figure are the cubic spline fits of the f_2-f_1 DTC's of Cat 47. It is evident here that the frequence dependence of the DT is different from that of the CDT*

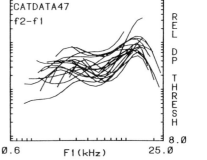

between cats for the DT, whereas all of our cats with good thresholds showed a fairly similar threshold for the CDT.

While we were measuring the DTC we also made ear canal pressure measurements in several animals with a calibrated Bruel and Kjaer ½ inch microphone terminating a 2 cm long probe tube. The probe microphone was used to ascertain the level of distortion in the external auditory meatus and in a closed acoustic cavity. In the acoustic cavity the level of the distortion products was always more than 70 dB below the level of the primaries (and near the distortion floor of the driver).

In Fig. 4 we show the FTC of a neural unit along with traces of two different
Fourier components of the ear canal pressure. The Fourier component of the ear
canal pressure at frequency f_1 is symbolized by the curve with the shorter dashes.
The curve with the longer dashes represents the pressure Fourier component at frequency $2f_1-f_2$. Both components are plotted as a function of f_1. In Fig. 4(a) the
Fourier components were measured while using the Kiang-Moxon paradigm to hold the
neural measure of the CDT constant. Note that the f_1 pressure Fourier component
follows the DTC trajectory while the $2f_1-f_2$ component remains constant at the
threshold of the FTC at CF. In Fig. 4(b) the ear canal pressure has been measured
with the Kiang-Moxon paradigm disabled (full output to the acoustic driver). In
this case the f_1 Fourier component follows the "cavity" response of the animal
outer and middle ear system while the $2f_1-f_2$ pressure Fourier component increases
in magnitude as f_2 approaches f_1. Notice that the $2f_1-f_2$ Fourier component curve
in Fig. 4(b) is almost the mirror image of the f_1 Fourier component in 4(a). This
is expected if the level dependence of the CDT is less marked than the dependence
upon relative frequency. The implication of Fig. 4 and of the data acquired from
several other units, is that the level of the distortion product as it is detected
in the ear canal, is sufficient to drive the unit directly.

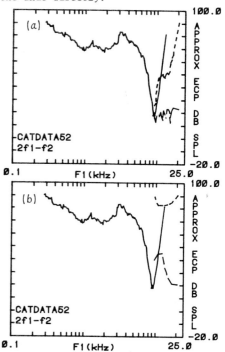

*Fig. 4. Here is an FTC of a neural
unit pictured with the Fourier component of the ear canal pressure at frequency equal to f_1 (short dashes) and
the Fourier component of the ear canal
pressure at frequency equal to
$2f_1-f_2=CF$ (longer dashes). In (a) the
DTC paradigm is enabled; hence, the
f_1 amplitude follows the DTC trajectory, while the $2f_1-f_2$ amplitude
remains relatively constant (and near
the threshold at CF). In (b) the DTC
paradigm is disabled and the f_1 component increases. Note that the
$2f_1-f_2$ trajectory in (b) approximately
mirrors the f_1 trajectory in (a).
Usually when the distortion product
was being generated most efficiently
the difference between the level of
the f_1 primary and the level of the distortion product was on the order of
40 dB for most units studied*

TWO-TONE SUPPRESSION

We also used a modified version of the Kiang-Moxon paradigm for our measure
of two-tone suppression. In this study we found the FTC's of several units along
with suppression threshold curves (STC's). The suppression threshold curve was
defined by the following measure.
     During one 50 ms interval we present a suppressor tone at the suppressor
frequency, f_s. During the adjacent 50 ms interval, we simultaneously presented
two tones; one was at the frequency equal to CF, usually 6 to 10 dB in level
above the FTC at CF (these CF tones are symbolized by the triangles in Fig. 5),
while the other tone was a repeat of the suppressor tone. The level of the suppressor tone was scanned until the number of spikes generated during the single-
tone 50 ms interval was one less than the number of spikes generated during the
two-tone 50 ms interval. The trajectory of the levels of the suppressor tones
found in this way in frequency-amplitude space is the suppression threshold
curve. In Fig. 5 we show suppression thresholds for two different units. The

triangle shows the excitor tone and the dashed line is the STC. For suppressor tones above the dashed line but below the FTC threshold the unit fires at its spontaneous rate. This way of measuring the STC is consistent with an alternative measure of two-tone suppression shown in Fig. 6.

In Fig. 6 the FTC (near CF) is remeasured, using the standard Kiang–Moxon paradigm, in the presence of a second subthreshold suppressor tone. The levels and frequencies of the suppressor tones are symbolized by the geometric figures and the suppressed FTC's are the curves nested within the FTC. The larger the

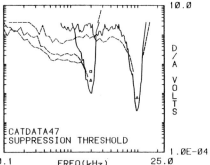

Fig. 5. In this figure we show two FTC's (solid curves) along with the suppression threshold curves (dasehd lines). The tone that is being suppressed is marked by a triangle or a square. In the unit with the two different excitor tones the higher STC corresponds to the higher excitor tone

suppressor the larger the corresponding FTC threshold at CF.

The results of Figs. 5 and 6 are also consistent in the following sense. If the level of a "suppressed" FTC threshold at CF in Fig. 6 is taken as the CF excitor tone level to be used in an STC experiment such as described by Fig. 5, then the corresponding suppressor tone level, A_s, at f_s of Fig. 6 is at a level such that it will lie on the suppression threshold curve in Fig. 5.

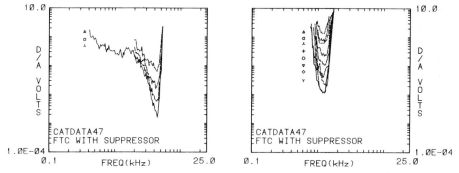

Fig. 6. We show here FTC's for two units. The FTC's were remeasured in the presence of a suppressor tone, with the frequency and amplitudes of the suppressors indicated by the geometric symbols. The higher the level of the suppressor tone the correspondingly higher the level of the tip of the FTC

One unit pictured in Fig. 5 (f_{CF}=2 kHz) shows two suppression threshold curves and two different excitor tones. From this unit and from the data in Fig. 6, we see that the neural excitatory threshold increases as the (subthreshold) suppressor increases. From Fig. 6 it appears that for excitatory tones at CF, an increase of 6 dB in suppressor tone level results in a 10–12 dB increase in the suppression. This seems to be true over a fairly large level range—as long as the suppressor is neither so low as to be ineffective nor so high as to drive the unit.

Also in Fig. 5 one can see some of the general features of the frequency dependence of suppression. The suppression threshold curves are fairly level independent over a broad frequency range for the high CF units. These thresholds generally range between 60 and 80 dB in level (10.0 volts corresponds to approximately 100 dB). Moreover, in units where we have measured the low frequency tails of the FTC, the suppression threshold parallels the low frequency tail. One can also note from Fig. 5 that there is negligible suppression (as defined here) at frequencies above CF in the units pictured. We found this to be generally true in

that the amount of suppression observed above CF was much less (or was absent)
relative to that seen below CF. For units having CF's below 1 or 2 kHz no suppression effect was observed using our measure.

DISCUSSION

     Several features of the data reported here have been observed by others in
different kinds of experiments. Buunen and Rhode (1978) have observed the CDT on
the auditory nerve in cats and have shown both the non-monotonic frequency dependence of the CDT and the slight increase in efficiency of generation of the CDT
at the higher frequencies. Buunen *et al.* (1977) and Smoorenburg *et al.* (1976)
have also observed frequency dependence of the CDT similar to our auditory nerve
studies in their AVCN studies in cat. Moreover, Smoorenburg *et al.* (1976) have
shown that the DT is much less frequency dependent than the CDT when detected at
the AVCN. Comparison of Figs. 2 and 3 shows that on the auditory nerve the DT is
also less frequency dependent than the CDT.
     The levels of the distortion products in the external auditory meatus that
we observed are consistent with what has been observed by others (Kim *et al.*, 1980;
Zurek *et al.*, 1982). Distortion products 40 dB below the primaries (thresholds
40 dB above) are easily and routinely detectable. Most importantly, the level
of these distortion products as found in the ear canal appears to be of a magnitude sufficient to drive the neural units.
     With regard to two-tone suppression we have found that the threshold of
suppression follows the middle ear response (the tuning curve tail). This result
was also found by Schmiedt (1982) using a slightly different threshold criterion
and by Allen (1981). Because the low spontaneous units usually have higher
thresholds, these units show a larger two-tone suppression effect since the
suppression effect does not seem to depend on the unit's CF threshold. When most
of the FTC is above 80 dB SPL, the response at CF can be more easily suppressed.
The suppression effect is largest for low spontaneous units having high thresholds.
     Another finding, in the majority of our units, was that the suppression
effect above CF was not as strong as that below CF. Indeed, only for units with
high threshold at CF did we find substantial suppression by a tone above CF. It
might be noted that Abbas and Sachs (1976) found substantial suppression above
CF using a fractional rate response measure. Their data indicates that the units
showing these suppression effects generally had thresholds at CF of 40 dB SPL and
greater. Hence, their results showing substantial suppression above CF are not
inconsistent with the data presented here.

CONCLUSION

     We have found that the level of distortion products, as seen in the external
auditory meatus, appears to be sufficient to drive any neural unit having a CF at
the distortion product frequency. This result is one interesting conclusion of
this study. Since we have ruled out distortion product generation by the acoustic
delivery system, it appears that there are two possibilities for the source of
these distortion products. First, the distortion products could be generated
within the middle ear structure itself. Second, the distortion could be generated
within the cochlea and could propagate backward (via the middle ear) into the
external auditory meatus. Indeed, given the strong frequency dependence of the
CDT and given that a plot of the DTC versus log (f_2/f_1) (Fig. 3) seems to be
more uniform over the frequency range than the DTC versus f_1 (Fig. 2), it appears
that the cochlea is a more likely source of the CDT than the middle ear. Moreover, the non-monotonicities in the DTC have been explained by Hall (1981) as the
interference of the primary distortion product wave with a wave that has been
propagated back toward the stapes and then reflected back into the cochlea.
Certainly, a wave propagated toward the stapes and partially coupled into the
middle ear is consistent with our observation of substantial distortion product
levels in the ear canal.
     Although the suggestion by Hall (1981) that the non-monotonicities are due to
the interference of a reflected wave is supported by the observation of the distortion product in the ear canal, an alternative explanation of the non-monotoni-

cities by Zwicker (1981) is also supported by some of our data as well as by the data of Kim *et al.* (1980). Zwicker has described the non-monotonicities in terms of a strongly level dependent superposition, at the distortion product place, of wavelets generated on the basilar membrane in the vicinity of the f_1 and f_2 places. We have taken data (not shown) where we have changed the gain of the neural detector by setting the distortion product frequency off of CF. For sharply tuned units this can change the gain by 10 dB while only changing the distortion product frequency by a factor of 0.9. Occasionally, but not always, this has smoothed out the nonmonotonic behavior of the DTC. At this time, we do not have enough systematic data to rule out one explanation of the non-monotonicities in favor of the other. Indeed, on physical grounds it would seem that both explanations would have validity.

Our observation of the relative independence of the suppression threshold curve with frequency (for frequencies below CF) has also been observed recently by Schmiedt (1982) in Mongolian gerbils. The effect both in cats and in Mongolian gerbils seems to become noticeable when the suppressor tones have levels on the order of 70 dB SPL. This relative independence of and the 70 dB SPL threshold for suppression is also evident in the cat rate response data of Abbas and Sachs (1976).

It is important to note that in this study, by using a Kiang-Moxon tuning curve paradigm and its various adaptations to generate the several different types of data reported here, we have been able to avoid the non-linearity of the rate-level response function and we have been able to build a data base of consistent measurements.

REFERENCES

Abbas, P.J. and Sachs, M.B. (1976). "Two-tone suppression in auditory-nerve fibers: Extension of a stimulus-response relationship." *J. Acoust. Soc. Am.* **59**, 112-122.

Allen, J.B. (1981). "Neural tuning thresholds in the presence of a second sub-threshold tone." *J. Acoust. Soc. Am.* **69**, S53.

Allen, J.B. (1983). "Magnitude and phase frequency response to single tone in the auditory nerve." *J. Acoust. Soc. Am.*, in press.

Buunen, T.J.F., ten Kate, J.H., Raatgever, J., and Bilsen, F.A. (1977). "Combined psychophysical and electrophysical study on the role of combination tones in the perception of phase changes." *J. Acoust. Soc. Am.* **61**, 508-519.

Buunen, T.J.F. and Rhode, W.J. (1978). "Responses of fibers in the cat's auditory nerve to the cubic difference tone." *J. Acoust. Soc. Am.* **64**, 772-781.

Hall, J.L. (1981). "Observation on a nonlinear model for motion of the basilar membrane." In *Hearing Research and Theory.* Volume 1, pp. 1-61, Academic Press, New York.

Kim, D.O., Molnar, C.C., and Matthews, J.W. (1980). "Cochlear mechanics: Non-linear behavior in two-tone response as reflected in cochlear-nerve-fiber responses and in ear-canal sound pressure." *J. Acoust. Soc. Am.* **67**, 1704-1721.

Kim, D.O. (1980). "Cochlear mechanics: Implications of electrophysiological and acoustical observations." *Hearing Research* **2**, 297-317.

Liberman, M.C. (1978). "Auditory-nerve response from cats raised in a low-noise chamber." *J. Acoust. Soc. Am.* **63**, 442-455.

Schmiedt, R.A. (1982). "Boundaries of two-tone rate suppression of cochlear-nerve activity." *Hearing Research* **7**, 335-351.

Smoorenburg, G.F., Gibson, M.M., Kitzes, L.M., Rose, J.E., and Hind, J.E. (1976). "Correlates of combination tones observed in the response of neurons in the anteroventral cochlear nucleus of the cat." *J. Acoust. Soc. Am.* **59**, 945-962.

Zurek, P.M., Clark, W.W., and Kim, D.O. (1982). "The behavior of acoustic distortion products in the ear canals of chinchillas with normal and damaged ears." *J. Acoust. Soc. Am.* **72**, 774-781.

Zwicker, E. (1981). "Cubic difference tone level and phase dependence on frequency and level of primaries." In *Psychophysical, Physiological and Behavioral Studies in Hearing.* (v.d. Brink and Bilsen, eds.). Delft Univ. Press, Netherlands.

GENERAL DISCUSSION:

BIALEK:
The sound pressure level of a distortion product in the ear canal must depend upon the impedance "looking out" of the eardrum into the earphone coupler. Thus the equality of observed sound pressure and effective sound pressure at the neuron (asserted by your Fig. 4a) is coincidental. Such studies with variable impedance couplers would be very useful.

FAHEY:
Indeed the sound pressure of the distortion product in the ear canal depends upon the impedance looking out. The distortion product activating the unit depends upon both the wave that reaches the unit directly from the point of generation and the wave present in the "resonator" consisting of the outer ear (closed by the sound delivery system) and middle ear and cochlea. Certainly using the neural unit as the detector of the distortion product guarantees that the sound pressure in the ear canal can be no more than the threshold of the unit at the distortion product frequency. It could, conceivably be less (depending upon the impedance looking out of the cochlea) but it is not.

PERIPHERAL AUDITORY ADAPTATION AND FORWARD MASKING

H.Duifhuis and A.W.Bezemer

*Biophysics Department, Rijksuniversiteit Groningen, and
Institute for Perception Research, Eindhoven, the Netherlands*

1. INTRODUCTION

Adaptation in responses in primary auditory nerve fibers is a well document-
ed phenomenon. There is little or no evidence that it is present at the level of
the hair cell receptor potential. Therefore, it is quite plausible that the underlying mechanism(s) originate at the synapse. An attractive model for this
mechanism is implied in the several "depletion" models, which have in common
that transmitter aspects (-substance, or channels) can be employed at a higher
rate than at which they are replenished (e.g., Schroeder and Hall, 1974;
Eggermont, 1975; Furukawa et al., 1978). These models lead to a multiplicative
adaptation model: the reduced response is the result of a reduced gain factor of
the system. Several theoretical studies had proposed to treat adaptation as an
aspect of an automatic gain control (Siebert and Gambardella, 1968; Duifhuis,
1972; Johannesma and Koldewijn, 1973; De Jongh, 1978). However, neurophysiological follow-up studies, in particular those examining responses to brief increments on a pedestal signal, casted serious doubt on the validity of this interpretation (e.g., Smith and Zwislocki, 1975; Harris, 1977; Prijs and
Eggermont, 1981). These data are, insofar as envelopes are concerned, described
more accurately with an additive adaptation model. Since neither interpretation described all aspects of the data it is a fortunate development that recent
theories present attempts to incorporate both mechanisms (Furukawa et al., 1982;
Smith and Brachman, 1982; Schwid and Geisler, 1982).

Since the discovery of auditory forward masking (de Maré, 1940) it was realized that this psychophysical phenomenon was related to adaptation effects, that
was likely to be caused by recovery from the state of adaptation at the masker
offset. Evidence in support of this view was presented by Harris (1977) and Bauer
(1978). The problem of relating the two is that visual inspection of the recorded
data does not lead to more than a qualitative relation of adaptation and forward
masking. The quantitative relation requires the quantification of (central) decision rules. For simple psychophysical detection tasks these rules have been described succesfully with optimum detectors operating on peripheral neural data
(starting with Siebert, 1965).

The present study is limited to an examination of the implications of the
antithetical models of adaptation (multiplicative or additive) regarding temporal
masking. This analysis should be followed up with the examination of the predictions of the more recent theories, which, however, still contain several assumptions that need further verification.

2. PREDICTING SIMULTANEOUS AND FORWARD MASKING

The first step in the analysis is to describe the responses in peripheral
auditory nerve fibers mathematically. As a basic frame-work we use De Jongh's
(1978) model, a synthesis of many concurrent models of the peripheral auditory
system. Figure 1a presents the (slightly modified) model. It is a multichannel
model in wich nonlinear interaction between channels is neglected. The model exhibits multiplicative adaptation, for the ease of analysis drawn here as a feed-
forward process. The modification towards additive adaptation is given in Fig.1b.
The major difference is that instead of multiplying $q_i(t)$, the output of G2, by
a factor $a_i(t)$, one decreases $q_i(t)$ by subtracting the quantity $d_i(t)$ (cf Smith,
1973; Prijs and Eggermont, 1981).

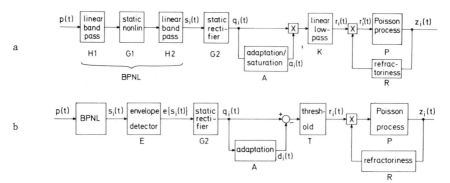

a

b

Fig.1a. *One channel of De Jongh's model of the peripheral auditory system, but with feed-forward instead of feed-back adaptation/saturation, and a Poisson spike-generator rather than a trigger process (to simplify the analysis). The BPNL-section models cochlear filtering and nonlinearity; G2 is a half-wave rectifier; K limits synchronisation at high frequencies; Poisson process plus refractoriness actually constitute a Markov process. By taking* $a_i(t) = (1+\alpha<q_i(t)>_\tau)^{-1}$, *where* $<..>_\tau$ *implies averaging over a window* τ, *the multiplicative adaptation model produces saturation. Fig.1b. The additive adaptation model, specified for the envelope of the response but not for the fine structure; hence E; T prevents the rate function* $r_i(t)$ *from being negative (linear half-wave rectifier). For* d_i *one might take* $d_i(t) = \beta<q_i(t)>_\tau$ *with* $0<\beta<1$ *(e.g., Smith, 1973)*

Next we analyse the response to a probe in the vicinity of a masker. In this paper we limit ourselves to tonal stimuli: a masker M of duration T and amplitude A_M, and a probe P with duration ΔT and amplitude A_P, presented at t_p after masker onset, and masker as well as probe at $f=f_0$.

It is useful to make serveral other approximations in order to gain transparency, albeit at the cost of losing details. These simplifications do not alter the main conclusions which we will reach. The first approximation is to take

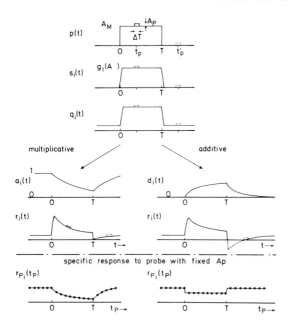

Fig.2. *Responses at successive points in the multiplicative and additive models to a tonal masker of duration T and amplitude* A_M *and a brief probe of duration* ΔT *and amplitude* A_P, *presented either simultaneously at* t_P, *or in the forward masking position* t_P'. *The bottom line shows the incremental responses to the probe as a function of its temporal location with respect to the masker. (The decrement in* $r_{Pi}(t_P)$ *in the simultaneous additive case is caused by the nonlinearities G1 and G2, not by adaptation.)*

rectangular bandpass filters which innervate N_e afferent neurons. Thus, given the tonal stimuli, N_e channels convey equivalent, but stochastically independent, information on P and M. Secondly, we neglect the effect of refractoriness because the refractory period is significantly smaller than the average inter-spike-interval at saturation. The envelopes of the responses at different points in the multiplicative and additive models are shown in Fig.2, for simultaneous and non-simultaneous probes.

The optimum use of information across the stochastically independent channels can be characterized by the rms sum of the relative distances d_i' for each channel (Green, 1958). Setting

$$d_{Ne}' = \{\underset{N_e}{\Sigma}(d_i')^2\}^{\frac{1}{2}} = N_e^{\frac{1}{2}} \cdot d_i' = 1 \qquad (1)$$

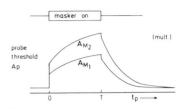

as a detection criterion, as usual, provides the equation from which the probe threshold can be solved. Optimum detection requires also optimization in the time domain, i.e. setting a detection window of duration ΔT at $t=t_P$. Because of the fixed frequency f_0, the information is contained in the spike rate. The Poisson process specifies the stochastic response, and leads to simple expression for average rate and its variance. Thus, d_i' can be evaluated, and the probe threshold can be predicted.

The results are:
a) for the multiplicative model and simultaneous masking

$$A_P(t_P) = \left[N_e \Delta T \frac{a_M(t_P)}{q_M} \left(\frac{\partial q_M}{\partial A_M} \right)^2 \right]^{-\frac{1}{2}} = \frac{1}{\sqrt{a_M(t_P)}} A_P(0). \qquad (2)$$

Note that $a_M(t_P)$ decreases as t_P goes from 0 to T, implying that A_P *increases* over this interval (see Fig.3).

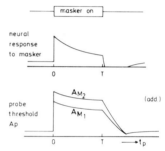

b) for the multiplicative model and forward masking

$$A_P(t_P) = g_2^{-1} \left[2N_e \Delta T \, a_M(t_P) \right]^{-1} \qquad (3)$$

immediately after masker offset $(q=g_2(A)=g_2\{g_1(A)\})$. If the spontaneous response begins to play a role the expression is more complicated. $A_P(t_P)$ monotonically approaches the threshold-in-quiet value.
c) for the additive model and simultaneous masking

$$A_P(t_P) = \left[1 - \beta(t_P) \right]^{\frac{1}{2}} A_P(0), \qquad (4)$$

with $A_P(0)$ as in Eq.2. Here $\beta(t_P)$ is an increasing function of t_P and A_P decreases as t_P goes from 0 to T (see Fig.4). (The definition of $\beta(t_P)$ relates to the earlier definition in the legend of Fig.1b, where β was a constant, as follows: $\beta(t_P) \cdot q_i(A_M) = \beta < q_i(A_M) >_T$.)
d) for the additive model and forward masking

$$A_P(t_P) = g_2^{-1} \left[\beta(t_P) \, g_2(A_M) \right] \qquad (5)$$

during the interval in which spontaneous activity is suppressed entirely by adaptation. Beyond this range $A_P(t_P)$ increases to its asymptotic value.

3. DISCUSSION

Using a concurrent model for peripheral auditory processing and a count statistic on cn information subjected to optimum detection rules we arrived at the prediction of certain trends in simultaneous and forward masking. Although the model parameters have not yet been specified in detail, the results for additive and multiplicative adaptation differ significantly, and the differences are not very sensitive to model parameters.

The most striking difference is found in the predictions for simultaneous masking (cf. Figs.3 and 4). Psychophysical data show at best a small overshoot effect at the makser onset (3 to 6 dB), but definitely not a rising behaviour such as is predicted by the multiplicative model (Fig.3). This increment reaches values of over 10 dB. Thus, on the basis of this analysis, as well as of the analysis of neural data (Smith and Zwislocki, 1975), the multplicative adaptation model has to be rejected. The additive model, on the other hand, gives a reasonable account of psychophysical and neural data. For simultaneous masking an overshoot of the order of 3 dB is expected (see also Smith and Zwislocki, 1975).

The additive model predicts forward masking only over the interval over which spontaneous activity is completely suppressed. Threshold is reached as soon as the probe elicits a spike, because the "noise background" is absent. Where the spontaneous activity begins to recover the probe threshold increases slightly, because the specific probe response is independent of t_p but the noise increases so that S/N decreases. The predicted local minimum in the transition disappears if it would occur at slightly different times in different fibers. The above mechanism predicts forward masking to stop abruptly at 30 to 70 ms after masker offset (see e.g., Harris and Dallos, 1979). In older psychophysical data such a breakpoint is found, but approximately at 200 ms after masker offset. Some recent data, however, indicate that hardly any forward masking is found beyond $t_p = T + 50$ ms (e.g., Stout, 1982). The rejected multplicative model would predict forward masking over a longer interval.

The above results were obtained using a count statistic, for which expectation and variance are proportional. It is conceivable that instead of this, the almost optimum interval statistic would be employed, based on a fixed small number of inter-spike-intervals rather than on a number of counts during a fixed window. The interval statistic leads to the following predictions: no adaptation effects at all for the multiplicative model, but for the additive model the adaptation effects are very similar to those obtained with the count statistic.

Note that the model potentially allows prediction of the Weber function. As this is an amplitude characteristic, it depends on the shape of G1 and G2. The combined effect may be approximated with a power function over a considerable dynamic range. For the additive model G1 and G2 have to cause saturation, so that the power than approaches 0.

In conclusion, the additive adaptation model appears adequate insofar as predictions based on signal envelopes are concerned. The multiplicative model is untenable. A firm physiological bases for the additive model may be emerging but is not yet complete (e.g. Furukawa et al., 1982). For the model of Fig.1b the restriction that it described envelope behaviour can be removed by deleting block E and reinserting block K before, or possibly after, block T. The additive model relates forward masking and the overshoot effect directly to peripheral auditory adaptation, hereby supporting de Maré's original interpretation.

Acknowledgement. *A part of this study was supported by the Netherlands organization for the advancement of pure research ZWO.*

REFERENCES

Bauer, J.W. (1978). Tuning curves and masking functions of auditory-nerve fibers in cat. *Sensory Processes* 2, 156-172.
Duifhuis, H. (1972). *Perceptual analysis of sound.* PhD thesis. Eindhoven, Univ. of Technology.

Eggermont, J.J. (1975). Cochlear adaptation: a theoretical description. *Biol. Cybernetics* 19, 181-189.

Furukawa, T., Hayashida, Y. and Matsuura, S. (1978). Quantal analysis of the size of excitatory post-synaptic potentials. *J.Physiol.* 276, 211-226.

Furukawa, T., Kuno, M. and Matsuura, S. (1982). Quantal analysis of a decrementa-response at hair cell afferent fibre synapses in the goldfish sacculus. *J.Physiol.* 322, 181-195.

Green, D.M. (1958). Detection of multicomponent signals in noise. *J.Acoust.Soc.Am.* 30, 904-911.

Harris, D.M. (1977). *Forward masking and recovery from adaptation in single auditory-nerve fibers*. PhD thesis. Northwestern University.

Harris, D.M. and Dallos, P. (1979). Forward masking of auditory-nerve fiber responses. *J.Neurophysiol.* 42, 1083-1107.

Johannesma, P.I.M. and Koldewijn, G.J.R. (1973). Model study of the peripheral auditory system. Described in: H.R.de Jongh (1978), Ch.III-3.

Jongh, H.R.de (1978). *Modelling the peripheral auditory system*. PhD thesis, University of Amsterdam.

Maré, G.de (1940). Fresh observations of the so-called masking effect of the ear and its possible diagnostic significance. *Acata Otolaryngol.* 28, 314-316.

Prijs, V.F. and Eggermont, J.J. (1981). Narrow-band analysis of compound action potentials for several stimulus conditions in the guinea pig. *Hearing Research* 4, 23-41.

Schroeder, M.R. and Hall, J.L. (1974). Model for mechanical to neural trans-duction in the auditory receptor. *J.Acoust.Soc.Am.* 55, 1055-1060.

Schwid, H.A. and Geisler, C.D. (1982). Multiple reservoir model of neurotrans-mitter release by a cochlear inner hair cell. *J.Acoust.Soc.Am.* 72, 1435-1440.

Siebert, W.M. (1965). Some implications of the stochastic behaviour of primary auditory neurons. *Kybernetik* 2, 206-215.

Siebert, W.M. and Gambardella, G. (1968). Phenomenological model for a form of adaptation in primary auditory-nerve fibers. *MIT RLE Quarterly progress report* 88, 330-334.

Smith, R.L. (1973). *Short-term adaptation and incremental responses of single auditory-nerve fibers*. Special Report LSC-S-11, Laboratory of Sensory Communication, Syracuse University.

Smith, R.L. and Brachman, M.L. (1982). Adaptation in auditory-nerve fibers: A revised model. *Biol.Cybernetics* 44, 107-120.

Smith, R.L. and Zwislocki, J.J. (1975). Short-term adaptation and incrementa-response of single auditory-nerve fibers. *Biol.Cybernetics* 17, 169-182.

Stout, N.K. (1982). *Psychoacoustical observations on frequency resolution in simultaneous and forward masking*. PhD thesis, Oxford.

PITCH AND COCHLEAR NERVE FIBRE TEMPORAL DISCHARGE PATTERNS

E.F. Evans

*Department of Communication & Neuroscience, University of Keele,
Keele, Staffordshire, ST5 5BG, U.K.*

1. INTRODUCTION

     Controversy still exists concerning the role played by the temporal
discharge patterns of cochlear nerve fibres in determining the pitch assigned to
complex stimuli (see Evans, 1978 for review). Recently, attention has been
focussed on a stimulus, similar to one originally used by Seebeck, consisting of
a pulse train having alternate intervals of 4.7 and 5.3 ms (Whitfield, 1979,
1980; Moore, 1980). This stimulus, when heard unfiltered has an ambiguous pitch
of 100 or 200 Hz. In contrast, Whitfield (1979, 1980) reported intervals
corresponding to the 4.7 and 5.3 ms intervals in the stimulus to predominate in
the interspike interval histograms (ISIH) of cochlear nerve fibres having
characteristic frequencies (CFs) from 0.55 to 2 kHz, in the guinea pig. He
consequently raised the questions why the pitches corresponding to these
intervals were not heard, and conversely why the 200 Hz pitch heard appeared to
have no corresponding interval in the neural discharge patterns. In response,
Moore (1980) has argued that neural intervals corresponding to the pitches heard
should be present in the discharge patterns of cochlear fibres of CFs corresponding to the *dominant region* for the pitch heard, usually some 3 - 5 times the
frequency matching the pitch.
     The present experiments were carried out in an attempt to clarify the situ-
ation, and to provide information on an underlying secondary question. This is
how well do cochlear fibres, having narrow-band filtering properties to continuous single- and multiple-component stimuli, in terms of the weighting of their
phase-locking properties (Evans, 1978, 1980b, 1981), behave as filters in
response to impulsive stimuli? Experiments were carried out on single fibres of
the cat's cochlear nerve and also on an electronic analogue of a cochlear nerve
fibre, having linear band-pass filtering properties (Evans, 1980a).

2. METHODS

     The stimulus in all experiments was a pulse train of rectangular pulses,
100 μs in width and having alternate intervals of 4.7 and 5.3 ms (see Fig. 1),
synthesized by computer, and presented closed-field to the ear by a Bruel &
Kjaer 4134 condenser-driver system (with compensation for distortion). ISIH and
autocorrelation histograms were obtained from cochlear fibres at several sound
levels in steps of 10-20 dB from below threshold to the stimulus up to about
60 dB above. In addition, the frequency threshold curve (FTC) of each fibre was
determined by computer.
     The details of the stimulation and recording techniques, physiological con-
trols, and of plotting the FTCs are given in Evans (1979). Briefly, micropipettes are used for recording the activity of single fibres in the cochlear
nerve of pentobarbitone anaesthetized cats. The cats were selected for freedom
from middle ear disease and great care was taken to minimise noise exposure
during the surgical preparation by avoiding drilling and bone snipping. The
threshold of the gross cochlear action potential to tone pips from 0.5-40 kHz was
monitored at intervals throughout the experiments and did not deteriorate. The
bulla was intact but vented to atmospheric pressure.
     ISIH and autocorrelation histograms were computed on- and off-line by a
Computer Automation Alpha 2/40 minicomputer system used for the synthesis of the
stimuli. A 'silo' DAC and hardware spike clock (Cambridge Electronic Design Ltd.

502 system) enabled synthesis of stimuli to be effected while logging spike data
with a resolution of 1 µs. Each histogram was computed on 4096 spikes, with 512
bins of width 60 µs for fibres with CFs below 1 kHz, and 30 µs for those above
(e.g. Fig. 1). Fast Fourier transforms (FFTs) were computed from autocorrelation
histograms constructed with bin widths of 100 µs (e.g. Fig. 2). FTCs were
obtained by an on-line up-down threshold tracking method described in Evans
(1979) in response to 50 ms tone bursts having 5 ms rise-fall times.

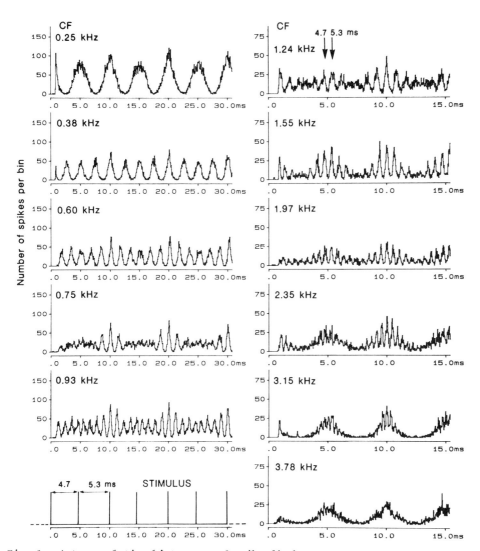

Fig. 1. Autocorrelation histograms of spike discharge patterns of 11 cochlear fibres with CFs indicated in response to a click train stimulus with alternate intervals of 4.7 and 5.3 ms (see lower left of Figure).
For CFs: 0.25-0.93 kHz, bin width was 60 µs; 1.24-3.78 kHz, 30 µs. 512 bins in each histogram, 4096 spikes. All fibres, with the exception of that with CF of 0.6 kHz, are from one cat. Stimulus level: constant in terms of electrical signal to the earphone at -40 dB (about 20-30 dB above response threshold of the fibres)

3. RESULTS

ISIH and autocorrelation histograms were obtained to the pulse train stimulus from 52 cochlear fibres in 2 cats, with CFs ranging from 0.25 to 5.9 kHz. The data for the 2 cats were virtually identical.

a) *Effect of fibre CF*

Fig. 1 illustrates the systematic changes in the autocorrelation histograms obtained with change in fibre CF from 0.25 to 3.78 kHz. Fibres with CFs below about 0.7 kHz yielded histograms dominated by a periodicity corresponding to the predominantly even harmonics of the 100 Hz fundamental. The histograms therefore included peaks at 5 and 10 ms. For CFs above about 0.7 kHz, the histograms became more complex. The 5 ms peak tended to split into two peaks corresponding to the stimulus intervals of 4.7 and 5.3 ms. However, these peaks were prominent only for CFs above 1 kHz, becoming comparable in size with the 10 ms peak for fibres with CFs in the 2 kHz region. For fibres with CFs above 2 kHz, the splitting of the 5 ms peak became progressively less prominent; eventually, at CFs of about 3 kHz, it divided into 3 sub-peaks at 4.7, 5 and 5.3 ms. Above about 3.5 kHz, the fine structure of the histograms became lost, a 200 Hz periodicity remaining.

b) *Effect of stimulus level*

Over the range of levels investigated, from threshold to 40-60 dB above, the forms of the autocorrelation histograms were relatively invariant (eg Fig. 2).

To quantify the effects of level, FFTs were taken of the histograms (eg Fig. 2, right half). The levels of the spectral peaks were then corrected for the levels of the corresponding components in the stimulus, and were plotted so that comparison could be made of their relative weighting (by the cochlea's filtering action) with the FTC of the fibre. Fig. 3 shows the results for 3 fibres, that with a CF at 1.08 kHz being the fibre illustrated in Fig. 2.

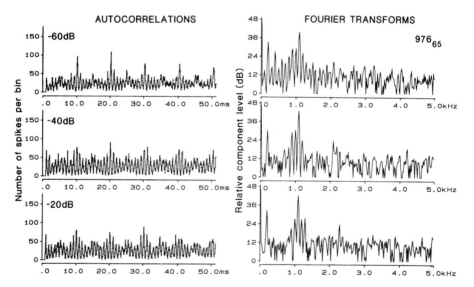

Fig. 2. *Autocorrelation histograms of a fibre with a CF of 1.08 kHz to the click train at three sound levels, (separated by 20 dB), at approximately 10, 30 and 50 dB above response threshold.*
Bin width 100 μs. Right half shows Fourier transforms of histograms on left

In the case of every fibre, at most stimulus levels there was relatively good agreement between the weighting functions and the pure tone FTC. Most deviations were systematic, as follows. The weighting function at stimulus levels nearest to threshold tended to diverge from the FTC, becoming wider than the FTC at 10-20 dB from the tip. In a few cases, (eg fibre 976_{65}, Fig. 3), the functions for the higher stimulus levels were somewhat narrower than the FTC. For fibres with the highest CFs (eg fibre 976_{70}, Fig. 3), the weighting function became displaced at the highest levels, towards lower frequencies, with a reduction in the slope of the low-frequency cut-off.

Rarely, and only at certain stimulus levels, individual frequency components were unexpectedly missing from the FFTs.

4. DISCUSSION

Over a wide range of fibre CFs, the strongest periodicities in the temporal discharge patterns are at multiples of 5 ms. Only for fibres with CFs between about 1 and 2.5 kHz, do peaks corresponding to the stimulus intervals of 4.7 and 5.3 ms become substantial. They become comparable in size with the peaks corresponding to 10 ms only at CFs between about 1.5 and 2 kHz, as would be expected from the predominance of the odd harmonics in that region of the stimulus spectrum. If the dominant region for the pitch of this stimulus is about 3-4 times the frequency matching the pitch, and if the pitch is determined by the discharge periodicities of fibres with CFs in this region (o.3-0.4 kHz; 0.6-0.8 kHz respectively), then the findings are not inconsistent with the ambiguous pitch of 100 and 200 Hz, although the dominant region for the 200 Hz pitch must not extend much beyond three times its matched value. A choice of other stimulus intervals might be more conclusive.

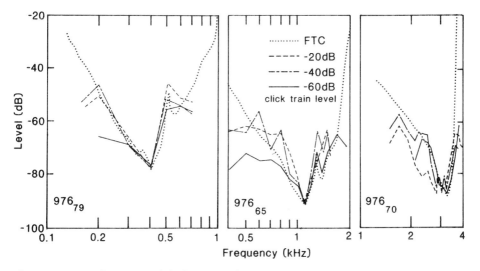

Fig. 3. *Comparison of weighting functions derived from the Fourier transforms of the autocorrelation histograms in response to the click train (see text), with the pure-tone FTCs, for 3 fibres with CFs of 0.37, 1.08 and 3.15 kHz respectively at 3 stimulus levels in each case.*
FTCs indicated by dotted lines; -60 dB level (about 10 dB above response threshold): continuous line; -40 dB level: dashed-dotted line; -20 dB level (about 50 dB above threshold): dashed line

Pitches corresponding to intervals of 4.7 and 5.3 ms are, however, heard if the stimulus is octave-band filtered at frequencies of 2 and 4 kHz, although at the latter frequency the pitch is weak (B.C.J. Moore, personal communication, 1981) Fibres with CFs in the 2 kHz region have a strong representation of these intervals in their discharge patterns. The present data are therefore not inconsistent with the pitches heard.

By the same token, the data are not in agreement with those reported by Whitfield (1979, 1980) in that substantial periodicities corresponding to intervals of 4.7 and 5.3 ms were encountered only over a restricted range of CFs, in the present data. Simulations with an electronic analogue of the cochlear nerve (Evans, 1980a) gave close correspondence to the histograms of Figs. 1 and 2 with linear filter Q factors (CF/-3 dB bandwidth) of the order of 10-20 for fibres with CFs above 0.6 kHz. In order to match Whitfield's illustrated data, however, (Figs. 3b and 1 of Whitfield, 1979 and 1980 respectively), Q factors of the order of 1-2 were required. This implies that the frequency selectivity of Whitfield's units were much less than those studied here. Two possible explanations are possible to account for this discrepancy. The first is that the cochleas from which Whitfield's data were obtained, were in a pathological condition as a result of the effects of anaesthesia and surgical preparation, not uncommon in the guinea pig (Evans, 1972). The second explanation arises from evidence that rodent cochlear nerve fibre tuning deteriorates more than that of the cat at high stimulus levels. With noise stimuli and reverse correlation techniques, the derived filter functions for cochlear nerve fibres in the cat are remarkably stable up to 40-60 dB above stimulus threshold (Evans, 1977; de Boer & de Jongh, 1978). In the rat (Møller, 1977) and guinea pig (Harrison & Evans, 1982), however, the frequency selectivity for broad-band stimuli appears to decrease monotonically with increasing noise level above threshold. Therefore, if Whitfield's stimulation was made at stimulus levels substantially above threshold, this could account for his findings.

The present results, obtained with impulsive stimuli, concerning the effects of stimulus level on the filtering properties of cat cochlear fibres, are in substantial agreement with previous data using broad-band noise stimuli (Evans, 1977), and continuous harmonic complexes (Evans, 1980b, 1981). In terms of the weighting of the phase-locked components of the fibre discharge patterns, the weighting functions correspond relatively closely to the pure-tone FTC. At threshold stimulus levels, the weighting function with harmonic complexes is sometimes slightly wider than the FTC (Evans, 1981, Figs. 4 and 5). At stimulus levels up to about 40-60 dB above threshold, however, the correspondence is close, particularly for fibres with CFs below about 1.5 kHz. For higher stimulus levels, the weighting function tends to shift towards lower frequencies for fibres with CFs above about 1 kHz (Fig. 3, fibre 976_{70}; Evans, 1977, Fig. 5; Evans, 1981, Fig. 4) together with a progressive decrease in the slope of the low frequency cut-off.

In experiments using paired click stimuli and recording in the rat cochlear nucleus, Møller (1970) concluded that the peripheral frequency-selective analyzer showed a bandwidth for impulse stimuli that was narrower than for pure tones. It has been argued elsewhere (Evans, 1975) that the assumption of a *comparable* bandwidth would have given a more satisfactory fit to the data. In any case, there may be difficulties associated with the theory underlying Møller's procedure (Pick & Narins, 1980). The present data, with the possible exception of fibre 976_{65} in Fig. 3 do not support the view that the frequency selectivity of the cochlea is sharper for impulsive than for continuous stimuli. Nor do they support the suggestion (Whitfield, 1982) that the cochlear frequency selectivity, as reflected in the temporal discharge patterns of cochlear fibres, is substantially *less* than that for continuous stimuli. While the effects of cochlear non-linearities do make themselves felt at stimulus levels above 40-60 dB above threshold, to a first approximation in the cat, the cochlear filtering behaves remarkably linearly to continuous wideband noise (Evans, 1977) and harmonic complexes (Evans, 1981), and to impulsive stimuli.

Acknowledgements. *This study was supported by grants from the Medical Research Council. I am grateful to Drs. J.P. Wilson, D.J. Parker and G.F. Pick for helpful comments on the manuscript, to Ms. M. Hodgson for typing and to Mssrs. R.C. Brunt and A.J. Heath for technical assistance.*

REFERENCES

de Boer, E. & de Jongh, H.R. (1978). On cochlear coding: potentialities and limitations of the reverse-correlation technique. *J. Acoust. Soc. Am.* 63, 115-135.

Evans, E.F. (1972). The frequency response and other properties of single fibres in the guinea pig cochlear nerve. *J. Physiol.* 226, 263-287.

Evans, E.F. (1975). Cochlear nerve and cochlear nucleus. In: *Handbook of Sensory Physiology.* Vol V/2. (W.D. Keidel and W.D. Neff, eds.). pp 1-108. Heidelberg, Berlin, New York, Springer-Verlag.

Evans, E.F. (1977). Frequency selectivity at high signal levels of single units in cochlear nerve and nucleus. In: *Psychophysics and Physiology of Hearing.* (E.F. Evans and J.P. Wilson, eds.). pp 185-192. London, Academic Press.

Evans, E.F. (1978). Place and time coding of frequency in the peripheral auditory system: some physiological pros and cons. *Audiol.* 17, 369-420.

Evans, E.E. (1979). Single unit studies of the mammalian auditory nerve. In: *Auditory Investigations: The Scientific and Technological Basis.* (H.A. Beagley, ed.). Chapter 15. pp 324-367. Oxford, Oxford University Press.

Evans, E.F. (1980a). An electronic analogue of single unit recording from the cochlear nerve for teaching and research. *J. Physiol.* 298, 6-7P.

Evans, E.F. (1980b). 'Phase-locking' of cochlear fibres and the problem of dynamic range. In: *International Symposium on Psychophysical, Physiological and Behavioural Studies in Hearing.* (G. v.d. Brink and F. Bilsen, eds.). pp 300-309. Delft, Delft University Press.

Evans, E.F. (1981). The dynamic range problem: Place and time coding at the level of cochlear nerve and nucleus. In: *Neuronal Mechanisms of Hearing* (J. Syka and L. Aitken, eds.). pp 69-85. New York, Plenum Press.

Harrison, R.V. & Evans, E.F. (1982). Reverse correlation study of cochlear filtering in normal and pathological guinea pig ears. *Hearing Research* 6, 303-314.

Møller, A.R. (1970). Studies of the damped oscillatory response of the auditory frequency analyzer. *Acta physiol. scand.* 78, 299-314.

Møller, A.R. (1977). Frequency selectivity of single auditory nerve fibres in response to broadband noise stimuli. *J. Acoust. Soc. Am.* 62, 135-142.

Moore, B.C.J. (1980). Neural interspike intervals and pitch. *Audiol.* 19, 363-365.

Pick, G.F. & Narins, P.M. (1980). Quantitative investigation of the 'paired-click' method: some limitations and insights. *Hearing Research* 3, 181-187.

Whitfield, I.C. (1979). Periodicity, pulse interval and pitch. *Audiol.* 18, 507-512.

Whitfield, I.C. (1980). Theory and experiment in so-called pulse-interval pitch. *Audiol.* 20, 86-88.

Whitfield, I.C. (1982). Series or parallel filtering in the cochlea? *J. Acoust. Soc. Am.* 70, 888-890.

GENERAL DISCUSSION:

This paper was followed by an extensive discussion between I.C. WHITFIELD (represented by P.E. STOPP), E.F. EVANS and B.C.J. MOORE. Because of its length the editors regret that they cannot include it in the proceedings.

TYLER:

One of the predictions of your model is that hearing-impaired listeners with poor frequency resolution would hear a different pitch than normal listeners would hear. I believe John Brandt published some work on periodicity pitch detection in hearing-impaired children, but I can't recall the nature of the results. Any comments?

EVANS:

I am very glad to hear that. I have argued for several years that it should be possible to provide a useful test of the rôle "straightforward" temporal coding might play in pitch perception by exploiting "naturally" occurring differences in auditory filter bandwidth, ideally in patients with unilateral cochlear hearing impairment. A different pitch could be looked for in an ambiguous residue pitch situation, or merely an abnormally enhanced pitch where harmonics fell in an area of impaired frequency resolution, i.e. abnormally wide spectral integration and therefore component interaction.

SUPPRESSION IN NEURAL RESPONSE OF THE AUDITORY SYSTEM TO CLICK PAIRS AND TO COSINE NOISE

J.H. ten Kate and G. Bloothooft

Biophysics Group, Applied Physics Department
Delft University of Technology
Delft, The Netherlands

I. INTRODUCTION

A number of observations (Thurlow 1957, Haye 1970, Eland 1974) was reported concerning an interesting asymmetry in the perceptibility of the socalled repetition pitch RP. (Bilsen & Ritsma 1970), when one pulse of a click pair is made less intense than the other. Thresholds for the perceptibility of RP differ in both cases notwithstanding similar power spectra of the two kind of click pairs, the one with the small pulse preceding and the other one with the small pulse following. The value of attenuation of the small pulse (in dB) with respect to the unvaried large pulse appears to be lower in obtaining the threshold sensation of RP on the first click pair than on the second one. Its value depends also on the delay between both pulses (Eland 1974). The assumed direct correspondence between the perception and the power spectrum of the stimulus does not seem valid for click pair perception in contrast to data with cosine noise. No asymmetry in RP is present on pseudonoise (MLS series) added with its attenuated repetition (cosine noise). Direct evidence of the representation of the described click pairs on the basilar membrane and in the nervous system is needed for a further understanding of this phenomenon. A number of studies in the following is presumably related to this asymmetry in RP. A non-linear pulse response of the basilar membrane in the 7 kHz area was measured with the Mössbauer technique in squirrel monkey (Robles and Rhode 1974, Rhode and Robles 1974). Goblick and Pfeiffer (1969) showed a temporal- and an amplitude non-linearity in the click pair response of eighth nerve of cat with a nulling method in socalled compound PST histograms. Kim et al (1973) modeled the BM motion with a system of non-linear differential equations, giving a number of auditive non-linear phenomena, including two-tone suppression above CF, the temporal-and amplitude non-linearity in response to click pairs. Eland (1974) described the neural data of the study by Goblick and Pfeiffer (1969) with a simulation model in which the pulse response $h(t)=G_1(t/T)^2 e^{-t/t_1} \sin 2\pi t/_T$, its amplitude dependence is determined by $t_1=(1+G_1/100)/(1+G_1/25)$ and the temporal non-linearity by suppressing the second pulse of the click pair by a factor $b=0.75+0.005 k$ in a time-interval ≤ 25 ms. $b=1$ for >25 ms. G_1=intensity of the click, t_1=time constant, $T=1/CF$. k=number of intervals $T/2$. Computed delay-histograms of the click pair stimulation with the small pulse preceding in comparison with those to click pairs with the small pulse following appear to be deeper modulated in this stimulation. Duifhuis(1973)presented data on nonsimultaneous masking of clicks, showing also asymmetry in backward and forward masking. The masking effect of the first pulse is lost after 25ms. Pluymert(1979)measured a decreasing influence of the first click on the N_1 amplitude of CAP to the second click in the interval 1-20ms. Møller (1970) measured delay-histograms to click pairs with equally intensive pulses in the CN of the rat. He computed a frequency selectivity for CN neurons to click pairs, which is about twice that derived from the tuning curve TC. This sharpening was ascribed to an effect of inhibition during broad-band stimulation. Ten Kate et al (1973, Bilsen et al 1975) determined (τ-diagrams) delay-histograms from the neural responses under influence of lateral inhibition in cat. A maximum value of the top-valley ratio was found between the third valley and the third top of the delay histograms for 60% of the neurons to <-5dB deep modulated cosine noise. No signs of a maximum in modulation of the delay-histogram were present in the remaining part of the CN neurons. Weighting functions of the neurons were computed from the delay-histograms with aid of spike-intensity relations to white noise. It was assumed, that both spike-intensity relations to cosine noise in the valley and to

cosine noise on the top are the same. Eighth nerve data however show a clear frequency dependence in the slopes of spike-intensity relations around CF (Evans 1974,
Sachs and Abbas 1974). Therefore experiments are needed to study spike-intensity
relations to cosine noise and to click pairs at different delays τ. Watanabe (1979)
succeeded in the separation of lateral inhibition of CN neurons and lateral suppression of eighth nerve cn by reversibly poisoning inhibitory synapses on the neurons during two-tone stimulation. The contribution of cn seems less effective than
the contribution of the inhibitory synapses to the two-tone suppression in his data.
Wilson et al (1974) have not found an influence of lateral suppression on the peak-
valley ratio as a function of the delay τ in cn response to 100% modulated cosine
noise. Ruggero (1973), Rhode et al (1978) and Schalk and Abbas (1980) measured clear
lateral suppression effects in the response to noise bands and in the pure tone response during the presence of noise bands. It is expected, that the cn with a valley
of the cosine noise spectrum on its CF is affected by its surrounding tops lying at
the suppression-areas of the nerve fibre. Three questions have been put in this
study: 1) Is there a difference between the neural responses to both kinds of click
pairs? 2) Are the frequency selectivities to these broadband stimuli equal to the
frequency selectivity of the neuron to pure tone? (ten Kate & Bloothooft 1978). 3)
Do the neural responses in the delay histograms to click pairs and to cosine noise
show nonlinearities and if present, in what way are they linked to well-known auditive nonlinearities?

2. METHODS

The animal preparation (cat), the response recording, the acoustical system,
the data collection and processing have been previously reported (Bilsen et al.
1975). The absence of adaptation effects on the recording are checked by requiring,
that the spike-intensity relations during pure tone, cosine noise, pulse and click
pair stimulation are symmetrical for increasing and decreasing intensity levels
over an equal range. The normal course of the spike-intensity relation is a monotonic function with a linear part in a kind of a S-shape between the threshold at the
spontaneous activity and the saturation. The output power of the auditive filter on
basis of the linear part of the spike-intensity relation is described by:

$$R_o^2(\omega) = R_{o,r}^2(\omega) \; 10^{(s-s_{rp})/10c} \tag{1}$$

s_{rp}=spontaneous rate, c=slope of the linear part of the spike-intensity relation.
s=spike rate, r=reference point, ω=frequency. The output power of the auditive filter for cosine noise and for click pair stimulation with one component attenuated
by a factor g is:

with the same polarity $\quad R_+^2(\tau) = \int_{-\infty}^{\infty} W(\omega) \; (1 + g^2 + 2g \cos(\omega\tau)) \; d\omega \tag{2}$

with opposed polarity $\quad R_-^2(\tau) = \int_{-\infty}^{\infty} W(\omega) \; (1 + g^2 - 2g \cos(\omega\tau)) \; d\omega \tag{3}$

$W(\omega)$=an even weighting function representing the auditive filter, τ=delay line.
Møller (1970) derived the autocorrelation function $A_c(\tau)$ of the pulse response of
the auditive filter:

$$A_c(\tau) = \frac{R_+^2(\tau)-R_-^2(\tau)}{R_+^2(\tau)+R_-^2(\tau)} = \frac{2g}{(1+g^2)} \frac{\int_{-\infty}^{\infty} W(\omega)\cos\omega\tau \; d\omega}{\int_{-\infty}^{\infty} W(\omega) \; d\omega} \tag{4}$$

$W(\omega)$ can be computed on basis of (2), (3) or (4). The denominator of (4) is constant for a linear system. It is also possible to prove the existence of a nonlinearity and to study its dependence of τ with aid of the next formula:

$$R_+^2(0). \; A_c(\tau) = f(\tau).4g \int_{-\infty}^{\infty} W(\omega) \; \cos\omega\tau \; d\omega \tag{5}$$

$$\text{with } f(\tau) = R_+^2(0)/\{R_+^2(\tau)+R_-^2(\tau)\} \tag{6}$$

RESULTS AND DISCUSSION

Delay histograms to cosine noise (left part of the upper panel of Fig. 1) and
to click pairs were recorded from 24 neurons out of a class of 71 sustained, primary-like neurons in the AVCN of cat. The remaining part was lost during the period

of extensive recording. The spontaneous firing rate of all neurons except one was below 10 spikes/sec. The computed value of the slope c of the spike-intensity relation showed the well-known frequency-dependence during tone-burst stimulation. The slope c of the spike-intensity relation during cosine noise burst and during click pair stimulation varied with delay time τ having the smallest value in the valley of the delay histogram. An example for cosine noise is given in the right part of the upper panel. c=5.4 spikes/dB s in the valley instead of 7.9 spikes/dB s at τ=0. The values of the output power $R_+^2(\tau)_1$ computed with the variable $c(\tau)$ appeared to be more symmetrically oscillating around a mean than the values of $R_+^2(\tau)_2$ calculated with c=7.9 sp./dB s.

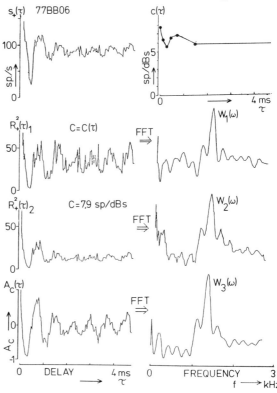

Fig. 1. Neuron 77 BB06. CF=1.3 kHz. The delay-histogram $\{S_+(\tau)\}$, the computed output power of the auditive filter $R_+^2(\tau)_2$ and the autocorrelation function $A_c(\tau)$ against the delay τ are successively presented from the top to bottom in the left part of the figure. Note that the tops and valleys of $R_+^2(\tau)_1$ and of $A_c(\tau)$ are lying more symmetrical around a mean value than those of $R_+^2(\tau)_2$. The slopes $c(\tau)$ of the spike-intensity relations to cosine noise are presented versus τ in right part of the upper panel. Three computed weighting functions $W_1(\omega)$, $W_2(\omega)$, $W_3(\omega)$ are compared in the right part of the figure. No significant difference between them is observed

$A_c(\tau)$ waxes and wanes also symmetrically around a mean value having less stochastic variation because of the addition of $R^2(\tau)$. The computed weighting functions, obtained by FFT from $R_+^2(\tau)_1$, $R_+^2(\tau)_2$ and $A_c(\tau)$, do not show significant differences. Similar results were collected from delay histograms to click pairs. The value of $f(\tau)$ appeared to be constant for all computed $A_c(\tau)$ from the delay histograms to click pairs. But the value of $f(\tau)$ is increasing in the range $0<\tau<5$ms with the increase of τ for all computed $A_c(\tau)$ to cosine noise. Since the firing rate of neurons to cosine noise bursts (5.4-7.9 sp/dBs in Fig. 1) is much higher than response of about 1 spike per pulse pair sp/pp with repetition frequency of 25 Hz (Fig. 2) and interval histograms had shown an evident contribution of small intervals <5ms during cosine noise bursts, this increase of $f(\tau)$ is ascribed to the refractory period.-Two examples of asymmetrical delay histograms to click pair stimulation with one pulse 6dB attenuated are presented in Fig. 2. More tops and valleys to positive delay τ are discernible than those to negative delays τ for neuron 77 PB 04 at 29-38 dB SPL eq. This asymmetry with a better modulation in the delay histogram to the click pair with the attenuated pulse preceding is present for the majority of the neurons (20). Some of the neurons (4) did not show an asymmetry or had a weak asymmetry to click pair stimulation with the attenuated pulse following (77 FD 04 in Fig. 2). Though the number of peaks and valleys is diminishing with increasing intensity levels, the asymmetry is more obvious with a larger intensity level. No asymmetry was found in delay histograms to click pairs with equal intensive pulses. But the number of peaks and valleys was smaller than in delay histograms to click pairs with the attenuated pulse preceding (see Fig.3). - This is demonstrated with the autocorrelation functions in top panel of Fig. 3

for neuron 77 PB04 with G=0dB and
G=6dB at 29 dB SPL. The computed
weighting functions (middle panel
of Fig. 3) appear to be different
in width. Also a small shift of
the best frequency occurs for the
weighting function from the click
pair with the attenuated pulse
following. Isorate TC's calculated from these weighting functions
are compared to the determined TC

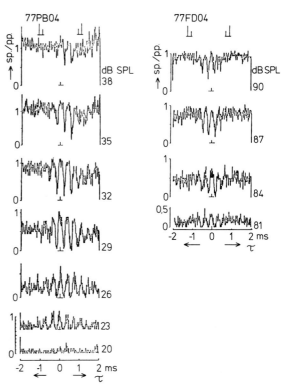

*Fig. 2. Delay-histograms for two
neurons to click pairs with one
pulse attenuated with a factor
G=6dB are presented at different
intensity levels (expressed in
dB SPL equivalent). Neuron 77
PB04 (CF=2.2 kHz, pulse width=
200 μs) appears to have asymmetrical delay histograms with
increasing level (left part of
the fig.). More peaks and valleys are discernible to the click
pair with the attenuated pulse
preceding (right part of the
curve) than to the click pair
with the attenuated pulse following (left part of the curve).
Neuron 77 FD04 (CF=2.5 kHz) appears to possess a weak asymmetry opposite to the neuron
77 PB04*

*Fig. 3. Top panel: Two autocorre-
lation functions against the delay
time τ of neuron 77 PB04 resp. to
click pairs with equally intensive
pulses (left curve, G=0) and to
click pairs with one pulse attenuated by 6dB (the stimulus configuration is indicated with vertical lines above the curves).
Middle panel: The three computed
weighting functions (fast Fourier
transformation FFT from the above
autocorrelation function) are resp.
to click pairs with equally intensive pulses (left), to click pairs
with the attenuated pulse following (centre) and to click pairs
with the attenuated pulse preceding (right). Lower panel: Isorate
TC's computed from the three kind
of click pair responses to the
click pairs compared with the pure
tone TC*

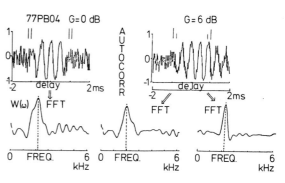

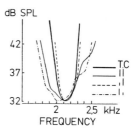

tone in the bottom panel of Fig.3.
Apparently the isorate TC to the
click pair stimulation with the
attenuated pulse preceding is about

Fig. 4. Compound PST histograms of neuron 77 PB04 (CF=^{1}/T=2.2 kHz, level of the pulse =28 dB SPL equivalent, repetition frequency of pulses and of click pairs = 64 Hz, 6dB attenuated pulse) to pulse- and click pair stimulation. The stimulus configuration is indicated by vertical lines under the curves. The firing probability P (the same to condensation- and rarefaction stimuli) is presented at the curves. The pulse responses alone (a and b) are given in the top panel. The click pair responses presented in the second, third and bottom panel are resp. to T/2, 3T/2, 5T/2. Note in the third panel the nulling of the response to click pairs with the attenuated pulse preceding. Vertical axis in spikes/ stimulus (=pulse or click pair).

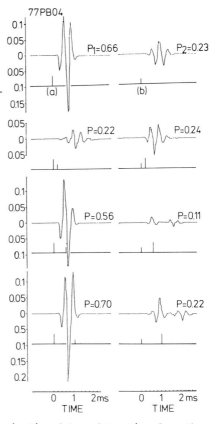

equally wide as the TC to pure tone. The two other isorate TC's are significantly broader than the pure tone TC. No sharpening of iso- rate TC's derived from click pair response with respect to the pure tone TC was found for all neurons in contrast to Møller (1970). - Compound histograms were measured for the same neuron 77 PB04 (Fig. 4) at delays of T/2, 3T/2, 5T/2 (T=^{1}/cF) at the level of 28 dB SPL eq. to two kinds of click pair stimulation with one pulse attenuated. The firing proba- bility P is presented at the corresponding curve and is equally large to condensation or to rarefaction stimulation. The response to the click pairs at T/2, 3T/2, 5T/2 should be reduced because of the opposite phase of the pulse responses (a and b in Fig. 4). It ap- peared impossible to obtain the click responses in Fig. 4 by subtraction from the pulse responses in a and b. The amplitude of the click pair response (T/2 for ex- ample) appeared to be suppressed indicating the same amplitude non-linearity as for eighth nerve data (Goblick and Pfeiffer 1969). A nulling of the peaks in the PST- histogram also occurred in case of 3T/2 for the click pair with the attenuated pulse preceding. Note that the firing probability P for 5T/2 to the click pairs with the attenuated pulse following is of the same order of magnitude like the one of the pulse response (a). No visible contribution of the attenuated pulse is ob- served anymore. The other kind of click pair at τ=5T/2 showed evident influence of the preceding, attenuated pulse on the second pulse. The shown amplitude-non- linearity in the compound PST histograms appeared to correspond to the asymmetry in delay-histograms (Fig. 2, 3) to click pairs with one pulse attenuated. This fact is predicted by Eland (1974) from data of Goblick and Pfeiffer (1969).

Though the number of neural responses in the sample is small, we felt confi- dent to draw the next conclusions: 1) The slopes of the spike-intensity for click pair and cosine noise burst stimulation are dependent on the delay time τ. 2) The delay-histograms of the majority of the AVCN neurons to click pair stimulation with one pulse attenuated appear to be asymmetric above a certain intensity level. The asymmetry in RP and in delay-histograms both may be related. 3) The nonlinearity shown for the autocorrelation A_c from the delay-histograms to cosine noise by the factor f(τ) is dependent on the refractory period of the neuron. 4)Computed isorate TC's to click pair stimulation of AVCN neurons appear to be equal or larger than pure tone TC in contrast to data[') of Møller (1970). 5) The amplitude-nonlinearity in compound histograms to clicks (Goblick & Pfeiffer 1969) and the asymmetrical delay-histograms to click pairs with one attenuated pulse are epiphenomena.

')*Recalculation from his data gives about equally wide TC's to click pair & tone.*

Acknowledgement. Mrs J.M.W. van Middelkoop-Hoek, Mrs S. Senduk-Tan, Mr. E.E.E. Frietman are thanked for their technical assistance and Mrs M. Mulder-van Nouhuys for typing the manuscript.

REFERENCES

Bilsen, F.A., Ritsma, R.J. (1970). Some Parameters Influencing the Perceptibility of Pitch. *J.Acoust.Soc.Am.* 47, 2, 469-475.

Bilsen, F.A., Kate, J.H. ten, Buunen, T.J.F., Raatgever, J. (1975). Responses of single units in the cochlear nucleus of the cat to cosine noise. *J.Acoust.Soc.Am.* 58, 4, 858-866.

Duifhuis, H. (1973). Consequences of peripheral frequency selectivity for non-simultaneous masking. *J.Acoust.Soc.Am.* 54, 1471-1488.

Eland, A.P. (1974). A model describing the neural response to click pairs. *Intern Report. Delft University of Technology*.

Evans, E.F. (1974). Auditory frequency selectivity and the cochlear nerve. *In Facts and models in hearing*, 118-129, Zwicker E. and Terhardt, E. (eds). Springer-Berlin.

Goblick, T.J. and Pfeiffer, R.R. (1969). Time domain measurements of cochlear non linearities using combination click stimuli. *J.Acoust.Soc.Am.* 46, 924-938.

Haye, A.C. (1970). Perception of repetitive pulse pairs. *Intern Report. Delft University of Technology*.

Kate, J.H. ten, Bilsen, F.A. and Raatgever, J. (1973). Spectral properties of single unit responses in the cochlear nucleus to noise and its repetition. *Delft Progr. Rep.* A1, 17-24.

Kate, J.H. ten, Bloothooft, G. (1978). Neural response to pairs of differently intensive clicks in the antero-ventral cochlear nucleus of the cat. *19th Dutch Federative Meeting, Rotterdam*.

Kim, D.O., Molnar, C.E., Pfeiffer, R.R., (1973). A system of non linear differential equations modeling basilar membrane motion. *J.Acoust.Soc.Am.* 54, 6, 1517-1529.

Møller, A.R. (1970). Studies of the damped oscillatory response of the auditory frequency analyzer. *Acta Physiol. Scand.* 78, 299-314.

Pluymert, N. (1979). C.A.P. of cat and human to pulse and click pair stimulation. *Intern Report. Delft University of Technology*.

Rhode, W.S., Robles, L. (1974). Evidence from Mössbauer experiment for non linear vibration in the cochlea. *J.Acoust.Soc.Am.* 55, 3, 588-596.

Rhode, W.S., Gleisler, C.D., Kennedy, D.F. (1978). Auditory Nerve Fiber Response to Wide-Band Noise and Tone Combinations. *J.Neurophysiol* 41, 3, 692-704.

Robles, L., Rhode, W.S., (1974). Non linear effects in the transient response of the basilar membrane. *In Facts and Models in Hearing*, p 287-298. Zwicker E. and Terhardt E. eds. Springer-Berlin.

Ruggero, M.A., (1973). Responses to Noise of Auditory Nerve Fibers in the Squirrel Monkey. *J.Neurophysiol.* 36, 569-587.

Sachs, M.B., Abbas, P.J. (1974). Rate versus level functions for auditory nerve fibers in cats: tone burst stimuli. *J.Acoust.Soc.Am.* 56, 1835-1847.

Schalk, F.B., Sachs, M.B. (1980). Non linearities in auditory-nerve fiber responses to band-limited noise. *J.Acoust.Soc.Am.* 67, 3, 903-913.

Thurlow, W.R. (1957). Further Observation on Pitch Associated with a Time Difference between Two Pulse Trains. *J.Acoust.Soc.Am.* 29, 12, 1310-1311.

Watanabe, T. (1979). Funneling Mechanism in Hearing. *Hearing Res.* 1, 111-119.

Wilson, J.P., Evans, E.F., Rosenberg, J. (1974). Linearity of the cochlear nerve fibre filter response: test for the influences of two-tone suppression. *8th Int. Congr. Acoust. London* p. 80.

GENERAL DISCUSSION

MØLLER:[*]

You stated in your paper that the tuning properties of AVCN units as determined using pure tones (iso-rate contours) were different from those determined
using the response to paired clicks. You mentioned that this is in contrast to my
earlier results (Møller, Acta Physiol. Scand. 78: 299, 1970) which showed a sharper tuning in response to paired clicks compared to iso-rate contours obtained
from stimulation with pure tones. You also point out that recalculating tuning
curves using my data shows tuning to be about equally wide in response to click
pairs and tones. I believe the difference between your results and mine are mainly
due to the different ways we have calculated the frequency transfer function from
the autocorrelation functions that were derived from the responses to paired
clicks.

My conclusion, that the tuning in cochlear nucleus cells is sharper in response to paired clicks than it is in response to pure tones, was based on the observation that the autocorrelation function obtained from the response to paired
clicks had a slower rate of decay than the autocorrelation function computed from
the iso-rate function obtained in response to pure tones. This strongly indicates
that paired click stimulation yields a narrower bandwidth than does pure tone stimulation. The duration of the autocorrelation function that was available is only
about 1 msec. Since the autocorrelation function still has a substantial amplitude
at a delay of 1 msec, the power spectrum determined from the autocorrelation using
a 1-msec window becomes a poor estimate of the transfer function because of a too
narrow data window. The estimated bandwidth becomes too large. In my 1970 paper I
therefore used a different method for estimating the bandwidth. I estimated the
tuning in response to click pairs - not by Fourier transforming the derived autocorrelation function - but by comparing the autocorrelation function computed from
a tuning curve of the same shape as the iso-rate function, and by varying the
width of these "iso-rate functions" until the autocorrelation functions computed
from these "iso-rate functions" had the same rate of decay as the autocorrelation
function obtained from the paired click experiments (see p. 305, Møller, 1970).

Thus, the difference between your calculation of frequency transfer functions
and my calculation seems to lie in the fact that you have used a narrow time window and, because of this, obtained a too broad frequency transfer function.

I am aware that nonlinearities affect the results. This is indicated by the
fact that $R_+^2(t) + R_-^2(t)$ is not constant. However, as was shown by Pick and Narins
(Hear. Res. 3: 180, 1980), the resulting transfer functions are affected by nonlinearities but it takes a relatively strong nonlinearity to produce a significant
error when only the bandwidth is studied.

The main point I showed in my 1970 paper, namely, that the selectivity of the
periphery of the auditory system is available instantaneously and thus cannot rely
on a neural (second filter) interaction, is valid. That the frequency selectivity
obtained using the paired click method, which was presumed to reflect the oscillation of the basilar membrane, was even greater than that of cochlear nucleus units
was only pointed out to indicate that there is neural convergence toward these
neurons. My main point was that the frequency selectivity in response to clicks is
at least as good as it is to tones, which I took to be a strong indication that
frequency sharpening does not occur by neural interaction. Although this has since
been confirmed many times, at the time the work on paired clicks was published
(1970) it was not at all clear that the high selectivity seen in single nerve fibers was a result of basilar membrane tuning alone.

---

[*]Submitted in written form by Prof. A.R. Møller, Pittsburgh, USA

TEN KATE:
It seems to me arbitrary to approach the autocorrelation function (your fig.3 B)
obtained from broad band stimulation with aid of a modified tuning curve (TC, dotted curve) to that from a pure tone having half of
its original bandwidth (solid line in present fig.
modified from Møller's Fig. 3D). Physical methods
are available in order to extrapolate partly measured auto-correlation functions in a correct way.
These methods were developed for the extrapolation
of the correlation function beyond the maximum lag
in order to improve the spectral resolution in
the classical measurements of power spectra.
(Burg, 37th Annu. Meeting Soc. of Exploration
Geophysicists Oklahoma, Oklahoma City, 1967.
van den Bos, IEEE Trans. Inform. Theory, 15,
493, 1971). In a first approximation we have
extrapolated the auto-correlation function by one period. Results from it by FFT
are indicated by triangles in the figure. The dots are values obtained from your
original auto-correlation function without extrapolation. Additional results are:
1) The bandwidth is somewhat smaller than the solid line, the original TC.
2) The best frequency appeared to be 5.6 kHz instead of 5.4 kHz (dotted modified
TC). 3) The dynamic range is only about 20 dB (because of noise in the data). The
isorate tuning curve (triangles) is only about 5% smaller than that obtained without extrapolation (black dots). Inverse Fourier transform delivers a nearly exact
replica of the original auto-correlation (your Fig. 3B) with one period added.

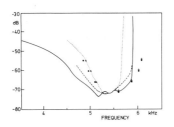

PICK:
It does not surprise me that you find deviations between FTC's and filter functions
derived from click-pair data. Narins and I (Hear. Res. 3, 181, 1980) reported some
limitations of Møller's transformation of click-pair data. We demonstrated analytically, and by simulation, using what we felt were realistic data for auditory-
nerve-fibre responses, that severe errors could contaminate the derived auditory
filter.

TEN KATE:
It was expected by us that a calculated W (f) should only represent the auditive
filter in a qualitative sense because of the presence of nonlinearities (Goblick
and Pfeiffer, 1969). The main result of the present paper is the difference between delay histograms for click pairs with either the first or the second pulse attenuated. It should be recommended by us to study the underlying theory for the
calculation of W (f) from the paired click method (Pick and Narins, 1980) with a
model containing nonlinearities (in the sense of Goblick and Pfeiffer, 1969) for
less deeply modulated spectra than only click pairs with equally intensive pulses.
Our hypothesis (Bilsen et al., 1975) should be checked that "the activity of a
particular unit is the result of signal power in a restricted response area around
the unit CF". A possible conclusion that can be drawn from the presented data is
that the nonlinearity and/or the filter preceding the nonlinearity is dependent
on the type of the stimulus used.

AUDITORY-NERVE FIBRE CORRELATES OF THE CRITICAL BANDWIDTH
AS DETERMINED BY LOUDNESS ESTIMATION

J.O. Pickles

Department of Physiology, University of Birmingham,
Birmingham B15 2TJ, U.K.

1. SUMMARY

The firing of guinea pig auditory nerve fibres was measured in response to
bands of noise of variable bandwidth, centre frequency, and intensity. The total
firing rate in the auditory nerve fibre array was calculated as a function of
stimulus bandwidth. As the bandwidth increased, the total firing rate increased
steadily for stimuli of constant total intensity. There was no sign of a constant
portion followed by a break-point, as appears in psychophysical estimates of
loudness with similar stimuli (Zwicker et al., 1957). The results cast doubt on
the theory (i) that loudness is a direct correlate of the total firing in the
auditory nerve, and (ii) that the critical bandwidth is revealed in the activity
of auditory nerve fibres. Changes in the form of the firing rate function with
cochlear pathology are described.

2. INTRODUCTION

It has often been suggested that the sensation of loudness is a direct function of the total amount of activity in the auditory nerve (e.g. Wever, 1949;
Bekesy, 1960; Scharf, 1978). If this is the case, the total number of action
potentials should vary in ways similar to loudness estimates when the stimulus
parameters are varied. Zwicker et al. (1957) showed that when the stimulus bandwidth was varied, but the total power was kept constant, the psychophysical estimate of loudness was constant for stimulus bandwidths less than the critical
bandwidth, and increased for wider stimulus bandwidths. On the above suggestion
the total number of action potentials in the auditory nerve should vary in a
similar way. They should therefore provide an estimate of the critical bandwidth,
and this would agree with suggestions that the critical bandwidth is set in the
cochlea (e.g. Fletcher, 1940).
    In the experiments described here, the hypothesis was tested. The firing of
single fibres of the guinea pig auditory nerve was measured in response to noise
bands of different widths. In estimating the firing in the whole auditory nerve
fibre array, the rates were not however integrated over many different fibres.
Rather, the stimuli were presented in many different frequency relations to the
CF of one fibre. The rates were then integrated over all frequencies of presentation, to give the mean rate in an array of fibres uniform in properties with
the fibre being measured.

3. METHODS

Guinea pigs (300-550g) were anaesthetised with urethane (1.5 g/kg IP), and
auditory nerve fibres recorded by the approach of Gilbert and Pickles (1980),
using a Bruel and Kjaer 4134 microphone as a sound source, driven via a compensation network (Evans, 1979). Bands of noise (noise floor 60 dB below level in
passband, other characteristics as described by Pickles, 1975) were produced in
a balanced modulator, and sinusoids were produced by two Farnell DSG1 frequency
synthesisers.
    The experiment was completely automated. When a fibre was isolated (crite-
ria as described by Evans, 1979), the FTC was determined in detail by a rapid
automated method, and then noise bands of eight widths (50, 100, 200, 500, 1000,

2000, 5000, 10000 Hz) were presented at three intensities, and at 11 centre frequencies in relation to the CF (0.2, 0.4, 0.6, 0.8, 0.9, 1.0, 1.1, 1.2, 1.4, 1.6,
2.0 x CF), making 264 possible stimuli in all. If a noise band overlapped 0 Hz
at any centre frequency, it was not presented. The stimuli were presented in
balanced pseudorandom order (300 ms on, 300 ms off). Firing rates to each stimulus were accumulated and the whole stimulus set was for most fibres repeated
six times. Later, for each bandwidth and stimulus intensity, the firing rate was
integrated over all frequencies of stimulus presentation, weighted by the frequency interval between adjacent stimuli.

     In addition, rate-intensity functions were determined at the CF.

4. RESULTS

     Fig. 1c shows the tuning curve of a high-spontaneous firing, low-threshold,
fibre. Since the spontaneous firing rate was high, the rapid FTC routine used a
high rate criterion (increment of 60 spikes/sec). The threshold for an increment

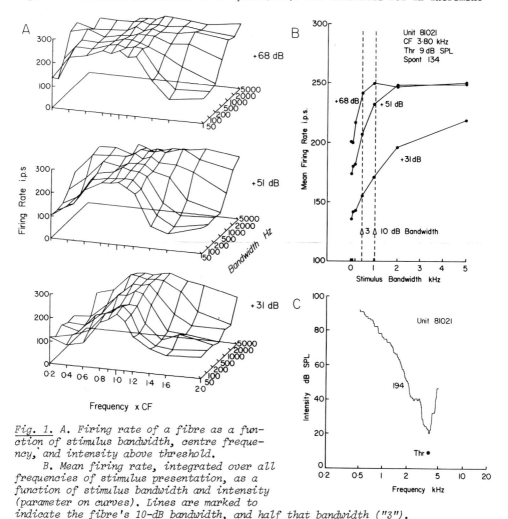

*Fig. 1. A. Firing rate of a fibre as a fun-
ction of stimulus bandwidth, centre frequency, and intensity above threshold.
     B. Mean firing rate, integrated over all
frequencies of stimulus presentation, as a
function of stimulus bandwidth and intensity
(parameter on curves). Lines are marked to
indicate the fibre's 10-dB bandwidth, and half that bandwidth ("3").
     C. FTC determined at a firing rate criterion of 194 ips, and the threshold
("Thr") determined at an increment of 20 ips above spontaneous*

of 20 spikes/sec, as determined from the rate-intensity function, was 9 dB SPL.
Fig. 1a shows the firing to each of the noise bands, as a function of the centre
frequency of the band, its width, and the intensity with respect to the fibre's
threshold. Whereas narrowband stimuli at low intensity produced a large increment in firing only when near the CF, narrowband stimuli at higher intensities,
and wideband stimuli at all intensities, produced a large increment in firing
over a wide range of frequencies. Fig. 1b shows the net firing rate as a function of stimulus bandwidth, for each of the three intensities. The rate here was
integrated over all frequencies of presentation, to give the mean firing rate in
a conceptual fibre array, where each fibre is similar to the one being measured.

In agreement with the psychophysical data of Zwicker et al. (1957), the integrated firing rate of Fig. 1b was higher for wider stimulus bandwidths, total
stimulus power being constant. However, unlike the psychophysical data, the integrated firing rate did not show an invariant region followed by a break point,
but increased steadily as the stimulus bandwidth increased. Also unlike the psychophysical data, the slope of the relation increased with intensity, until the
maximum rate was reached.

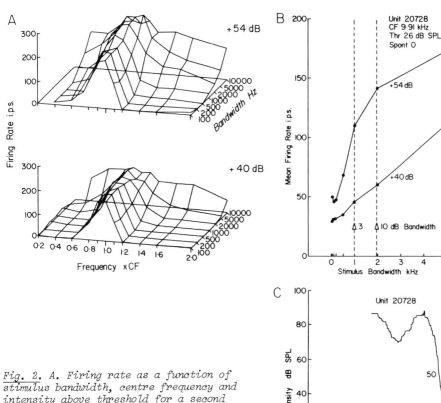

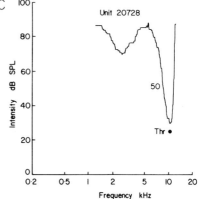

*Fig. 2. A. Firing rate as a function of
stimulus bandwidth, centre frequency and
intensity above threshold for a second
fibre.*

*B. Integrated firing rate as a fun-
ction of stimulus bandwidth and intensity
(parameter on curves). Dotted lines at
the fibre's 10-dB bandwidth, and at half
that bandwidth ("3").*

*C. FTC determined at 50 ips criterion,
and threshold at 20 ips criterion*

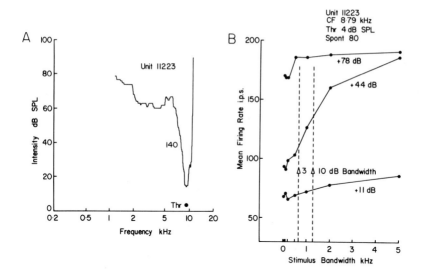

Fig. 3. A. FTC at 140 ips criterion, and threshold at increment of 20 ips.
B. Integrated firing rate function (see text and Fig. 1 caption).

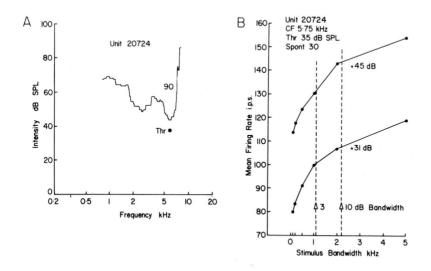

Fig. 4. A. Pathologically wide FTC (90 ips rate criterion).
B. Integrated firing rate function (see text and Fig. 1 caption).

Fig. 2b shows similar results for a fibre of slightly higher threshold and low spontaneous firing rate. Although a small invariant region followed by a breakpoint was seen at one intensity, it was within experimental error and the bandwidth at which it occurred (about 200 Hz) was only about 10% of the fibre's 10-dB bandwidth. Fig. 3b shows similar results for a further low threshold fibre. Results like these were without exception seen in all fibres displaying FTCs of normal shape.

Fig. 4 shows results from a fibre with a pathologically wide FTC, recorded in an animal with depressed respiration and raised round-window N_1 thresholds. As in normal fibres, the integrated firing rate increased steadily with stimulus bandwidth, without showing a breakpoint. However, in contrast to normal fibres, the initial slope of the function did not increase with increasing stimulus intensity.

5. DISCUSSION

The results show that the total firing rate in an array of uniform nerve fibres is greater for wide than narrow band stimuli, even if the total stimulus power is kept constant. The reason may be understood from the shape of the rate-intensity function. Over all except the lowest part of the intensity range, neural rate-intensity functions are negatively-accelerated functions of stimulus intensity, if intensity is plotted on linear rather than logarithmic or dB scales. Functions of such shape have the property that the greatest mean output is obtained if the input energy is spread as evenly as possible over all input channels, rather than concentrated in only a few (see e.g. Pickles, 1982, p. 277). As the intensity is raised, and the rate-intensity function becomes flatter, this phenomenon is accentuated, until we reach a maximum limited by fibres being driven nearly to saturation for all frequencies of stimulation (e.g. Fig. 1b, +51 and +68 dB, 1-5 kHz bands).

What is unexpected is that the functions do not show any breakpoint, corresponding to the critical bandwidth, similar to that seen in psychophysical estimates of loudness when the stimulus bandwidth is varied (Zwicker et al., 1957). This casts doubt on the generally-accepted direct relation between loudness and the total amount of activity in the auditory nerve. It also casts doubt on the idea that the critical bandwidth in this task is set in the cochlea, an idea that has been challenged for a variety of other tasks (e.g. Pickles, 1976, 1979, 1980; Pickles and Comis, 1976).

The lack of any gross difference in the functions for normal and pathological fibres suggests that this task is not suitable for assessing changes in neural integration bandwidth with cochlear pathology, as has already been found (Bonding, 1979). The small difference in the behaviour of the slope of the integrated firing function in pathological fibres may be ascribed to the early widening of the FTC in those fibres.

Acknowledgements: this work was supported by the Medical Research Council (UK).

REFERENCES

Bekesy, G. von. (1960). Experiments in Hearing. New York, Wiley.
Bonding, P. (1979). Critical bandwidth in loudness summation in sensorineural hearing loss. *Brit. J. Audiol.* 13, 23-30.
Evans, E.F. (1979). Single unit studies of mammalian cochlear nerve. In: *Auditory Investigation: The Scientific and Technological Basis.* (H.A. Beagley, ed.). pp 324-367. Oxford, Clarendon Press.
Fletcher, H. (1940). Auditory patterns. *Revs Modern Phys.* 12, 47-65.
Gilbert, A.G. and Pickles, J.O. (1980). A stereotaxic approach to the auditory nerve of the guinea pig. *J. Physiol.* 301, 3-4P.
Pickles, J.O. (1975). Normal critical bands in the cat. *Acta Otolar.* 80, 245-254.
Pickles, J.O. (1976). Role of centrifugal pathways to cochlear nucleus in determination of critical bandwidth. *J. Neurophysiol.* 39, 394-400.

Pickles, J.O. (1979). Psychophysical frequency resolution in the cat as deter-
    mined by simultaneous masking and its relation to auditory-nerve resolution.
    J. Acoust. Soc. Amer. 66, 1725-1732.
Pickles, J.O. (1980). Psychophysical frequency resolution in the cat studied with
    forward masking. In: *Psychophysical, Physiological and Behavioural Studies
    in Hearing.* (G. van den Brink and F.A. Bilsen, eds). pp 118-126. Delft, Delft
    University Press.
Pickles, J.O. (1982). *An Introduction to the Physiology of Hearing.* London, Acad-
    emic Press.
Pickles, J.O. and Comis, S.D. (1976). Auditory-nerve fiber bandwidths and critical
    bandwidths in the cat. *J. Acoust. Soc. Amer.* 60, 1151-1156.
Scharf, B. (1978). Loudness. In: *Handbook of Perception*, Vol. 4. (E.C. Carterette
    and M.P. Friedman, eds). pp 187-242. New York, Academic Press.
Wever, E.G. (1949). *Theory of Hearing.* New York, Wiley.
Zwicker, E., Flottorp, G. and Stevens, S.S. (1957). Critical band width in loud-
    ness summation. *J. Acoust. Soc. Amer.* 29, 548-557.

GENERAL DISCUSSION

SCHARF:
1. As stimulus bandwidth increased, overall intensity was kept constant. Consequently, spectrum level went down. Should not firing rate to a noise centered
on the characteristic frequency decrease with increasing bandwidth, especially
at the widest bandwidths?
2. Do you have any feeling about the coding for loudness other than by total
number of spikes per time unit? For example, your analysis, based on a single
fibre, would miss changes in patterns of synchrony over a large group of fibers.

PICKLES:
1. As the stimulus bandwidth is increased, the spectral density decreases. However, the effect on neural firing rate to stimuli at the CF is less than might
otherwise be thought. (i) The driving stimulus to the fibre changes only when
the stimulus bandwidth is spread beyond the neural integration bandwidth. So,
for example, if the fibre has an integration bandwidth of 1 kHz, increasing
the stimulus bandwidth to 5 kHz will reduce the driving stimulus by only 7 dB,
compared with the narrowest bandwidth. (ii) In most cases the stimulus intensities
were such that the narrowband stimulus at CF saturated the fibre. The rate therefore did not vary with small changes in intensity. (iii) Very narrowband stimuli
(e. g. 50-100 Hz wide) produce lower mean firing rates than wider stimuli of
equal total power, within the neural integration bandwidth. This is presumably a
result of the amplitude fluctuations in the narrowband stimulus. Under conditions
where these three effects are not important, the expected decline in firing rate
with stimulus bandwidth is indeed seen.
2. My interest in these experiments was to test the classical hypothesis that the
correlate of loudness was the mean net firing rate. Now that seems not to be true
in detail, it is worth looking at other hypotheses. I did not measure the synchrony of the firing. However, at first sight it is difficult to see how changes
in patterns of synchrony should produce a breakpoint corresponding to the critical bandwidth. But you never know till you look !

MERZENICH:
In studies conducted in a cochlear implant patient, we have recently found that
with intracochlear electrical stimulation with bipolar electrodes we can generate
loudnesses over the full dynamic range, with the excited nerve fibre population
not extending over more than about 2 - 3 mm. Moreover, parallel animal studies
have revealed that at supra-threshold stimulus levels at which intolerably loud
sounds are evoked in man, unit discharge rates in cats do not usually exceed
250 discharges/second (i.e., the normal saturation rates). Further, loudness is
strongly affected by changing stimulus waveform in a manner that alters the local
temporal dispersion of auditory nerve fiber discharges without substantially al-

tering (we believe) the overall quantity of evoked input or the length of the
auditory nerve array sector excited. Such studies strongly indicate that:
1. Consistent with the conclusions of Dr. Pickles' studies, overall activity does
not likely signal loudness; 2. local temporal features of response patterns play
a role in loudness representation and 3. in at least the electrical stimulation
case (in which synchronization of inputs can be artificially exaggerated) the full
dynamic range of loudness can be signalled by a highly restricted population of
eighth nerve fibres.

PICKLES:
These results are even worse for the traditional model than mine. Concerning the
limited spread of activity needed for the full sensation of loudness: I can only
say that if I integrate firing rates over a limited range of frequencies of presentation around the CF, the resulting bandwidth rate functions look less, rather
than more, like the psychophysical functions.

DYNAMIC MAINTENANCE AND ALTERABILITY OF CORTICAL
MAPS IN ADULTS; SOME IMPLICATIONS

Michael M. Merzenich and William M. Jenkins

*Departments of Otolaryngology & Physiology, University of California
Coleman Laboratory, San Francisco, CA 94143*

1. INTRODUCTION

Recent studies conducted principally in the somatosensory nervous system of
primates have revealed that cortical maps are alterable as a function of experience in adults. The specific nature of this evident dynamism of cortical representations bears a series of important implications for consideration of the
significance of features of sensory system organizations. In this report, we
shall a) briefly summarize the basic conclusions drawn from these studies on
the dynamics of cortical map structure, b) outline by example the results of
studies from which these conclusions have been drawn, and c) then specifically
consider some implications of these studies for our understanding of the significance of special organizational features of the auditory system.

2. CORTICAL FIELDS ARE DYNAMICALLY MAINTAINED AND ARE ALTERABLE IN ADULT PRIMATES

According to the dominant contemporary view of cortical organization,
cortical representations are established early in life through a "critical
period" before which there is a pruning of anatomical projections to a fixed,
adult form. Cortical representations have been believed by most investigators to
be static in adults, with their functional structure defined by a static projection system anatomy. That basic view of sensory system organization has been
particularly reinforced by studies on the origins of ocular dominance columns
within visual cortical fields (see Movshon and Van Sluyters, 1981; and Sherman
and Spear, 1982 for review) and in studies of "barrels" representing individual
vibrissae within the somatosensory cortex of rodents (see Kaas, et al., 1983
for review). In both of these carefully studied systems, alterations of ocular
dominance column or barrel boundaries and structure are possible during the
first days of postnatal life, for example by sensory deprivation. However, at
later times no anatomical alteration of projections into these zones is seen.
Thus, the neuroanatomical connections establish functional cortical maps early
in life, and after that early stage (goes the current dominant view) substantial
map alterations can not occur.
    Recent studies conducted principally within the somatosensory projection
system challenge that view. They reveal that: a) There is great individual
variability in the details of representation of the skin surfaces in adult
primates. This variability must, in part, be accounted for by the different
individual tactile experiences of the animal. b) A rapid reorganization of
cortical maps occur after peripheral nerve injury (Merzenich, et al., 1983a;
Merzenich and Kaas, 1983) or digit amputation (Merzenich, et al., 1983b).
Following such lesions, the representation of the skin surfaces in the border-
ing cortical map regions rapidly expand, to "reoccupy" the deprived cortical
sector. By that reorganization, representations of surrounding skin surfaces
are topographically enlarged. With that enlargement, there is a corresponding
reduction in receptive field sizes, i.e., the expanded representations are
finer-grained. c) This reorganization is progressive, and occupation of a
deprived zone several millimeters across is initially completed in roughly 2-3
weeks (Merzenich, et al., 1983c). However, even after initial complete
territorial "reoccupation", further substantial map changes are recorded, over
time. d) There is also a rapid reorganization of cortical maps after induction

of a cortical lesion completely destroying the representation of a part of the body surface (Jenkins, et al., 1982). In this reorganization, all of the skin surfaces formerly represented within a small infarcted zone are later found to be represented in the cortical region surrounding it. With this reestablishment of representation, the mapping of skin surfaces formerly represented in this surrounding zone is degraded, i.e., is of a coarser grain. e) Substantial local alteration of cortical maps have been recorded following changes of the use of the hand in normal monkeys. Thus, for example, dramatic map alterations have been recorded in the cortical representation of a finger struck several thousand times/day for several months in a bar-press task. Almost equally remarkable changes were seen in the patterns of representation of surrounding skin surfaces (W. Jenkins, M. Merzenich, J. Zook, and M. Stryker, unpublished observations).

These studies indicate that the detail of cortical maps is established by use, and is alterable throughout life. They have established a series of "rules" on the reorganization process which indicate, in part, the nature and purposes of this alterability. Those rules (see Merzenich, et al., 1983c; 1983d) include: a) During the course of map alteration, map topography is continuously maintained. b) During map alteration, the normal overlap "rule" (percentage overlap of receptive fields is a nearly linear function of cortical distance, and the distance over which fields no longer overlap is roughly constant at 500-600 microns) defined by Sur and colleagues (1980) is at least roughly maintained. c) There is apparently a distance limit to map reorganization. In Area 3b (the somatosensory konicortex) it is roughly 600 microns. That is, a given skin surface site can be represented anywhere over a zone roughly 1200 in diameter, with the actual site of representation defined by the monkey's functional use of his skin surfaces over the long term.

It is almost certain that temporal coincidence or sequencing of inputs and levels of temporally appropriate activity constitute the basis of the dynamic maintenance and alteration of these maps (see Merzenich, et al., 1983d; Edelman and Finkel, 1983). The reason is simple: There are no other realistic alternatives. Since the original postulation of Hebb (1949), there have been several proposed models of how cortical maps might be created (the issue has usually been addressed as a developmental one) by such response correlations (e.g., see Malsburg, 1973; Swindale, 1980; 1982; Willshaw and Malsburg, 1976).

We have hypothesized that map alterations by use constitute the basis of acquisition of skill, and have drawn several correlates between observed map changes and the neurological consequences of corresponding lesions (see Merzenich, et al., 1983b; 1983d). Our results are consistent with a "group selection" theory for pattern recognition, formally proposed by Edelman (1978; 1982).

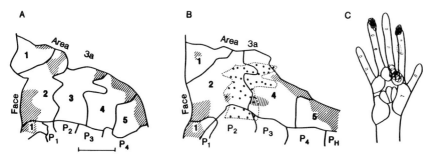

Fig. 1. Maps of hand surface representations within cortical Area 3b in a normal adult owl monkey (A), and 64 days after amputation of digit 3 (B). Representational areas of dorsal hand surfaces are shaded. The cortical zone originally representing digit 3 is outlined by a dotted line in B. Receptive fields defined for neurons in microelectrode penetrations into the former digit 3 representational zone in the second map (dots in B) were on adjacent skin surfaces on digits 2, 4 and palmar pads; all are drawn in C

3. SOME EXPERIMENTAL EXAMPLES

An example of the kind of study upon which these conclusions are based is illustrated in Figure 1. There, cortical maps are shown for the representation of the hand surface before and 64 days after amputation of the third digit. Before surgical amputation, the nerve innervating the surfaces of the finger were located, and the proximal nerve stumps sutured to prevent their regeneration.

Two months after amputation in this and in all other studied adult monkeys (Merzenich, et al., 1983c), the territory formerly representing the now-missing digit was occupied by inputs from the adjacent digits and palms. The skin surfaces found to be represented within this zone are indicated in the hand drawing in the right of Figure 1.

In all such cases, receptive fields for neurons in the former zone of representation of the missing digit(s) were found to be smaller as the representation of adjacent digits and palmar surfaces expanded into it, i.e., the digit came to be represented in finer grain. Changes in receptive field sizes and topography were also recorded in the always-innervated surrounding cortex. These rather striking changes are especially clear in two-digit amputation cases (Figure 2). There is an up to severalfold change in the cortical magnification for the skin surfaces that expand to occupy the "deprived" cortical sector, and a concommitant roughly inverse change in receptive field sizes across this zone. This manifests the fact that the normal shifted overlap rule is maintained through the time course of representational expansion. Also note (Figure 2) the unresponsive zone in the core of the reorganized cortex. Such zones appear to be permanent, and manifest the before-mentioned distance limit for this reorganizational process.

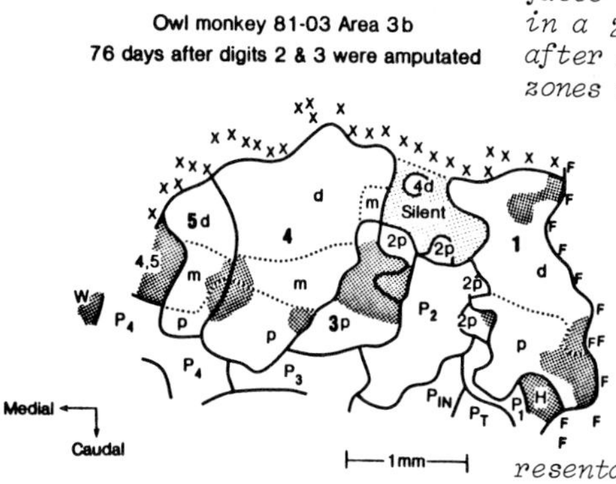

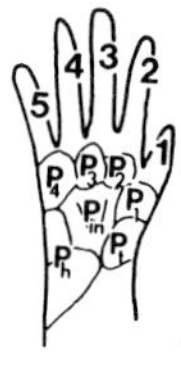

Fig. 2. Map of the representation of the surfaces of the hand in cortical Area 3b, derived in a 284 penetration site map obtained 76 days after digits 3 and 2 were amputated. Outlined zones represent skin areas indicated in the hand drawing at the right. Representational territories for dorsal hand surfaces are shaded. At sites labelled X, no cutaneous inputs were recorded; receptive fields were on the face at sites labelled F; d, m and p refer to distal, middle and proximal digital segments. Fields on 3 and 2 were on amputation stumps. The representations of adjacent digits 4 and 1 were about 1.8 and 1.7 times normal size. Redrawn from Merzenich, et al., 1983b

During reorganization in this and all other models, cortical map features that are usually thought to be determined by the organization of anatomical projections are found, in fact, to be the consequence of functional processes, and are subject to change. Thus, for example, the normally discontinuous borders between the representations of the digits (as a rule, receptive fields do not extend onto facing surfaces of adjacent digits) progressively *move* as representations of adjacent digits expand. New, representationally discontinuous borders form, where normally non-adjacent digits become apposed in the reorganized map. The locations of submodality column boundaries (Sur, et al., 1981b; Dykes and Gabor, 1982) almost certainly shift within the map. Thus, along with the receptive field sizes and the sites of representation of different skin surfaces, these second-order map features are also dynamically maintained and are adjustable. They are the product of physiological processes, and are not merely a simple consequence of the anatomical organization of terminal projections.

4.   WHAT FUNCTIONAL PROCESSES UNDERLY THE DYNAMIC MAINTENANCE AND ALTERATION OF
     CORTICAL MAPS?

     From a review of the literature and from a consideration of the nature of
recorded map reorganization, we have concluded that cortical map alteration
probably involves a strengthening of pre-existing synapses, i.e., that cortical
fields are normally degenerately wired, and that the map recorded at any point
in the animal's history is the product of a selection of inputs based on the
animal's idiosyncratic experiences to that point in life (Merzenich, et al.,
1983c,d). There is considerable evidence in all sensory systems that the spreads
of terminal arbors are much greater than would be expected from a consideration
of the functionally manifest detail of cortical maps (see Merzenich, et al., 1983
d for review). That is especially the case in the auditory cortex, which receives
remarkable convergent-divergent connections from the medial geniculate body
(Colwell, 1977; Merzenich, et al., 1979; 1981; Merzenich and Kaas, 1980;
Merzenich, et al., 1983e; Middlebrooks and Zook, 1982) (see Figure 3). In the
somatosensory case, in which terminal arbors have been studied (Pons, et al.,1981;
Landry and Deschenes, 1981), the distance limits recorded for reorganization are
consistent with the observed spreads of arbors (Merzenich, et al., 1983c,d).

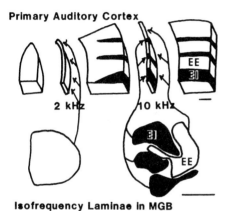

Primary Auditory Cortex

2 kHz   **10 kHz**

Isofrequency Laminae in MGB

*Fig. 3. Schematic illustration of pro-
jections from the ventral division of the
MGB (below) to Al (above) in the cat.
Projections from 2 and 10 kHz MGB isofrequency laminae to corresponding iso-
frequency strips in Al are depicted. From low
frequency excitatory-excitatory zones of
the MGB, afferents distribute in a nearly
all-to-all fashion all along low frequency
Al strips. For higher frequency zones, projections from and to MGB and Al EE and EI
sectors are segregated; each thalamic source
projects in a nearly all-to-all fashion to
their corresponding cortical subdivisions.
By contrast, afferent inputs are very restricted in the orthogonal (frequency representational) axis. Bars=1mm. Redrawn
from Middlebrooks and Zook, 1983*

5.   IMPLICATIONS FOR CONSIDERATIONS OF AUDITORY SYSTEM ORGANIZATION

     It is almost certain that the dynamic alterability of somatosensory cortical
maps will apply generally. In fact, we have hypothesized that the alteration of
the details of cortical maps by experience is *the* principal cortical process
(Merzenich, et al., 1983d). What general implications does it bear for interpretation of the significance of features of organization of the auditory
projection system?
     First, it indicates that cortical maps are of functional continua, and are
refined by experience. This is in contradistinction to a view of the system as
a fixed-in-place algorithmic feature extractor analytically resolving sound
parameters. A self-organizing system is representational. It does not extract
information parameter by parameter, performing a computerlike measurement of
those parameters. Rather, it *creates* details of representations from physical
continua, and fine-tuning of that creation is a life long process. A self-
organizing system necessarily maintains those inputs which overlap temporally
in the sound field in representational adjacency. At the same time, it can
represent any given continuum in any number of highly individual forms; and it
can be expected to make territorial adjustments as dictated by experience and
by the vicissitudes of life as they inflict on either the auditory nervous
system or the auditory periphery.
     The complex convergent-divergent projections from the auditory thalamus
into Al constitute a clear example of a degenerately wired cortical zone, capable
of supporting many forms of what it "maps". The fact that neurons have highly

site-specific responses despite this highly degenerate pattern of connection constitutes evidence that effective inputs at each site are selected from a large
repertoire of possibilities. The mixing of input in the auditory projection
system from manifold brainstem sources reflects the multidimensional nature of
sound localization (by our view, a principal concern of the main-line system),
i.e., information from a number of sources signalling sound location by
different cues is converged, and representational maps are created by response
correlation of this converged information.

Each auditory cortical zone will be organized by experience, and the order
of each determined by the nature of projecting inputs and their potentials for
response correlation. In every cortical zone, map structure and alterability
will necessarily be limited by the spreads of terminal arbors.

In the auditory projection system, we have specifically hypothesized that
the tonotopic organization in the main-line system is largely dictated by the
organization of anatomical projections, which are quite strict in this representational dimension of the system (see Merzenich, et al., 1983e). In this
dimension, experience leads only to fine-tuning. However, in the orthogonal
isofrequency dimension, projections are highly convergent and divergent at every
level, and in this dimension, the representation itself must be established by
response correlation. We now have strong evidence that Al is necessary and
sufficient for the localization of brief sounds in the cat (Jenkins and Merzenich,
1981). We have hypothesized that: 1) sound source location must be represented,
in some form, across this isofrequency dimension; and 2) its representation must
be organized by experience and alterable throughout life (Merzenich, et al.1983c).

*Acknowledgements. This work was supported by NIH Grant NS-10414, the Coleman
Fund and Hearing Research, Inc.*

REFERENCES

Colwell, S.A. (1977) *Corticothalamic Projections from Physiologically Defined
    Loci Within Primary Auditory Cortex in the Cat: Reciprocal Structure in
    the Medial Geniculate Body.* Thesis U.C.S.F. San Francisco.
Dykes, R.W. & Gabor, A. (1981). Magnification factors and organization of sub-
    modality-specific bands in SI cortex of the cat. *J. Comp. Neurol.* 202,
    497-520.
Edelman, G.M. & Mountcastle, V.B. (1978). *The Mindful Brain.* MIT Press,
    Cambridge.
Edelman, G.M. (1982). Group selection as a basis for higher brain function.
    In: *The Organization of the Cerebral Cortex.* (F.O. Schmitt, F.G. Worden,
    G. Adelman & S.G. Dennis, eds.) MIT Press, Cambridge, pp. 535-563.
Edelman, G.M. & Finkel, L. (1983). Neuronal group selection in the cerebral cortex.
    In: *Dynamic Aspects of Neocortical Function* (G.M.Edelman, et al, eds) In Press.
Hebb, D.O. (1949). *Organization of Behavior.* J. Wiley, New York.
Jenkins, W.M. & Merzenich, M.M. (1981). Lesions of restricted representational
    sectors within primary auditory cortex produce frequency dependent sound
    localization deficits. *Soc. Neurosci. Abstr.* 7:392.
Jenkins, W.M., Merzenich, M.M., Zook, J.M., Fowler, B.C. & Stryker, M.P. (1982).
    The Area 3b representation of the hand in owl monkeys reorganizes after
    induction of restricted cortical lesions. *Soc. Neurosci. Abstr.* 8:141.
Kaas, J.H., Merzenich, M.M. & Killackey, H.P. (1983). The reorganization of
    somatosensory cortex following peripheral nerve damage in adult and
    developing mammals. In: *Annual Review of Neuroscience* (W.M. Cowan, ed.)
    6:325-356, Palo Alto, CA.
Landry, P. & Deschenes, M. (1981). Intracortical arborizations and receptive
    fields of identified ventrobasal thalamocortical afferents to the primary
    somatic sensory cortex in the cat. *J. Comp. Neurol.* 199:345-371.
Malsburg, C. von der (1973). Self organization of orientation sensitive cells
    in the striate cortex. *Kybernetik* 14:85-100.
Merzenich, M.M., Andersen, R.A. & Middlebrooks, J.C. (1979). Functional and
    topographic organization of the auditory cortex. *Exptl. Brain Res.*

Supp. 2:61-75.

Merzenich, M.M. & Kaas, J.H. (1980). Principles of organization of sensory-
    perceptual systems in mammals. In: *Progress in Psychobiology and
    Physiological Psychology* (J.M. Sprague & A.N. Epstein, eds.) Academic
    Press, N.Y. 9:1-42.

Merzenich, M.M. & Kaas, J.H. (1982). Reorganization of somatosensory cortex
    in mammals following peripheral nerve injury. *TINS* 5:(12):434-436.

Merzenich, M.M., Colwell, S.A. & Andersen, R.A. (1982). Thalamocortical and
    corticothalamic connections in the cat. In: *Cortical Sensory Organi-
    zation, Vol. 3. Multiple Cortical Areas* (C.N. Woolsey, ed.) Humana
    Press, Clifton, N.J.

Merzenich, M.M., Nelson, R.J., Stryker, M.P., Cynader, M., Schoppmann, A., &
    Zook, J.M. (1982b) Somatosensory cortical map changes following digit
    amputation in adult monkeys. *J. Comp. Neurol.* In Press.

Merzenich, M.M., Kaas, J.H., Wall, J.T., Sur, M., Nelson, R.J., and Felleman,
    D.J. (1982c). Progression of change following median nerve section in
    the cortical representation of the hand in Areas 3b and 1 in adult owl
    and squirrel monkeys. *Neuroscience.* In Press.

Merzenich, M.M., Edelman, G.M., Sur, M., & Kaas, J.H. (1983). The selection
    and dynamics of cerebral cortical maps. *Science.* Submitted.

Merzenich, M.M., Jenkins, W.M., & Middlebrooks, J.C. (1983). Observations and
    hypotheses on special organizational features of the central auditory
    nervous system. In: *Dynamic Aspects of Neocortical Function* (W.E. Gall
    & S. Hassler, eds.) Rockefeller University Press.

Merzenich, M.M., Kaas, J.H., Wall, J.T., Nelson, R.J., Sur, M. & Felleman,
    D.J. (1983a). Topographic reorganization of somatosensory cortical
    Areas 3b and 1 in adult monkeys following restricted deafferentation.
    Neuroscience. 8:33-55.

Middlebrooks, J.C. & Zook, J.M. (1983). Segregated medial geniculate body inputs
    to subunits of auditory cortex. *J. Neurosci.* 3:203-224.

Movshon, J.A. & Van Sluyters, R.C. (1981). Visual neural development. *Ann. Rev.
    Psychol.* 32:477-522.

Pons, T., Sur, M. & Kaas, J.H. (1981). Axonal arborizations in Areas 3b of
    somatosensory cortex in the owl monkey, Aotus Trivirgatus. *Anat. Rec.*
    202:151A.

Sherman, S.M. & Spear, P.D. (1982). Organization of visual pathways in normal
    and visually deprived cats. *Physiol. Rev.* 62:738-855.

Sur, M. (1978). *Some Principles of Organization of Somatosensory Cortex.*
    Thesis, Vanderbilt University, Nashville, TN.

Sur, M., Merzenich, M.M. & Kaas, J.H. (1980). Magnification, receptive field
    area, and "hypercolumn" size in Areas 3b and 1 of somatosensory cortex
    in owl monkeys. *J. Comp. Neurol.* 44:295-311.

Swindale, N.V. (1980). A model for the formation of ocular dominance stripes.
    Proc. Roy. Soc. B. 208:248-264.

Swindale, N.V. (1982). A model for the formation of orientation columns. *Proc.
    Roy. Soc. B.* 215:211-230.

Willshaw, D.J. & Malsburg, G. von der (1976). How patterned neural connections
    can be set up by self-organization. *Proc. Roy. Soc. B.* 194:431-445.

GENERAL DISCUSSION

LANGNER:
In our laboratory we found clear evidence for plasticity in the field L of
chickens in the first days after hatching. Shifts were observed for 2-deoxy-
glucose markings with pure stimuli indicating that the same units are activated
by different frequencies at different times of the ontogenetic development.

MERZENICH:
The cortical map alterations we have described were all recorded in adult monkeys. A number of studies have revealed a "plasticity" of connectivity in deve-

lopment. The dynamic site-by-site selection of specific inputs from a large input repertoire constitutes a second class of hitherto unappreciated dynamic processes, operating throughout life.

PALMER:
What is the functional basis for this cortical plasticity - axon/dendrite growth and death or simply change or effectiveness of connections ?

MERZENICH:
For a variety of reasons (see Merzenich et al., 1983 a-c) we believe it most likely that cortical map alterations are a consequence of changes in synaptic effectiveness. However, it is not yet possible to completely rule out a sprouting or movement of terminal arbors as an underlying mechanism(s) for effecting some (not all) features of cortical map dynamics.

TEMPORAL RESOLUTION OF AMPLITUDE MODULATION AND COMPLEX SIGNALS IN THE AUDITORY CORTEX OF THE CAT

Chr. Schreiner, J.V. Urbas and S. Mehrgardt*

*Max-Planck-Institut für biophysikalische Chemie and *Drittes Physikalisches Institut, Universität Göttingen, D-3400 Göttingen, Germany*

1. INTRODUCTION

Studies of the neuronal response along the auditory pathway to repetitive acoustic stimulation and to phase locking have revealed a loss of temporal resolution in higher stations (Ribaupierre et al., 1972; Rouiller et al., 1979). In particular, the auditory cortex seems to be limited in its ability to follow repetitive temporal changes in the input signal. On the other hand, cortical responses to fast changes in the spectral content or in the amplitude of signals, i.e. 'transients', seem to be rather good, as long as they do not follow each other too rapidly (Creutzfeldt et al., 1980).

Most of the above mentioned studies of the auditory cortex were done in the primary auditory field A I, however, without a clear description of the location of the measurements. With the redefinition of the auditory cortical fields by Merzenich and colleagues (1975, 1979) and Reale and Imig (1980), a more precise picture of several aspects of signal representation has been established, however, not with respect to temporal properties. Therefore, to pursue more detailed information about temporal resolution we measured the response in various auditory cortical fields to amplitude modulated (AM) signals and to certain harmonic complexes. The results presented here focus mainly on the processing of temporal features in harmonic complexes as a function of their phase composition. The representation of AM signals across some areas of the auditory cortex is described briefly. A more detailed description of the AM results is in preparation (Schreiner and Urbas).

2. METHODS

The experiments were performed on adult, anesthetized cats (pentobarbital 1.75 mg/(kg.hr). The animals were ventilated through a tracheal cannula. Exhaled CO_2 concentration, EKG and temperature were monitored and kept at physiological levels. The stimuli were delivered via calibrated headphones (Sennheiser HD 424). The burst duration of the AM signals and the harmonic complexes was one second. The interstimulus interval was 800-1000 ms. The stimuli could be presented monaurally and binaurally. Multiple unit activity was recorded with glass-coated carbon fibers (impedance approx. 1MOhm) in depths between 500 and 1200 microns. Prior to the presentation of the complex stimuli, tone bursts were used to determine thresholds, CF, Q_{10dB} and the binaural interaction type. For the responses to AM signals and harmonic complexes PST histograms were constructed (binwidth 1 ms, 20 averages). As a measure of the synchronization of the responses with the input signal, the amplitude spectrum of the PSTH was calculated and the amplitudes of the first and second harmonic of the response relative to the dc component of the histogram were determined.

3. RESULTS

3.1 AMPLITUDE MODULATION

A tone at the CF of the recording place served as the carrier for the AM. The modulation depth was 100 %. For rectangular and sinusoidal modulation from 2 Hz to 150 Hz modulation transfer functions (MTF's) have been constructed out of the total rate and out of the degree of synchronization of the response. More than 95% of the MTF's measured in the primary auditory field (A I), the second

auditory field (A II) and the anterior auditory field (AAF) were 'tuned', i.e.
a certain modulation frequency rate and/or synchronization showed a clear maximum.
This 'best modulation frequency' (BMF) provides a reliable characterization of the
AM representation since there were only relatively small differences between the
BMF obtained from rate or synchronization and from rectangular or sinusoidal modulation, respectively. When Ribaupierre et al. (1972) studied the coding of repetitive clicks in the auditory cortex, they were not able to demonstrate a 'BMF', but
rather decreasing synchronization with increasing repetition rate of the clicks.

In general, rectangularly modulated tones appear to be more effective as
stimuli than sinusoidal modulation. This is the case in A I, A II, AAF, the
posterior auditory field (PAF), and ventro-posterior field (VPAF). However, there
are clear differences between the auditory fields in the representation of AM
signals. In A I, for example, the degree of the synchronization to rectangular
modulations was more than two times larger than the synchronization to sinusoidal
modulation. In AAF, on the other hand, the response to sinusoidally modulated
tones was almost as good as to rectangular modulation.

Table 1. BMF of synchronization to rectangular modulation.

	AAF	A I	A II
BMF(Hz)	22.3+13.7	11.9+6.5	8.0+3.9

Another parameter which revealed differences between auditory cortical fields
is the (averaged) BMF. Table 1 shows the values of the BMF for the synchronization
of rectangular modulation for AAF, A I and A II. It is apparent that the BMF's
in AAF are higher than in A I and A II. In other words, responses in AAF can
follow higher repetition/modulation rates of the input signal than A I or A II.

In addition, there is another characteristic property in the representation
of AM which distinguishes AAF from A I and A II. It seems that there is no clear
relationship between the CF of the neurons and the BMF of the MTF in A I and A II,
however, we could find a clear gradient of the BMF of sinusoidal modulation across
the tonotopically organized AAF. In portions of AAF with high CF's higher BMF's
are represented than in portions with low CF's.

In conclusion, it is evident that the anterior auditory field in the cat
shows a better temporal resolution of repetitive and modulated signals than A I
and A II, and, furthermore, contains a spatial distribution (or even 'map') of
BMF's or repetition rates. Therefore, AAF has unique functional properties which
are connected with the representation/processing of temporal features of an auditory input.

3.2 HARMONIC COMPLEXES

We found that harmonic complexes can produce strong and well-synchronized
cortical responses and also allows a more precise parametric description of signal
conditions than is usually possible for AM, FM or click stimuli. Therefore, we
applied harmonic complexes to study the relationship between signal conditions and
strengths of neuronal responses. The signals consisted of from 133 to 533 harmonics centered around the CF of the considered cortical location. The frequency
separation of the harmonics was chosen as 15 Hz or higher, corresponding, as far
as possible, to the BMF of the neuronal response to AM signals. By changing the
phase of components of the harmonic complex differently shaped wave forms could be
produced, which had identical long-term power spectra and well-defined short-term
spectra. The two extremes of the temporal shape of the signals were 'click' of
less than 0.5 ms duration when all components were in cosine phase, and for random
distribution of the phase angles an impulse of nearly constant amplitude for the
duration of one repetition period. The continuum between cosine phase and random
phase of the partial tones was covered by using a phase formula published by
Schroeder (1970): $\varphi_n = 2\pi\, n^2\, P\, /\, C$ (φ_n is the phase of the n 'th harmonic;
P is a phase factor; C = 64000).

A special property of the phase formula is that the formed impulse contains a frequency sweep across the entire bandwidth of the harmonic complex. Positive phase factors yield sweeps from high to low frequencies, negative phase factors sweep from low to high frequencies. The sweep velocities were between 25 and 1600 kHz/second.

The difference in the response of cortical cells to harmonic complexes with different phase compositions is striking. Usually the highest rate and synchrony of the response was found for the zero-phase condition ('click'). For a random phase condition synchronization could not be found. Ribaupierre et al. (1972) classified the coding properties of cortical neurons to repetitive acoustic pulses. They defined three different response classes: 'locker', 'grouper' and 'special responder' according to whether the spikes were time-locked, loosely synchronized or not at all synchronized to the individual clicks. During our experiments with harmonic complexes similar response types could be identified. However, it was revealed that with variation of the parameters of the harmonic complex, like phase composition, bandwidth, and frequency separation, the response type could be altered. For example, the response to a complex of 8 kHz bandwidth, zero-phase and 15 Hz repetition rate, clearly suggested classification of the neuron(s) as 'locker'. An increase of the frequency separation of the partial tones resulted in a decrease of the total rate, but the precision of the time locking was not altered significantly, supporting the classification as a 'locker'. Decreasing the bandwidth of the complex to about 2 kHz, however, resulted in a clear loss in synchronization, although the total rate was almost uninfluenced. The response to this stimulus constellation corresponded to 'grouper' neurons. Change of the phase composition also influenced the synchronization of the spikes and, finally, led to a response only compatible with a classification as 'special responder'. Therefore, spectro-temporal changes of the stimulus may result in an ambiguous classification of the neuron according to the classification given by Ribaupierre et al. (1972).

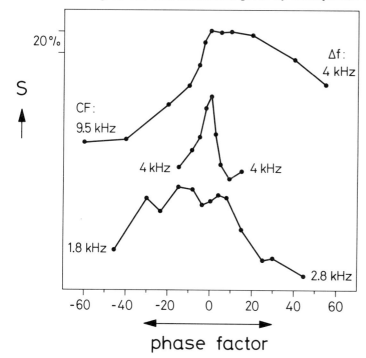

<u>Fig. 1.</u> *Synchronization of cortical responses to harmonic complexes as a function of the phase composition. (AAF; f_{rep}=15 Hz)*

In other words, the functional classification of neurons using click stimulation may be valid only for that special signal and may not be useful as a description of the general temporal response aspects of the neuron.

Some other effects produced with phase changes in the neuronal response to harmonic complexes will be briefly illustrated in the following section. The selectivity of cortical neurons to the direction of the frequency sweeps has been reported previously (Whitfield and Evans, 1965; Suga, 1965). Our findings of similar results with harmonic complexes , i.e. with a steady state long-term spectrum, underscores the meaning of short time windows for the analysis of the wave-form of the incoming signal (Schroeder and Mehrgardt, 1982; Mehrgardt and Schroeder, this volume). In Figure 1, three different response types to harmonic complexes found in AAF are shown under different phase constellations. In the upper curve the synchronization of the response to the 15 Hz periodicity of the complex is best for phase factors which produce fast sweeps from high to low

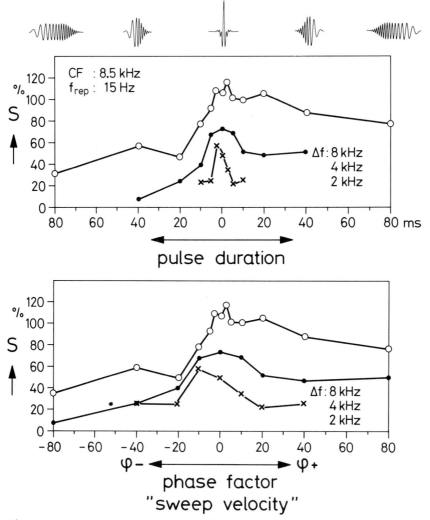

Fig. 2. Synchronization of cortical responses to harmonic complexes as a function of pulse duration and sweep velocity. At the top sample waveforms are displayed. Parameter: bandwidth of the harmonic complexes

frequencies only. The lower curve shows a response more sensitive to sweeps from
low to high frequencies. The middle trace shows a response sharply tuned to fast
frequency sweeps in either direction, or to very short impulse durations.

Figure 2 illustrates the dependence of the synchronization on the pulse duration and sweep velocity. Changes of the phase factor result in alterations of the
pulse duration and, consequently, of the sweep velocity within a 'click' or burst.
At the top of Figure 2, five portions of the harmonic complexes are shown for
different phase factors. The connection of sweep rate to pulse duration can be
easily seen. By changing the bandwidth of the harmonic complex this relationship
can be further explored. The upper part of Figure 2 shows the synchronization of
a response (A I, CF: 8.5 kHz, Q_{10dB}: 1.85, EE, BMF: 10 Hz; 15 Hz repetition rate)
for different pulse durations. Positive phase factors are plotted to the right,
negative phase factors to the left. Parameter is the bandwidth of the complex.
For a large bandwidth the response documents a high synchronization and a selectivity for positive phase factors (sweep from high to low frequencies). This
preference is lost when the bandwidth decreases and the area of good synchronization is restricted to very short pulse durations. A better description of the
response is given in the lower part of Figure 2. Here the synchronization for the
three complexes is plotted as a function of the sweep velocity (expressed as phase
factor). Still the decrease of synchronization with decreasing bandwidth is obvious, however, the shape of the three curves resemble each other far more than in
the plot for the pulse duration. This points to a close relationship between
synchronization and sweep velocity rather than pulse duration. A more precise
analysis of the connection between synchronization and frequency sweeps, e.g. the
shift of the curve for 2 kHz bandwidth (Fig. 2), requires detailed information
about FTC, inhibitory areas, time constants, etc., and is therefore beyond the
scope of this paper.

Figure 3 shows the synchronization to harmonic complexes (zero-phase) as a
function of the level of the partial tone at the CF of the neuron(s). At 0 dB the
component has the same level as all other components. With increasing level the
synchronization of the response deteriorates. This result can be explained by
considering again not the spectrum, but the temporal course of the signal. The
added tone at CF fills up the valley between consecutive 'clicks' in the signal.
When the amplitude difference between peak and valley is too small, the synchronization mechanism fails. Therefore, increasing the bandwidth of the signal requires
a higher level of the CF tone to fill the valley (see Figure 3). Figure 4, however, demonstrates that the simple connection between synchronization and
peak/valley ratio is not enough to explain all cases. The synchronization shows
a clear maximum for a specific enhancement of the CF component, or in other words,
an increase of a certain component of the harmonic complex may increase or decrease
the synchronization of the neural response.

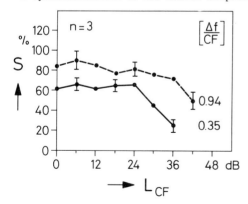

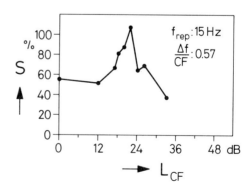

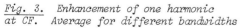

Fig. 3. Enhancement of one harmonic   Fig. 4. Enhancement of one harmonic
at CF. Average for different bandwidths at CF (7 kHz)

Psychoacoustic experiments have been done with similar signals concerning masking properties and audibility of single harmonics which revealed interesting corresponding elements to our findings (Duifhuis, 1971; Schroeder and Mehrgardt, 1982; Mehrgardt and Schroeder, this volume).

In conclusion, it becomes clear that the response characteristics of cortical cells to moderately complex stimuli is far from being well-described, not to mention understood. The short examples given above illustrate that the classification of the temporal properties of cortical responses cannot be solely based on one kind of stimulus (e.g. click or tone burst). The complexity of the spectro-temporal interaction in determining the neuronal response at the cortical level makes it necessary to use for its exploration a highly variable and well-defined stimulus. Harmonic complexes seem to fulfill these requirements satisfactorily.

Acknowledgement: We would like to express our gratitude to Mr. H. Alrutz for providing the highly adaptable apparatus for producing the harmonic complex signals. This study was supported by the Deutsche Forschungsgemeinschaft (SFB 33).

REFERENCES

Creutzfeld, O.D., Hellweg, F.-C., Schreiner, Chr. (1980). Thalamocortical transformation of responses to complex auditory stimuli. *Exp. Brain Res.* 39, 87-104.
Duifhuis, H. (1971). Audibility of high harmonics in a periodic pulse. II. Time Effect. *J. Acoust. Soc. Amer.* 49, 1155-1162.
Merzenich, M.M., Knight, P.L., Roth, G.L. (1975). Representation of cochlea within primary auditory cortex in the cat. *J. Neurophysiol.* 38, 231-249.
Merzenich, M.M., Andersen, R.A., Middlebrooks, J.H. (1979). Functional and topographic organization of the auditory cortex. *Exp. Brain Res., Suppl. II,* 61-75.
Ribaupierre, F. de, Goldstein, M.H., Yeni-Komshian, G. (1972). Cortical coding of repetitive acoustic pulses. *Brain Res.* 48, 205-225.
Reale, R.A., Imig, T.J. (1980). Tonotopic organization in auditory cortex of the cat. *J. Comp. Neurol.* 192, 265-291.
Rouiller, Ribaupierre, Y. de, Ribaupierre, F. de (1979). Phase-locked responses to low frequency tones in the medial geniculate body. *Hearing Res.* 1, 213-226.
Schroeder, M.R. (1970). Synthesis of low-peak-factor signals and binary sequences with low autocorrelation. *IEEE Trans. on Information Theory* IT-16, 85-89.
Schroeder, M.R., Mehrgardt, S. (1982). Auditory masking phenomena in the perception of speech. In: *The Representation of Speech in the Peripheral Auditory System,* Eds. R. Carlson and B. Granström, pp. 79-87, Amsterdam, New York, Oxford, Elsevier Biomedical Press.
Suga, N. (1965). Analysis of frequency-modulated sounds by auditory neurons of echo locating bats. *J. Physiol.* 179, 26-53.
Whitfield, I.C., Evans, E.F. (1965). Responses of auditory cortical neurons to stimuli of changing frequency. *J. Neurophysiol.* 28, 655-672.

GENERAL DISCUSSION

STOPP:
Have your cortical neurones displayed any lability, and if so, have you been able to select another stimulus adequate to drive them in their new state ?

URBAS:
Yes, we often observed response lability in the cortical recordings. Sometimes we were again able to obtain good responses by changing to a new stimulus; sometimes by merely waiting a short time (several minutes) and then resuming stimulation with the "old" stimulus; sometimes we had no further success and finally moved the electrode to a new location.

SYKA:
In the written version of your paper you mentioned that you are recording multiple unit activity. Do your results represent responses of single units or more units recorded at the same time? The question is because in the inferior colliculus in rat we often observe that adjacent cells have very different rates of following to repetitive click stimuli. Do all neurons recorded at one position of the electrode (in the cortex) display the same synchronization to amplitude modulation? Do they all belong either to EE or EI types of interaction?

URBAS:
Our results were obtained from multiple cells, recorded simultaneously from a low impedance microelectrode. The average recording involved the activity of 3 - 4 neurons and we did not isolate the individual cell spikes. In other experiments which I have made, using single neuron recordings, I too found neighbouring neurons in the cortex that have quite different "best modulation frequencies". Thus our MTFs are probably a little broader than would be found from single cell' recordings. We believe our multiple-cell recordings have been made from cells which belong to a "column" structure in the cortex; however, this does not mean that all of the neighbouring cells necessarily have identical binaural, or other, properties.

LANGNER:
From my recordings in the forebrain of the guinea fowl I can support these findings of relatively low best modulation frequencies. In the field L these frequencies were typically lower than about 100 Hz, in contrast to the best modulation frequencies of up to about 1000 Hz in the midbrain of the guinea fowl.

THE DISTRIBUTION OF THE OLIVO-COCHLEAR BUNDLE AND ITS POSSIBLE ROLE IN FREQUENCY/INTENSITY CODING

Phyllis E. Stopp

Sub-department of Neurocommunications within the Department of Pharmacology
The Medical School, University of Birmingham, Birmingham B15 2TJ, England.

There are two methods by which sensory systems signal changes in the stimulus intensity -- by an increase in the pulse rate within a fibre and by an increase in the number of fibres activated. There may also be a change from low threshold to high threshold channels. In general, as we proceed along a sensory pathway towards the cortex, the relationship between stimulus strength and discharge rate becomes less strong (Hilali and Whitfield, 1953; Katsuki *et al.*, 1959) and may cease to be monotonic; thus the number and identity of the fibres becomes relatively more important.

In the auditory system Allanson and Whitfield (1955) originally proposed the CN as the site of a major change from predominantly rate coding of intensity to a code in which intensity is signalled almost entirely in terms of the number of active fibres. One of the problems that such a transformation brings in its train is that of preserving the separate identity of stimuli when two or more are simultaneously present. The existence of mutual inhibition in the CN appears to be the mechanism by which inhibitory gaps are maintained between the blocks of activity due to each stimulus, and hence their separateness preserved (Whitfield, 1956).

With more sophisticated studies of the properties of single auditory nerve fibres, two facts became evident. First that <u>most</u> auditory nerve fibres of a given characteristic frequency all have thresholds within 20-30 dB of each other (see however Evans, 1975). Secondly, many different workers in several species (Kiang *et al.*, 1965; Rose *et al.*, 1971) have found that the discharge rates of fibres stimulated at their characteristic frequencies saturate at levels of 60-80 dB above their threshold. Thus we cannot account for the dynamic range of hearing purely in terms of fibre discharge rate, and unless we postulate some new mechanism altogether, we have to assume that the width of the array of stimulated fibres is an important coding factor even at this level. As soon as we do so, however, we are brought face to face again with the problem of the maintenance of the separation of multiple stimuli.

The problem was highlighted by Viemeister in 1974 in experiments with band-stop noise. Vietmeister showed that a signal located in the gap in noise spectrum exhibited normal loudness increments even at high intensities. However this experiment merely demonstrates rather elegantly a problem inherent in the whole mechanism. If we simply saturate the system with white noise at, say 80 dB, then no signal should be able to get through. This difficulty is got around at the cochlear nucleus level at least in part by the action of mutual inhibition, but the evidence for a similar process at the cochlear level is rather tenuous (Tasaki, 1954; Rupert *et al.*, 1963; Nomoto *et al.*, 1964). However, whereas the existence of lateral inhibition at the hair cell level is doubtful, the existence of <u>centrifugal</u> inhibition of hair cells is well established (Fex, 1967).

CENTRIFUGAL INFLUENCES

Centrifugal influences appear to play a role in fixing the excitation levels of auditory neurones at all stages of the pathway. Comis and Whitfield (1968) showed that stimulation of the centrifugal pathway from the superior olive can alter the excitation thresholds of cells in the ventral cochlear nucleus, and the effects of stimulation of the olivo-cochlear bundle on hair cell excitability has already been referred to. It is probable that a centrifugal mechanism as well as the originally postulated mutual inhibition mechanism plays a role in the cochlear nucleus transformation, and it further seems that the centrifugal pathway plays the major role at the periphery.   Certainly it is known that interference with the centrifugal pathway impairs that phenomenon -- the detection of signals in noise -- whose mechanism we are seeking, both at the cochlear nucleus (Pickles and Comis, 1973) and cochlear (Dewson, 1968) levels.

There are two ways in which the centrifugal pathway could act (Whitfield, 1978).   One is by an inhibitory action at the edges of the array, as originally proposed for the cochlear nucleus.   The other is by adjusting the thresholds of the receptors to some new level so that they no longer saturate.   A combination of these two effects is obviously not ruled out.   No recordings from single auditory nerve fibres in unanaesthetized preparations have been reported, so that the finding of a 70 dB dynamic range for individual neurones, which is the basis of our difficulty, is in the absence of any normal centrifugal activity.   There is one published account of single neurone activity in the cochlear nucleus, that of Moushegian et al., (1962), and it is noteworthy that these workers found much more widespread inhibition in the ventral nucleus than is commonly seen in anaesthetized preparations.

ANATOMICAL CONNECTIONS

Because of the difficulty of making worthwhile recordings from the periphery of normally functioning animals, it seemed that a detailed anatomical approach might be helpful.   It is well-known that the afferent pathway is very strongly cochleotopic, that is to say the cochlea is projected in an orderly way not only on the cochlear nucleus but also on the lateral superior olive, with which latter nucleus the origins of the uncrossed olivo-cochlear bundle (OCB) are associated.

If the OCB is concerned to adjust the general level of activity of the whole cochlea then we might expect the distribution of the centrifugal fibres to be rather diffuse.   If it is concerned with controlling activity in particular parts of the array (edges) then we might expect a more limited distribution.   A further question would be whether the efferent fibre returns to the same part of the cochlea, or is systematically displaced.   We have started to investigate this problem by means of retrograde tracer techniques.

HORSERADISH PEROXIDASE

Following previous workers (e.g. LaVail and LaVail, 1974) we started our study using horseradish peroxidase (HRP).   We found that we could reproduce Warr's results (1975) if the HRP was introduced via the round window, but not if introduced through perfusion holes in the wall of scala tympani, unless the round window was at the same time open (Stopp and Whitfield, 1981).   We were forced to the conclusion that HRP is taken up only by centrifugal nerve endings in the hook region of the basilar membrane, and that suggests that these particular fibres may be in some way different from those in the rest of the cochlea.   We have no suggestions as to the functional implications of this.

TRUE BLUE

The fluorescent dye, True Blue (TB), is also transported retrogradely (Bentivoglio et al., 1979), and unlike HRP appears to be taken up by efferent endings throughout the cochlea.   It is therefore highly suitable for our purpose. In order to determine the distribution of the fibres it was necessary to limit the region of the cochlea perfused, and this was done by introducing plugs made of Reprosil, a silicone dental impression material, into scala tympani at different points (Stopp, 1983).   After suitable survival time the guinea pigs were perfused; frozen sections of brainstem were mounted and when dry examined uncovered with a Leitz ultraviolet microscope using UG 1 and BG 38 barrier filters and K 435 excitation filter.

Labelling of cells was found most predominantly in the lateral superior olive (LSO) ipsilateral to the perfused cochlea, with a lesser amount of staining

178   STOPP

occurring in the contralateral periolivary areas.   The position of labelling in
the LSO was related to the area of cochlea treated.   Thus, basal turn perfusion
resulted in labelling in the medial portion, while apical perfusion caused
labelling in the dorsolateral region.   Figure 1 summarizes the distribution.

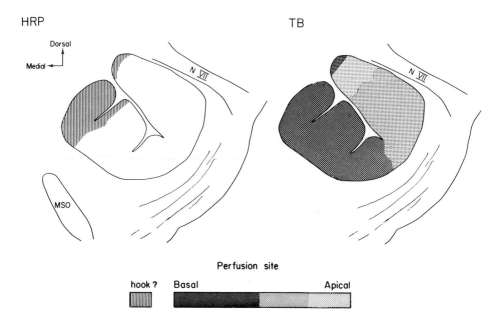

*Fig. 1.   Schematics of the LSO showing the distribution of cells labelled
(left) by perfusion of the entire cochlea (round window patent) with HRP;
(right) by perfusion of segregated regions of the cochlea with TB.*

The basal turn has the greatest representation but this agrees with the finding
that it has the highest density of efferent nerve endings (Smith and Sjöstrand,
1961).
        The orderly relationship between the positions of the labelled cells in the
nucleus and the parts of the cochlea perfused does suggest at least a general
segregation of different fibres of the system to different frequency regions,
though it is not yet possible to say how detailed the separation might be.
Unfortunately, there is at present no information available about the frequency
distribution of afferents in the guinea pig superior olive.   However, analogy
with the cat (Guinan *et al.*, 1972), where the high frequencies are found medially
and low frequencies laterally, would suggest that the position of the cells of
origin of efferent fibres innervating a particular cochlear region may be closely
related to the site of termination of afferents from that region.

Acknowledgements.
        *Thanks are due to Miss Karen Hewlett for her unstinting technical and artistic
help.   The author is also grateful to Dr. Harold Wilson of the Birmingham Dental
School for recommending and supplying the impression materials.*

REFERENCES

Allanson, J.T., Whitfield, I.C. (1955).   The cochlear nucleus and its relation to
        theories of hearing.   In: *Third London Symposium on Information Theory*,
        (C. Cherry, ed).   pp 269-286.   London, Butterworth.

Bentivoglio, M., Kuypers, H.G.J.M., Catsman-Berrevoets, C.E., Dann, O. (1979).
     Fluorescent retrograde neuronal labeling in rat by means of substances
     binding specifically to adenine-thymine rich DNA. *Neurosci. Letters* 12,
     235-240.
Comis, S.D., Whitfield, I.C. (1968).   Influence of centrifugal pathways on unit
     activity in the cochlear nucleus.   *J. Neurophysiol.* 31, 62-68.
Dewson, J.H. III (1968).   Efferent olivocochlear bundle: Some relationships to
     stimulus discrimination in noise. *J. Neurophsiol.* 31, 122-130.
Evans, E.F. (1975).   Cochlear nerve and cochlear nucleus.   In: *Handbook of
     Sensory Physiology*, (Vol. V, part 2) (W.D. Keidel and W.D. Neff, eds). pp.
     1-108, Berlin, Heidelberg, Springer-Verlag.
Fex, J. (1967).   Efferent inhibition in the cochlea related to hair-cell dc
     activity: Study of postsynaptic activity of the crossed olivocochlear fibres
     in the cat.   *J. acoust. Soc. Amer.*, 41, 666-675.
Guinan, J.J. Jr., Norris, B.E., Guinan, S.S. (1972).   Single auditory units in the
     superior olivary complex II: Locations of unit categories and tonotopic
     organization.   *Internat'l J. Neurosci.*, 4, 147-166.
Hilali, S., Whitfield, I.C. (1953).   Responses of the trapezoid body to acoustic
     stimulation with pure tones.   *J. Physiol.* 122, 158-171.
Katsuki, Y., Watanabe, T., Maruyama, N. (1959).   Activity of auditory neurons in
     upper levels of brain of cat.   *J. Neurophysiol.*, 22, 343-359.
Kiang, N.Y.S., Watanabe, T., Thomas, E.C., Clark, L.F. (1965).   *Discharge
     Patterns of Single Fibers in the Cat's Auditory Nerve*.   Cambridge, Mass.
     M.I.T. Press.
LaVail, J.H., LaVail, M.M. (1974).   The retrograde intraaxonal transport of
     horseradish peroxidase in the chick visual system: A light and electron
     microscope study.   *J. comp. Neurol.* 157, 303-358.
Moushegian, G., Rupert, A., Galambos, R. (1962).   Microelectrode study of ventral
     cochlear nucleus of the cat.   *J. Neurophysiol.* 25, 515-529.
Nomoto, M., Suga, N., Katsuki, Y. (1964).   Discharge pattern and inhibition of
     primary auditory nerve fibers in the monkey.   *J. Neurophysiol.* 28, 768-787.
Pickles, J.O., Comis, S.D. (1973).   Role of centrifugal pathways to cochlear
     nucleus in detection of signals in noise.   *J. Neurophysiol.* 36, 1131-1137.
Rose, J.E., Hind, J.E., Anderson, D.J., Brugge, J.F. (1971)   Some effects of
     stimulus intensity on response of auditory nerve fibers in the squirrel
     monkey.   *J. Neurophysiol.* 34, 685-699.
Rupert, A., Moushegian, G., Galambos, R. (1963).   Unit responses to sound from
     auditory nerve of the cat.   *J. Neurophysiol.* 26, 449-465.
Smith, C.A., Sjöstrand, F.S. (1961).   Structure of the nerve endings on the
     external hair cells of the guinea pig cochlea as studied by serial section.
     J. Ultrastruct. Res. 5, 523-556.
Stopp, P.E., Whitfield, I.C. (1981).   Differential sensitivity in the guinea-
     pig olivocochlear bundle.   *J. acoust. Soc. Amer.* 70(1), S28(A).
Stopp, P.E. (1983).   Cochleotopic organization of the olivo-cochlear bundle in
     the guinea pig as demonstrated by the fluorescent retrograde tracer, true
     blue.   *J. Physiol.* In Press.
Tasaki, I. (1954).   Nerve impulses in individual auditory nerve fibers of guinea
     pig.   *J. Neurophysiol.* 17, 97-122.
Viemeister, N.F. (1974).   Intensity discrimination of noise in the presence of
     band-reject noise.   *J. acoust. Soc. Amer.* 56, 1594-1600.
Warr, W.B. (1975).   Olivocochlear and vestibular efferent neurons of the feline
     brain stem: their location, morphology and number determined by retrograde
     axonal transport and acetylcholinesterase histochemistry.   *J. comp. Neurol.*
     161, 159-182.
Whitfield, I.C. (1956).   Electrophysiology of the central auditory pathway.
     Brit. med. Bull. 12, 105-109.
Whitfield, I.C. (1978).   The neural code.   In: *Handbook of Perception*. Vol. IV.
     (E.C. Carterette and M.P. Friedman, eds).   pp 163-183. New York, Academic
     Press.

GENERAL DISCUSSION

CAIRD:
When recording from the Superior Olivary Complex of the cat the very few "efferent type" recordings I got seemed to be spatially separate from the "afferent type" cells, i.e. the data supported Warr's findings. How do you know that your marked cells are efferents and not afferent cells stained by transynaptic transport and where do the axons run ?
Secondly, you say you saw a similar marked cell body distribution to that found by Warr, i.e. outside the LSO, when HRP staining with opened round window. Did you see these cells when staining with TB ?

STOPP:
1) This technique has been used in other systems in the nervous system and has been shown not to be transported across the synapse; the dye accumulates at the cell body. Also, we have found that these fluorescing cell bodies are very small, compared with the majority of cells in the LSO, so you might not be able to so easily isolate these small cells with a microelectrode.
2) No, what we found, applying HRP to the whole cochlea with the round window patent, was that the labelling on the ipsilateral side was confined to a small region, i.e. the dorsomedial quadrant - within the LSO, whereas on the contra-lateral side the cells were more diffusely located (as Warr described) in the periolivary nuclei and trapezoid body. With True Blue the difference was that now many more labelled cells were scattered throughout the whole LSO. The contralateral picture remained much the same as with HRP. Lengthening the survival time did not alter the amount or pattern of labelled cells on the contralateral side, nor did it result in fluorescence being seen in the larger (afferent?) cell bodies in the ipsilateral LSO.

Section III
Binaural Interaction

REVIEW PAPER: PSYCHOACOUSTIC BINAURAL PHENOMENA

J. Blauert

Lehrstuhl für allgemeine Elektrotechnik und Akustik
Ruhr-Universität, 4630 Bochum, Fed. Rep. of Germany

The human hearing apparatus extracts substantial information from specific
differences between the acoustic inputs to the two ears. In this paper, some of
the more important features of binaural hearing are reviewed from a psychoacoustical point of view.

1. INTRODUCTION

The auditory system has two peripheral input ports, namely, the ears. The
acoustic input signals to the two ears differ under almost all "natural" sound
stimulation conditions. Each sound signal, impinging on a listeners eardrum, is
subject to linear distortions by the transfer functions of the external ear.
Among other factors, these transfer functions depend upon the direction of sound
incidence. For a given sound source position the different transfer functions of
the two ears will produce position-specific interaural signal differences. In this
way, information about the geometry of the sound field is encoded in interaural
differences of the ear input signals, e.g., information about the positions of
sound sources and reflecting surfaces. The auditory system is capable of decoding
a great deal of this information by evaluating these interaural signal differences.
The information is primarily used to establish the spatial positions and ex-
tents of auditory events, to better detect and recognize desired signals in the
presence of interfering noise, and to discriminate between signals from different
sources.

2. LATERALIZATION AND IMAGE SPLITTING

One of the most important effects of interaural differences of the ear input
signals is that they determine the lateral deviation at which a listener's auditory events occur with respect to his median plane. A rough outline of the psychoacoustics of lateralization is as follows: When the two ear input signals are
sufficiently correlated, as in the case of one single sound source in a free
sound field, usually one spatially distinct auditory event will occur, whose lateral displacement is determined by the interaural signal differences. This is
called "binaural fusion".

It is a reasonable assumption that one of the first steps in auditory signal
processing is spectral decomposition, or in other words a running Fourier transform is applied to the signal at each ear. From the physiological evidence we
know that this takes place mainly in the peripheral ear. One of the next steps is,
then, that the spectral components coming from each ear are compared with respect
to their interaural differences. It has been shown that narrow band signals only
lead to fusion if the spectral contents at both ears are within a range which is
roughly equal to the well known critical bands. We may therefore concede that the
evaluation of interaural signal differences is performed in "bands" such that
only components in the same critical band are compared interaurally.

What are, then, the interaural signal differences which are evaluated in each
band and used as cues by the auditory system? These interaural cues are interaural
level difference, interaural phase delay, and interaural group delay. Interaural
level differences are evaluated in the whole frequency range of hearing. To explain the range in which phase and group delay are effective, a preliminary re-
mark is necessary: A narrow band signal, like a critical band signal, can be regarded as a sinusoidal carrier wave which is AM and FM modulated. The arrival time
differences of two correlated signals of this kind can, under some mathematical
restrictions, be described in the following way: Interaural phase delay describes

the time difference of the fine structure of the signals, i.e., of the carrier. Interaural group delay gives the time difference of the modulation of the signal. In the case of a purely AM modulated signal, the modulation signal is the envelope. It has been found that the evaluation of interaural phase delay is restricted to spectral components up to about 1,5 kHz. Group delay is evaluated for all components above this limit, but also to a certain extent below.

In "natural" hearing interaural level differences and arrival time differences always occur in a forced combination. By means of earphones, however, the different interaural cues can be manipulated independently. The use of such experimental conditions have produced many interesting results. It has been established, for example, that, for most of the "realistic" signals, there is a monotonic relationship between the lateral displacement of the auditory event and either the interaural level difference, the interaural phase delay, or the interaural group delay. Maximum laterality is achieved for about $\pm$ 10 dB level difference, or about $\pm$ 1 ms interaural delay. The just noticable differences are approximately 1 dB and 10 µs. Another interesting result is that, for critical band noise signals with a fixed interaural arrival time difference, the lateral deviation decreases with increasing centre frequency above about 1,5 kHz.

One can try to evaluate the lateralization potency of the different interaural cues by "trading"-experiments. In an experiment of this type the auditory event is displaced laterally, e.g., by an interaural level difference. Then, the lateral displacement is compensated by, e.g., an interaural phase delay. It is concluded thereafter that the two opposite cues are of the same lateralization potency. Such conclusions must, however, be treated with scepticism. One of the reasons is that in many trading experiments and other experiments with earphones a splitting up of the auditory event into one or more components has been observed, these components often behaving differently with respect to the interaural cues. It is not always clear which of the components has been traced by the experimental observer, or whether some kind of a "center of gravity" of the multiple components has been taken to describe the lateral displacement.

We must admit that our knowledge about the relative importance of the different interaural cues is still very incomplete, although a great amount of experimental data can be found in the literature. These data have, however, almost exclusively been collected with highly unnatural signals delivered through earphones. Nevertheless, we may anticipate that some crucial experiments will be repeated in the near future with more natural signals, e.g., those collected with dummy head microphones.

A question that has only been touched superficially is that of the integration times of the lateralization mechanism. At the present time, we have some indication that at least two time constants are necessary to explain the spatial persistence of an auditory event, when the interaural cues are changing. One is of the order of 10 ms, the other typically in the 100 to 200 ms range.

It has been mentioned above that the ear input signals are dissected in critical band components and thereafter separately examined with respect to the interaural cues. At the end we still have, at least in most cases with a single sound source, one homogeneous auditory event. This leaves us with the following queries: Do all frequency components contribute equally to the lateral displacement, or are certain bands more dominant than others? What happens when the interaural cues in the different bands do not fit each other? The answer to the first question is that the region around 600 Hz is of particular importance as far as arrival time differences are concerned. Further details are largely unknown. As to the second question: if the constellation of interaural cues is such that they do not fit between the different bands, the auditory event may disintegrate into multiple components, each representing a certain frequency range, and having its individual lateral displacement. Unexperienced listeners may not be able to identify the separate components, but have one diffusely localized, spatially extended auditory event instead.

At the end of this section, it must be stated that, although the psychoacoustics of lateralization have been examined extensively in the past, many problems remain unanswered.

3. THE PRECEDENCE EFFECT AND BINAURAL SUPPRESSION OF COLOURATION

"Precedence effect" is not a well defined term, although very commonly used. To make the psychoacoustic phenomena behind this term more clear, we shall sub-divide the matter into two effects, namely, "summing localization" and "the law of the first wave front".

Let two or more sound sources send out well correlated signals. Under certain conditions of signal arrival time and level only one auditory event may appear. The spatial position and extent of this auditory event may depend on the positions of all contributing sound sources and the signals they deliver. This effect is called "summing localization". Its best known technical application is in stereophony. Typically, all those signals which reach the listener within an interval of 0 to 1 ms after the first signal will contribute to the effect but, given adequate level adjustments, this span may reach up to 50 ms.

Now let the first signal arrive at the listener with a time lead that is so large, typically above 1 ms, that the further signals no longer contribute to the position and extent of the auditory event. These are, consequently, determined by the "first wave front": giving this effect the name "law of the first wave front". The best known occurrence of the effect is in architectural acoustics: in an enclosed space the auditory event normally appears in the direction of the sound source. Reflected and, therefore, delayed sounds are disregarded with respect to the perception of the auditory event's direction.

There is, though, an upper time limit for disregarding the lagging sounds. If they come in later than the echo threshold interval, they will be perceived as distinct echoes: normally at their own direction of sound incidence. The echo threshold lies, as a rule, at about 50 ms for speech, and 80 ms for music. For brief sound impulses it may be as low as 10 ms.

It may be said that the precedence effect, in general, is fundamental to acoustical orientation in space. The ability to merge information from a number of correlated, incoming sound waves, and to form one single auditory event, is the key to finding the position of sound sources in the presence of reflected sounds, as in enclosed spaces. However, there is yet another interesting binaural effect, binaural suppression of colouration.

Consider the input signal to one ear in the case of one first wave and a reflected, thus delayed, wave. Both waves will add, and, as they are highly correlated, will interfere in such a way that their spectrum will be modified as if they had passed through a comb filter. In other words: the modified spectrum will have sharp spectral dips and peaks superimposed on the original spectrum. Listening to such a signal with one ear only (monotic) or over one single microphone (monophonic) will reveal an auditory event with unnaturally "coloured" timbre. The tones will, for example, sound "boomy" or "hollow" if the delay of the reflected wave is on the order of 1 to 2 ms, as, e.g., easily produced by a desk top reflection. Listening to the same sound field with two ears will, surprisingly, end up with a far less coloured auditory event. An explanation of this effect may start with the finding that the spectral arangement of dips and peaks is different at the right and left ear input signals. The hearing apparatus is obviously capable of merging the left and right ear signals, such as to produce a smoother "internal spectrum".

Precedence effect and suppression of colouration have been reinvestigated recently. One of the more interesting results is the following: it is not, in the case of the law of the first wave front, that the directional information of the reflected sounds is completely inhibited. Rather, the just noticeable angular difference for the direction of sound incidence is set to a higher value for a certain period, e.g. some milliseconds, after the first wave front has arrived.

4. AUDITORY SPACIOUSNESS

We have explicated in the preceding section that, when the law of the first wave front applies, the reflected sound waves do not or only slightly contribute to the direction of the auditory event. This does by no means imply that the reflections are imperceptible. For example, the reflections contribute to the loudness, and they may cause some colouration. Also there is another sensory outcome: due to the reflections the auditory event will be more extended in space – more "spacious" – than if we only had the direct, unreflected wave.

This effect of spatial spreading of the auditory events in the presence of reflections has recently drawn attention. The reason for this is that it has been discovered by multidimensional psychoacoustic evaluations that the typical auditory spaciousness of auditory events due to reflections, is a highly esteemed component of "good acoustics" in concert halls.

Auditory spaciousness, being one of the factors of the spatial impression of a listener in a concert hall, is a genuine binaural effect. It can be explained psychoacoustically in the following way: subsequent to the reflected sounds reaching each ear with different time delays and levels, the interfering effect on the direct sounds is not the same at each ear. Thus, interaural differences of the ear input signals are produced. They lead to interaural cues that are, according to the combfilter-spectra of the input signals, varying distinctly with frequency. In addition to that, since musical signals have nonstationary running spectra, these frequency-dependent interaural cues also vary as a function of time. Consequently, we have an auditory event split up into components which appear at different positions and, additionally, change their positions continuously. The result is a spatially spread out, or diffusely localized auditory event: auditory spaciousness.

Auditory spaciousness increases with the amount of reflected sound energy that reaches the listener from lateral directions. Low frequency components of the reflection can cause the sensation that the listener is completely enveloped by "sound". The effect of auditory spaciousness increases dramatically with overall level, partly as a consequence of the nonlinear level-to-loudness function.

Another way of looking at the psychoacoustics of spaciousness is as follows: by interfering with the direct sound in a different way at each ear, the reflected sounds cause a reduction of the interaural correlation of the ear input signals. Decrease of interaural correlation leads, however, to a broadening or spatial spreading of the auditory event. This is a well known psychoacoustic relationship.

Maximum interaural decorrelation of the ear input signals is observed in diffuse sound fields. In concert halls, for example, diffuse sound fields may occur due to reverberation after sudden stops or sudden attenuation of the sound signals radiated by the orchestra. The associated auditory events fill large portions of the concert hall. Listeners, consequently, report a sensation of envelopment. The auditory effect of diffuse, reverberant sound field is, nevertheless, not the same as the one produced by strong discrete reflections. Experts disagree whether the spatial effect of reverberant fields should be included in the concept of auditory spaciousness, although it surely contributes to the spatial impression.

5. BINAURAL LOCALIZATION IN A NOISY ENVIRONMENT

Most auditory localization in nature and in civilization must be performed in the presence of interfering noise. The influence of such noise on the ability to identify the position of a sound source is an issue of extreme practical importance: just imagine acoustical orientation of pedestrians in road traffic. Unfortunately, up to the present time, only a few researchers have examined this field.

One of the troubles with noise is that the definition of what the target-signal, and what the interfering noise is, may differ considerably depending on the individual situation. For example, in a conversation among several persons the target sound source may be different for each participant. Also: depending on the circumstances the reflected sound waves in an auditorium may be useful to enhance the "rich" sound of music, however, with respect to speech transmission, the same reflections may degrade intelligibility.

Some results for simple paradigms are at hand: one is that the mechanism which evaluates interaural phase delay is more robust against noise than the one which evaluates group delay. As a rule, it may be said that localization blur of a broadband signal is hardly effected as long as the noise level is on the order

of 10 dB below the level of the target signal. This is a very rough value, valid
for binaurally uncorrelated noise and a point source for the target-signal.

6. BINAURAL SIGNAL DETECTION AND DISCRIMINATION

When, several years ago, stereophonic sound reproduction became popular, one
of the marketing arguments was, that, by the use of this technique, sound localization would become more natural than from a monophonic system. More careful evaluation of the reasons of preference for this new technique showed, however, that
another benefit rates ever higher than improved localization. Most esteemed is
what listeners sometimes call auditory "transparency". When listening to music,
for example, it becomes easier to concentrate on one instrument and disregard the
rest, or to discriminate between different instruments.

What has been observed with stereophony seems also to be a good point with
respect to binaural hearing in general: even more important than the contribution
of binaural hearing to localization may be its ability to improve detection and
recognition of target-signals in interfering noise, as well as discrimination of
different target-signals from one another.

A popular way of looking at these abilities of binaural hearing starts with
the concept of interaural crosscorrelation. It is reasonable to state that most
binaural signal detection and discrimination capabilities can be modelled quantitatively by signal processing algorithms that include a running interaural
cross-correlation process.

The improvement of binaural signal detection as compared to the monaural one
is measured by means of binaural masking level differences (BMLD's). A BMLD describes the increase of the noise level that can be taken in a binaural detection
experiment with respect to a reference condition. Reference condition may be
monaural and/or diotic presentation of both target-signal and interfering noise.

Some typical results are: if the signal is presented to one ear only, and
the noise to both ears simultaneously and in phase, the BMLD will be on the order
of 6 to 9 dB. The highest BMLD's - up to 15 dB - are observed for a condition in
which the noise is presented with no interaural phase difference, whereas the
signal is interaurally phase reversed. In free sound fields BMLD's up to 9 dB
are found if both signal and noise are radiated from individual sound sources
which are situated at different directions relative to the listener.

Binaural signal detection is, undoubtedly, that area of the psychoacoustics
of binaural hearing which has been screened most extensively. There are hundreds
of relevant papers in the literature. One might suspect that this is partly due
to the relatively simple experimental equipment which is needed to this kind of
research.

Instead of going into more details in the course of this review, I shall
rather finish this section with an interesting curiosity which is however, well
understood: let both lateralization blur and BMLD be examined in experiments
where the interaural phase of the noise signal can be set to different values.
The outcome seems to be surprising at first: the conditions under which lateralization blur is greatest are those under which the target-signal is most easily
detected, and vice versa. The explanation is as follows: the noise interferes with
the target-signal components at both ears, thus, eventually causing stochastic
changes of the lateral displacement of the auditory event corresponding to the
signal. The listeners can use these spatial fluctuations as a clue for the presence of noise. At the same time, however, these fluctuation will increase the
lateralization blur.

7. THE COCKTAIL-PARTY EFFECT

Consider the following every days situation: in a room there are a number of
persons engaged in a lively conversation. A listener is, nonetheless, able to
pay attention to one individual speaker, even without turning towards him. If
the listener plugs one ear, the speech becomes much more difficult to understand.
The same holds e.g., if the listener is bilaterally hard of hearing, but has only
one hearing aid. This psychoacoustical effect is called the "cocktail-party effect".

Speech recognition in the presence of interfering noise – e.g., unwanted speech signals – is easier with two ears than it is monaurally. Evaluation of the gain of binaural hearing is performed in a similar way as in detection experiments: for quantitave description of the effect "binaural intelligibility level differences" (BILD's) are measured. They denote the increase of the level of the unwanted noise that can be taken in a binaural speech recognition experiment with respect to a monaural reference condition, so, that the same degree of intelligibility is maintained: e.g., a 50 % score of correctly recognized test words or syllables, usually from a phonemically balanced list.

For broadband noise at both ears, simultaneously and in phase, but a speech signal at one ear only, we may get a BILD of about 3 dB. For both speech and noise to both ears, but the noise interaurally phase reversed, a BILD as high as 6 dB may be found. In free fields with one source for the speech and another one, at a different direction, for the noise, BILD's of 8 dB and more have been measured. In general, the BILD's tend to be smaller than the corresponding BMLD's, but this finding depends on the characteristics of the noise signals used. It should be noted that a speech signal at one ear cannot be masked by noise at the other one; in other words, there is no contralateral masking.

It has been mentioned in the preceding section that reverberation can degrade the intelligibility of speech. This is due to the "slurring" effect of reverberation on the characteristic features of speech signals. But even in highly reverberant surroundings, binaural hearing may improve intelligibility though the possible improvement decreases with increasing reverberation time.

The improvement of speech recognition in reverberant fields due to binaural hearing is, undoubtedly, linked somehow to another psychoacoustical effect that shall be dealt with in the next paragraph. Their quantitative relationships are however, as yet unknown.

8. BINAURAL INHIBITION OF REVERBERANCE

It has been known for some time that an acoustic presentation in a room sounds less reverberant, when a person listens with both ears than when one ear is plugged. The same effect occurs when we switch from monophonic to stereophonic sound transmission.

One way of demonstrating this effect quantitatively is as follows: broadband noise, amplitude-modulated to give a sinusoidal envelope, is radiated into a reverberant room. The sound field in the room is listened to: (a), by direct binaural listening, (b), by observation via a single microphone and a pair of earphones, connected in parallel. The modulation depth is then set such, that a fluctuation of the noise level in accordance with the sinusoidal modulation function can just be perceived. For condition (a), this just perceptible modulation depth is lower than for condition (b).

9. BINAURAL PITCH

All binaural effects that we have commented on hitherto are obviously directly useful for everyday hearing tasks. There are, however, further binaural effects whose practical benefits are less obvious or even not existent. Such effects may still be of profound scientific interest, as they may provide insights into the functions of binaural hearing. One class of such effects are those, generally called "binaural pitch" or, more precisely, "dichotic pitch".

Binaural pitch denotes pitch phenomena that arise solely as a consequence of presentation of signals to both ears in a dichotic manner such that the ear input signals differ in interaural phase resp. arrival time. Presenting the ear input signals separately does not give rise to the effect – a sometimes very faint and sometimes more distinct sensation of pitch. Studies on binaural pitch play an important role in the efforts to construct more general models of the processes by which interaural time differences are evaluated in the hearing system. Indeed, it seems that models based on continuous interaural correlation in bands or related processes may be able to meet many of the necessary requirements. I shall now describe some of the stimulus configurations causing

binaural pitch. For simplicity, let a noise with a flat power spectrum be the
test signal, to make sure that no pitch would be heard in a monaural presentation.

   Binaural pitch was first discovered in the following situation: noise is presented to one ear directly and to the other ear through an all pass phase shifting
network introducing a phase-shift of 360° in a narrow frequency band. Thus, the
interaural phase is zero below the frequency band where the phase shift occurs,
and 360° in the region above it. The pitch sensation is similar to that of a
fluctuating tone at a frequency corresponding to the center frequency of the all-
pass, superimposed by noise which nearly masks it. To create the effect, the
all-pass must be positioned in the range between roughly 250 and 1500 Hz. The
effect is quite robust against additional interaural level differences.

   Another experimental situation giving rise to binaural pitch is when a constant interaural arrival time difference in the range of 2 to 10 ms is introduced. The effect is extremely faint in this case, but can be considerably reinforced by presenting a second noise, uncorrelated to the first one with a different interaural delay which must be smaller than about 3 ms.

   Further binaural pitch experiments are, e.g., characterized by an interaural
phase that changes 360° at a fundamental frequency and again by 360° at the first
harmonic or, additionally, once more at every higher harmonic frequency.

10. FURTHER EFFECTS AND CONCLUSION

   The potpourri of binaural psychoacoustic effects that has been mentioned so
far is far from being complete. In this last paragraph I shall shortly quote some
additional effects; our list of effects must, however, remain open. One reason
for this is that new effects will turn up as long as experimental work on binaural hearing goes on.

   An issue that has attracted the interest of many researchers is "binaural
loudness summation". In general, the loudness of the corresponding auditory event
is greater, when a signal is presented binaurally instead of monaurally; the
signal being kept at a constant level. The rules for the loudness increase are
more complicated than one would expect at a first glance. For instance the increase cannot simply be explained by power summation of the two ear input signals.
At higher levels, nonlinear effects like neural recruitment may come into play,
also acoustic reflex, contractions of middle ear muscles that effect the transfer function of the middle ear, may play a role: the acoustic reflex is obviously stimulated by the loudness sensation. At levels at or close to the absolute threshold, internal noise inside the hearing apparatus - interaurally
correlated as well as uncorrelated - adds to the ear input signals in a complicated manner. The situation is different for earphone presentation as compared
to the free field, due to the occlusion effect.

   Let us now, once more, return to "binaural fusion": the term "fusion" has
a broader meaning in some fields of binaural research other than lateralization.
For example, it is also called fusion when auditory events are accepted conceptually as to stem from one source, even if they appear in a diffusely localized
or spatially split manner. If some spectral components of a speech signal are
presented to one ear and the rest to the other, fusion may occur in such a way
that the auditory event is clearly understandable speech even if each ear input
signal is completely incomprehensible when presented separately. In this sense,
fusion may also occur when a speech signal is switched periodically in time between the two ears, provided that the switching intervals do not interfere with
basic perceptual units of the speech.

   Experiments in which the signals to the two ears are varied in time, either
by appropriate experimental synthesis, or because they originate from moving
sound sources, have been reported more often recently. These experiments are,
on the one hand, helpful in determining the integration times of the auditory
system and, consequently the spatial persistence of the auditory events. On the
other hand, experiments with moving sources and/or varying ear input signals
will, undoubtedly, uncover further properties of the binaural system that cannot
be observed with "static" signals.

   The "octave-illusion" is a good example for an unexpected effect that has been found with a paradigm of interaurally switched signals: in the original study, two sinusoids - 400 Hz and 800 Hz - were presented repeatedly and in alteration to one ear, without pauses in between. The same sequence was presented to the other ear, with the exception that the 400 Hz signal was on when the 800 Hz was on at the first ear, and vice versa. Thus the listeners were presented with a single, continuous two-tone chord, but each component repeatedly switched between the two ears. The switching interval was 250 ms. A typical percept was that only one auditory event appeared, jumping from ear to ear and simultaneously changing its pitch from high to low, and vice versa. Commonly, it was not realized that a chord rather than a tone was the stimulus. Right-handed subjects, by the way, used to hear the high pitch at their right ear, whereas the left-handed did not show such preference.

At the end of this paper, I want to recall that binaural hearing as well as hearing in general is no isolated process; rather, information from all senses is used by the central nervous system when forming a perceptual event. So it is no surprise that a considerable amount of research has been undertaken to explore the aspects of "heterosensory, spatial complication" with regard to binaural hearing. Since our two ears are mounted on a holder - the head - that can be moved rather freely with respect to the surroundings, the interaction of interaural cues with information about the actual position and movement of the head is of crucial importance. Further, the interaction of visual and auditory cues is a most important feature in many tasks of binaural hearing.

For more detailed and comprehensive representations of the subject matter of this paper as well as extensive bibliographies refer to the list of books below.

REFERENCES

Tobias, J.V., ed. (1972). *Foundations of Modern Auditory Theory*, Vol.II, Academic Press, New York and London: see especially the contributions of A.W. Mills, L.A. Jeffress and J.V. Tobias.
Carterette, E.C. and Friedman, M.P., eds. (1978). *Handbook of Perception*, Vol. IV, Academic Press, New York and London: see especially the contributions of Colburn, H.S. and Durlach, N.I. and Durlach, N.I. and Colburn, H.S.
Raatgever, J. (1980). *On the Binaural Processing of Stimuli with Different Interaural Phase Relations*, Dutch Efficiency Bureau, Pijnacker (NL).
Blauert, J. (1983). *Spatial Hearing - The Psychophysics of Human Sound Localization*, MIT-Press, Cambridge (Mass.), (in print).

RECENT DEVELOPMENTS IN BINAURAL MODELING

H. Steven Colburn

Biomedical Engineering Department, Boston University
Boston, MA 02215.   U.S.A.
and
Research Lab of Electronics, Massachusetts Institute of Technology
Cambridge, MA 02139.   U.S.A.

1. INTRODUCTION

The goal of a mathematical model is to express a hypothesis for understanding natural phenomena in such a manner that assumptions are stated explicitly and quantitative predictions can be evaluated for measureable phenomena. The value of a particular model is generally related to the number of phenomena that are successfully described within a small set of assumptions, the degree to which the assumptions are consistent with fundamental physical principles, and the degree to which the model captures the current understanding of the field.

Our goal in binaural hearing is to develop a mathematical model that is consistent with available physiological data and that describes a broad set of psychophysical phenomena. Unfortunately, we are far from this goal, even though binaural hearing models have received considerable attention for a long time. Previous psychophysical modeling efforts that have explicitly incorporated physiological phenomena have been either general but non-quantitative (Bekesy, 1930; Jeffress, 1948), quantitative but restricted to a small number of stimuli or phenomena (Hall, 1965), or quantitative and general but so complex that critical evaluations in particular applications were obscured by details and approximations (Colburn, 1973, 1977; Stern and Colburn, 1978; Blauert, 1982).

Part of the difficulty that must be overcome by models that encompass both physiological and psychophysical data arises from our ignorance about how the psychophysical judgement process is reflected in neural firing patterns. Even when conscious aspects of subjects' behaviors are ignored, issues of strategy and a priori information remain and are too complicated to include as neural networks in a model. On the other hand, the physiological data from the periphery should be incorporated explicitly as neural networks or mechanisms.

The modern approach to this problem is to separate the issues of judgement and decision from issues of available information. This is accomplished with statistical communication theory. In communication-theoretic models, available information can be represented by "decision variables" and performance can be calculated under the assumption that these variables are processed optimally. This approach requires that the decision variables be random variables; thus, the decision variables reflect explicitly the internal randomness (internal noise) of the auditory system.

Our previous applications of this approach (e.g., Colburn, 1977) have included the constraint that the final decision variable be expressed explicitly as the output of a neural mechanism. The consequence of this unnecessary constraint is that complex, non-optimum aspects of binaural processing must be modeled explicitly with a neural mechanism or simply ignored. This has limited both the phenomena addressed by our models and the comparisons with other approaches.

In the present paper we formulate an outline for models that incorporate available physiology, that apply to a broad range of psychophysical experiments, and that can be directly compared with most black-box models of binaural processing. After outlining the constraints that we adopted as a starting point, we suggest a general formulation, and briefly outline how several categories of data would be addressed within this formulation.

2. MODELING CONSTRAINTS

In addition to the general issues addressed above, there are several specific constraints that have influenced our formulation of binaural processing models. Since some of these constraints are based on conclusions that may not be uniformly accepted, we make them explicit here.

The peripheral mechanisms within the model should be consistent with the most important attributes of available physiological data from the auditory system, including the auditory nerves, cochlear nuclei, and superior olivary nuclei. Judgements about which aspects of the data are important for binaural phenomena are very difficult. Since increases in the complexity and level of detail in a model generally reduce the insight provided by the model, judgements about what aspects of the data can be ignored or simplified are of central importance. In the binaural modeling case these judgements are complicated by the fact that prominent aspects of the data may be of great importance for auditory phenomena generally but of little significance for binaural interaction. Also, available data are quite limited and some of the physiological factors involved are poorly characterized, most notably anesthesia effects, interspecific differences, and efferent pathways. It is evident that the modeling of the peripheral physiology requires continual modification as we learn more about the functioning of the human auditory periphery.

Interaural time differences and interaural intensity differences are assumed to be processed by separate peripheral mechanisms. Further, as we have argued previously (Ruotolo et al., 1979; Colburn and Hausler, 1980), the combination of these differences is non-optimum and can be influenced by the strategy chosen by the experimental subject. Thus, we incorporate time-intensity interactions in the central, non-neural part of the model.

The processing of both the temporal and spectral aspects of the interaural differences is also non-optimum, complex, and relegated to the non-neural part of the model. As temporal examples, consider target-duration and masker-fringe effects (Trahiotis et al., 1972, 1978), non-simultaneous masking phenomena (e.g., Yost and Walton, 1977), and the experiments demonstrating "binaural slugishness" (Grantham and Wightman, 1978, 1980). Spectral examples include the lack of an apparent critical band in interaural correlation discrimination (Gabriel and Colburn, 1981).

For binaural masking experiments, the random variability due to the external stimulus is assumed to be comparable to the internal variability generated by the randomness in the transduction from stimulus waveforms to patterns of firing on the auditory nerve fibers. This assumption is contrary to our earlier assumption (Colburn, 1977) that the external variance is negligible. Although there were a variety of arguments in favor of our earlier assumption, subsequent experiments (Siegel, 1979; Gilkey et al., 1981) that were designed to test this hypothesis directly concluded that the internal and external noise contributions to the variance are comparable in binaural detection situations. The consequence of the new assumption is that the model must be formulated such that the contribution of the external variance can be meaningfully evaluated. (Our earlier models did not satisfy this condition. In these cases, the variance of the decision variable in the model is dominated by extremely rare samples of the noise waveform, samples so rare that they would occur only once every few hundred trials. We believe that this is a consequence of approximations in the auditory-nerve description; calculations based on other models of the auditory nerve activity were either excessively complex or excessively arbitrary.)

3. SUGGESTED FORMULATION

The model comprises four sections. The first section describes the peripheral physiology explicitly. The second section is an optimum estimator that processes the neural patterns of the first section to generate a temporal sequence of estimates of interaural time difference and interaural intensity difference for each frequency band. (Each estimate is based upon the neural

activity over the brief time interval between estimates, roughly ten
milliseconds.) The third section specifies the non-optimum combination of these
estimates to form a set of decision variables. The last section is assumed to
process optimally the decision variables from the third section to make the
final psychophysical decision.

Note that this formulation is not a complete model. To specify a complete
model requires specific assumptions for the first and third sections. (The
second and fourth are specified by the optimum assumption.)

Note, second that the assumptions for the first section are chosen to match
physiological data and those for the third section are chosen to match
psychophysical data. This separation of physiology and psychophysics has the
benefit that the third and fourth sections of the model are directly analogous
to black-box psychophysical models (e.g., Jeffress et al., 1956; Hafter, 1971)
and many psychophysical modeling issues can be considered independent of the
peripheral physiology.

Note, third, that the internal noise (internal random variability) in this
formulation is determined by the peripheral physiology and is reflected in the
fact that the estimates generated by the second section are random variables.

Note, fourth, that the stimulus variability is primarily represented in the
time sequence of external interaural differences that are estimated in the
second section of the model (i.e., the expected values of the estimates). Since
the nerve fibers are sensitive to a relatively narrow range of frequencies and
estimates are made separately for each band, the interaural differences are
approximately constant over the small time interval between samples. (This
formulation automatically avoids the problem mentioned above, namely the
excessive influence of unlikely smaples of noise.)

4. MODELING OF PHYSIOLOGICAL DATA

Our modeling of the peripheral physiology is the same as before (Colburn
and Moss, 1981). Specifically, the auditory nerve patterns are assumed to be
relayed through the cochlear nuclei to the olivary nuclei with no substantial
change in the firing pattern description. These patterns are assumed to be
processed in the superior olive by two mechanisms, one called the interaural
time displayer (imagined to correspond to the medial superior olive) and one
called the interaural intensity displayer (imagined to correspond to the lateral
superior olive).

The interaural time displayer is modeled as a coincidence network with a
fixed distribution of internal interaural delays (consistent with suggestions of
Jeffress, 1948). Estimates of interaural time (or phase) delay are based on the
activity in the network during each sampling interval. At low frequencies,
these estimates would be based on the ongoing fine structure of the filtered
stimulus waveform; at high frequencies, the bandwidth becomes sufficient to
allow estimates based on the ongoing envelope timing differences.

The interaural intensity displayer is modeled as population of "EI cells".
The EI cells receive excitatory and inhibitory (via the medial nucleus of the
trapezoid body) inputs to a generator potential that decays toward the resting
potential and that stimulates an output firing when threshold is exceeded. In
addition to a sensitivity to interaural intensity differences in the stimulus,
this type of mechanism is also sensitive to interaural onset or offset delays
(since an effective interaural intensity difference is present in this case).
The analysis of the interaural intensity display has not been pursued to any
significant degree.

5. APPLICATION TO PSYCHOPHYSICAL DATA

Some psychophysical tests, such as interaural time discrimination, are
based on information about the expected value of the interaural differences.
Other tests, such as NOSPI detection, must be based on the width of the
distribution of the interaural differences. Thus, tests from these two
categories require fundamentally different central processing of the estimates.
It is interesting to note that this distinction (between sensitivity to mean

values of interaural parameters on the one hand and sensitivity to the scatter
of interaural parameter values on the other hand) places experiments in coherent
masking in the first category. It follows from this point of view that coherent
masking (e.g., masking of a tone by a tone or a noise by a coherent noise)
should be considered as a discrimination experiment and not a detection
experiment.

The application of this model to interaural discrimination is relatively
straightforward. The estimates of the interaural time or intensity can simply
be averaged for an optimum use of the display information, and interaural
discrimination results can be used to specify the internal variability of the
estimates without reference to the physiology. When the model for the
physiological data (the first section of the overall model) is specified
mathematically, interaural discrimination can be predicted quantitatively. Most
available interaural time and intensity discrimination data are generally
consistent with these predictions; a notable discrepancy is in the degree to
which an interaural intensity difference interferes with interaural time
discrimination as outlined in Colburn (1973). In the present formulation, this
problem would have to be resolved within the central processor.

The application of the model to binaural detection phenomena and to
interaural correlation discrimination are based on the scatter of the estimates
(cf., Webster, 1951). Although the function of the central processor is less
obvious in these tasks, it is relatively easy to predict correlation
discrimination from the detection data. Also, the source within the model for
some of the dependencies seen in the data can be specified for detection. For
example, the observed dependence on target interaural parameters is a
consequence of the properties of stimulus waveform (Domnitz and Colburn,
1976); the observed dependence on the masker interaural delay is a consequence
of the peripheral processor as in Colburn (1977); the dependence on the
bandwidth of the masker and the frequency of the target are related to multiple
factors (cf., Zurek et al., 1983) including both peripheral and central parts of
the model; and the interesting temporal effects mentioned above must be
accounted for by the central processor.

The application of this model to interaural time discrimination in a noise
background could be based on the average value of the interaural time difference
estimates, consistent with the model suggested by Ito et al. (1982). Her data
and those of Cohen (1981) are generally consistent with a model based upon
samples of interaural delay in the stimulus. A model that includes effects of
interaural intensity difference has been developed by Stern et al. (1983).

The application of this model to subjective phenomena, such as pitch,
lateralization, and spaciousness, requires a different formulation of section
four of the model since optimum performance is not easily defined in these
cases. Many aspects of binaural pitch phenomena appear to be related to a
network like the interaural time displayer (Bilsen, 1977). In the context of
the present formulation, these pitch phenomena could be analyzed in terms of the
estimates of interaural delay as a function of frequency. (From the point of
view of the external time delay, this is equivalent to the original time
displayer.) Subjective position judgements are clearly based on both interaural
time and intensity estimates; however, algorithms for predicting position
judgements from these estimates are difficult to specify. In our formulation,
this processing would be in section three of the model and would presumably
relate to constraints on objective judgements about combinations of time and
intensity differences (cf., Stern and Colburn, 1978). The spaciousness or
spatial extent of the image have been addressed by Blauert (1982) and his
students (Lindemann, 1982) with promising results. They suggest that the
distribution of interaural time estimated (or possibly position estimates) as a
function of frequency (including temporal variation of the estimates) may be
directly related to the spaciousness of an image.

6. FUTURE WORK

Since the formulation that we have presented here is only an outline for a model, the work is just beginning. More specific assumptions for both the physiological and psychophysical parts of the model are required for most quantitative predictions. Nevertheless, we hope that this formulation will lead to accessible, while still rigorous, models and that interaction between physiologists and psychophysicists will be stimulated by these models. Also, models that incorporate both physiological and psychophysical phenomena explicitly will help us to understand better the functioning of imparied auditory systems.

Acknowledgments.

Many of the ideas in this paper were developed in close collaboration with R. Siegel, Y. Ito, K. Gabriel, N. Durlach, and P. Zurek. On the other hand they should not be held responsible for my extrapolations, speculations, and possible distortions of their ideas.
(This work was supported by the National Institutes of Health (NINCDS) Grant No. NS10916.)

REFERENCES

Bekesy, G. von (1930) Zur Theorie des Hörens. *Physikalische Zeitschrift* 31, 857-868.

Bilsen, F.A. (1977) Pitch of noise signals: Evidence for a "Central Spectrum". *J. Acoust. Soc. Am.* 61, 150-161.

Blauert, J. (1982) Binaural localization: Multiple images and applications in room- and electroacoustics. in *Localization of Sound: Theory and applications* R.W. Gatehouse (Ed.) Amphora Press: Groton, CT.

Cohen, M.F. (1981) Interaural time discrimination in noise. *J. Acoust. Soc. Am.* 70, 1289-1293.

Colburn, H.S. (1973) Theory of binaural interaction based on auditory-nerve data. I. General strategy and preliminary results on interaural discrimination. *J. Acoust. Soc. Am.* 54, 1458-1470.

Colburn, H.S. (1977) Theory of binaural interaction based on auditory-nerve data. II. Detection of tones in noise. *J. Acoust. Soc. Am.* 61, 525-533.

Colburn, H.S., and Hausler, R. (1980) Note on the modeling of binaural interaction in impaired auditory systems. in *Psychophysical, Physiological, and Behavioural Studies in Hearing* G. van den Brink and F. A. Bilsen (Eds.) Delft University Press.

Colburn, H.S. and Moss, P.J. (1981) Binaural interaction models and mechanisms. in *Neuronal Mechanisms of Hearing* J. Syka and L. Aitkin (Eds.) Plenum Publishing Corporation.

Domnitz, R.H., and Colburn, H.S. (1976) Analysis of binaural detection models for dependence on interaural target parameters. *J. Acoust. Soc. Am.* 59, 598-601.

Gabriel, K.J., and Colburn, H.S. (1981) Interaural correlation discrimination: I. Bandwidth and level dependence. *J. Acoust. Soc. Am.* 69, 1394-1401.

Gilkey, R.H., Hanna, T.E., and Robinson, D.E. (1981)Estimates of the ratio of external to internal noise obtained using repeatable samples of noise. *J. Acoust. Soc. Am.* 69(S1), S23.

Grantham, D.W., and Wightman, F.L. (1978) Detectability of varying interaural temporal differences. *J. Acoust. Soc. Am.* 63, 511-523.

Grantham, D.W., and Wightman, F.L. (1980) Detectability of a pulsed tone in the presence of a masker with time-varying interaural correlation. *J. Acoust. Soc. Am.* 65m 1509-1517.

Hafter, E.R. (1971) Quantitative evaluation of a lateralization model of masking-level differences. *J. Acoust. Soc. Am.* 50, 1116-1122.

Hall, J.L. (1965) Binaural interaction in the superior-olivary nucleus of the cat. *J. Acoust. Soc. Am.* 37, 814-823.

Ito, Y., Colburn, H.S., and Thompson, C.L. (1982) Masked discrimination of
    interaural time delays with narrow-band signal. *J. Acoust. Soc. Am.* 72,
    1821-1826.
Jeffress, L.A. (1948) A place theory of sound localization. *J. Comp. Physiol.
    Psychol.* 41, 35-39.
Jeffress, L.A., Blodgett, H.C., Sandel, T.T., and Wood, C.L., III (1956) Masking
    of tonal signals. *J. Acoust. Soc. Am.* 28, 416-426.
Lindemann, W. (1982) Evaluation of interaural signal differences. in *Binaural
    Effects in Normal and Impaired Hearing* O.J. Pederson and T. Poulsen (Eds.)
    Scand. Audiol. Suppl. 15.
Ruotolo, B.R., Stern, R.M., Jr., and Colburn, H.S. (1979) Discrimination of
    symetric, time-intensity traded binaural stimuli. *J. Acoust. Soc. Am.* 66,
    1733-1737.
Siegel, R.A. (1979) Internal and external noise in auditory detection. S.M.
    Thesis, M.I.T.
Stern, R.M., Jr., and Colburn, H.S. (1978) Theory of binaural interaction based
    on auditory-nerve data. IV.A model for subjective lateral position.
    J. Acoust. Soc. Am. 64, 127 - 140.
Stern, R.M., Jr., Slocum, J.E., and Phillips, M.S. (1983) Interaural time and
    amplitude discrimination in noise. *J. Acoust. Soc. Am.,* in press.
Trahiotis, C., Dolan, T.R., and Miller, T.H. (1972) Effect of "backward" masker
    fringe on the detectability of pulsed diotic and dichotic tonal signals.
    Percept. and Psychophys. 12, 335-338.
Trahiotis, C., Hanna, T., and Bernstein, N. (1978) Effects of duration and
    interaural delays of masking noise of detectability under homophasic and
    antiphasic signal conditions. *J. Acoust. Soc. Am.* 61, S29.
Yost, W.A., and Walton, J. (1977) Hierarchy of masking-level differences
    obtained for temporal masking. *J. Acoust. Soc. Am.* 61, 1376-1379.
Webster, F.A. (1951) The influence of interaural phase on masked thresholds.
    I. The role of interaural time-deviation. *J. Acoust. Soc. Am.* 23, 452-462.
Zurek, P.M., Durlach, N.I., Colburn, H.S., and Gabriel, K.J. (1983) Masker
    bandwidth and the MLD. *J. Acoust. Soc. Am.* 73, S1.

GENERAL DISCUSSION

CAIRD:
I think you should be careful with your model not to assume that LSO and MSO code
interaural intensity and time differences respectively. This assumption seems to
be implicit in most papers on the Superior Olivary Complex and has led to a great
deal of confusion. It is true that the LSO is sensitive to intensity differences
but both LSO and MSO are affected by interaural time differences, but in different ways (LSO - "group delay", MSO - "phase delay"). Also the physiological evidence for the presence of "characteristic delay" MSO cells is very poor and there
is no evidence for sequential sampling of interaural time in the MSO as you propose. Such sampling may first take place higher in the CNS.

LATERALIZATION OF TRANSIENT SIGNALS AND TYPES OF DELAY

G. B. Henning

Department of Experimental Psychology, Oxford University
South Parks Road, Oxford OX1 3UD, England

Lateralization of narrow-band, low-frequency transient signals can be based on phase delay; however, narrow-band low-frequency signals cannot be lateralized on the basis of group delay. Good lateralization performance with broadband signals apparently based on group delay is determined by phase-delay cues extracted from frequency bands remote from the centre frequency of the signal. Performance is significantly influenced by the magnitude and sign of the interaural phase delay near 650 Hz.

1. INTRODUCTION

Transients provide important cues for locating sound sources (Wallach, 1940; Stevens and Newman, 1936; David, Guttman, and van Bergeijk, 1959); but until recently it has been possible to manipulate only the simplest of their acoustic characteristics. Digital-to-analogue converters (DAC's) with sufficient dynamic range now make it feasible to produce transients to virtually arbitrary specifications. The signals used here to study lateralization had their constraints specified in the frequency doman: centre frequency, bandwidth, and type of interaural delay were manipulated (Henning, 1983).

A. TYPES OF DELAY Consider two waveforms $h_\ell(t)$ and $h_r(t)$, one for each ear with identical energy-density spectra $H(\omega)$. The waveforms differ in their phase spectra, $\phi_\ell(\omega)$ and $\phi_r(\omega)$, where phase, in radians, is given as a function of radian frequency, ω. If one waveform is a delayed version of the other – $h_r(t)$ is equal to $h_\ell(t-\Delta t)$, say – then the difference in phase at each frequency, the phase difference spectrum, is a linear function of frequency. The phase difference spectrum, $\Delta\phi(\omega)$, is given by

$$\Delta\phi(\omega) = \phi_r(\omega) - \phi_\ell(\omega)$$

$$= -\omega\Delta t. \qquad\qquad 1.$$

When the waveforms differ by a simple shift or pure delay, that delay, $-\Delta t$, is given by the slope of the phase difference spectrum. The slope of the phase difference spectrum, $\frac{d\Delta\phi(\omega)}{d\omega}$, by extension of the more conventional definition, might be called interaural group delay and denoted Δt_{gr} (Papoulis, 1962). For a simple time shift, or pure delay, the delay is also given by the ratio of the phase difference at a given frequency to that frequency: $\frac{\Delta\phi(\omega)}{\omega}$. This is sometimes called the phase (or carrier) delay and denoted Δt_{ph}. Like the group delay, phase delay is independent of frequency for simple time shifts. In general, however, group and phase delay may differ at any frequency or, indeed, be different functions of frequency.

In this experiment interaural group and phase delay were manipulated in low-frequency transients in order to determine which of the two properties of the stimulus is used by the auditory system and how our sensitivity to different types of delay depends on the centre frequency and bandwidth of the transients containing the cue.

A fourth type of delay, wavefront delay, is defined as the limit, if it exists, approached by the phase delay as frequency increases indefinitely. No attempt was made to manipulate interaural wavefront delay in this study; it was always zero.

2. METHOD

The signals were impulse responses of ideal bandpass filters truncated by a Hamming window (Rabiner and Gold, 1975). The ideal filters had a constant gain within their bandwidth, ω_{bw} and complete attenuation outside that band. Both the bandwidth and centre frequency, ω_c, of the filter could be adjusted. The phase response of the filter was linear so that the filter's frequency domain representation, $H(j\omega)$, was given by

$$H(j\omega) = \begin{cases} Ao\ e^{-j\ [\Delta t_{gr}\ \omega\ +\ \Delta t_c \omega_c]} & |\omega - \omega_c| \leq \omega_{Bw}/2 \\ 0 & \text{otherwise.} \end{cases} \qquad 2.$$

In the standard waveform (presented to alternate ears in the two observation intervals of each trial) Δt_{gr} and Δt_c were set to zero. To produce a "delayed" waveform with a pure delay or time shift for the other ear, Δt_c was set to zero and Δt_{gr} fixed to the delay required. To produce group delay only, Δt_c was set to have the same magnitude as, but opposite sign from, Δt_{gr}. Thus the group delay, $\frac{d\Delta\phi(\omega)}{d\omega}$, was $-\Delta t_{gr}$ but the phase delay at the carrier was zero. To produce a waveform with zero group delay, Δt_{gr} was set to zero and Δt_c set to give the required delay at ω_c. All frequencies had the same phase shift as the carrier thus leading to zero group delay but phase delays that were slightly different at each frequency in the signal. Since the phase spectrum of the standard signal nominally was zero, the interaural phase difference spectrum is that of the "delayed" waveform.

The impulse response of the filter, $h(t)$, is given by

$$h(t) = \frac{2Ao}{\pi} \left\{ \sin[(\omega_{Bw}/2)/(t-\Delta t_{gr})] \text{ X } \sin[\omega_c(t-\Delta t_{gr})-\omega_c\Delta t_c] \right\}, \qquad 3.$$

where the envelope and carrier of the signal are readily seen. The signals for a given condition were generated from 2048 samples of the waveforms described, sampled at 20 µs intervals and weighted by a Hamming window. The weighted

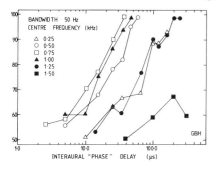

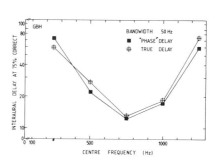

Fig. 1 shows the percentage of correct lateralization judgements as a function of interaural phase delay. The bandwidth of the transient signals was 50 Hz and centre frequency is shown as a parameter. Each point is based on 200 judgements from a single observer

Fig. 2 summarizes the results of Fig. 1 and shows the interaural phase delay corresponding to 75% correct judgements (logarithmic scale) as a function of centre frequency

sample values were rounded to fill the dynamic range of the 14-bit DAC's used to produce the analogue waveforms and stored. Signals for the ears were generated simultaneously, passed through matched low-pass filters set at 10 kHz to matched pairs of TDH-39 earphones driven in phase.

A trial consisted of two observation intervals. In the first, the standard
waveform was presented to one ear and the "delayed" waveform presented to the
other. In the second observation interval (which followed after a pause of
about 600 milliseconds) the signals to the ears were interchanged. The
observers were required to indicate the interval in which the signal appeared to
lie farther to the left.

3. RESULTS

Fig. 1 shows the percentage of correct lateralization judgements (linear)
as a function of interaural phase delay (logarithmic). The transients had a
bandwidth of 50 Hz and their centre frequency is shown as the parameter. Since
the functions are parallel on these coordinates the data can be summarized
conveniently by specifying the delay corresponding to one performance level –
75% correct, say.

Fig. 2 shows the phase delay (logarithmic scale) corresponding to 75%
correct judgements as a function of the centre frequency of the 50-Hz wide
filter specifying the signal. The results, based on a single observer (the
author) are similar to those Zwislocki and Feldman (1956) obtained with tones;
there is a broad minimum near 700 Hz and lateralization on the basis of phase
delay in a 50-Hz wide signal is impossible if the centre frequency of the band
exceeds about 1500 Hz.

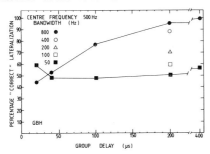 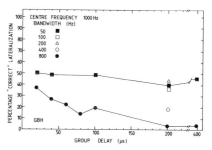

*Fig. 3 shows percent correct laterali
zation as a function of interaural
group delay. Each point is based on
200 observations from a single
observer and the parameter is bandwidth. Signals were centred on 500 Hz*

*Fig. 4 shows percent correct latera-
lization as a function of interaural
group delay. Each point is based on
200 observations from a single
observer and the parameter is bandwidth. Signals were centred on 1 kHz*

Fig. 3 shows the percentage of correct lateralization judgements for the
same observer as a function of group delay. The signal was centered on 500 Hz
and the parameter is the bandwidth. The observer is unable to use group delay
with signals 50 Hz wide even with very large interaural delays. When the delay
was fixed at 200 μs, however, and bandwidth increased, lateralization improved
so that at a width of 800 Hz nearly errorless lateralization was achieved.
Performance even with this bandwidth, however, is much worse than with phase
delay.

Fig. 4, however, shows the percentage of correct lateralization judgements
obtained with 1 kHz centre frequency; lateralization is again impossible with
signals of narrow bandwidth. Increasing bandwidth for a fixed 200-μs delay
yields consistent but unusual lateralization; with 800-Hz bandwidth, the
observer reliably lateralizes the signal towards the ear receiving the waveform
with group delay. Similar results for two additional observers are shown in
Henning (1983).

Fig. 5 shows results extending the observations of Figs. 4 and 5 to
different centre frequencies. The percentage of "correct" lateralization for
signal of 800 Hz bandwidth and 100 s group delay as a function of the centre
frequency of the band. Performance is almost errorless for low-frequency

signals and is in the sense one might expect; the sound is heard from the side of the head away from the "delayed" signal. Lateralization performance decreases to 50% correct for signals centred near 650 Hz (observers can, of course, achieve 50% correct by guessing). Consistent lateralization occurs for signals greater than 650 Hz but it is lateralization in the opposite sense; that is, sources are heard on the side receiving the "delayed" signal. Virtually errorless performance (0% correct) is obtained over a wide frequency region up to 1.5 kHz where performance begins to deteriorate towards 50% correct (the guessing level).

4. DISCUSSION

The results of Figs. 3 and 4 make it clear that the observer is unable to lateralize narrow-band, low-frequency transients on the basis of interaural group delay. Although the results (Fig. 3) with 800 Hz wide signals centered on 500 Hz seem to suggest that group-delay based lateralization is possible with wideband signals, the results with identical bandwidths centered on 1 kHz (Fig. 4) make this interpretation unlikely; lateralization based on group delay would yield similar results at both centre frequencies.

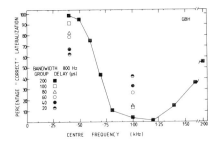

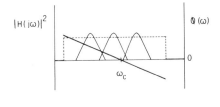

Fig. 5 shows the percentage of "correct" lateralization judgements based on a group of 200 μs in an 800-Hz wide signal as a function of centre frequency. Each point is based on 200 judgements from one observer

Fig. 6 is a schematic representation of group delay in a signal that has a bandwidth greater than the local critical bandwidth. The signal has both group and phase delay in the band above the centre frequency of the signal and group delay but phase advance in the band centred below the centre frequency of the signal

A plausible explanation of the results may be found by noting that the signals of 50 Hz bandwidth are narrower than the narrowest estimates of the critical bandwidth in the low-frequency region. And group delay is ineffectual with this bandwidth. The signals of 800 Hz bandwidth are much wider than the critical bandwidth so that bands centred below and above the centre frequency of the signal have significant levels of stimulation. For bands that are not centred on the centre frequency of the signal there is both group <u>and</u> phase delay as examination of Fig. 6 readily shows. Bands centred above the centre frequency of the signal have the group delay of the signal together with a phase delay; critical bands centred below the centre frequency of the signal have the group delay of the signal but a phase advance at their centre frequency. There are thus conflicting lateralization cues based on phase delay in different regions. The resultant lateralization appears to be a compromise in which information from the band near 650 Hz is heavily weighted (Bilsen and Raatgever, 1973).

The results of this study with transients, then, are consistent with inferences drawn earlier (Henning and Ashton, 1981) from experiments using amplitude-modulated tones: observers can use phase delay, but not group delay, in extracting information about the direction of a source of low-frequency signals.

Acknowledgements: Figures 1, and 3 - 5 are published with the kind permission of Elsevier Biomedical Press. The research was supported by an N.I.H. Grant to Dr. E.R. Hafter and the Medical Research Council of Great Britain.

REFERENCES

Bilsen, F.A., Raatgever, J, (1973). Spectral dominance in binaural lateralization. *Acustica* **28**, 131-132.

David, E.E., Guttman, N., van Bergeijk, W.A. (1959). Binaural interaction of high frequency stimuli. *J.Acoust.Soc.Am.* **31**, 774-782.

Henning, G.B., Ashton, J. (1981). The effect of carrier and modulation frequency on lateralization based on interaural phase and interaural group delay. *Hearing Res.* **4**, 185-194.

Henning, G.B. (1983). Lateralization of low-frequency transients. *Hearing Res.* **6** 153-172.

Papoulis, A. (1962). *The Fourier Integral and its Applications,* New York, McGraw-Hill.

Rabiner, L.R., Gold, B. (1975). *Theory and Application of Digital Signal Processing,* Englewood Cliffs, N.J., Prentice-Hall.

Stevens, S.S., Newman, E.B. (1934). The location of actual sources of sound. *Am.J.Psychol.* **119**, 297-306.

Wallach, H. (1940). The role of head movements and vestibular and visual cues in sound localization. *J.Exp.Psychol.* **27**, 339-368.

Zwislocki, J.J., Feldman, R.S. (1956). Just-noticeable differences in dichotic phase. *J.Acoust.Soc.Am.* **28**, 860-864.

GENERAL DISCUSSION

DE BOER:
In the case of true interaural delay there are phase delays in the various frequency bands. Do I correctly interpret your results when I conclude that in the case of true delay lateralization is determined by interaural phase delay in the individual bands?

HENNING:
For both pure delays and carrier (or phase) delays it appears that lateralization is indeed based on a band-by-band comparison of interaural phase delays. Some bands are more important than others, however, and a rough idea of their relative contribution can be gained from Fig. 2. In the high-frequency region, of course, it is a different matter.

KIM:
Is there any observed physiological correlate of the binaural dominance effect around 750 Hz that you just described?

CAIRD:
In the Superior Olivary Complex of cat cells seem to be sensitive to interaural phase of signals only below about 1 kHz (unpublished data) so this may be the physiological correlate you seek. As soon as you have more than one cycle in your low frequency signal, you will have mostly phase locked information in the discharge of your auditory nerve fibres, so I think that the dominance of phase delay at low frequencies is a peripheral phenomenon.

RAATGEVER:
We think the spectral dominance of the 600-700 Hz region cannot be understood completely as a peripheral process. The weighting of the low-frequencies probably is the result of some peripheral processes decreasing the synchronization of the spike generation. However, the dominance is sharper than can be expected on the basis of this weighting alone. Most likely we are dealing with a more central process like focussing the attention at that frequency region where the binaural time processing seems to operate optimally. Our data concerning unharmonic dichotic pitches also confirm this rather sharp dominance of the 600 Hz region. (Bilsen, J.A.S.A. 61, 150, 1977; Raatgever, Dissertation, Delft University, 1980)

LATERALIZATION OF TRANSIENTS PRESENTED AT HIGH RATES:
SITE OF THE SATURATION EFFECT

E. R. Hafter, and E. M. Wenzel

Dept. of Psychology, Univ. of California
Berkeley, Calif. 94720, USA.

1. INTRODUCTION

There is a growing concensus among those who study sound localization that
an assertion of the classic duplex theory, the insensitivity to Interaural Differences of Time (IDTs) in frequencies above about 1200 Hz, is fundamentally wrong.
Although the theory is true for sinusoids, studies using amplitude modulation (AM)
have shown that temporal information can be extracted from the stimulus envelopes
of high frequencies (e.g., Leakey *et al*., 1958; Bielek, 1975; Henning, 1974;
Nuetzel and Hafter, 1976, 1981; McFadden and Passanen, 1976; McFadden and Moffitt,
1977). While there are cautionary demonstrations that observers may, in some
cases, be listening for IDTs in the highly attenuated, low-frequency skirts of a
nominally high-frequency signal (Yost *et al*., 1971; Bernstein and Trahiotis, 1981),
the fact remains that with AM, the region below 1500 HZ can be masked without
destroying the ability to detect an IDT. Thus one may conclude that envelope
timing is indeed coded and available to the central nervous system for binaural
interaction.
     Why is the binaural system deaf to IDTs in high-frequency tones but not in
AM? In seeking an answer to this question, we have employed a form of pulse modulation consisting of a train of filtered clicks. Unlike the wideband stimuli of Yost
(1976), the center frequencies (cf's) of our clicks are restricted to high frequencies. With trains of clicks, cf is analogous to the carrier frequency of sinusoidal AM; the analogue of modulation frequency is the inverse of the Interclick Interval (ICI). Of primary interest in these experiments has been the joint effect of
the ICI and the number of clicks in a train (n) on the interaural threshold (ΔIDT).
Following an approach derived from Houtgast and Plomp (1968) we have measured the
effect on binaural thresholds of increasing n, with the modulation frequency as the
critical parameter. The assumption is that, if each click in the train is equally
effective in conveying information, there should be a $1/\sqrt{n}$ reduction in the standard deviation of the internal noise which limits detection. If true, the relation
between thresholds for n clicks (ΔIDT_n) and that for only 1 click should be

$$\Delta\text{IDT}_n = \Delta\text{IDT}_1 / \sqrt{n} \tag{1}$$

In logarithmic form, this predicts a linear function with a slope of -0.5:

$$\log \Delta\text{IDT}_n = \log \Delta\text{IDT}_1 - 0.5 \log n \tag{2}$$

At the symposium in Noordwijkerhout (Hafter *et al*.,1980) we presented data for modulation frequencies varying from 100/s to 1000/s and trains of 1 to 32. With an ICI
of 10 ms, the slopes of the log functions approach the hypothetical value of -0.5.
For shorter ICIs, the functions remain linear but their absolute slopes move toward
0.0. In subsequent papers (Hafter and Dye, 1983; Hafter *et al*., 1983), we have
argued that none of the three causes commonly thought to limit high-frequency

1. *Some of the data in Expt. I were presented at a meeting of the Acoustical*
   Society of America (Hafter and Wenzel, 1982).

neural coding can account for this decrease in the absolute slopes. The rejected
models include: (a) loss of information due to limited bandwidths in the auditory
system, i.e., a reduction in the depth of modulation;   (b) loss due to neural refractoriness, i.e., a reduction in the number of evoked events when clicks occur
during the absolute refractory periods of relevant neurons; (c) loss due to lack of
independence between successive samples of the added internal noise. Each, it is
argued, leads for all values of n to a stationary process in which the probability
of encoding information derived from the jth click equals that from $(j - 1)$.
Obviously, for all of these models, the overall efficiency of transduction of the
envelope cues must be lower at high rates. An example of this is easily seen in the
case where the frequency of modulation is so high that the sidebands fall outside
of an auditory filter, turning what is AM at the earphones into a high-frequency
tone in the nervous system. What is important, though, is that for stationary processes, the loss translates into an upward shift in the intercept of the log plots,
leaving the slopes at $- 0.5$.
   An alternative model offered to explain the effects of high rates of stimulation envisions a form of neural saturation. Noting that a change in slope of the
log functions is achieved by raising the denominator of Eq. (1) to a power less
than 1.0, we proposed that n should be replaced by N, a hypothetical number proportional to the neural representation of the n stimulus events. If N is a compressive power function of n,

$$n \propto N^k \qquad \text{where } 0.0 \leq k \leq 1.0 \qquad \text{and } k = f(\text{ICI}) \qquad (3)$$

the log function becomes

$$\log \Delta \text{IDT}_n = \log \Delta \text{IDT}_1 - 0.5 \, k \, \log n \qquad (4)$$

   The relation in Eq. (3) suggests that saturation at high rates makes each
click in a train less effective than the one before, with the probability of
evoking a neural event on the jth click defined by the relation

$$P(j) = (j)^k - (j - 1)^k \quad \text{where} \quad 0.0 < k < 1.0 \quad \text{and} \quad k = f(\text{ICI}) \qquad (5)$$

For values of the compressive power, k, less than 1.0, this process is non-stationary, describing a decline in efficiency as the train progresses. The notion that
lateralization may be more influenced by the initial portion of a dichotic signal
than that which follows is not a new one; it is essentially a statement of binaural
"precedence" or the "law of the first wavefront" (Wallach et al., 1949; Blauert,
1971; Zurek, 1980). What is different about the relation in Eq. (3) is that the
strength of the compression is dependent on the modulation frequency so that the
reduction in the importance of ongoing sound is a function of the information rate.
   A most intriguing aspect of the loss of information at high rates is seen if
a similar logic is applied to lateralization of interaural differences of intensity
(IDIs). It is well known that listeners can detect IDIs in high-frequency tones.
Thus, it is somewhat surprising to find that when listeners were asked to detect
IDIs in trains of clicks, the results were virtually indistinguishable from those
with IDTs. That is, for higher click rates, the log threshold vs. log n plots produce linear functions whose slopes grow more shallow with shorter ICIs. This suggests the possibility of a common mechanism for saturation, perhaps in regions peripheral to the binaural system, through which all information presented at a high
rate is subject to compression. Arguments concerning why this might be advanta-
geous to a nervous system trying to conserve effort are presented in Hafter (1983).

2. THE SITE OF THE SATURATION

   In the research to be described, the intent was to illuminate the neural
site(s) of the proposed saturation. Once again, listeners lateralized trains of di-

chotic clicks, only this time, the trains consisted of two types of clicks that differed on a single dimension, for example, carrier frequency. Figure 1 illustrates the logic of these experiments, showing hypothetical time-lines for trains of clicks. Each mark represents a dichotic click with an interaural difference to be detected. The two types of clicks are labelled A and B and what is shown are the experimental designs for three basic conditions. In the first, depicted in

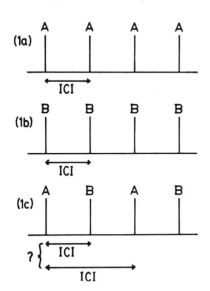

Fig. 1a, the clicks were all of type A, that is, identical to one another. As before, performance was measured as a function of ICI and n, with reductions in the absolute slopes of the log-threshold vs. log-n plot taken as the sign of saturation. Figure 1b shows a similar condition except that the clicks were all type B. The condition shown in Fig. 1c was meant to get at the question of site. In this case, the two types of click were alternated within a single train. Listeners reported hearing these trains as single percepts, suggesting treatment of them as unitary stimuli at some level in the binaural process. Implicit in Eqs. (4) and (5) is an assumption that the clicks are alike except for their positions in the train. The question then was whether the mechanism of saturation would treat type A and type B clicks as being alike? More specifically, would the *effective* ICI be the interval between adjacent clicks, regardless of the A-B dimension, or the interval between alternates, with type A's interacting only with A's and B's with B's?

Fig 1. Schematic representation of the logic of Expts. I and II. Each vertical mark represents a dichotic click (see text)

In the experiments to be described, the A-B dimension was defined in two ways. In the first, it referred to the carrier frequencies of the clicks, with the interest being in whether the saturation was cross-spectral or within individual bands. In the second, A-type clicks contained an IDT while B-types contained an IDI. Here, the question was whether the process of saturation acts across interaural information *per se*.

3. PROCEDURE

Stimuli were generated by a PDP-11/34 computer at a sampling rate of 50 kHz, low-pass filtered through 10 kHz filters (Frequency Devices 901F) with 48 dB/octave skirts and presented through STAX SR-5 electrostatic headphones. Each click was the product of a cosine at the frequency of the carrier and a Gaussian whose ±1 sigma points were .455 ms. Thus, the duration between points 40 dB below the peak was 1.39 ms. Trains were made by repeating the clicks at the rate 1/ICI. For the carriers used, the spectrum was symmetric about the carrier, down by 40 dB at ±2250 Hz.

Percentage of correct responses, P(C)s, were based on 100-trial runs in a two-alternative, forced choice (2AFC) task. Each trial presented one train that sounded to the left of center and one that sounded to the right. Listeners indicated the direction of lateral movement between alternatives and visual feedback was given after each trial. Subjects received at least 30 hours of practice before testing began.

4. EXPERIMENT I: ALTERNATION OF CARRIER FREQENCIES

In this experiment the A-B dimension referred to the center frequencies of the individual clicks, with A and B being 4000 and 6000 Hz respectively. In order to compensate for differences of detectability between the two types, preliminary testing with each subject was done to determine the absolute thresholds for single clicks. Lateralization was tested with clicks set to be 60 dB SL. For both kinds of conditions, *single-carrier* and *mixed*, every click in a train contained the same value of interaural delay. Obviously, the mixed conditions required even numbers of clicks and for these, the first click in the train was chosen to be 4000 Hz. The ICIs tested were 2.5 ms and 5 ms. One or more points were used to obtain performance estimates both below and above the target value of P(C) = 76% and a threshold for interaural time, ΔIDT, was computed by interpolation.

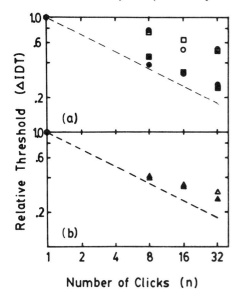

Fig. 2. Relative thresholds (see text) for trains of clicks plotted as functions of n. Carrier frequencies are: 4000 Hz (circles); 6000 Hz (squares); Alternating (triangles). ICIs are: 2.5 ms (open symbols); 5 ms (closed)

The results of Expt. 1, averaged across three subjects, are shown in Fig. 2. Interaural thresholds and the numbers of clicks are plotted logarithmically. Since our primary interest is in the slopes, the intercepts were made identical before averaging by first dividing the obtained values of each ΔIDT by the listener's own ΔIDT for 1 click.[2] The dashed lines have slopes of – 0.5. They represent stationary performance as defined by a k of 1.0 in Eq. (5). The parameter is the ICI.

Data from the single-carrier conditions are shown in Fig. 2a. For both the 4000-Hz and 6000-Hz clicks, depicted by circles and squares respectively, the slopes for ICIs of 5 ms were more shallow than the value of – 0.5 that would imply no saturation. Specifically, they were –.41 and –.40, suggesting that some saturation was present even at this slower rate. For ICIs of 2.5 ms, the absolute slopes declined further, as expected, in these cases to 0.19 and 0.18 respectively. Fig. 2b shows the data with alternating carrier frequencies. Here, the slopes of the two functions are nearly identical, –0.37 and –0.40. Thus, it would seem that the nominal 2.5-ms ICI of the mixed condition was treated by the auditory system as though it was a 5 ms interval.

A comparison of the upper and lower halves of the figure shows that high stimulus rates reduced the informational effectiveness of the ongoing train at either 4000 or 6000 Hz but that there was no compression across bands. This interaction with carrier frequency clearly indicates that the mechanism of saturation is within individual frequency channels.

5. EXPERIMENT II: ALTERNATION OF TIME AND INTENSITY

In Expt. II, the *A-B* dimension referred to the nature of the interaural difference to be detected. Thus, for the *single-type* conditions, each click in a train contained either an IDT or an IDI. Figure 3 illustrates an example of a *mixed* condition in which the alternation was between clicks having an IDT and those with an IDI. The first click in the train was chosen at random to have either an IDT or an IDI. To eliminate monaural spectral cues introduced by the presence of an IDT on alternate clicks, those with an interaural difference of time were made by inserting a lead of 1/2 IDT in one channel and a delay of 1/2 IDT in the other. Similarly, clicks with a difference of intensity were 40 dB + 1/2 IDI in one

2. *Stimulus values used by the 3 subjects for the single-click conditions were for 4000 Hz, 116, 68 and 118 us; for 6000 Hz, 118, 144 and 198 us.*

channel and 40 - 1/2 IDI in the other. Throughout,
the carrier frequency was 4000 Hz and levels were
set to 40 dB SPL. ICIs were 2.5 and 5 ms.

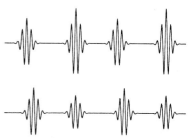

   While the psychophysical technique remained
2AFC, the P(C)s so obtained were converted to the
detection index d'. We assumed that, just as with
the log-threshold plots above, for a single
value of the stimlus (an IDT, an IDI or a combination of both), a stationary process would predict
slopes of + 0.5 in the log-d' vs. log n functions
while saturation would lead to a reduction in the
slope. The decision to use d's instead of thresholds was based on the belief that it would be impossible to obtain psychometric functions for the
mixed cases since there would be no way to pick
appropriate pairs of values. Instead, psychometric

*Fig. 3.   An example of alter-
nating IDTs and IDIs.   Shown are
signals to the left and right
ears*

functions were first obtained for the single-type conditions at $n = 4$. Then, the
IDT or IDI that produced a d' of 0.50 for each subject was used for the remainder
of the tests, both with IDTs and IDIs alone and mixed.
   The results of this experiment, averaged across two subjects, are shown in
Fig. 4 as logarithmic plots of d' vs. n. The intercepts were made identical before
averaging, in this case by dividing each d' by that listener's d' for 4 clicks.[3]
Here, the dashed line has a slope of + 0.5. The parameter is the ICI. Solid symbols
are for an ICI of 5 ms, open for 2.5 ms.

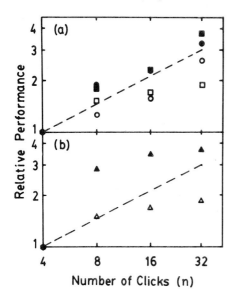

An immediately apparent difference between these data and the results of Expt.
I is the fact that for long ICIs, the
slopes are in excess of the presumed optimum of + 0.5. We have no ready explanation for this except perhaps to note that
both subjects seemed to have special difficulty with the low levels of performance that defined the conditions with
trains of 4 clicks. It may be that attention played a larger role in determining
d's of around 0.50, depressing those
points relative to the others.
   Fig. 4a shows results from the
single-type conditions. For ICIs of 5 ms,
the slopes are 0.59 for IDTs (circles)
and 0.63 for IDIs (squares). As in Expt.
I, reducing the ICI to 2.5 ms led to apparent saturation, with the slopes falling to 0.41 and 0.34 respectively. Fig.
4b shows the data obtained with alternating IDTs and IDIs. For an ICI of 5 ms,
the slope was 0.76 while for 2.5 ms it
fell to 0.28. Thus, unlike the results
of Expt. I, reducing the ICI with alternating As and Bs had an effect qualita-

*Fig. 4.   Relative performances (see
text) for trains of clicks plotted as
functions of n.   Interaural differences
are: IDTs (circles); IDIs (squares);
Alternating (triangles). ICIs are :
2.5 ms (open symbols); 5 ms (closed)*

tively similar to that obtained with s
and s alone. If every click in the
train acted to reduce the effectiveness
of its successor, regardless of the interaural information to be conveyed, it
suggests that the hypothetical neural
site where compression of binaural signals
takes place is a region which makes no
distinction between information derived from interaural time and intensity.

3. *Stimulus values used by the 2 subjects for the four-click conditions were:
    for an ICI of 2.5 ms, 104 us and 1.60 dB; 136 us and 1.40 dB;
    for an ICI of 5 ms, 60 us and 1.24 dB; 88 us and 1.04 dB.*

6. CONCLUSION

Expt. I showed that saturation takes place within individual frequency bands while Expt. II found no distinction on the basis of the type of interaural difference. When these results are taken together, they form the basis of a preliminary theory for the site of the mechanism, suggesting that the process takes place in the channels that feed into the binaural system. Segregated as these channels are by frequency, they do not compress information at high rates except for signals whose spectra overlap. However, by the point in the binaural chain where interaural differences have been encoded and turned into a perception of lateral space, the effects of saturation are complete and rate has no effect.

We wish to thank our colleague Ginny Richards for her valuable contributions toward developing the techniques for stimulus generation. This work was supported by a Grant from the National Institutes of Health, NS 07787.

REFERENCES

Bernstein, L.R. & Trahiotis, C. (1982). Detection of interaural delay in high-frequency noise. *J. Acoust. Soc. Am.* 71, 147-152.
Bielek, K. H. (1975). Sectrale Dominanz bei der interauralen Signalanalyse. Diploma Thesis, Ruhr-University, Bochum cited in Blauert, J. (1981) Lateralization of jittered tones. *J. Acoust. Soc. Am.* 70, 694.
Blauert, J. (1971). Localization and the law of the first wavefront in the median plane. *J. Acoust. Soc. Am.* 50, 466-470.
Blauert, J. (1982). Binaural localization: multiple images and applications in room- and electroacoustics. In: R. W. Gatehouse (Ed.) *Localization of Sound: Theory and Applications.* Amphora Press: Groton, 65-83.
Hafter, E. R. & Dye, R. H. Jr. (1983). Detection of interaural differences of time in trains of high-frequency clicks as a function of interclick interval and number. *J. Acoust. Soc. Am.* (in press).
Hafter, E. R., Dye, R. H., Jr., & Nuetzel, J. M. (1980). Lateralization of high-frequency stimuli on the basis of time and intensity. In: G. van den Brink & F. A. Bilsen, (Eds.) *Psychophysical, Physiological, and Behavioral Studies in Hearing.* Delft: Delft, 393-400.
Hafter, E. R. Dye, R. H. Jr. & Wenzel, E. M. (1983). Detection of interaural differences of intensity in trains of high-frequency clicks as a function of interclick interval and number. *J. Acoust. Soc. Am.* (in press).
Hafter, E. R. & Wenzel, E. M. (1982). Lateralization of trains of clicks having alternating center frequencies. *J. Acoust. Soc. Am.* 70, S81.
Henning, G. B. (1974). Detectability of interaural delay in high-frequency complex waveforms. *J. Acoust. Soc. Am.* 55, 84-90.
Houtgast, T. & Plomp, R. (1968). Lateralization threshold of a signal in noise. *J. Acoust. Soc. Am.* 4, 807-812.
Leakey, D. M., Sayers, B. McA. & Cherry, C. (1958). Binaural fusion of low- and high-frequency sounds. *J. Acoust. Soc. Am.* 30, 222-223.
McFadden, D. M. & Moffitt,C. M. (1977). Acoustic integration for lateralization at high frequencies. *J. Acoust. Soc. Am.* 61, 1604-1608.
McFadden, D. & Pasanen, E. (1976). Lateralization at high frequencies based on interaural time differences. *J. Acoust. Soc. Am.* 59, 634-639.
Nuetzel, J. M. & Hafter, E. R. (1976). Lateralization of complex waveforms: Effects of fine structure, amplitude, and duration. *J. Acoust. Soc. Am.* 60, 1339-1346.
Nuetzel, J.M. & Hafter, E. R. (1981). Lateralization of complex waveforms: Spectral effects. *J. Acoust. Soc. Am.* 69, 1112-1118.
Wallach, H., Newman, E. B., & Rosenzweig, M. R. (1949). The precedence effect in sound localization. *Am. J. Psychol.* 62, 315-336.
Yost, W. A. (1976). Lateralization of repeated filtered transients. *J. Acoust. Soc. Am.* 60, 178-181.
Yost, W. A., Wightman, F. L. & Green, D. M. (1971). Lateralization of filtered clicks. *J. Acoust. Soc. Am.* 50, 1526-1531.
Zurek, P. M. (1980). The precedence effect and its possible role in the avoidance of interaural ambiguities. *J. Acoust. Soc. Am.* 67, 952-964.

GENERAL DISCUSSION

MOORE:
The interpretation of your experiment II may be more complicated than you suggest.
The mechanisms coding time or intensity differences might initially act separately. Each might not be able to "ignore" the alternate clicks which contain no relevant disparity. Hence a train of clicks with alternating IDTs of Δt and 0 would
be treated as a train with $0.5\Delta t$. The saturation could still occur in the time
or intensity mechanisms separately, before their information is combined.

HAFTER:
You are absolutely correct in noting that Experiment II is based on the strong
and possibly incorrect assumption that non-informative events do not directly affect the detection. A non-informative event is one which is identical in the two
halves of the forced-choice trial. An example is the zero-value interaural delays
in the clicks with interaural differences of intensity. In a sense, such events
cannot be avoided, regardless of paradigm. Since any stimulus has a value on
every dimension, one must assume that identity across comparison makes these
events unimportant. However, that assumption is improven and I think your point
is well taken. Thus, I intend to reexamine our data with a close eye to an alternative solution which includes an averaging of the non-informative events with
the informative.

LANGNER:
In the auditory midbrain of the guinea fowl I found units with intrinsic oscillations which may be triggered by various kinds of amplitude fluctuations. The minimal period of these neuronal oscillations is 0.8 ms corresponding to 1250 Hz.
These intrinsic oscillations may be entrained by the periodicities of the acoustic
signals, e.g. by amplitude modulations. Would you agree that the properties of
these units may be important for lateralization of transients?

HAFTER:
In your paper you point out that the intrinsic oscillation is dominated by the
imposed AM for modulation frequencies as high as 1250 Hz but no higher. Our experience with psychophysical measurement suggests that your units have far more
accuracy than is needed to model lateralization. With sinusoidal AM, performance
shows rapid deterioration for modulation much above 600 Hz, a number only slightly exceeded using trains of high carrier-frequency impulses. If your question relates to the effect of neural activity uncorrelated with the information that our
listeners are using to lateralize, then I must assume that such intrinsic oscillation would act simply as a form of internal noise against which the interaural
delay must be detected.

DE BOER:
You are effectively studying a kind of cooperative phenomenon. In doing studies
on bandwidth effects, I found it necessary to monitor the shape of psychometric
function - just to avoid what Green has described as uncertainty. Therefore my
question: did you measure psychometric functions?

HAFTER:
We have done a systematic study of the slopes of the psychometric functions for
detection of interaural delay in trains of clicks. However, Yost and Dye have
studied the psychometric functions for various train lengths and rates where the
detection is of an interaural difference of intensity and they find no apparent
difference between slopes.

SCHARF:
Please comment on strong effect of intensity on lateralization threshold that you
found, since literature doesn't show, in general, that lateralization threshold
decreases very much with increasing stimulus level.

HAFTER:
You are referring to Dye's results which show a parallel shift of each log-ΔIDT v.
log-n function with a change of click level. We have found that lateralization on
the basis of interaural delay is rather strongly affected by level for weak to
moderate stimuli. This is true for both tones and impulses. The stimuli used here
are in that region, ranging from 20 to 60 dB SPL per click.

DYNAMIC CUES IN BINAURAL PERCEPTION

Richard M. Stern and Stephen J. Bachorski

Department of Electrical Engineering and Biomedical Engineering Program
Carnegie-Mellon University
Pittsburgh, Pennsylvania 15213 USA

1. INTRODUCTION

The binaural system is exquisitely sensitive in its ability to resolve very small interaural differences of arrival time for signals presented to the two ears. It is at first surprising, then, that the system is relatively poor at processing temporal changes in these interaural time differences. In recent years there has been an increased interest in the perception of binaural stimuli with time varying interaural time delays (ITDs), interaural intensity differences (IIDs), and interaural correlation. In this paper we review some of the results of psychoacoustical experiments using stimuli with time-varying interaural differences, and we present some new theoretical predictions to describe some of these data.

2. PERCEPTION OF STIMULI WITH TIME-VARYING INTERAURAL DIFFERENCES

In this brief review we will consider only experiments with stimuli using constantly changing interaural differences, presented through headphones. This excludes, for example, the literature on the precedence effect, as well as experiments using moving loudspeakers as sound sources.

First insights into the dynamics of the binaural system came largely from subjective reports of the perceptual images of stimuli presented with time-varying ITDs. For example, the presentation of two monaural pure tones with slightly different frequencies, one to each ear, establishes an interaural time difference that varies linearly as a function of time. Licklider, et al. (1950), Perrott and Musicant (1977), and others have noted that the presentation of two tones with frequencies below about 1 kHz causes the perception of a "rotating tone" that smoothly traverses the head in a quasi-sinusoidal function of time. As the IFD is increased, the dominant perception becomes one of a change in binaural loudness. Still greater IFDs cause the perception of a roughness in the sound and, ultimately, two difference smooth monaural tones.

Time-varying ITDs and IIDs are also established when two *binaural* tones of slightly different frequencies are presented simultaneously. It is easy to show that the instantaneous ITDs and IIDs produced by these stimuli [which we refer to as $\tau(t)$ and $\alpha(t)$], are complex periodic waveforms, with a shape that depends on the ITD, IID, and overall amplitude of each of the components. The fundamental frequency of $\tau(t)$ and $\alpha(t)$ is equal to the difference between the frequencies of the component tones.

Pairs of binaural tones have been used as stimuli in the detection experiments of McFadden et al. (1972), and in recent unpublished interaural time discrimination experiments by Kaiser and Stern. McFadden et al. measured $N_m S_m$ and $N_0 S_\pi$ detection using 400-Hz tonal maskers, varying the frequency of the tonal target as an experimental parameter. They found that the masking level differences (MLDs) for the two conditions were a nonmonotonic function of target-to-masker frequency separation, and that the greatest improvement in detection performance provided by the binaural system occurs when target and masker differ both by about 10 to 15 Hz. As McFadden et al. point out, it is probable that detection of the target in the $N_0 S_\pi$ configuration is affected by perception of motion of the brief target-masker complex, at least for small target-masker frequency separations.

Kaiser and Stern measured interaural time jnds for 500-Hz tonal targets in the presence of tonal maskers as a function of target-to-masker ratio and masker frequency, with the stimuli presented in the N_0S_0 and $N_\pi S_0$ configurations. They observed very little difference between jnds obtained in the presence of the N_0 versus the N_π maskers. In contrast, Cohen (1981), Ito et al. (1982), and Stern et al. (1983), all of whom measured interaural time and amplitude jnds in the presence of broadband maskers, observed that time jnds in the presence of the N_0 maskers were much smaller. These comparisons are interesting because if we assume that the peripheral auditory system includes a narrowband filtering operation, the probability distributions of $\tau(t)$ and $\alpha(t)$ for these experiments are identical for the tonal and broadband maskers. We believe that these two sets of jnds are different in form because $\tau(t)$ and $\alpha(t)$ for the combined target and masker vary much more slowly with the filtered broadband maskers than with the tonal maskers.

More recently, Grantham has studied various aspects of the dynamics of the binaural system in a series of experiments using forced-choice paradigms. For example, Grantham and Wightman (1977) measured the ability to discriminate broadband stimuli with sinusoidally varying ITDs from spectrally-matched diotic stimuli. Their results indicate that the binaural system is extremely "sluggish" in its response to the time-varying stimuli, as the discrimination performance becomes progressively worse as the frequency of the ITD is increased above about 5 Hz. In a later experiment Grantham and Wightman (1979) measured the detectability of short-duration tonal targets in the presence of narrowband maskers with sinusoidally varying interaural correlation, and they found that the binaural system is similarly slow to respond to temporal variations in the interaural correlation. From these results Grantham and Wightman estimated the effective integration time of the binaural system to be between approximately 45 and 140 ms for 500-Hz stimuli. Blauert, in an earlier (1972) study reported similar phenomena, but he used an experimental method that required the listeners to adopt a subjective criterion in forming their jnd.

3. BINAURAL MODELS FOR TIME-VARYING STIMULI

All of the above results are consistent with the general hypothesis that the binaural system can perfectly track the perceptual images of binaural stimuli with very slowly changing ITD, IID, or interaural correlation, but that the system is very slow to respond when the rate of change of these stimulus parameters exceeds a few Hz. However, the exact mechanism in the binaural system that limits the perception of temporally fluctuating stimuli has not yet been identified.

Most of the models that have been developed to describe and to predict the subjective perception of binaural stimuli are composed of similar structural components, which include peripheral bandpass filtering of the signals to the two ears, mechanisms for the estimation of ITD and IID, and a mechanism for the formation of spatial percepts from the estimated ITD and IID (cf. Colburn and Durlach, 1978). The slow temporal response that "blurs" the perception of time-varying ITDs and IIDs could occur after the level of, the peripheral filtering, the extraction of ITD and IID, or the percept-formation mechanism, or any combination of these levels of the system.

a) The Running Crosscorrelation Model

The earliest binaural model that could explicitly describe the perception of stimuli with time varying ITDs is that of Sayers and Cherry (1957). In the simplest formulation of this model, interaural timing information of the stimulus is obtained via a short-term or "running" crosscorrelation operation of the form

$$R_s(t,\tau) = \int_{-\infty}^{t} s_L(\alpha)\ s_R(\alpha-\tau)\ W(t-\alpha)\ d\alpha \tag{1}$$

where $s_L(t)$ and $s_R(t)$ are the inputs to the two ears, and $W(t)$ is a short-duration pulse that serves to cause more recent events to be more heavily weighted in the computation of the crosscorrelation function. Sayers and Cherry

used the temporal window $W(t) = e^{-kt}$ in their calculations, and proposed that
6 ms was a reasonable value for the integration time constant (Cherry, 1961).
Sayers and Cherry also proposed a method by which the inputs to the cross-
correlator could be weighted by the IID of the stimulus, and a mechanism for
judging the subjective laterality of the signals. They also proposed, in a subsequent elaboration of the model, a peripheral frequency analysis that could be
performed by autocorrelation of the signals to the two ears.

The running crosscorrelation model implicitly assumes that the lowpass
operation is part of the ITD estimator, since the expression for $R_s(t,\tau)$ is
mathematically equivalent to the output of a causal lowpass filter with impulse
response e^{-kt} when the signal $s_L(t)s_R(t-\tau)$ is the input. Since the expanded
Sayers and Cherry model also includes a time-intensity conversion that takes
place before the running crosscorrelation operation, temporal variations in IID
would be lowpass filtered as well. Unfortunately, Sayers and Cherry never compared the predictions of their model to experimental results using stimuli with
time-varying interaural differences. Blauert and Cobben (1978) did apply a
similar model to transient stimuli that produced the precedence effect, using a
value of 5 ms for the integration time.

*b) Extension of the Position-Variable Model to Describe Time Varying Binaural
Phenomena*

The position-variable model (Colburn, 1973; Stern and Colburn, 1978) was
developed to describe the lateralization, discrimination, and detection of
binaural stimuli in terms of firing patterns of the auditory nerves. In this
model information related to the ITD is contained within a timing function, the
IID information is contained within an intensity function, and a position vari-
ble $\hat{P}$ is generated by computing the centroid (or center of mass) of the product
of the timing and intensity functions. The firing times of the auditory nerve
are modeled as sample functions of nonhomogeneous Poisson processes. The timing
function, which is related to the interaural crosscorrelation of the stimuli, is
obtained from the outputs of hypothetical units which record coincidences of
this auditory-nerve activity, after a deterministic interaural delay. Specifically, the timing function is defined to be the total number of counts of a network of such units as a function of their interaural delay. This function may
be regarded as a quantification of earlier theories suggesting crosscorrelation
mechanisms (Jeffress, 1948; Sayers and Cherry, 1957; Licklider, 1959). The
intensity function is assumed to be a Gaussian-shaped pulse of constant width,
with a location that depends on the IID of the stimulus.

In the original formulation of the position-variable model, it was assumed
that all coincidences occurring during the presentation interval of the stimulus
tone contribute equally to the timing function. Stern and Colburn (1978)
represent the number of coincidences occurring over a stimulus interval by the
random function $L_m(\tau)$, where τ is the characteristic interaural delay parameter.
It can be shown that if the duration of the coincidence window, T_W, is sufficiently short, the expected value of $L_m(\tau)$ is approximately

$$E[L_m(\tau)] = T_W \int_0^{T_S} r_L(t)\, r_R(t-\tau)\, dt \qquad (2)$$

where T_S is the duration of the stimulus. The functions $r_L(t)$ and $r_R(t)$ are
the rate functions of the Poisson processes characterizing the auditory-nerve
response at a given characteristic frequency to the signals presented to the
two ears.

This model can easily be modified to produce a time-varying representation
of interaural timing information by allowing more recent coincidences to be
given greater weight in the formation of the timing function. The expected
value of this new time-varying function, which we refer to as $R_m(t,\tau)$ is

$$E[R_m(t,\tau)] = T_W \int_{-\infty}^{t} r_L(\alpha)\, r_R(\alpha-\tau)\, W(t-\alpha)\, d\alpha \qquad (3)$$

where the weighting function $W(t)$ in our calculations is of the form $W(t) = e^{-kt}$
for t greater than zero. This expression is obviously very similar to the

original running crosscorrelation function proposed by Sayers and Cherry (Eq.1), except that in the present model we are, in effect, crosscorrelating auditory-nerve rate functions rather than the acoustical stimuli themselves. If T_W is sufficiently small, the occurrences of coincidences of auditory-nerve activity can also be modeled as Poisson processes. It is then easy to verify that the function $R_m(t,\tau)$ can be modeled as a filtered Poisson process (Parzen, 1962). Because of this, the variance of $R_m(t,\tau)$ resulting from the variability of the auditory-nerve patterns is

$$\text{Var}[R_m(t,\tau)] = T_W \int_{-\infty}^{t} r_L(\alpha) \ r_R(\alpha-\tau) \ W^2(t-\alpha) \ d\alpha \qquad (4)$$

Given $E[R_m(t,\tau)]$ and $\text{Var}[R_m(t,\tau)]$, time-varying predictions for the mean and variance of the subjective lateral position, $\hat{P}$, may be obtained using the assumptions stated in Stern and Colburn (1978). Specifically, we obtain the expected value and variance of $\hat{P}(t)$ from the equations

$$E[\hat{P}(t)] = \frac{\int_{-\infty}^{\infty} \tau L_I(\tau) \ p(\tau) \ E[R_m(t,\tau)d\tau}{\int_{-\infty}^{\infty} L_I(\tau) \ p(\tau) \ E[R_m(t,\tau)]d\tau} \qquad (5)$$

and

$$\text{Var}[\hat{P}(t)] = \frac{\int_{-\infty}^{\infty} \tau^2 L_I^2(\tau) \ p(\tau) \ \text{Var}[R_m(t,\tau)]d\tau}{\{\int_{-\infty}^{\infty} L_I(\tau) \ p(\tau) \ E[R_m(t,\tau)]d\tau\}^2} \qquad (6)$$

where $p(\tau)$ is a function describing the relative number of fiber pairs as a function of their characteristic interaural delay, and $L_I(\tau)$ is the weighting function reflecting the stimulus IID, as discussed in Stern and Colburn (1978).

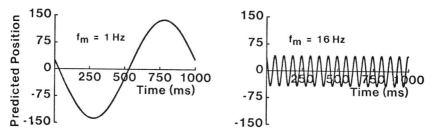

Fig 1. *Sample position predictions of the expanded position-variable model for stimuli with sinusoidally-varying ITDs of 1 and 16 Hz*

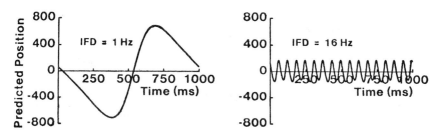

Fig 2. *Position predictions for binaural stimuli with interaural frequency differences of 1 and 16 Hz*

Figure 1 shows sample predictions for $E[\hat{P}(t)]$ for stimuli presented with sinusoidally varying ITDs of frequencies 1 and 16 Hz. Figure 2 shows similar predictions for a "rotating-tone" stimulus (producing a linearly increasing ITD) presented with IFDs of 1 and 16 Hz. Both sets of predictions were obtained using the same exponential temporal weighting used by Sayers and Cherry and Blauert and Cobben, with k equal to $(2\pi)(5)$ radians/s. This weighting function may be thought of as a lowpass filter with cutoff 5 Hz, or as a leaky integrator with a time constant of about 32 ms. We have found that the peak amplitude of excursion of $E[\hat{P}(t)]$ rolls off at about 6 dB/octave above 5 Hz for both sets of stimuli, which is consistent with the shape of $W(t)$. The units of the vertical axis are arbitrary, but consistent over the four sets of stimuli.

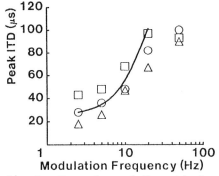

Fig. 3. *Comparison of theoretical predictions (curve) and data (symbols) of Grantham and Wightman (1978) from an experiment measuring the smallest "amplitude" of a sinusoidally-varying ITD needed for discrimination from a diotic stimulus*

In Figure 3 we compare predictions of the extended position-variable model to some of Grantham and Wightman's (1978) results describing the ability to discriminate targets with sinusoidally varying ITDs from diotic targets. These predictions were obtained by modelling the observed performance as that of an ideal receiver discriminating between two time-varying signals of the form $E[\hat{P}(t)]$ in the presence of an additive Gaussian noise process with average power equal to the average value of $Var[\hat{P}(t)]$. This is an oversimplified realization of the model, since it ignores the possibility that subjects may make use of temporal fluctuations in $Var[\hat{P}(t)]$ in forming their judgments. The theoretical predictions in Figure 3 are only relative, as the absolute predictions were freely adjusted to roughly describe the average of the data points at the modulation frequency of 2 Hz. Since the average variance of $\hat{P}(t)$ was found to be approximately constant over all ITDs and modulation frequencies of interest in the Grantham and Wightman experiment, predicted discrimination performance depends primarily on the "energy" of the function $E[\hat{P}(t)]$ for the stimuli with the sinusoidally varying ITDs. It is seen that, at least with the above assumptions, the model provides a reasonable description of the discrimination data for low modulation frequencies.

We presently believe that this type of model has the ability to characterize experimental phenomena incorporating dynamically changing ITDs, IIDs, and interaural correlations, although it is clear that many details remain to be worked out. For example, while the present calculations assume poor (running) temporal resolution only at the level of the interaural timing processor, it is also quite possible that the mechanisms producing the intensity functions and/or the mechanisms generating the subjective position percept are similarly limited in their ability to process binaural stimuli with dynamic interaural cues. We are currently attempting to gain greater insight into these phenomena and classes of models by comparing predictions and data for other discrimination experiments of Grantham and Wightman, McFadden et al., and Kaiser and Stern, under the assumption that performance in these experiments is limited by the variability of the auditory-nerve activity.

Acknowledgements. This research was partially supported by NIH grants 5 R01 NS14908 and 1 T32 GM07477. We also thank Stuart Meyer for assistance in some of the original theoretical calculations.

REFERENCES

Blauert, J. (1972). On the Lag of Lateralization Caused by Interaural Time and Intensity Differences. *Audiology* 11, 265–270.
Blauert, J. and Cobben, W. (1978). Some Consideration of Binaural Cross-correlation Analysis. *Acustica* 39, 96–103.
Cherry, C. (1961). Two Ears – but One World. In: *Sensory Communication.* (W.A. Rosenblith, ed.). pp. 99–117. Cambridge, MIT Press.
Cohen, M.F. (1981). Interaural Time Discrimination in Noise. *J. Acoust. Soc. Amer.* 70, 1289–1293.
Colburn, H.S. (1973). Theory of Binaural Interaction Based on Auditory-Nerve Data. I. General Strategy and Preliminary Results on Interaural Discrimination. *J. Acoust. Soc. Amer.* 54, 1458–1470.
Colburn, H.S., and Durlach, N.I. (1978). Models of Binaural Interaction. In: *Hearing.* Vol. IV of Handbook of Perception (E.C. Carterette and M.P. Friedman, eds.) New York, Academic Press.
Grantham, D.W. and Wightman, F.L. (1978). Detectability of Varying Interaural Temporal Differences. *J. Acoust. Soc. Amer.* 63: 511–523.
Grantham, D.W. and Wightman, F.L. (1979). Detectability of a Pulsed Tone in the Presence of a masker with Time-Varying Interaural Correlation. *J. Acoust. Soc. Amer.* 65, 1509–1517.
Ito, Y., Colburn, H.S., and Thompson, C.L. (1982). Masked Discrimination of Interaural Time Delays with Narrowband Signal. *J. Acoust. Soc. Amer.* 72, 1821–1826.
Jeffress, L.A. (1948). A Place Theory of Sound Localization. *J. Comp. Physiol. Psychol.* 41, 35–39.
Licklider, J.C.R. (1959). Three Auditory Theories. In: *Psychology: A Study of a Science, Study 1.* Vol. 1 (E.S. Koch, ed.). New York: McGraw-Hill.
Licklider, J.C.R., Webster, J.C., and Hedlun, J.M. (1950). On the Frequency Limits of Binaural Beats. *J. Acoust. Soc. Amer.* 22, 468–473.
McFadden, D.M., Russell, W.E., and Pullman, K.A. (1972). Monaural and Binaural Masking Patterns for a Low-Frequency Tone. *J. Acoust. Soc. Amer.* 51, 534–543.
Parzen, E. (1962). Stochastic Processes (Holden-Day, San Francisco).
Perrott, D.R., and Musicant, A.D. (1977). Rotating Tones and Binaural Beats. *J. Acoust. Soc. Amer.* 61, 1288–1292.
Sayers, B. McA., and Cherry, E.C. (1957). Mechanism of Binaural Fusion in the Hearing of Speech, *J. Acoust. Soc. Amer.* 29, 973–987.
Stern, R.M., Jr., and Colburn, H.S. (1978). Theory of Binaural Interaction Based on Auditory-Nerve Data. IV. A Model for Subjective Lateral Position. *J. Acoust. Soc. Amer.* 64, 127–140.
Stern, R.M., Jr., Slocum, J.E., and Phillips, M.S. (1983). Interaural Time and Amplitude Discrimination in Noise. *J. Acoust. Soc. Amer.* (in press).

GENERAL DISCUSSION

LINDEMANN:
In order to model the non-stationary behaviour of the binaural system in frequency bands I have proposed an extension to the crosscorrelation models which is
based on a lateral inhibition mechanism along the crosscorrelation axis.

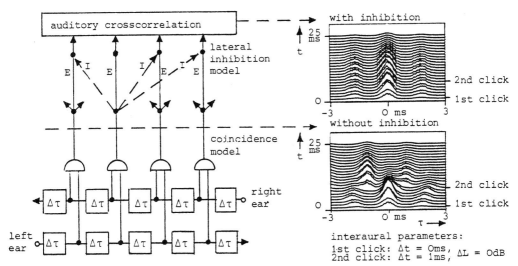

*Structure of the model and running auditory crosscorrelograms demonstrating the
Law of the first wavefront for clicks in a critical band centered at 500 Hz.*

The required EE- and EI-gates may be combined in different ways to achieve good
results. The proposed model has been matched to psychoacoustic data by choosing
the optimal time constants, especially for the inhibition mechanism, the spike
coincidence window and the spike firing process. The information about the onset
characteristics of the signal will be saved in this system with a time constant
which depends on the signal statistics within the corresponding frequency band.
For stationary signals this model not only evaluates interaural time differences
but also interaural level differences as well without further assumptions, and
trading curves can be computed from the model results. For non-stationary signals
the model can explain the law of the first wavefront and related psychoacoustical
effects (Lindemann and Blauert, DAGA/FASE, Göttingen, 1982; to be published).

STERN:
I thank you for calling your work to my attention, and look forward to seeing the
detailed predictions of your model. Bachorski and I have concentrated more on
simple stimuli with continually changing interaural differences because we can
characterize the neural response to these sounds with a little more confidence.
We haven't yet looked carefully at transient phenomena such as the law of the
first wavefront, although they clearly are important as well.

CAT SUPERIOR OLIVARY COMPLEX (SOC): THE BASIS OF BINAURAL INFORMATION PROCESSING

D. Caird and R. Klinke

Zentrum der Physiologie, J.W. Goethe-Universität Frankfurt
D-6000 Frankfurt/Main 70, Germany

The SOC is the first station in the ascending auditory pathway where binaural interactions occur and lesions of the pathway to and from the SOC result in impaired sound localization ability (Jenkins and Masterton 1982). The two major cues for localization of a sound source are differences in time of arrival at the two ears (Δtime) and interaural intensity differences due to sound shadowing by the head (Δint). Sound shadowing by the head is frequency-dependent, in the cat a maximum Δint of 15–20 dB is shown at and above 2 kHz, declining to around 0 below 1 kHz (Wiener et al., 1966). Conversely interaural phase differences (Δpha) are only important below about 1 kHz where a significant amount of phase-locked information is present in the discharge of primary auditory fibres. The two main binaural nuclei are the lateral (LSO) and medial (MSO) superior olivary nuclei. The main cell type in the LSO is high CF ipsilateral excitatory/contralateral inhibitory (EI) i.e. sensitive to Δint (Tsuchitani 1977) and the main MSO cell type is low frequency binaural excitatory (EE), often with ipsi (Ee) or contra (eE) ear dominant (Guinan et al., 1972). It has been suggested that the LSO codes high frequency Δint and the MSO low frequency Δtime/Δpha (Masterton and Diamond, 1967). This assumption is implicit in studies of Δtime processing in the SOC which have been confined to the MSO. This study is the first to look at the effect of Δtime on LSO cells. This point is important as high frequency signals can be localized on the basis of Δtime provided some form of amplitude modulation is present (McFadden and Pasanen, 1976). One can thus make a distinction between Δpha, ongoing time differences of a continuous periodic signal and Δtime, transient time differences in the envelope of any signal.

METHODS

Recordings were made from single units in the SOC of the Nembutal anaesthetized cat using a dorsal stereotactic approach. End-tidal CO_2 and blood pressure were monitored throughout each experiment. Electrodes were glass micropipettes filled with 3M KCL or Alcian Blue (Harnischfeger, 1979) or Fast Green (Woolf, 1981) dye solutions. Electrode tracks were reconstructed histologically from serial sagittal frozen sections. Both dye marking methods proved unreliable with fine electrodes under our recording conditions. In most cases unit location along a given track was to the reversal point of the click evoked field potentials (FPs). This point was taken to be the level of the MSO centre (Galambos et al., 1959; Guinan et al., 1972; Caird, unpublished). Sound stimuli (continuous tones, tone and noise bursts) were delivered through closed sound systems using 1" B & K 4145 condenser microphones. A digital bucket brigade delay line (based on Intersil TAD32A) was used to provide different interaural signal delays (1 µs steps, max. Δtime 2048 µs). Attenuation of left and right channels were independently varied to provide Δint. Left and right click evoked CAPs were recorded and Δint was adjusted to give the same hearing level at each ear.

RESULTS

a) LSO cells

Fig. 1 shows ipsilateral and contralateral Frequency Response Plots FRPs) obtained from an EI cell in the LSO with a pseudorandom stimulus programme (Caird et al., 1980). Typically, the FRPs are sharp and primarylike and the same on both sides, although complementary. In this spontaneously active example it can be seen

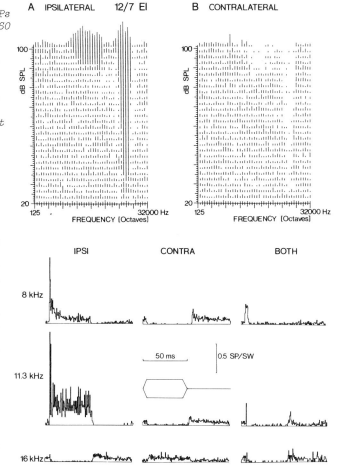

Fig. 1. Ipsilateral (A) and contralateral (B) FRPs from an EI cell in the LSO of 11.3 kHz CF. In this and subsequent figures the header number refers to experiment and unit. The FRPs were obtained with a pseudorandom stimulus programme (Caird et al., 1980); the height of each bar shows the number of spikes evoked by a tone burst at that frequency/intensity value. Note that the frequency characteristics of the ipsilateral excitatory and contralateral inhibitory response are identical, but complementary. This is more clearly seen in the PSTHs below (stimulation level = 80 dB SPL, nspikes = 1024). Not only do the main excitation and inhibition responses complement each other but the inhibitory ipsilateral side bands correspond to contralateral excitatory (or disinhibitory) sidebands, particularly clearly seen in the 16 kHz PSTH. This ipsi- and contralateral mirror image response is typical of LSO EI cells, although the inhibitory sidebands could only be seen in such spontaneously active cells. In all PSTHs 512 μs bins were used, the calibration SP/SW indicates the spikes/bin divided by the number of stimulus presentations

that this extends even to the inhibitory ipsilateral sidebands which correspond to excitatory contralateral sidebands (see 16 kHz PSTHs in Fig. 1. The PSTHs produced by LSO EI cells in response to CF (11.3 kHz in this case) tone burst stimulation consists of 5 - 8 ms latency "On" response, followed by a plateau (primary-like or "fast chopper" response). This response was strongly inhibited by contralateral stimulation (11.3 kHz PSTH in Fig. 1. The 'On' response was sensitive to Δtime of dichotic stimulation (Fig. 2). The response was progressively inhibited as contralateral time delay was decreased towards zero from values well outside the physiological range (400 - 500 μs maximum, see Blauert 1974, 1983). Shifting of the carrier signal within the fixed tone burst envelope (Δpha only) gave, as would be expected at these frequencies, no effect on cell response (dotted line in Fig. 2 B). An exception was shown by a 560 Hz LSO cell, which will be discussed later. Stimulation of these cells with noise bursts or noise masked tone bursts produced similar Δtime/response curves, i.e. these units were not affected by the spectral content of the signal provided that enough energy was present in the unit response area (Caird and Klinke, 1983). In summary, LSO EI cells show an inhibito-

Fig. 2 A. Δ*time response of an LSO EI cell when stimulated binaurally with CF tone burst. In this case max. delay range was used (contralateral from 4096 to 0 μs in 512 μs steps, ipsilateral delay constant 2048 μs) and 256 spikes counted at each delay step. Note that the initial "ON" response is progressively*

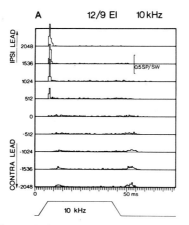
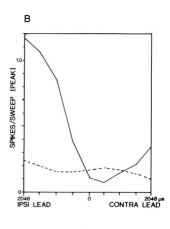

inhibited as contralateral delay reduces to zero Δtime.

B. This peak response (the highest peak plus its 4 neighbours) is plotted against Δtime (solid line). Shifting of the carrier alone (dotted line) had no effect. This one sided decline in response is typical of LSO cells. As contralateral lead increases, this response may show some recovery, as here or remain inhibited. The overall discharge rate (spikes/stimulus) was not affected by Δtime (contrast Fig. 4). The latency of the peak response is not significantly altered by contralateral inhibition (2048 – 0 μs ipsilateral lead in A). Where a recovery peak is seen, this appears to be a disinhibitory peak (0 – 2048 μs contralateral lead in A) with much longer latency. The stimulus envelope is shown below A.

ry Δtime response to signal envelope transients. This response is highest (least inhibited) when ipsilateral lead is greatest and decreases to a minimum around zero Δtime. In Fig. 3 a series of time curves at different contralateral SPLs shows the effect of Δint on an LSO EI cell. This effect is essentially the same as that of Δtime in that increasing "ipsilaterality" (i.e. ipsi sound pressure increase or time lead) gives a less inhibited response. In the area around zero interaural difference (cross in Fig. 3) the responses are complementary. Time intensity trading ratios calculated from 6 of these cells in the range from 0 – 512 μs ipsi lead gave values between 99 and 550 μs/dB.

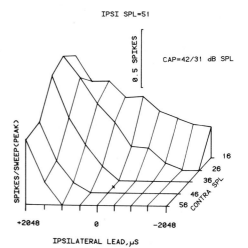

Fig. 3. The effect of changing contralateral SPL on Δtime curves from an LSO EI cell. The cross indicates the point where the two ears are stimulated at the same hearing level. Both Δint and Δtime response decline as the stimulus moves away from ipsilateral dominance (ipsi time lead or intensity increase) to reach a minimum around the zero point where the stimuli to both ears are equal

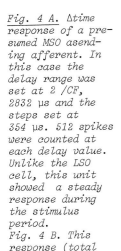

Fig. 4 A. Δtime response of a presumed MSO asending afferent. In this case the delay range was set at 2 /CF, 2832 μs and the steps set at 354 μs. 512 spikes were counted at each delay value. Unlike the LSO cell, this unit showed a steady response during the stimulus period.

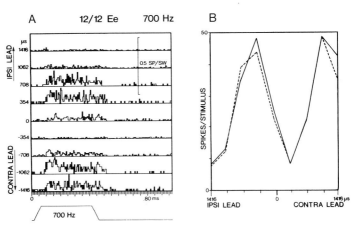

Fig. 4 B. This response (total spikes/stimulus presentation during the 45 ms stimulus period) for whole signal (solid line) and carrier only (dotted line) shifts is plotted against time. Note that the two curves are very similar and that there is a strong CF component in the response

b) MSO cells.

We found it difficult to record from MSO cells, as noted by other authors (Goldberg and Brown, 1968; Guinan et al., 1967). This is probably due to the thinness of the MSO and the very large FPs it generates. Nevertheless some data were obtained from units in or near the MSO and units ventrolateral to the LSO which we assume to be ascending MSO efferent fibres (see Caird and Klinke, 1983). MSO type cells had lower CFs, broader FRPs and mostly bilateral excitatory inputs (2:8:7:4 EE:eE:Ee:EI). A typical Δtime response from such an MSO type cell is shown in Fig. 4. Note that the response shows a 1/CF component and is the same to carrier only (dotted line) or whole signal shifts, i.e. the cell is responsive to Δpha. All the low CF (below 2 kHz) cells tested (n=6, including one LSO EI cell of 560 Hz CF) showed "characteristic delays" (Moushegian et al., 1971). A "characteristic delay" neuron was defined as one that shows a cyclic Δtime response as in Fig. 4 when stimulated with noise bursts or one that shows a cyclic Δtime response only at certain stimulation frequencies. In all cases however these "characteristic delays" were 1/CF and we could find no evidence that cells possessed "characteristic delays" in the physiological range, i.e. were sensitive to particular sound source angles. Time intensity trading measured in 2 cells gave much lower values (11 and 26 μs/dB) than those obtained from the LSO cells.

DISCUSSION

The LSO/MSO Δint/Δtime coding theory of Masterton and Diamond (1967) is not supported by the evidence presented here although LSO and MSO cells appear to code Δtime and Δint in different ways. LSO cells are affected by transient Δtime/Δint differences in signal envelopes whereas MSO cells are sensitive to Δpha and appear to be relatively unaffected by Δint. This would be expected from a mechanism that repeatedly samples Δtime, i.e. every carrier cycle, as opposed to the transient Δtime sampling in the LSO. In both cases further information processing higher in the CNS would be necessary before the direction of a sound source could be unambiguously coded.

Nevertheless the two separate psychophysical 'group delay' (Δtime) and 'phase delay' (Δpha) localization mechanisms (see Blauert, this volume) are clearly already present in LSO and MSO. Perhaps two distinct binaural nuclei have been evolved in the brainstem because the neural substrates needed for two types of

information processing are fundamentally different. If the bases of these interactions are indeed set by the characteristics of these SOC nuclei, then further
psychophysical research into the 'group delay' (LSO, binaural difference) and
'phase delay' (MSO, binaural addition) mechanisms combined with physiological
studies in the SOC would provide a unique combined approach to an important
problem in auditory physiology.

*Acknowledgement. This work was supported by the Deutsche Forschungsgemeinschaft
            (SFB 45).*

REFERENCES

Blauert, J. (1974). Räumliches Hören. Hirzel Verlag, Stuttgart. English version:
    Spatial Hearing. MIT Press, Boston, Mass. (1983, in press).
Caird, D.M., Göttl, K.-H., Klinke, R. (1980). Interaural attenuation in the cat,
    measured with single fibre data. *Hearing Res.* 3, 257 - 263.
Caird, D.M., Klinke, R. (1983) Processing of binaural stimuli by cat superior
    olivary complex neurons. *Exp. Brain Res.* , submitted
Galambos, R., Schwartzkopf, J., Rupert, A. (1959). Micro electrode study of
    superior olivary nuclei. *Am. J. Physiol.* 197, 527 - 536.
Goldberg, J.M., Brown, P.B. (1968). Functional organisation of dog superior
    olivary complex: Functional and anatomical study. *J. Neurophysiol.* 27,
    706 - 794.
Guinan, J.J., Norris, B.E., Swift, S.H. (1967). A paucity of unit responses in
    the accessory superior olivary nucleus of barbiturate anaesthetized cats.
    J. Acoust. Soc. Am. 41, 1585 - 1967.
Guinan, J.J., Norris, B.E., Guinan, S.S. (1972). Single auditory units in the
    superior olivary complex II. Locations of unit categories and tonotopic
    organisation. *Intern J. Neurosci* 4, 147 - 166.
Harnischfeger, G. (1979). An improved method for extracellular marking of
    electrode tip positions in nervous tissue. *Neuroscience Methods* 1, 195 -
    200.
Jenkins, W.M., Masterton, R.B. (1982). Sound localization: Effects of unilateral
    lesion in central auditory system. *J. Neurophysiol.* 47, (6) 987 - 1016.
Masterton, B., Diamond, I.T. (1967). The medial superior olive and sound locali-
    sation. *Science* 155, 1696 - 1697.
McFadden, D., Pasanen, E.G.(1976). Lateralisation at high frequencies based on
    interaural time differences. *J. Acoust. Soc. Am.* 59, 634 - 639.
Moushegian, G., Stillman, R.D., Rupert, A.C. (1971). Characteristic delays in the
    superior olivary complex and inferior colliculus. In: *Physiology of the
    Auditory System.* (Sachs, M.B. ed.) pp. 245 - 254. Baltimore National Education-
    al Consultants.
Tsuchitani, C.(1977). Functional Organisation of Lateral Cell Groups of Cat
    Superior Olivary Complex. *J. Neurophysiol.* 40, (2) 296 - 318.
Wiener, F.M., Pfeiffer, R.R., Bachus, A.S.N. (1966). On the sound pressure
    transformation by the head and auditory meatus of the cat.*Acta Otolaryngol.*
    61, 255 - 269.
Woolf, N.K. (1981). Precise extracellular marking in the auditory nerve with
    high impedance micropipettes. *Hearing Res.* 4, 121 - 125.

GENERAL DISCUSSION

KIM:
For neurones in an iso-CF strip of MSO, what physiological properties of the neurones vary? About how many neurones are there over an iso-CF axis? What percentage of neurones is EE, or EI type?

CAIRD:
I'm afraid that I do not have enough data to answer that. It is very difficult to
record from MSO units and I have not been able to systematically sample MSO units
in the longitudinal (iso-frequency) direction. The number of neurones in both LSO

and MSO is about 4000 and they seem to be about equally distributed in iso-frequency (longitudinal) and tonotopic (transverse) directions. The number of LSO (EI) and MSO cells is about equal in the cat. About one quarter of the MSO cells are EI and those we tested show the same Δpha propertics as the MSO EE cells.

COLBURN:
I have three comments about your interesting paper. First, I note that your example LSO cells seem to respond to the onsets and offsets of the stimulus when the intensity difference is zero. Since the stimuli are sinusoids of constant amplitude except for the onsets and offsets, you have not demonstrated a response to interaural group delay generally, only to interaural onset and offset time delays. Second, would you clarify what you mean by characteristic delay neurones and by the characteristic delays in the low-CF MSO cells. Your paper suggests you mean the period of the cyclic response versus the interaural delay; I do not believe that this is common usage. Finally, I don't understand why you choose to characterize the LSO cells as a "group delay localization mechanism" and at the same time to criticize Masterton and Diamond for their characterization as an interaural intensity mechanism. The cells are sensitive to both interaural onset delay and to interaural intensity difference. This is reasonable, of course, since a stimulus with an interaural onset delay has a large interaural intensity difference at the beginning of the stimulus.

CAIRD:
Using their tone bursts, the offset response in the LSO cells was always much smaller than the onset response. This would be expected as it was a disinhibition of the lower plateau region of the PSTH rather than an inhibition of the shown 'On' response. I accept your point that group delay in this case would imply a continuous AM modulation of the stimulus rather than just onset and offset ramps. Perhaps it is best to call it 'envelope Δtime'. As I said in the talk, though not in the paper, the peaks and dips of these cyclic MSO cells are also fairly randomly distributed and most are outside the physiological range. You are quite correct in saying that a tone burst cannot have an interaural delay without transient intensity differences. This is also true for any AM modulated signal or a pure Δpha low frequency sinusoid. What I wanted to criticize in Masterton and Diamond's theory was the assumption that Δtime and Δint are coded separately in the auditory system. I also think that psychophysical modellers should be careful not to make this assumption.

BROWNELL:
Your demonstration of ipsilateral inhibitory sidebands in an EI cell is a welcome confirmation of Goldberg's (Handb. Sensory Physiol. Vol. V/2, 1975) report of their existence in a few spontaneously active LSO units recorded in barbiturate anaesthetized animals as well as our own (Brownell et al., Brain Res. 177, 189, 1979) report of their presence in LSO units recorded in unanaesthetized decerebrate cats. How many of your units were characterized by ipsilateral inhibitory sidebands? The presence of contralateral disinhibitory sidebands is quite exciting. Again, how many of your units could be characterized by this feature? In our own studies of histologically confirmed LSO units similar disinhibitory sidebands were not a conspicuous feature. Is it possible that the EI unit shown in Fig. 1 may have been recorded outside the LSO? You have made a welcome and significant contribution to our understanding of binaural interactions by demonstrating that the response characteristics of LSO and MSO units is most likely richer than previously thought. In your presentation, however, you seemed to imply certain limitations in their response characteristics because they were not present in your preparation. By implying such limitations you may be guilty of perpetuating yet another set of simplifications. We have demonstrated that barbiturate anaesthesia can increase the latency of response to tonal stimuli, and decrease the coefficient of variation of their interspike interval distribution (Brownell et al., as above) suggesting that barbiturate anaesthesia may effect temporal processing. We have also noted that binaural stimulation, in the unanaesthetized decerebrate preparation, within the physiological range of interaural intensity differences, results in strongly non-monotonic rate intensity functions at CF and frequency intensity response maps that are dominated by inhibition. The response maps re-

semble those of type IV units originally described by Evans and Nelson (Exp. Brain Res. 17, 402, 1973) and Young and Brownell (J. Neurophys. 39, 282, 1976) in the cat DCN. It would seem that the richness of response characteristics of LSO units is indeed greater than previously thought and that we may not have reached the limits of their binaural processing capabilities.

CAIRD:
All spontaneously active units seemed to have inhibitory sidebands. I think that you should be careful not to assume that non-spontaneous units do not have inhibitory sidebands just because you can't see them with pure tone stimuli. I did not systematically look for contralateral disinhibitory sidebands, so I don't know how many cells have them. Your work in the Trapezoid Body where inhibitory sidebands are already present (Brain Res. 94, 413, 1975) suggests to me that you could find inhibitory ipsilateral/disinhibitory contralateral sidebands in most, if not all, LSO units if you systematically looked for them. I'm fairly certain that the unit in Fig. 1 was in the LSO. I'm sure that you're right in saying that barbiturate anaesthesia will suppress complex features of SOC cell responses. This is particularly true of any modulation due to descending influence. However, we are only 2 or 3 synapses away from the VIIIth nerve and I think that the relatively simple effects that I showed are qualitatively not affected by anaesthesia.

MERZENICH:
There is, in fact, strong but largely indirect evidence that: MSO neurones are strongly driven by binaural stimulation (nearly all have response maxima) across the behavioural range of interaural delays; MSO neurones have "characteristic delays"; and those characteristic delays do not necessarily fall at response minima or maxima. Most unit population studies have been conducted within the MSO projection zone of the ICC, with perhaps the most relevant series being those of Rose and colleagues, Roth, and Yin and colleagues. The limited data presented by Caird and Klinke does not constitute a clear challenge to the "LSO/MSO delta intensity/delta time coding theory", as they suggest. The basic role of these nuclei for intensity difference and time difference coding are well established by both intranuclear evoked response and unit studies. The authors' data do suggest a possible contribution of LSO neurones to the encoding of "group delay". However, without a more careful analysis of response properties of populations of neurones across the behavioural range of delays, and with AM stimuli, their possible contribution to group delay encoding is uncertain. It is likely that group delays are encoded, at least in part, in the MSO (along with phase delays).

CAIRD:
I do not understand how you define a "characteristic delay" which is not a maximum or minimum. I assume that this is the point of greatest slope of the Δpha function which would support my point that the information from the MSO must be processed elsewhere to unambiguously encode sound source direction. In this case systematic variation of this Δpha function across cells in a given iso-frequency band will give neurones with "characteristic delays". These neurones will, however, be higher in the CNS - perhaps the MSO projection zone in the Inferior Colliculus. I agree that our (and other published) results on the MSO cells are not sufficient to test this hypothesis properly. I do think that our data present a clear challenge to, or rather modification of, the MSO/LSO Δtime/Δint coding theory. We show that these two nuclei are both coding Δtime and Δint but in different ways which correspond nicely to the psychophysical data on lateralization of low and high frequency signals. I also do not think that the MSO codes group delays as phase delays as the psychophysical data presented by Blauert and Henning show that the CNS cannot localize sound sources on the basis of low frequency group delays.

PICK:
I have been attempting to record brain-stem evoked responses, in man, to interaural time differences in a continuous white-noise stimulus. This produces a very compelling percept. Although my investigations are not complete, it would appear that little, or no, evoked response is elicited in the latency range 0-16 ms. This might be interpreted as suggesting that there is no strong phasic response within the brain-stem to this stimulus, possibly because of the broadband nature of the stimulus.

CAIRD:
We have been comparing Brain Stem Evoked Response (BSER) in cat to intracranially
recorded Field Potentials (IFPs) in the cat during dichotic stimulation with
clicks and noise bursts (Caird and Sontheimer, Naunyn-Schmiedeberg's Arch. Pharma-
col. Suppl. 322, R102, 1983). We have found strong interaction in waves IV and V
of the BSER at physiological interaural time delays of less than a few hundred
microseconds. The wave IV interaction arises in the Superior Olivary Complex and
wave V in the Inferior Colliculus. However, neither the correlations between IFPs
and BSER nor between IFPs and unit activity are simple. In particular tonic unit
responses in the brainstem to continuous stimuli show up neither in the IFPs nor
in the BSER, so any lack of effect may be due to using continuous stimulation.
Broadband stimuli evoke phasic responses in the brainstem, just as strongly as
pure tone stimuli.

STRUCTURE AND FUNCTION OF CROSSED AND UNCROSSED PATHWAYS
TO THE INFERIOR COLLICULUS IN THE RAT

J. Syka, J. Popelář and R. Druga

*Institute of Experimental Medicine, Czechoslovak Academy
of Sciences, 128 08 Prague 2, Czechoslovakia*

The relatively large nucleus within the auditory pathway in mammals, the inferior colliculus (IC), represents a unique auditory structure which apparently not only plays a role of a relay station but serves as an important integrating centre. The stream of information emerging from several nuclei lying lower in the auditory pathway, is funneled to the IC and transmitted to the cortex through a single channel via the medial geniculate body. The close connection of the IC with the superior colliculi, an intriguing centre for representation of the external world in the mammalian brain indicates the important role of the IC in spatial hearing.

The auditory system of the rat reflects typical properties of small head animals: due to small interaural distance the interaural amplitude differences are the predominant cue for sound source localization. This is in agreement with the fact that the rat belongs to animals with high frequency hearing. The present paper summarizes our recent data concerning the connections and response properties of IC neurones in the rat with the aim of elucidating the neural encoding in this structure. The emphasis is placed on the properties important for auditory localization.

1. ASCENDING PATHWAYS TO THE INFERIOR COLLICULUS

The results of studies with the HRP technique give evidence for complicated multichannel inputs to the IC in rat (Beyerl, 1978; Syka et al., 1981; Druga and Syka, 1983). The main ascending inputs to the IC in the pigmented Sprague-Dawley rat originate in contralateral cochlear nuclei, the lateral superior olive of both sides, the contralateral medial superior olive, contralateral superior paraolivary nucleus, the dorsal nuclei of the lateral lemniscus of both sides and the ipsilateral ventral nucleus of the lateral lemniscus. Essentially the same structure of pathways ascending to the IC has been described in the cat (Roth et al., 1978; Adams, 1979) with the exception that the input from the medial superior olive is more powerful in the cat. The MSO in the rat is relatively small as in other small head animals (Harrison and Feldman, 1970).

Because in the rat IC the majority of nerve cells is excited by contralateral ear stimulation and inhibited by ipsilateral ear stimulation, we may tentatively assume that the direct pathway from the contralateral cochlear nuclei is an excitatory pathway. Several crossings of auditory fibres at the level of the superior olive do not permit straightforward interpretation of the function of pathways connecting the superior olive and the lateral lemniscus with the IC. It is known that cat neurones of the lateral superior olive (LSO) are excited by stimulation of the ipsilateral ear and inhibited by the stimulation of the contralateral ear (Tsuchitani, 1977). Inhibition is probably mediated through the medial nucleus of the trapezoid body which never project to the IC either in the cat or in the rat. The excitatory-inhibitory interactions typical for the rat IC should reflect the properties of cells in the contralateral LSO. The role of the powerful input from the ipsilateral LSO still remains to be explained in the light of the fact that IC neurons are not excited from the ipsilateral ear at all.

2. DESCENDING CONNECTIONS AND CONNECTIONS WITHIN THE TECTUM

The temporal auditory cortex is a source of a powerful pathway descending mainly to the dorsomedial part of the IC central nucleus. Fibres originate in pyramidal cells of layer V and project bilaterally to the IC. The ipsilateral projection is, however, more extensive and also terminates in the dorsolateral parts of the central IC nucleus (Syka et al., 1981; Druga and Syka, 1983). In contrast to the distinct topographic projection of several auditory nuclei to the central IC nucleus there does not exist any systematic topographic projection from the auditory cortex to the IC, which can be demonstrated with the HRP technique. The functional organization of the auditory cortex in the rat resembles the organization found in other mammals (recent review by Goldstein and Knight, 1981). Using microelectrode mapping we observed two auditory fields in the rat which have opposite frequency progression in the rostrocaudal direction.

Strong commisural topographically organized connections between both inferior colliculi were also evident from results of studies with HRP injection into the IC. Besides the connections between external nuclei of the IC many fibres connect basolateral parts of the central IC nucleus. Of interest are also connections of the IC with the superior colliculus (SC). SC contains many multimodal neurones especially in middle and deep layers, the properties of which are in register with the projection of the visual space and body surface on the SC (Harris et al., 1980). Although the main auditory input to the SC in the rat is represented by the pathway from the ipsilateral dorsal nucleus of the lateral lemniscus (Druga and Syka, 1982) there are numerous neurones which project mainly from the basal parts of the central IC nucleus and from the external nucleus to caudal parts of the SC. It is probable that these pathways, similarly as in the cat (Syka and Straschill, 1970), transmit auditory information to the multimodal cells in the SC.

3. RESPONSE PROPERTIES OF NEURONES

In the absence of controlled auditory stimulation, few cells of the IC in Sprague-Dawley rats anaesthetized with pentobarbital are spontaneously active. The predominant type of response to short duration tones (100 ms with 5 ms rise and decay time) is an onset or phasic response which consists of one or a few spikes appearing shortly after beginning of the stimulus. The latency to clicks, which usually are effective in exciting neurones with the onset response to tonal stimuli, varies in the range of 6-15 ms. The latency characteristically decreases with increasing sound intensity and frequency. 64% out of 256 IC neurones in our study displayed the onset response to short duration tones. The distribution of neurones within the inferior colliculus is homogenous and no clustering of cells with the onset response was observed during vertical penetrations through the cortex or during horizontal penetrations through the cerebellum. There was also no evidence of any prevalence of the onset response with respect to the characteristic frequency (CF) of neurones (Fig. 1). The hearing range in the rat extends from 1 kHz to 60 kHz when CF of IC neurones are taken into account. No units with the CF lower than 1 kHz were found in our material.

The other type of response to tonal stimuli may be characterized as a sustained excitation or a tonic response. This response usually consists of a few initial spikes which are followed by an inhibitory pause and then by continuous firing lasting up to the end of the tone burst. In other cases the firing occurs throughout the total duration of the tone burst without the inhibitory intermission. The sustained response thus comprises the "primary-like" and the "pauser" type of response pattern according to the classification by Pfeiffer (1966) and Kiang et al. (1965). We never observed IC neurones in the rat with the firing pattern characterized as "chopped". The sustained excitatory response was found in 36% out of 256 IC neurones. The occurrence of the sustained type of response seems to be related to the unit CF. Fig. 1 shows that many units with the low CF (up to 4 kHz) responded to tonal stimuli with the sustained type of response, whereas such a relationship is not evident for units with the onset type of response. Because units in the rat inferior colliculus are similarly as in other mammals organized in isofrequency layers with low frequencies represented dorsally and high frequencies represented basally (Syka et al., 1981), units with the sustained response are mostly encountered in vertical penetrations at the beginning of the penetration whereas in horizontal penetrations the clustering corresponds to the inclination of isofrequency layers. The higher occurrence of sustain-

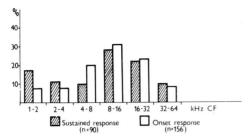

Fig. 1. Distribution of neurones with sustained and onset pattern with respect to the characteristic frequency

ed excitatory responses in low frequency neurones may correspond to the specific properties of auditory localization at low frequencies. For encoding of binaural disparities in time and phase which are dominant for low frequency signals continuous firing of units is probably more relevant. We may suppose therefore that units in the rat MSO (which play an important role in the coding of binaural time disparities) would display the sustained type of response more frequently than units in the rat LSO.

The binaural properties of IC neurones were studied in pigmented Sprague-Dawley rats by Silverman and Clopton (1977). Our data are consistent with their findings. The mostly observed response is characterized by excitation from the contralateral ear and inhibition from the ipsilateral ear (EI type of response). 70% out of 127 investigated neurones were classified as EI neurones. The predominance of the EI type of interaction is not surprising since the rat as an animal with the high frequency hearing mainly utilizes the intensity cue in the auditory localization. The EI units sensitively reflect small binaural differences in intensity. The efficiency of the ipsilateral ear to suppress the firing to zero level was studied in detail in 18 units. It was mostly necessary to increase the intensity in the ipsilateral.ear by 15-30 dB in order to suppress the excitation evoked from the contralateral ear. However, in some cases even a 5 dB increase in the ipsilateral ear fully inhibited the firing. The 15-30 dB difference between ears necessary to inhibit the activity is in good agreement with the interaural intensity differences in the rat found by Harrison and Downey (1970) at frequencies higher than 4 kHz.

Other two types of binaural interaction were encountered less frequently in the rat IC. The excitatory-excitatory type of interaction (excitation from both ears-EE type) was found in 13% of units and the monaural excitation from the contralateral ear (without any influence from the ipsilateral ear) in 17% of units. Semple and Atkin (1979) demonstrated that units with monaural excitation (which probably represent targets of fibres from the contralateral cochlear nuclei) are distributed mainly in the caudal parts of the IC in the cat. We were not able to extend their finding to the rat IC, however, the small sample of neurones with monaural excitation (n=22) makes our conclusion only tentative.

4. RESPONSES TO AMPLITUDE MODULATED SOUNDS

The high frequency hearing range and prevailing excitatory-inhibitory type of binaural interaction speaks in favour of utilization of the intensity cue in space hearing of the rat auditory system. Precise differentiation of small changes in amplitude of sounds should be inherent, therefore, to the rat auditory system. We have investigated responses of IC neurones in rats to 5 second lasting series of amplitude modulated tones and clicks (the amplitude decreased and increased once in 5 s from the intensity 20 or 30 dB above the threshold at the CF or above the threshold for clicks).

Units with the response pattern denoted as sustained excitation were mostly driven by the tone at CF for the total period of stimulation (48 units out of 120 units). Units with the onset response pattern reacted either to click series (33

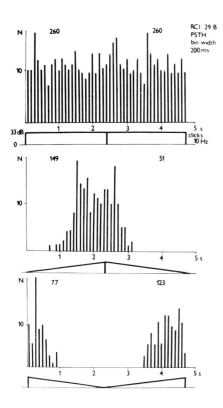

Fig. 2. *Responses of an IC neurone to 10 Hz click series with a constant amplitude (top), with amplitude modulation starting at zero SPL (middle part), and with amplitude modulation starting at 33 dB SPL (bottom). Sum of 10 responses*

units) or did not respond either to the tone or to the click series (39 units). The optimum repetition rate for clicks usually did not exceed 10 Hz; in some units, however, even 100 Hz repetition rate activated the unit. (Neurones excited with the tone or click series are comparable with movement sensitive neurones in the visual system.) Fig. 2 shows an example of a unit excited by 10 Hz click trains in the contralateral ear. Typically, the response is larger during the amplitude increase than during the amplitude decrease (number of spikes for each period is indicated above the corresponding halves of histograms). This rule holds independently whether the sound intensity at first decreases or increases. The a-symmetry of the response is expressed to a different extent in different neurones. Interestingly, such asymmetry is present when the ipsilateral inhibitory input is amplitude modulated (amplitude in the contralateral ear is held constant). The a-symmetry is opposite in this case, i.e. the firing is more suppressed during the ipsilateral amplitude increase than during the decrease. In fact, these effects are complementary, i.e. during binaural amplitude modulation the response is more asymmetrical.

On the basis of these preliminary data, we may assume that neurones in the rat IC which react more vigorously to sounds with increasing amplitude represent a system which may detect the direction of a moving sound source precisely. The movement of the sound source from the midline to the contralateral ear will result in a higher firing rate than the opposite movement. The comparison with the direction sensitive neurones in the visual system is conspicuous, however, more data are necessary for a serious interpretation.

5. SUMMARY

     Information from several brain stem auditory nuclei is integrated in the in-
ferior colliculus of the rat and delivered via the medial geniculate body to the
auditory cortex. The inferior colliculus is under the influence of pathways descending from the auditory cortex and has numerous connections with the opposite
IC and with the superior colliculi. IC neurones in the rat discharge predominantly during the onset of a tone stimulus, the sustained excitation is present only
in one third of neurones. The occurrence of a sustained excitatory pattern is
higher in units with low frequency CF. The majority of IC neurones is excited
from the contralateral ear and inhibited from the ipsilateral ear (EI units). IC
neurones are sensitive to small changes in the amplitude of sound and react more
vigorously during the amplitude increase. The amplitude increase also results in
more marked inhibition from the ipsilateral ear.

REFERENCES

Adams, J.C. (1979). Ascending projections to the inferior colliculus. *J. Comp.
     Neur.* 183, 529-538.
Beyerl, B.D. (1978). Afferent projections to the central nucleus of the inferior
     colliculus in the rat. *Brain Res.* 145, 209-223.
Druga, R. and Syka, J. (1982). Afferents to the superior colliculus demonstrated
     by retrograde axonal transport of HRP in the rat. *Physiol. Bohemoslov.* 31,
     260.
Druga, R. and Syka, J. (1983). Ascending and descending projections to the infer-
     ior colliculus in the rat. *In preparation.*
Goldstein, M.H., Jr. and Knight, P.L. (1980). Comparative organization of mammal-
     ian auditory cortex. In: *Comparative Studies of Hearing in Vertebrates.* (A.
     N. Popper and R.R. Fay, eds.), pp. 375-398, New York, Heidelberg, Berlin,
     Springer-Verlag.
Harris, L.R., Blakemore, C., and Donaghy, M. (1980). Integration of visual and
     auditory space in the mammalian superior colliculus. *Nature* 288, 56-59.
Harrison, J.M. and Downey, P. (1970). Intensity changes at the ear as a function
     of the azimuth of a tone source: A comparative study. *J. Acoust. Soc. Am.*
     47, 1509-1518.
Harrison, J.M. and Feldman, M.L. (1970). Anatomical aspects of the cochlear nuc-
     leus and superior olivary complex. In: *Contributions to Sensory Physiology.*
     Vol. 4. (W.D. Neff, ed.), pp. 95-142, London, New York, San Francisco, Aca-
     demic Press.
Kiang, N.Y.-S., Watanabe, T., and Thomas, E.C. (1965). Discharge patterns of sing-
     le fibres in the cat's auditory nerve. Res. monograph No. 35, Cambridge,
     Massachussetts, MIT.
Pfeiffer, R.R. (1966). Classification of response patterns of spike discharges
     for units in the cochlear nucleus: Tone burst stimulation. *Exp. Brain Res.*
     1, 220-235.
Roth, G.L., Aitkin, L.M. Andersen, R.A., and Merzenich, M.M. (1978). Some featur-
     es of the spatial organization of the central nucleus of the inferior colli-
     culus of the cat. *J. Comp. Neur.* 182, 661-680.
Semple, M.N. and Aitkin, L.M. (1979). Representation of sound frequency and late-
     rality by units in central nucleus of cat inferior colliculus. *J. Neuro-
     physiol.* 42, 1626-1639.
Silverman, M.S. and Clopton, B.M. (1977). Plasticity of binaural interaction. I.
     Effect of early auditory deprivation. *J. Neurophysiol.* 40, 1266-1274.
Syka, J. and Straschill, M. (1970). Activation of superior colliculus neurones
     and motor responses after electrical stimulation of the inferior colliculus.
     Exp. Neurol. 28, 384-392.
Syka, J., Druga, R., Popelar, J., and Kalinova, B. (1981). Functional organizati-
     on of the inferior colliculus. In: *Neuronal Mechanisms of Hearing.* (J. Syka
     and L. Aitkin, eds.), pp. 137-153, New York, London, Plenum Press.
Tsuchitani, C. (1977). Functional organization of lateral cell groups of cat sup-
     erior olivary complex. *J. Neurophysiol.* 40, 296-318.

GENERAL DISCUSSION

KLINKE:
Can you tell more about the localization of your cells?

SYKA:
Our data concern mostly units in the central nucleus of the inferior colliculus
(IC). We tried to localize units with the identical type of binaural interaction
as Semple and Aitkin (J. Neurophys. 42, 1626, 1979) did in cat. However, this
work is tedious due to the small size of the inferior colliculus in rat. We may
say that EO· units are mainly localized in dorsal and caudal parts of the IC.
Interestingly, three units which were sensitive to Δt changes (out of 60 units
investigated) were found in the pericentral or external nucleus, not in the central nucleus.

STOPP:
May I ask if, with your HRP tracing, you were able to establish any centrifugal
connections, as well as the centripetal pathways you described?

SYKA:
Our experience with efferent fibers in the auditory system concerns only efferents
descending from the cortex to the inferior colliculus, because we injected HRP into the IC. We found with the HRP only efferents descending from the ipsilateral
auditory cortex (layer V) mainly to the dorsomedial part of the central IC nucleus. However, in related studies, with degeneration techniques (Nauta and Gygax)
we found after lesions of the auditory cortex fibers descending to the IC also
from the contralateral cortex. Few cells labelled with HRP were found in the medial geniculate body.

MONAURAL AND BINAURAL CONTRIBUTIONS TO AN AUDITORY SPACE MAP IN THE GUINEA-PIG
SUPERIOR COLLICULUS

A.R. Palmer and A.J. King

National Institute for Medical Research,
The Ridgeway, Mill Hill, London NW7 1AA, UK.

1. INTRODUCTION

The superior colliculus (SC) is not part of the classical auditory pathway
but nevertheless receives direct projections from several auditory nuclei including the superior olive and the inferior colliculus (Edwards *et al.* 1979). We
have recently demonstrated that cells in the deep layers of the guinea-pig SC
respond more strongly or more reliably when sounds originate from a limited horizontal angle (Palmer and King 1982, King and Palmer, 1983). This 'spatial tuning'
was obvious in some cells only for near threshold stimuli whilst in others it was
maintained even when stimuli up to 35 dB above threshold were employed. Within
this nucleus the cells are organized so that those responding best to sounds
behind the animal are located at the caudal extreme and those responding to sounds
in front are located rostrally with intermediate sound locations represented at
appropriate positions in between. Thus, in the SC there is a topographical representation of at least the horizontal plane of auditory space similar to that
previously demonstrated directly in the midbrain auditory nucleus and optic tectum
of the barn owl (Knudsen and Konishi 1978, Knudsen 1982) and indirectly in the
superior colliculus of other mammals (e.g. Gordon 1973, Chalupa and Rhoades 1977,
Dräger and Hubel 1975).
     There are three cues which are used to discriminate the location of a sound:
interaural differences in intensity; interaural time differences; or monaural
spectral differences which arise due to reflections within the pinna and concha
(see Blauert this volume). Since cells in the SC do appear to be selective for
sound location, they are presumably responding to one or more of these cues.
Indeed, in the barn owl the elevation component of the auditory spatial receptive
fields is due to interaural intensity differences derived from comparison of the
monaural spectra. The azimuthal component is determined by these spectral intensity cues and also by ongoing time disparities between the signals reaching the
two ears (see Knudsen 1980).
     The present experiments represent the first stage in the elucidation of the
effective stimulus for the cells in the SC which are sensitive to sound location.
We have recorded responses under three conditions: 1) ipsilateral ear occlusion;
2) ipsilateral cochlear destruction; 3) ipsilateral ear occlusion or cochlear
destruction and removal of the contralateral pinna and concha. The results
indicate that the topographical representation of auditory space in the SC has
both monaural and binaural components and that the pinna is required for a normal
representation.

2. METHODS

Pigmented guinea-pigs (200-450g) were anaesthetized using a neuroleptic
technique (Evans 1979). The tracheae were cannulated and the core temperature
maintained at 37°C. Following a craniotomy above the cortex overlying the
superior colliculus, the animals were mounted on a minimal headholder consisting
of a metal bar with an annulus which surrounded the craniotomy. The pinnae were
repositioned with sutures and the headholder adjusted so that the head and ears
were in a normal position. The animals were placed on a small table at the centre
of an anechoic chamber and recordings were made with glass-coated tungsten microelectrodes remotely advanced through the cortex into the superior colliculus.
Electrolytic lesions were used to enable histological reconstruction of the

recording sites from cresyl violet stained frozen sections.
    Stimuli consisted of 100ms bursts of white noise presented from one of 11
loudspeakers positioned in a 1.1m arc in the horizontal plane at 22.5° intervals
around the centre of the animal's interaural plane. The noise bandwidth was
100-20000Hz (determined by the speaker responses) and its mean maximum r.m.s. level
was 83 dB SPL (s.d. 1.58 dB) measured at the position of the centre of the animal's
head. Discharges during a time window extending usually from 10-70ms after stimulus onset were electronically counted and summed over 32 repetitions.
    Reversible occlusion of the ipsilateral ear was achieved with a cotton/wax
plug sealed with Vaseline. Cochlear microphonic measurements indicated that this
block produced at least 10 dB of attenuation at low frequency (up to 2000Hz)
rising to more than 25 dB at higher frequencies, for all speaker positions.

3. RESULTS

a) *Reversible occlusion of the ipsilateral ear*

    We have investigated the effects of blocking the ipsilateral ear on the
responses of 41 cells. In each case, responses were measured as a function of
sound location before occlusion, during occlusion and after removal of the plug,

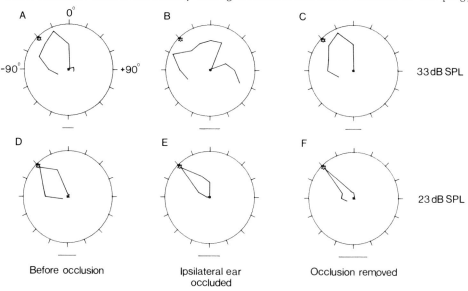

*Fig.1. Response of an SC cell to a 100ms burst of white noise as a function of
its horizontal location and level. Each value plotted on the radial axis is the
mean number of spikes elicited by 32 stimulus repetitions. The bar represents 0.5
counts per presentation. The star symbol shows the position of the visual
receptive field of cells in the superficial layers of the SC encountered in the
same electrode track*

at two or more noise levels. We obtained a full set of measurements on 20 cells
and a typical cell is shown in figure 1. Figures 1a and d show the normal response
to a noise burst as a function of its level and location. This cell was tuned to
45° azimuth at levels near threshold (23 dB SPL), with some broadening of its
specificity when the sound level was increased even by 10 dB above threshold.
When the ipsilateral ear was occluded (figures 1b and e) the threshold response
was unchanged, but the response to the 10dB higher level showed little indication
of preference for a particular sound location. Indeed, the exclusively contralateral response which was found for binaural noise stimuli was replaced by an
omnidirectional response extending into the ipsilateral hemifield. Removal of

the block gave the responses shown in figures 1c and f which are very like the pre-block data of figures 1a and d. Of the 41 cells investigated, 36 showed reversible broadening of their spatial receptive fields to high level stimuli. The remaining 5 were only examined with near threshold stimuli and showed no change. Eighteen cells were examined with both threshold and higher level noise and showed differential effects like those in fig.1. In general, the spatial tuning of cells to sounds within a few dB of threshold was unchanged by occlusion of the ipsilateral ear, whilst any preference for sound location shown at levels of more than 10-20dB above threshold was lost during ear blocking when strong responses to ipsilateral sound sources were found.

b) *Unilateral cochlear destruction*

Responses of 43 cells were investigated after destruction of the ipsilateral cochlea. Thirty-three of these were analysed with sounds exceeding 10-20dB above threshold and in every case the spatial receptive fields were extremely broad, extending into the ipsilateral field with little response attenuation. Thirty-eight units were analysed with near threshold stimuli which revealed well

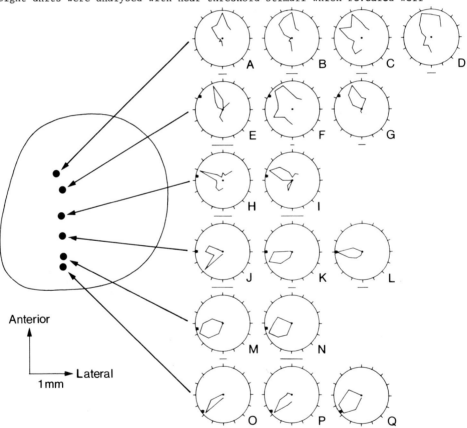

Fig.2. Surface view of the right SC in a guinea-pig in which the ipsilateral cochlea has been destroyed, showing the location of six electrode penetrations. Polar diagrams (as Fig.1) are shown for all cells in these six penetrations for which sufficient data was obtained. Each polar diagram shown is for a single sound level, near threshold, at which the cell's response was most sharply tuned for sound location

defined spatial tuning.

    Figure 2 shows the responses of 17 cells in 6 electrode tracks located over most of the rostro-caudal extent of the SC as indicated on the surface view. The majority of these polar diagrams show responses to noise stimuli within a few dB of threshold and indicate well defined spatial tuning. We have made no attempt to select these data, but have presented all units analysed in each track. A trend is quite clear: those cells responding best to sounds in front of the animal are located rostrally and progressively more posterior sound locations are represented at increasingly more caudal positions.

c) Ipsilateral ear occlusion or cochlear destruction and removal of the contralateral pinna and concha

    We have analysed the threshold responses of 43 units under monaural conditions and with the contralateral pinna removed. All of these units showed a preference for sounds located at 67.5-112.5° azimuth which is directly opposite the external auditory meatus. Figure 3 shows the responses of 13 units recorded in chronological order in 5 electrode tracks extending most of the length of the SC as indicated on the surface view. Figure 3a shows the threshold response of a unit recorded with the pinna intact and 3b shows the same unit after the pinna

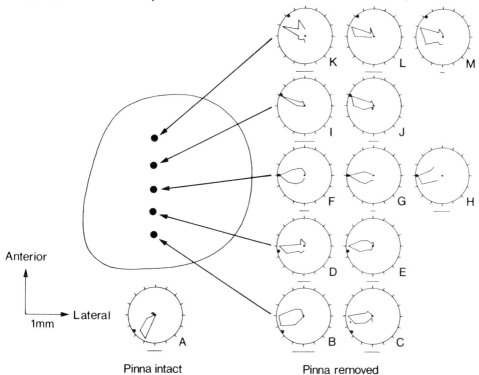

Pinna intact   Pinna removed

Fig.3. Surface view of the right SC in the guinea-pig in which the ipsilateral ear has been occluded and the contralateral pinna and concha removed, showing the location of five electrode penetrations. Polar diagrams (as Fig.1) are shown for all cells in these five penetrations for which sufficient data was obtained. Each polar diagram is for a single sound level, near threshold, at which the cell's response was most sharply tuned for spatial location. The responses in A and B are from the same cell obtained before and after pinna removal

was removed. The receptive field of this cell has been shifted by about 60°.
All of the cells had fields which were located within a 45° range opposite the
meatus despite the range of electrode positions which from previous experiments
we would expect to yield receptive fields covering the entire hemifield.

4. DISCUSSION

The data may be summarized as follows:- occlusion of the ipsilateral ear
does not affect threshold spatial tuning of SC cells, but destroys any location
preference at higher sound levels. Threshold spatial tuning is present in animals
with ipsilateral cochlear destruction and the distribution of the cells is such
as to produce a threshold space map. When the contralateral pinna and concha are
removed, in monaural animals, all cells recorded thereafter have threshold
spatial receptive fields in line with the external auditory meatus.

The data from the occlusion and cochlear destruction experiments are consistent and suggest that the threshold spatial tuning is a response to monaural cues.
The monaural threshold space map which we have demonstrated here is exactly
similar to that which we previously reported using binaural stimulus presentation
(King and Palmer 1983). Many of the cells in that study were spatially tuned
only near threshold and thus presumably also represent responses to monaural cues.
However, maintenance of spatial tuning to suprathreshold sound levels which
occurred in many cells, clearly requires input from both ears, and indeed the
activation of SC cells by ipsilateral sounds in monaural animals has been
demonstrated before (Dräger and Hubel 1975). We have previously shown that the
cells with sharp suprathreshold spatial receptive fields produce a space map
which is coincident with that at threshold, therefore binaural and monaural
information representing the same spatial location is conveyed to a single SC
locus. We do not as yet know what binaural cues these cells are responding to,
but both EE (excited by both ears) and EI (excited by one ear and inhibited by
the other) types of cell response have been reported in the SC of the cat
(Wise and Irvine 1981).

It has been repeatedly shown psychophysically that subjects can localize
complex sounds accurately using only one ear (e.g. Freedman and Fisher 1968,
Harris and Sergeant 1971). The cues which are used are a result of multiple
reflections of sound within the pinna and concha. In the present data it would
appear that, at threshold, the SC cells are responding differentially to such
cues, since removal of these structures causes compression of the threshold
spatial receptive fields to within ±20° of the presumed acoustic axis of the
external meatus.

*Acknowledgements: We thank Simon Caidan for his excellent technical assistance
and Dr M.J. Keating for helpful criticism of this manuscript.
A.J.K. is an M.R.C. Scholar.*

REFERENCES

Chalupa, L.M., Rhoades, R.W. (1977). Responses of visual, somatosensory, and
    auditory neurones in the golden hamster's superior colliculus. *J.Physiol.
    (Lond.)* 270, 595-626.
Dräger, U.C., Hubel, D.H. (1975). Responses to visual stimulation and relation-
    ship between visual, auditory, and somatosensory inputs in mouse superior
    colliculus. *J.Neurophysiol.* 38, 690-713.
Edwards, S.B., Ginsburgh, C.L., Henkel, C.K., Stein, B.E. (1979). Sources of
    subcortical projections to the superior colliculus in the cat. *J.Comp.
    Neurol.* 184, 309-330.
Evans, E.F. (1979). Neuroleptanaesthesia for the guinea-pig. *Arch.Otolaryngol.*
    105, 185-186.
Freedman, S.J., Fisher, H.G. (1968). The role of the pinna in auditory
    localization. In: *Neuropsychology of Spatially Oriented Behaviour.*
    (S.J. Freedman, ed.). Illinois, Dorsey Press.
Gordon, B. (1973). Receptive fields in deep layers of cat superior colliculus.
    J.Neurophysiol. 36, 157-178.

Harris, J.D., Sergeant, R.L. (1971). Monaural/binaural minimum audible angles
     for a moving sound source. *J.Speech Hear.Res.* 14, 618-629.
King, A.J., Palmer, A.R. (1983). Cells responsive to free-field auditory stimuli
     in guinea-pig superior colliculus: distribution and response properties.
     J.Physiol. (Lond.) In press.
Knudsen, E.I. (1980). Sound localization in birds. In: *Comparative Studies of
     Hearing in Vertebrates*. (A.N. Popper and R.R. Fay, eds.). pp.289-322.
     New York, Heidelberg, Berlin, Springer-Verlag.
Knudsen, E.I. (1982). Auditory and visual maps of space in the optic tectum of
     the owl. *J.Neurosci.* 2, 1177-1194.
Knudsen, E.I., Konishi, M. (1978). A neural map of auditory space in the owl.
     Science 200, 795-797.
Palmer, A.R., King, A.J. (1982). The representation of auditory space in the
     mammalian superior colliculus. *Nature* 299, 248-249.
Wise, L.Z., Irvine, D.R.F. (1981). Auditory response properties of neurones in
     intermediate and deep layers of cat superior colliculus. *Proc.Aust.Physiol.
     Pharmacol.Soc.* 12, 18P.

GENERAL DISCUSSION

KIM:
On which part of the superior colliculus are these space-selective neurons located? Do they respond to visual stimuli? Have you attempted to determine whether
there is a topographic representation of space-selective neurons in various subdivisions of the inferior colliculus? What are the effects of anaesthesia?

PALMER:
The auditory projection to the superior colliculus of the guinea pig extends over
most of the rostro-caudal axis except for a region at the rostral extreme. The
exact details of the projection are species specific. Space-selective neurons
were found throughout this projection area in the deeper layers 4-7. We do not
routinely test with visual stimuli but our sample definitely includes both uni-
modal auditory cells and bimodal auditory/visual cells. In an unpublished pilot
study 50 cells were analysed in the central nucleus of the inferior colliculus,
but no responses were found which were inconsistent with interaction of EI/EE responses with head shadow and pinna effects. We have no data from external or
pericentral nuclei. We have used urethane, halothane, and neuroleptic anaesthetic
techniques. We now routinely use the neuroleptic technique, since at least in our
hands the superior colliculus auditory cells were almost inactive when we used
either of the more convenient techniques.

CAIRD:
I think that the fact that these monaural effects are only seen at threshold can
be explained by EI cell information processing as seen in the LSO. Such cells are
seen up to the auditory cortex (as IE cells, due to the crossing of ascending
pathways from the SOC) where they are very sensitive along the pinna axis. Such
cells are sensitive to interaural differences rather then absolute level, and the
effect would be to stabilize the monaural effects that you have described over a
large range of absolute intensity (Middlebrooks et al., J. Neurosc. 1, 107, 1981).

PALMER:
I agree with this suggestion, especially since IE and EE type responses have been
reported in superior colliculus (Wise and Irvine, 1981, see paper).

KLINKE:
Can you tell us more about the frequency response of your cells? I'm thinking in
terms of directional bands.

PICKLES:
We would expect the pinna to emphasize high frequency sounds coming from the
front, and attenuate those coming from behind. Since you used wideband stimuli,
could your map be just a reflection of tonotopicity?

PALMER:

Our measurements of the guinea-pig pinna effects using both sound pressure and cochlear microphonics suggest that the pinna is not very directional. We have not directly looked for tonotopicity, but have measured frequency response areas for 46 cells. Some of these areas were narrow and 'V'-shaped but the majority were either very broad or complex with high and low frequency minima. If tonotopicity is present it cannot, therefore, be well defined and we do not think that our data are a consequence of such organization.

SYKA:

We have strong evidence from our HRP studies in rat that the main auditory input to the superior colliculus originates in the ipsilateral dorsal nucleus of the lateral lemniscus. There is also powerful input from the ipsilateral auditory cortex and from the ipsilateral inferior colliculus (see Syka et al., this volume). Also data available from many species clearly demonstrate that stimulation of the superior colliculus results in the movements of the contralateral pinna. I believe these facts should be incorporated into the interpretation of your data.

PALMER:

We do not know which is the auditory projection to the superior colliculus responsible for the data we obtain, but latencies are too short for a significant contribution from auditory cortex. One reason for choosing the guinea pig is its relatively immobile pinna, unlike the cat for example. Whilst in some species pinnae effects must certainly be included in interpretation, they are unlikely to be a large factor in the presented data.

BINAURAL HEARING AND NEURAL INTERACTION

J.J. Eggermont, W.J.M. Epping and A.M.H.J. Aertsen

Dept. of Medical Physics and Biophysics;
University of Nijmegen, Nijmegen, The Netherlands

INTRODUCTION

Binaural hearing in mammals relies on differences in spectrum (ΔS), intensity (ΔI), time (Δt) or phase ($\Delta\phi$) between the sounds processed by both ears. In birds and other lower vertebrates with small interaural distance only very minute ΔI and Δt differences are available. In cold blooded vertebrates especially, the slower pace of the central nervous system processing does not allow to resolve time differences below a few hundred microseconds (Feng and Capranica, 1976), in addition a small head does not cause intensity differences sufficiently large to be detected for the frequencies below 2 kHz. In frogs and toads, as well as in reptiles or birds, there is an open connection between the tympanic membranes and mouth cavity providing the animal with a mechanism not unlike that of a combined pressure-pressuregradient microphone. At low frequencies (< 300 Hz) a single ear shows a cardioid directional sensitivity and at higher frequencies (< 1500 Hz) there is still a useful displacement difference between both ears equivalent to ΔI values of more than 2-3 dB (Aertsen et al., in preparation) that can be detected by neurons in the torus semicircularis (Feng and Capranica, 1978). The minute phase differences at both ear drums and at the sound transparent mouth cavity thus cause movement differences of the tympanic membranes large enough for reasonably accurate directional hearing: about 10-15° as the resolving power (Rheinländer et al., 1979) determined by behavioural experiments.

Neurons that are sensitive to interaural intensity differences require input from both ears. It is known that binaural units in the auditory midbrain of the grassfrog receive input from fibers with equal spectral sensitivity but with distinctly different latencies (Hermes et al., 1982). Thus minute phase differences are transformed into detectable "equivalent-intensity" differences that are processed with quite large (up to 10 msec) differences in latency.

Neurons in the torus semicircularis interact with each other, this interaction has appeared to be stimulus dependent: tone-burst or continuous noise stimulation produce a different neural correlation even after a correction procedure for stimulus lock of the spikes (Eggermont et al., in preparation). Since ipsi-, contra-, or bilateral stimulation produce a difference in neural activity for torus semicircularis units it is worthwhile to investigate this effect upon the neural correlation. *This may indicate whether processing of binaural information can be done on the single unit level or that groups of interacting neurons are involved.* In the present paper we offer preliminary results of the investigation of binaural influences on neural correlation for units in the auditory midbrain of the grassfrog (Rana temporaria L.).

METHODS

Recordings were made from the torus semicircularis in the immobilized and locally anaesthetised grassfrog (Rana temporaria L.) using metal (tungsten or stainless steel) electrodes with an exposed tip of about 10 μm and a 1 kHz impedance in the 1-3 MΩ range (For details see Hermes et al., 1981).

The multi-unit spike train was separated into single-unit spike trains on basis of spike waveform by using the matched filter approach (e.g. Abeles and Goldstein, 1977). Four orthogonal templates were used to represent each waveform but the separation was carried out using the best set of two out of these four. By using a colour code to represent spike waveform we were able to construct MU dot displays where each single unit contribution had its own colour. This procedure

facilitates the problem of finding (neural) synchrony in the firings of the
different units and easily sorts out double and triple correlations which may be
obscured in standard correlation analysis procedures. To give an impression part
of a dot display for a four unit recording is represented; instead of colour we
use symbols (Figure 1) thereby giving up resolution.

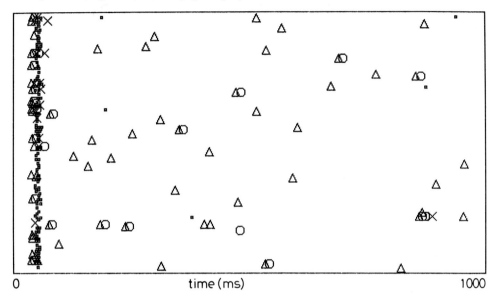

0   time (ms)   1000

*Fig. 1. Four-unit recording using single microelectrode. The responses of the
separated individual units are indicated with different symbols. Stimuli consisted of 127 tonebursts randomly selected in frequency and presented once per
second. One observes the onset response of all four units followed by spontaneous
activity from the units indicated by Δ and 0. It is easily observed that responses
of neuron 0 are likeli to be preceeded by firings of the unit indicated by Δ. A
firing of the unit X is in most cases preceeded by both firings of units Δ and 0*

Neural correlation under stimulus conditions contains a component due to
correlation with the stimulus (Perkel et al., 1967). For the purpose of correction
we present the stimulus ensemble twice (Aertsen et al., 1979) and calculate both
the simultaneous and non-simultaneous cross coincidence functions between two
spike trains from a multi-unit record (Eggermont et al., in preparation) (see
Fig. 2).

The difference is, under the assumption of an additive effect of the stimulus
on the number of spikes, a measure for the strength of the neural correlation. In
case the neurons are spontaneously active a direct measure for neural interaction
can be obtained.

Sound was presented using closed sound systems. Stimuli were presented
ipsilateral and contralateral with respect to the recording site as well as
binaural. No intensity or time differences were introduced. Three types of
stimulus ensembles were used:
a. Tonal stimuli with envelope $m(t) = c(t/\beta)^{\gamma-1} \exp(-t/\beta)$; $t \geq 0$; with parameter
   $\gamma=3$ and duration parameter $\beta=4.35$ leading to a 48 ms duration. Frequency range
   was 4 octaves: 125-2000 Hz or 250-4000 Hz depending on the frequency
   characteristics of the neuron. Frequency values were selected in random order
   from 127 values equidistant on log frequency scale. Peak amplitude was kept
   constant. Four sequences were used leading to tonal stimulus ensemble duration
   of 8 min 28 s.
b. Tonal stimuli with $\gamma=3$ but $\beta=1.45$ leading to 16 ms duration. Frequency values
   were selected from 255 frequency values with onset intervals of 128 ms. This

sequence was repeated 9 times, resulting in a duration of 4 min 54 s. for the
stimulus ensemble.
c. Noise generated by a pseudo-random binary-sequence generator. Sequence length
   was 1048575 steps, a sufficient number of feedback loops was provided to assure
   that the statistical properties of the noise, especially its second order autocorrelation function were satisfactory. Either 1.5 kHz or 5 kHz low pass noise
   was used with sequence duration of 34.95 s or 10.49 s. Generally 32 sequences
   were used.

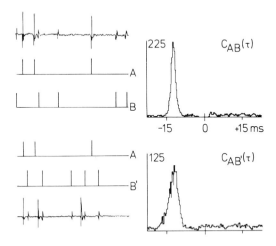

Fig. 2. Construction of simultaneous and non-simultaneous crosscoincidence histograms for a double unit recording. For the simultaneous crosscoincidence histogram $C_{AB}(\tau)$ the firings are taken from the same part of the double unit record. In case of the non-simultaneous histogram $C_{AB'}(\tau)$ one correlates the original A-train with B-spikes from a record to a repeated presentation of the stimulus sequence. The first histogram represents stimulus correlation as well as neural correlation, the second histogram only stimulus correlation

Spectro-temporal sensitivities of the single units were determined by
calculating the average pre-event stimulus intensity as a function of tonepip
frequency and time before the spike, and by calculating the average pre-event
CoSTID $\equiv (\omega, \tau)$ which can be considered as a single Fourier transform of the second
order Wiener-kernel for the noise stimulus. Further details in Hermes et al.
(1981, 1982).

RESULTS

Thirty-one double-unit pairs were recorded in the auditory midbrains from
eleven grassfrogs under ipsilaterally, contralaterally and binaurally presented
random tone-pip sequences and continuous noise sequences. Spectro-temporal
sensitivities (STS) were obtained for the separated single unit records. Two main
types of STS for the double-units were observed: either there was a close
resemblance with respect to the spectral properties and with only the response
latencies different, or the STS's were each others complement. In 14 cases we
found a close match of the STS's, while in the remaining 17 double-unit pairs the
STS were largely complementary with respect to the spectral sensitivity. In most
cases the STS for ipsilateral presentation was confined to the central part of
the STS under contralateral stimulation. This is illustrated in Fig. 3 where for
one neuron (X) out of the four-unit recording illustrated in Fig. 1 the STS are
shown for both ipsi- and contralateral stimulation with the three stimulus
ensembles described in the methods section. The other unit had nearly the same
STS.
The spike trains for these two units obtained by two times presenting the
same tonal or noise stimulus ensemble were used to compute coincidence histograms
(cf. Fig. 2) for the simultaneous and non-simultaneous conditions. An example of
such an analysis is shown in Figure 4 for ipsi- and contralateral stimulation.
The example again represents the same two units as in Fig. 3 and the spikes of
these two units are indicated in Fig. 1 using the symbols Δ and X. One observes
that for the ipsilateral stimulation with 48 ms duration tonepips presented once

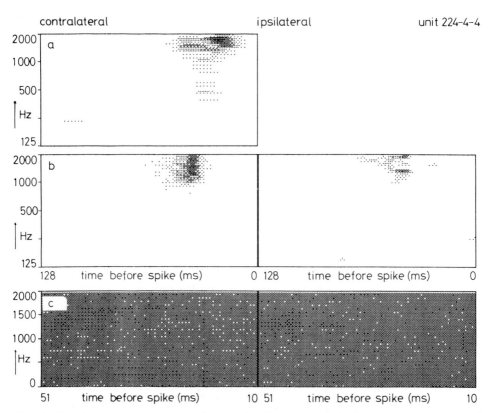

Fig. 3. Spectro-temporal sensitivities of unit 4-4 to stimulus sequences referred to as a, b and c in the methods section for both contralateral and ipsilateral presentation. Shown is the averaged pre-spike intensity in grey coding. For the tonal stimuli (a,b) the frequency scale is logarithmic, for the noise stimulus (c) linear. One observes that best frequency is between 1000 and 2000 Hz. The number of spikes are for contralateral respectively ipsilateral stimulation: a, 73-0; b, 391-45; c, 149-48

per second the coincidence histograms both are zero. This is due to the fact that unit 4-4 did not fire in that case. For the other stimulus conditions unit 4-2 generally fired more than unit 4-4. For contralateral stimulation one notes that the simultaneous and non-simultaneous coincidence histograms were the same for the long pause tonal sequence and that the difference is largest for the continuous noise stimulation. This indicates a stimulus dependent neural correlation. Comparing the ipsilateral and contralateral stimulus presentations one gets the impression that this does not so much influences the strength of the neural correlation (note the different scaling).

For the 31 double-unit pairs we observed in four cases a clear stimulus dependence and in another 4 cases some stimulus dependence. In none of these cases was an effect of stimulus presentation on the ipsilateral or contralateral side upon the strength of the neural correlation.

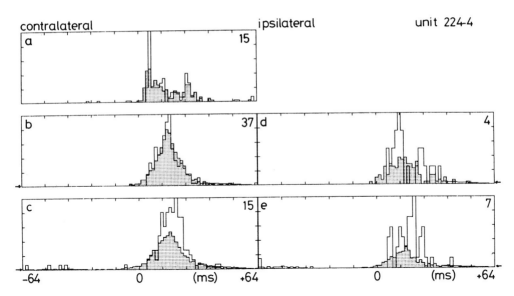

Fig. 4. Simultaneous and non-simultaneous cross coincidence histograms for units 4-2 and 4-4. In a, b and c the stimuli used were again as in Figure 3. One observes a larger difference between simultaneous and non-simultaneous cross coincidence histograms going from a to c. The numbers of spikes involved in the computation of the histograms are a: 237-73; b: 391-391; c: 516-149; d: 229-45; e: 416-48. The non-simultaneous histograms are dotted

DISCUSSION

Binaural hearing in frogs is probably based on mechanisms completely different from those attributed to mammals. First of all phase lock in the grassfrog at temperatures around 15°C is only present for best frequencies under 350 Hz as deduced from the measurement of reverse correlation functions (Hermes et al., 1981; Epping et al., in preparation). This excludes phase differences as a useful cue for directional hearing except at very low frequencies. However, in frogs in free field, small interaural phase differences are transformed by the tympanic-cavity, mouth-cavity system into quite large movement differences of the tympanic membranes. This is such that each ear acts as a pressure- pressure-gradient receiver having at low frequencies a cardioid direction characteristic. Secondly neurons in the auditory midbrain appear to be sensitive to small intensity differences between sounds applied using closed sound systems. Values of 2 dB are sufficient to change the firing rate of particular cells. Under natural conditions these differences arise only at the higher frequencies to which the frog is only marginally sensitive. When this sensitivity is combined with the peripheral pressure gradient transformer a large directional sensitivity results for the low frequencies but at the expense of an overall low sensitivity. EI cells in the auditory midbrain then are directional sensitive according to a figure-of-eight characteristic (EE cells would not show a directional preference). EI cells therefore can be seen as responding to quite large *effective* ΔI differences between both ears. The ears are most sensitive in free field around the resonance frequency of the mouth cavity, but at these frequencies (1000 - 1700 Hz) the directional sensitivity is poor. Quite a reasonable optimum combination of overall and directional sensitivity is present at the dominant frequencies found in the species own vocalisations (600 - 800 Hz), which is just below the tympanic membrane resonance.
Thirdly, on basis of evoked potential recordings from the midbrain of grassfrogs (Pettigrew et al., 1981) it is suggested that space (azimuth) is coded in the

midbrain such that rostral regions respond best to sound from the rostral aspect of the contralateral field and that caudal regions are best stimulated from tones presented in the caudal part of the contralateral field. This seems to be intermingled by a better representation of high frequencies in the rostral regions and low frequencies in the caudal regions of the midbrain (Pettigrew et al., 1981, Hermes et al., 1982).

Such spatial maps with relatively large receptive fields probably require the central reconstruction of target position on basis of the response of neural populations in order to obtain cue's for accurate source localisation. It is suggested that the synchrony within such a population of neurons plays an important role in the reliability of such a system. This synchrony will be enhanced by neural correlation. In this respect it might be of advantage that the strength of the neural correlation does not depend strongly on the site where the source is located, as is suggested by our measurements. On the other hand, our measurements suggest that neural correlation is strongly stimulus dependent, this could result in enhanced detectability in space of particular types of stimuli. The function of neural interaction would then be dominantly the enhancement of signal-to-noise ratio.

Acknowledgement. This investigation was supported by the Netherlands Organization for the Advancement of Pure Research (ZWO). Wim van Deelen and Jan Bruijns were indispensible for the computer analysis. Koos Braks prepared the animals and took part in the experimental procedure. Marianne Nieuwenhuizen prepared the manuscript.

REFERENCES

Abeles, M. and Goldstein, M.H. Jr (1977). Multispike train analysis. *Proc. IEEE* 65, 762-773.
Aertsen, A.M.H.J., Smolders, J.W.T., Johannesma, P.I.M. (1979). Neural representation of the acoustic biotope: on the existence of stimulus-event relations for sensory neurons. *Biological Cybernetics* 32, 175-185.
Feng, A.S., Capranica, R.R. (1976). Sound localization in anurans. I. Evidence of binaural interaction in dorsal medullary nucleus of bullfrogs (Rana catesbeiana). *J. Neurophysiology* 39, 871-881.
Feng, A.S., Capranica, R.R. (1978). Sound localization in anurans. II. Binaural interaction in superior olive nucleus of the green tree frog. *J. Neurophysiology* 41, 43-54.
Hermes, D.J., Aertsen, A.M.H.J., Johannesma, P.I.M., Eggermont, J.J. (1981) Spectro-temporal characteristics of single units in the auditory midbrain of the lightly anaesthetised grassfrog (Rana temporaria L.) investigated with noise stimuli. *Hearing Research* 5, 145-179.
Hermes, D.J., Eggermont, J.J., Aertsen, A.M.H.J., Johannesma, P.I.M. (1982) Spectro-temporal characteristics of single units in the auditory midbrain of the lightly anaesthetised grassfrog (Rana temporaria L.) investigated with tonal stimuli. *Hearing Research* 6, 103-126.
Perkel, D.H., Gerstein, G.L., Moore, G.P. (1967). Neuronal spike trains and stochastic point processes. II. Simultaneous spike trains. *Biophysical Journal* 7, 419-440.
Pettigrew, A.G., Anson, M., Chung, S.H. (1981). Hearing in the frog: a neurophysiological study of the auditory response in the midbrain. *Proc. R. Soc. Lond. B.* 212, 433-457.
Rheinlaender, J., Gerhardt, H.C., Yager, D.D., Capranica, R.R. (1979). Accuracy of phonotaxis by green treefrog (Hyla cinerea). *J. Comparative Physiology A.* 133, 247-255.

GENERAL DISCUSSION

KLINKE:
What is interaural attenuation in frogs with your sound system and do the terms
"ipsilateral" and "contralateral" then really apply?

EGGERMONT:
In our experiments we used closed sound systems (Hermes et al., Hear. Res. 5, 147,
1981), and ipsilateral respectively contralateral stimulation have the conventional meaning. However, since there exists an open connection between both tympanic
cavities, the effect upon the frogs' central nervous system may be different. We
have measured interaural attenuation using laser interferometry (De Vlaming et al.,
to be published) and found it to be frequency dependent: around 1 kHz the attenuation is only 6 dB, but it rapidly increases to both low and high frequencies (up
to 20 dB in mouth-closed condition).

NARINS:
Your results showing a range of CFs for high-frequency-sensitive neurones in the
torus semicircularis must be interpreted carefully with respect to the tuning of
the basilar papilla. This is a simple organ containing about 100-120 hair cells
in the bullfrog (Rana catesbeiana). We find that the basilar papillar fibers in
an individual animal are tuned to a small range of frequencies (400 Hz). Is it
possible that the spread of high-frequency CFs that you observe in the torus might
be of central origin?

EGGERMONT:
I believe that there is ample evidence that the basilar papilla in e.g. the bullfrog or leopard frog are singly tuned. The disparities that seem to originate
from our measurements in torus semicularis units in the grass frog deserve some
elaboration. First of all we did not measure tuning curves but the equivalent of
iso-intensity contours. So it may well be that the tuning curves indicate a single
CF, but that the iso-intensity contours show a shift of the BF to either lower or
higher frequency or even split up. It is difficult for me to conceive that this is
due to some central phenomenon, since we presented single tones (48 ms duration)
randomly selected in frequency at one-second intervals. In addition we often observe that the high frequency units we encounter show a different BF for ipsilateral and contralateral stimulation. It seems that roughly two BF regions exist:
one around 1250 Hz, the other around 1750 Hz.

DE BOER:
What would be the physiological significance of a unit's sensitivity to interaural
delays of up to 10 ms?

EGGERMONT:
The crosscoincidence functions that we show in Fig. 4 point to latency differences
between units 2 and 4 of 15 ms. This, however, holds for both contralateral and
ipsilateral presentation, so these units are not responding to interaural time
differences of 15 ms. The receptive fields (cf Fig. 3) indicate latency differences between ipsi- and contralateral stimulation of the same order of magnitude.
This will include one extra synaptic delay but still remains large. When using bilateral stimulation, we always presented the sounds with a $\Delta t = 0$, so we have no
evidence of units being actually sensitive to these large latency differences.

Section IV
Psychophysics

REVIEW PAPER: PSYCHOACOUSTICS OF NORMAL AND IMPAIRED LISTENERS

Brian C.J. Moore

*Department of Experimental Psychology, University of Cambridge,
Downing Street, Cambridge   CB2 3EB, England*

In this paper I will give a brief introduction to some basic concepts and methods in psychoacoustics. The topics have been chosen to help the reader to understand the following papers, although it is not possible to cover all the relevant material. Since hearing involves the analysis of sounds in both the frequency and time domains, I start with an introduction to methods of measurement of the frequency and time resolution of the ear.

1. THE MEASUREMENT OF FREQUENCY AND TIME RESOLUTION

a) *Frequency resolution*

     Frequency resolution is most commonly measured in masking experiments. The results can be interpreted with the concept of the auditory filter. It is assumed that the peripheral auditory system contains a bank of overlapping linear bandpass filters, and that in detecting a signal in the presence of a masker the subject "listens" to the output of the auditory filter giving the best signal-to-masker ratio. The auditory filter at a given centre frequency can be thought of as a weighting function, W(f), which is applied to the power spectrum of a sound to determine the effective output of the filter at that frequency. It may be similar to the neural tuning curve at that characteristic frequency (CF). If we assume that the power of a signal at threshold, Ps, is proportional to the noise power passing through the auditory filter at that frequency, then this model can be described by the following equation:

$$Ps = K. \int_0^\infty N(f)W(f)df, \qquad\qquad (1)$$

where N(f) represents the power spectrum of the masker, and K is a constant representing the efficiency of the detector mechanism following the filter.
     In principle, if the signal threshold is measured as N(f) is varied in a suitable way, then this equation can be used to derive the shape of the auditory filter at a given centre frequency. The methods for deriving auditory filter shape depend on choosing a form for N(f) which simplifies equation (1), and allows the evaluation of the integral. In practice there is a serious difficulty. The auditory filter has a rounded top and rather steep skirts. Hence for many maskers the optimum signal-to-masker ratio will occur for a filter which is not centred at the signal frequency. Performance can be improved by listening to the output of this filter, rather than the one centred at the signal frequency, a process known as off-frequency listening (Patterson, 1976). When the masker spectrum is altered, the optimum signal-to-masker ratio may occur at different centre frequencies. Thus the subject will listen through different filters as N(f) is altered, and equation (1) will be invalid.
     Off-frequency listening can have a marked influence on several commonly used methods of measuring frequency selectivity. Consider, as an example, the psychophysical tuning curve (PTC). In this method the signal frequency and level are fixed, and the masker is either a sinusoid or narrowband noise whose centre frequency and level are varied to determine threshold. The method is intended to give a measure analogous to the neural FTC (Zwicker, 1974). Just as only one neurone (and therefore only one CF) is involved in the measurement of an FTC so, if the signal is at a very low level, only one auditory filter

should be involved in the determination of a PTC. If this were true, then the
PTC would be like an inverted filter shape; this follows directly from
equation (1). In practice, even for signals only 10 dB above absolute
threshold, off-frequency listening does occur. The main result is that the
PTC is sharpened around its tip relative to the "true" filter (Johnson-Davies
and Patterson, 1979; O'Loughlin and Moore, 1981a,b). The slopes of the skirts
can also be affected by off-frequency listening (Verschuure, 1978).

Off-frequency listening can be minimized by using maskers whose spectra
are symmetrical about the signal frequency. Unfortunately, the use of such
maskers does not allow the measurement of asymmetries in the auditory filter.
There is evidence, however, that at moderate sound levels the filter is only
slightly asymmetrical (Patterson and Nimmo-Smith, 1980). A masker which works
well in practice is a noise with a spectral notch centred at the signal
frequency. The threshold of the signal is determined as a function of the
width of the notch. Patterson (1976) has described results obtained using
such a masker, and has shown how the results can be used, together with
equation (1), to give a direct estimate of auditory filter shape. Since then
the method has been widely used by Patterson and others. Rather than giving
details, the major findings applying to young, healthy ears are summarised
below:
1) The auditory filter has a rounded top, and skirts which are initially
quite steep (about 100 dB/oct). If we express frequency in terms of g, the
normalized frequency deviation from the filter centre frequency, f_c,
$(g = |f - f_c|/f_c)$ then the filter shape within 25 dB of the tip is well
approximated by the equation:

$$W(g) = (1 + pg) \, e^{-pg} \qquad (2)$$

where p is a parameter which determines the bandwidth and slope of the filter
(Patterson *et al.*, 1982). The equivalent rectangular bandwidth (ERB) of the
filter is $4f_c/p$. The slope decreases 25-30 dB down from the tip.
2) The ERB of the filter increases with increasing centre frequency. When
expressed as a proportion of centre frequency the bandwidth decreases slightly
with increasing centre frequency. Over the range 100 - 6500 Hz, and at
moderate sound levels, the ERB is well approximated by:

$$ERB = 6.23F^2 + 93.39F + 28.52 \qquad (3)$$

where F is centre frequency in kHz (Moore and Glasberg, 1983a).
3) The ERB tends to increase with increasing sound level (Weber, 1977).
4) The low-frequency skirt of the filter becomes shallower with increasing
level, whereas the high-frequency skirt becomes steeper (Lutfi and Patterson,
1983).

An alternative method of measuring filter shape uses a noise whose
spectrum has a sinusoidal ripple on a linear frequency scale (Houtgast, 1974a,
1977; Pick, 1980). Threshold is measured with the signal at a maximum in the
masker spectrum and with the masker spectrum "inverted", so that the signal is
at a minimum in the noise spectrum. When the spacing of the ripples is large
compared to the auditory filter bandwidth, the threshold difference between
the normal and inverted spectra is large. As the spacing of the ripples is
decreased the threshold difference decreases. By measuring the threshold
difference as a function of ripple density it is possible to derive the shape
of the auditory filter. This method appears to give a good estimate of the
tip of the filter characteristic, but it becomes inaccurate more than 10-15 dB
below the tip (Glasberg, Moore and Nimmo-Smith, 1983).

The measures described so far all use a fixed signal frequency, and
attempt to characterise frequency selectivity at that frequency (i.e. at a
particular CF or place). An alternative approach is to characterise the
distribution of excitation across frequency for a given masker; this
distribution has been referred to as the excitation pattern or internal

spectrum of the masker. In terms of the filter-bank analogy, the excitation pattern can be considered as the output of the auditory filters as a function of filter centre frequency. The excitation pattern of a masker can be determined by measuring signal threshold as a function of signal frequency (Zwicker and Feldtkeller, 1967), on the assumption that the signal threshold is directly proportional to the masker excitation at the signal frequency. Again, however, off-frequency listening may influence the form of the results (Verschuure, 1978). An alternative approach is to infer excitation patterns from filter shapes, by calculating the filter outputs as a function of filter centre frequency, using equations (2) and (3) (Moore and Glasberg, 1983a).

Simultaneous masking does not seem to show the effects of suppression, a nonlinear process which clearly operates in the auditory periphery. Houtgast (1972, 1974a) has suggested that this is because suppression in a particular frequency region does not change the signal-to-masker ratio in that region. Threshold in simultaneous masking appears to depend primarily on this ratio, so it will not be affected by suppression. Houtgast presented evidence that nonsimultaneous techniques could be used to demonstrate suppression, the most popular methods being forward masking and the pulsation threshold. His arguments have been widely accepted, although each method has certain difficulties associated with it.

Forward masking is complicated by the fact that large changes in threshold may be produced by changes in the cues available to the subjects. Many demonstrations of suppression seem to be confounded in this way (Moore, 1980). This problem can be minimized by using broadband maskers and sinusoidal signals. In addition, forward masking is complicated by the nonlinear relationship between signal threshold and effective masker level. This problem can be minimized by keeping signal level fixed, or by using a transform to compensate for the nonlinearity (Moore and Glasberg, 1981).

In the pulsation threshold method the "masker" and "signal" are alternated, and the subject is required to adjust the signal (usually its level) until it is on the borderline between sounding pulsating and sounding continuous. Unfortunately there is no adequate theory to account for the continuity effect, and the interpretation of the results is complicated by uncertainty as to the criterion adopted by the subject. The results are sometimes highly variable, and the method does not seem suitable for use with untrained subjects. Nevertheless, results from trained subjects do show suppression effects which parallel those observed in primary auditory neurones.

b) *Time resolution*

A wide variety of techniques has been used to estimate the temporal resolution of the ear. In all methods it is necessary to ensure that performance is based on temporal cues rather than on the detection of spectral changes. Some workers have analysed their results in terms of a temporal filter analogous to the frequency-domain filter discussed above. However, linear systems theory does not seem to work so well in this case, and it is not generally possible to describe the results of different experiments in terms of a single temporal filter characteristic.

Several workers have measured temporal modulation transfer functions (MTFs) for sounds which are amplitude modulated (Viemeister, 1979) or intensity modulated (van Zanten, 1980). The threshold depth of the modulation is determined as a function of modulation frequency. The threshold is lowest at low modulation frequencies, and increases progressively for modulation rates above about 10 Hz; thus the MTFs show a low-pass characteristic. The MTFs are roughly independent of overall level except at very low levels. When bandlimited noise is used, the time constant indicated by the MTF decreases with increasing centre frequency.

An approach which is similar to the measurement of MTFs involves measuring the threshold for brief probes (usually filtered clicks) at various temporal locations in an amplitude- or intensity-modulated noise (e.g. Fastl, 1977). An experiment similar to the rippled-noise experiments described in section 1(a) is obtained if the difference in masked threshold between signal-at-peak and signal-at-trough is measured as a function of modulation frequency (Festen and Plomp, 1981). The threshold difference decreases with increasing modulation frequency. The width of the temporal "window" or filter inferred from the data depends strongly on the form which is assumed for the window. The data have not generally been sufficiently precise to allow this form to be determined.

Temporal acuity has also been measured using gap-detection tasks. For broadband noise the minimum detectable gap is about 2-3 ms. For bandpass noise the minimum detectable gap decreases with increasing centre frequency (Fitzgibbons and Wightman, 1982; Shailer and Moore, 1983), reaching values of about 8 ms at 1 kHz and 22 ms at 200 Hz. Below 1 kHz the reciprocal of the gap threshold is proportional to the bandwidth of the auditory filter, implying that "ringing" in the filter limits performance at low frequencies (Shailer and Moore, 1983).

2.   FREQUENCY AND TIME RESOLUTION IN THE HEARING IMPAIRED

a)   *Frequency resolution*

There is now almost overwhelming evidence that in listeners with hearing impairments of cochlear origin there is a loss of frequency selectivity. This has been demonstrated primarily using masking techniques (rippled-noise, notched-noise and PTCs). However, the following cautions should be observed:
1)   There can be considerable variability among patients, even when the elevation in absolute threshold is similar. Although the bandwidth of the auditory filter is correlated with the threshold elevation (Pick *et al.*, 1977), some patients have broad filters and almost normal thresholds, while some have elevated thresholds but almost normal filters.
2)   The auditory filter bandwidth increases at high sound levels in normally-hearing subjects. Since measurements with patients usually have to be made at high sound levels, part of the broadening may be attributable to a normal level effect.
3)   The auditory filter tends to broaden with increasing age (Patterson *et al.*, 1982). Since many hearing-impaired patients are elderly, part of the broadening may be a "normal" age effect. However, the variability of the auditory filter bandwidth also increases with age, and abnormally broad filter bandwidths can be observed even in young hearing-impaired patients.

In spite of these cautions it seems clear that the frequency selectivity of the cochlea is physiologically vulnerable, and psychophysical frequency resolution is commonly reduced in listeners with cochlear impairments.

There is also evidence that the suppression mechanism may be damaged, or even completely inoperative in cases of cochlear hearing impairment. In normal subjects the auditory filter measured in nonsimultaneous masking is sharper than that measured in simultaneous masking, a difference which is commonly attributed to suppression (Houtgast, 1974a, 1977; Moore and Glasberg, 1981; Glasberg *et al.*, 1983). In patients with cochlear impairments the differences are reduced, and may even be zero (Festen and Plomp, 1983). We have found using a notch-noise masker (Moore and Glasberg, unpublished data) that in cases of moderate impairments (losses of 40 - 50 dB) the auditory filter measured in forward masking is still slightly sharper than that in simultaneous masking. However, the difference is seen mainly on the skirts of the filter, rather than around the tip. Thus suppression may operate weakly in these cases.

b)   *Time resolution*

The comparison of temporal resolution in normal and impaired listeners is somewhat more straightforward than the comparison of frequency resolution, since temporal resolution varies little with overall level, except at very low levels. Again, however, the results are characterised by considerable individual differences. On average, listeners with cochlear impairments show impaired temporal resolution in comparison with normal subjects. This has been shown clearly for gap-detection tasks (Irwin *et al.*, 1981; Fitzgibbons and Wightman, 1982; Tyler *et al.*, 1982). Measurements of temporal-window shape using intensity-modulated noise also tend to reveal poorer resolution in patients with cochlear impairments (Festen and Plomp, 1983), although there has been no direct comparison of normal and impaired subjects using exactly the same methods.

The reduced frequency resolution observed psychoacoustically in patients with cochlear impairments appears to correspond well with the reduced tuning of single primary neurones found in animals with abnormal cochleas (see, for example, Evans, 1975). However, the physiological correlate of impaired temporal processing is not so clear. Woolf *et al.* (1981) found that the frequency range over which a given neurone would phase lock was reduced in animals with cochlear damage induced by kanamycin treatment. In contrast Harrison and Evans (1979) found no deficit in phase locking in damaged animals, and Salvi *et al.* (1979) found no change in the latencies of single neurone or whole nerve responses.

3. PSYCHOACOUSTICAL ABILITIES AND SPEECH PERCEPTION IN THE HEARING IMPAIRED

For normally hearing persons speech is a highly redundant stimulus. Hence quite gross distortions or modifications can be tolerated without a large loss of intelligibility (see Moore, 1982 for a review). However, in impaired listeners this redundancy is considerably reduced, since the full range of acoustic cues available to the normal listener may not be usable by the impaired listener. As a result, speech intelligibility is impaired, particularly when background noise or competing speech is present. Indeed, difficulty in understanding speech in noise is one of the commonest complaints of hearing-impaired patients.

We may identify the following factors as potentially contributing to the difficulties in speech perception experienced by the impaired listener:
1) Reduced sensitivity: in normal conversation the weaker components in speech may reach levels of only about 40 dB SPL at middle to high frequencies. Hence if threshold elevations exceed 35 dB the weaker components may be inaudible unless they are amplified.
2) Recruitment: the threshold for detection is elevated, but the threshold for discomfort may be almost normal, i.e. the growth of loudness with intensity is more rapid than in a normal ear. Thus if the strong components in speech are at a comfortable level, the weak components may be inaudible. Recruitment alone may produce marked deficits in speech intelligibility (Villchur, 1977).
3) Reduced frequency discrimination: changes in the fundamental frequency of speech may be harder to hear (Hoekstra and Ritsma, 1977), so that the prosodic features of speech (such as intonation patterns) may be lost.
4) Reduced frequency selectivity: the auditory filter may be broader than normal, so that the spectral patterns of speech sounds will be harder to recognize and discriminate. In addition there will be an increased susceptibility to masking by background noise, since components in the noise far removed from the important speech frequencies will have a masking effect.
5) Poor temporal resolution: the gaps and rapid transitions in speech, which are important in the identification of consonants, may be harder to detect. Background noise may make discrimination of temporal features even worse.
6) A high susceptibility to, or a slow recovery from, temporal masking effects (e.g. Dreschler and Plomp, 1983). This means that weak consonants will be more easily masked by vowels.
7) A loss of binaural processing: the ability to compare and combine

information from the two ears may be reduced. Thus the normal advantages of directional listing and the binaural masking level difference (BMLD) may not be available (Laurence, Moore and Glasberg, 1983).

Many workers have attempted to determine whether the intelligibility of speech is strongly related to any particular psychoacoustical ability such as frequency resolution or temporal resolution. The results have been somewhat variable, and sometimes difficult to interpret, partly because of large individual differences and partly because patients may compensate for particular deficits by making greater use of residual abilities. For example, a patient with impaired frequency resolution but normal temporal resolution may partly compensate for the deficit by making greater use of temporal cues. In addition, some deficits tend to occur together (e.g. recruitment and reduced frequency resolution), so it is difficult to separate their effects.

A good deal of work has been done on the relationship between frequency resolution and speech perception. Experiments using vowel-like sounds as maskers have shown that in normal-hearing subjects the "internal spectrum" contains peaks and dips corresponding to the first three or four formants. Nonsimultaneous masking reveals that the internal representation of the formants is enhanced by suppression (Houtgast, 1974b; Moore and Glasberg, 1983b). In subjects with cochlear impairments the formants are much less well preserved, and suppression does not produce an enhancement (Bacon, 1979). We might expect therefore that speech intelligibility is impaired by reduced frequency resolution. This does appear to be the case, although a strong relationship is found only for speech intelligibility in noise (Festen and Plomp, 1983; Dreschler and Plomp, 1980, 1983).

There is also a relationship between temporal resolution and speech intelligibility in noise. Tyler *et al.* (1982) found that, for hearing-impaired patients, longer gap-detection thresholds were significantly correlated with reduced speech intelligibility in noise, even when the effects of pure-tone threshold loss were partialled out. However, Festen and Plomp (1983) found only a weak correlation between the width of the psychophysical temporal window and threshold for speech in noise.

The detection of modulation in speech also appears to be of considerable importance. Steeneken and Houtgast (1980) have shown that the speech-transmission quality of a communication channel can be accurately predicted from a physical measure based on the measurement of MTFs in seven octave bands. The physical measure, the Speech Transmission Index (STI), correlates highly with direct measures of speech intelligibility, and can be used to predict the effect of various types of distortions such as filtering, peak-clipping, reverberation, background noise and automatic gain control (AGC).

4. SIGNAL PROCESSING TO COMPENSATE FOR HEARING IMPAIRMENTS

Given what we know about the psychoacoustical characteristics of patients with cochlear impairments, to what extent is it possible to process sounds so as to compensate for the impairments? Unfortunately, the answer to this question appears to be "rather little", although there is some promise of progress. Signal processing to compensate for recruitment has been studied for many years. The commonest method is to use some form of AGC. A single AGC amplifier applied to the whole speech signal is of limited use, since the vowels of speech, which have the highest levels, will set the gain, and the weak high-frequency consonants will be inaudible. In addition, the amount of recruitment often varies considerably with frequency. An alternative is to split the speech signal into a number of frequency bands, each with its own AGC amplifier. The outputs of the different channels are then recombined. Such systems appear to work well in some situations, but if many channels are used speech intelligibility at high levels, or in background noise can actually be impaired (Lippmann, *et al.*, 1981). One reason for this is that the processing reduces the modulation depth of the speech envelope, and also

distorts the envelope. Schreiner and Lewien (1982) have reported that this
problem can be alleviated by filtering the speech envelope in each frequency
band to enhance modulations above 6 Hz. This improves intelligibility for
impaired patients. An alternative way of minimizing envelope distortion is to
use a small number of channels, and to use an initial AGC amplifier with a
long recovery time, operating on the whole speech signal (Laurence *et al.*,
1983).

It appears rather difficult to compensate for impaired frequency
resolution. For patients with this problem, narrowing the formant bandwidths
in synthetic speech does not improve speech intelligibility (Summerfield *et al.*,
1981). Presumably this is because the formant bandwidths in normal speech are
already narrow in comparison to the bandwidths of the auditory filters in the
impaired ear. Similarly, it appears difficult to compensate for impaired
temporal resolution. Perhaps the most promising approach lies in schemes to
enhance speech-to-noise ratios. Patients experience most difficulty in noisy
situations, and even small improvements in speech-to-noise ratio, say 3-dB,
can produce worthwhile improvements in intelligibility. One of the simplest
ways of enhancing speech-to-noise ratios is by using directional microphones;
if the microphone faces forward then the speech-to-noise ratio is improved
when the listener looks directly at the speaker. Unfortunately, the miniature
microphones used with hearing aids rarely give an improvement of more than 3
dB.

Hearing aids of the future might operate by extracting speech parameters
such as formant frequencies, presence or absence of voicing, and fundamental
frequency. Provided the parameters were accurately extracted, even in the
presence of background noise, the parameters could be used to re-synthesize
speech which was entirely noise free. In addition it would be possible to
transform the output in various ways to enhance the discriminability of speech
features. For example, the formants could be spread over a greater frequency
range to reduce mutual masking. Similarly the variations in fundamental
frequency could be enlarged (the frequency range expanded) to compensate for
deficits in frequency discrimination and enhance the perception of intonation.

*Acknowledgements: I am grateful to Roy Patterson, Brian Glasberg and Bob
Carlyon for helpful comments on an earlier version of this paper. Lorraine
Evans patiently typed several drafts of the paper. Part of the work reported
here was supported by the Medical Research Council.*

REFERENCES

Bacon, S.P. (1979). Suppression effects in vowel pulsation patterns:
    normal-hearing and hearing-impaired listeners. M.A. Thesis, University
    of Kansas.
Dreschler, W.A. and Plomp, R. (1980). Relation between psychophysical data
    and speech perception for hearing-impaired subjects.I. *J. Acoust. Soc.
    Am.*, 68, 1608-1615.
Dreschler, W.A. and Plomp, R. (1983). Relation between psychophysical data
    and speech perception for hearing-impaired subjects.II. *J. Acoust. Soc.
    Am.*, (submitted).
Evans, E.F. (1975). The sharpening of cochlear frequency selectivity in the
    normal and abnormal cochlea. *Audiology*, 14, 419-442.
Fastl, H. (1977). Roughness and temporal masking patterns of sinusoidally
    amplitude modulated broadband noise. In: *Psychophysics and Physiology of
    Hearing*, Eds. E.F. Evans and J.P. Wilson, pp. 403-414, London, Academic
    Press.
Festen, J.M. and Plomp, R. (1981). Relations between auditory functions in
    normal hearing. *J. Acoust. Soc. Am.*, 70, 356-369.
Festen, J.M. and Plomp, R. (1983). Relations between auditory functions in
    impaired hearing. *J. Acoust. Soc. Am.* (in press).

Fitzgibbons, P.J. and Wightman, F.L. (1982). Gap detection in normal and hearing-impaired listeners. *J. Acoust. Soc. Am.*, 72, 761-765.

Glasberg, B.R., Moore, B.C.J. and Nimmo-Smith, I. (1983). Comparison of auditory filter shapes derived with three different maskers. *J. Acoust. Soc. Am.*, (submitted).

Harrison, R.V. and Evans, E.F. (1979). Some aspects of temporal coding by single cochlear nerve fibers from regions of cochlear hair-cell degeneration in the Guinea Pig. *Arch. Otolaryngol.*, 224, 71-78.

Hoekstra, A. and Ritsma, R.J. (1977). Perceptive hearing loss and frequency selectivity. In: *Psychophysics and Physiology of Hearing*, Eds. E.F. Evans and J.P. Wilson, pp. 263-271, London, Academic Press.

Houtgast, T. (1972). Psychophysical evidence for lateral inhibition in hearing. *J. Acoust. Soc. Am.*, 51, 1885-1894.

Houtgast, T. (1974a). Lateral suppression in hearing. Thesis, Free University of Amsterdam.

Houtgast, T. (1974b). Auditory analysis of vowel-like sounds. *Acustica*, 31, 320-324.

Houtgast, T. (1977). Auditory-filter characteristics derived from direct-masking data and pulsation-threshold data with a rippled-noise masker. *J. Acoust. Soc. Am.*, 62, 409-415.

Irwin, R.J., Hinchcliffe, L.K. and Kemp, S. (1981). Temporal acuity in normal and hearing-impaired listeners. *Audiology*, 20, 234-243.

Johnson-Davies, D. and Patterson, R.D. (1979). Psychophysical tuning curves: restricting the listening band to the signal region. *J. Acoust. Soc. Am.*, 65, 765-770.

Laurence, R.F., Moore, B.C.J. and Glasberg, B.R. (1983). A comparison of behind-the-ear high-fidelity linear hearing aids, and two-channel compression aids, in the laboratory and in everyday life. *Brit. J. Audiol.*, (in press).

Lippmann, R.P., Braida, L.D. and Durlach, N.I. (1981). Study of multi-channel amplitude compression and linear amplification for persons with sensorineural hearing loss. *J. Acoust. Soc. Am.*, 69, 524-534.

Lutfi, R. and Patterson, R.D. (1983). On the mechanism of masking asymmetry. *J. Acoust. Soc. Am.* (submitted).

Moore, B.C.J. (1980). Detection cues in forward masking. In: *Psychophysical, Physiological and Behavioural Studies in Hearing*, Eds. G. van den Brink and F.A. Bilsen, pp. 222-229, Delft, Delft University Press.

Moore, B.C.J. (1982). *Introduction to the Psychology of Hearing*, 2nd Ed., London, Academic Press.

Moore, B.C.J. and Glasberg, B.R. (1981). Auditory filter shapes derived in simultaneous and forward masking. *J. Acoust. Soc. Am.*, 69, 1003-1014.

Moore, B.C.J. and Glasberg, B.R. (1983a). Suggested formulae for calculating auditory-filter bandwidths and excitation patterns. *J. Acoust. Soc. Am.*, (submitted).

Moore, B.C.J. and Glasberg, B.R. (1983b). Masking patterns for synthetic vowels in simultaneous and forward masking. *J. Acoust. Soc. Am.*, (in press).

O'Loughlin, B.J. and Moore, B.C.J. (1981a). Off-frequency listening: effects on psychoacoustical tuning curves obtained in simultaneous and forward masking. *J. Acoust. Soc. Am.*, 69, 1119-1125.

O'Loughlin, B.J. and Moore, B.C.J. (1981b). Improving psychoacoustical tuning curves. *Hear. Res.*, 5, 343-346.

Patterson, R.D. (1976). Auditory filter shapes derived with noise stimuli. *J. Acoust. Soc. Am.*, 59, 640-654.

Patterson, R.D. and Nimmo-Smith, I. (1980). Off-frequency listening and auditory-filter asymmetry. *J. Acoust. Soc. Am.*, 67, 229-245.

Patterson, R.D., Nimmo-Smith, I., Weber, D.L. and Milroy, R. (1982). The deterioration of hearing with age: Frequency selectivity, the critical ratio, the audiogram and speech threshold. *J. Acoust. Soc. Am.*, 72, 1788-1803.

Pick, G.F. (1980). Level dependence of psychophysical frequency resolution and auditory filter shape. *J. Acoust. Soc. Am.*, 68, 1085-1095.

Pick, G.F., Evans, E.F. and Wilson, J.P. (1977). Frequency resolution in patients with hearing loss of cochlear origin. In: *Psychophysics and Physiology of Hearing*, Eds. E.F. Evans and J.P. Wilson, pp. 273-281, London, Academic Press.

Salvi, R.J., Henderson, D. and Hamernik, R.P. (1979). Single auditory nerve fiber and action potential latencies in normal and noise-treated chinchillas. *Hear. Res.*, 1, 237-251.

Schreiner, C. and Lewien, T. (1982). Envelope filtering in speech processing for cochlear implants. Presented at the Symposium on Artificial Auditory Stimulation, Erlangen.

Shailer, M.J. and Moore, B.C.J. (1983). Gap detection as a function of frequency, bandwidth and level. *J. Acoust. Soc. Am.* (submitted).

Steeneken, H.J.M. and Houtgast, T. (1980). A physical method for measuring speech-transmission quality. *J. Acoust. Soc. Am.*, 67, 318-326.

Summerfield, A.Q., Tyler, R.S., Foster, J.R., Wood, E. and Bailey, P.J. (1981). Failure of formant bandwidth narrowing to improve speech reception in sensorineural impairment. *J. Acoust. Soc. Am.*, 70, S108-109.

Tyler, R.S., Summerfield, Q., Wood, E.J. and Fernandes, M.A. (1982). Psychoacoustic and phonetic temporal processing in normal and hearing-impaired listeners. *J. Acoust. Soc. Am.*, 72, 740-752.

Van Zanten, G.A. (1980). Temporal modulation transfer functions for intensity modulated noise bands. In: *Psychophysical, Physiological and Behavioural Studies in Hearing*, Eds. G. van den Brink and F.A. Bilsen, pp. 206-209, Delft, Delft University Press.

Verschuure, J. (1978). Auditory excitation patterns, Thesis, Erasmus University, Rotterdam.

Viemeister, N.F. (1979). Temporal modulation transfer functions based upon modulation thresholds. *J. Acoust. Soc. Am.*, 66, 1364-1380.

Villchur, E. (1977). Electronic models to simulate the effect of sensory distortions on speech perception by the deaf. *J. Acoust. Soc. Am.*, 62, 665-674.

Weber, D.L. (1977). Growth of masking and the auditory filter. *J. Acoust. Soc. Am.*, 62, 424-429.

Woolf, N.K., Ryan, A.F. and Bone, R.C. (1981). Neural phase-locking properties in the absence of cochlear outer hair cells. *Hear. Res.*, 11, 109-127.

Zwicker, E. (1974). On a psychoacoustical equivalent of tuning curves. In: *Facts and Models in Hearing*, Eds. E. Zwicker and E. Terhardt, Berlin, Springer-Verlag.

Zwicker, E. and Feldtkeller, R. (1967). *Das Ohr als Nachrichtenempfanger*, Stuttgart, Hirzel.

GENERAL DISCUSSION

PICK:
I would like to address myself to the difficulty for linear theory that in cochlear pathology both frequency and temporal resolution are impaired. I have been
investigating models involving linear filters with nonlinear feedback around them,
which stimulate a number of empirical measurements. Such models have faster settl-
ing times than linear filter with identical amplitude functions. If, in pathology,
the nonlinearity becomes less effective, as appears likely, then this phenomenon
might contribute to the deficit in temporal resolution.

MOORE:
I think that the temporal response of the peripheral filter will only affect temporal resolution in very restricted situations, when the filter has a narrow
bandwidth. This applies to healthy ears at low frequencies (below 1 kHz). The impairments in temporal resolution in some patients are probably related to processes other than ringing in their filters, since the filters are generally broader
in these patients. However, the type of effect you describe may play a role in a
few cases, particularly at low frequencies.

FASTL:
Recently we found suppression effects not only in nonsimultaneous masking (post
masking) but also in simultaneous masking (Fastl and Bechly, Acoustica 51, 242,
1982). Suppression in simultaneous masking is most prominent at the lower slope
of the masker and the suppressor. The magnitude of the suppression effect is
smaller in simultaneous masking (8 dB) than in post masking (14 dB).

MOORE:
I became aware of your experiments after my paper was completed. I think that we
should be cautious in attributing "unmasking" effects which we find psychophysically to physiological suppression. Psychophysical unmasking may sometimes have
other causes (e.g. Moore, 1980). Your results may, on the other hand, indicate
that the assumptions used to explain why suppression is not usually revealed in
simultaneous masking (as outlined in my paper) are not completely correct.

EVANS:
I have described effects of stimulus level on the cut-off slopes of cochlear fibre
filter functions (see Evans, 1977, 1980b, 1981 and the data in my paper) analogous
to those you describe for psychoacoustic filter functions: namely increase in high
frequency cut-off slope and decrease in low frequency cut-off slope, with increase
in level. However, in my cochlear fibre data this is true only for fibres with CFs
above 1 kHz. Fibres with lower CFs, if anything, show opposite effects. Is this
reflected in the psychophysics?

MOORE:
There is some evidence that the change of the filter slope with level are reduced
at low frequencies. For example the filter shapes obtained by Fidell et al. (1983)
using a noise spectrum level of 60 dB are similar to those that we obtained at a
level of 40 dB, at low frequencies. However, the decrease in low-frequency slope
of the filter with increasing level appears to occur at all frequencies; the masked audiograms of narrowband noise, as obtained by Zwicker and others, show a decreasing high-frequency slope with increasing level at all centre frequencies.

TYLER:
I would like to suggest that the perception of dynamic stimuli might be another
psychoacoustical ability that contributes to speech perception in the hearing impaired. For example, we have found that the discrimination of frequency transitions can be very poor in the hearing impaired. Although our data are of a preliminary nature, neither frequency discrimination nor frequency resolution was related
to the discrimination of frequency transitions. I think further investigation of
dynamic stimuli is fundamental to our understanding of and the remediation of
hearing impairment.

MOORE:
You may well be right.

KIM:

I have a question of terminology to our colleagues in psychoacoustics. Instead of the term "off-frequency listening", I suggest that "off-place listening" is a more appropriate term. This is beacuse the intention of the term appears to be that the brain pays attention to discharge activity of cochlear neurones located at a place slightly shifted from the normal place along the cochlear partition for a particular probe frequency. What is shifted is not frequency but place under this condition.

MOORE:

The frequency referred to in the phrase "off-frequency listening" is the centre frequency of the auditory filter used to detect a signal, not the frequency of the signal. I agree that this use can be confusing, and a phrase such as that suggested by Kim might be more appropriate. However, I doubt that we will be able to persuade our colleagues to adopt a new term after so many years of using the old one.

DUIFHUIS:

I want to raise a terminology point. You use the term the auditory filter as defined in sect.1a. This is a very general term, but you refer to a very specific measure of auditory frequency selectivity. The studies where broadband maskers are used will only show linear aspects of the auditory filter because broadband backgrounds tend to linearize a system for simultaneous small signals (narrowband strong backgrounds do the same, to a lesser extent). The linearizing effect provides a fortunate justification of the use of the linear analysis, which, as you mentioned, has been used by Patterson and by Houtgast. However, it seems to be quite generally accepted by now that the cochlear filter is markedly nonlinear, and for me "the auditory filter" refers to this nonlinear filter. I agree that this does not make life easier. It is not at all clear what "filter shape" one can use to depict this nonlinear filter. An iso-response criterion (tuning curve) appears to overemphasize selectivity, whereas an iso-input measure may lead to an underestimation (given the saturating nonlinear behaviour). So I admit that a linear description of the auditory filter is often practical and useful, but I want to maintain that this is not a complete characterization of the auditory filter.

MOORE:

The term auditory filter was used in my paper to describe the intensity weighting function which can be used to account for simultaneous masking data at a given centre frequency. I agree that it may not be appropriate to talk of the auditory filter, since different functions may be required to account for different types of data. We have found, however, that the filter shape derived using a notched-noise masker is almost the same as that derived with a two-tone masker (Glasberg et al., 1983). Hence the shape is not strongly dependent on using broadband maskers. For non-simultaneous masking it is not true that a single linear filter characteristic can explain a variety of data.

LOUDNESS ADAPTATION INDUCED INTERAURALLY AND MONAURALLY

B. Scharf, M.-C. Botte and G. Canévet

Auditory Perception Laboratory, Northeastern Univ., Boston, MA 02115, USA;
Laboratoire de Psychologie Expérimentale, CNRS, Paris, France;
Laboratoire de Mécanique et d'Acoustique, CNRS, Marseille, France

Loudness is unusually stable. Unlike most other sensations, it does not decline over time simply as the result of continued stimulation. The failure of
loudness to adapt under most listening conditions poses an intriguing question.
Just what keeps loudness from adapting? To help answer that question, we have investigated two of those conditions under which loudness does adapt, at levels below about 30 dB SL (Scharf, 1983) and in the presence of a contralateral intermittent sound (Botte et al., 1982). The present paper extends the latter investigation. First we review the phenomenon which we have called *induced loudness ad-*
aptation and present new data on the effect of intermittency. Second we examine
the reduction in the loudness of a continuous tone while a 10-s tone is present in
the contralateral ear; particular attention is paid to frequency selectivity.
Third we show that loudness adaptation can be induced by an intermittent tone in
the same ear(s) as the continuous tone, whether the tones are presented through
earphone(s) or from loudspeaker(s) in a free field.

1. GENERAL PROCEDURE

The method of successive magnitude estimation was used to obtain numerical
judgments of the loudness of a continuous sound over time. This method is derived
from Stevens's method of magnitude estimation (Stevens, 1956) whereby the observer
(O) assigns a number to represent the loudness of a sound. In our experiments the
O judged the loudness of a continuous sound at successive points in time, indicated by a visual signal. Generally, O was asked to judge loudness every 10 to 30 s.
He was free to choose any number whose magnitude he felt matched the loudness at
the moment the judgment was called for. Only the loudness of the continuous,
1000-Hz tone was to be judged and any other sound was to be ignored.

2. EXPERIMENT I. ADAPTATION INDUCED INTERAURALLY

Elsewhere (Botte et al., 1982), we have shown that an intermittent tone in
one ear induces a drop of about 50% (equivalent to 10 dB according to the sone
function) in the loudness of a continuous tone in the other ear after 2 to 3 min.
The loudness drop appears to reach an asymptote within that time. Surprisingly,
however, after the intermittent tone ends, the continuous tone does not return
to its initial, unadapted loudness but remains near its reduced loudness for at
least 5 min (Scharf et al., in press). Also surprising is that neither the level
nor the frequency of the intermittent tone matters much (Botte et al., 1982). Induced loudness adaptation of a continuous 1000-Hz tone at 60 dB was about the same
whether the level of the contralateral intermittent tone was 40, 60, or 80 dB and
whether its frequency was 400 or 6000 Hz or some value in between. The temporal
parameters of the intermittent tone also did not seem important, but we only briefly explored the effect of period and duty cycle. We now present some additional
data that confirm this last conclusion.

Both the continuous and intermittent sounds were 1000-Hz tones at 60 dB SPL.
The continuous tone began first in the right ear. The intermittent tone began
20 s later in the left ear and lasted 3 min. Intermittency was varied from .5 s

on, .5 s off to 10 s on, 20 s off. With the faster rates, the off periods were
too brief to permit a loudness judgment while there was no sound to the left ear
but with off periods of 5 s or longer, the loudness in the right ear could be
judged with no sound present in the left ear at that moment. In two control runs,
the continuous tone was presented entirely alone. In one control run the tone was at
60 dB throughout its presentation; in the other it began at 60 dB and then decreased
gradually to 50 dB during the next 3 min. Means are for 9 to 12 Os.

Figure 1 presents the results in the form of adaptation quotients (AQ), calculated as follows: AQ = {E(i) - E(t)}/E(i)   where E(i) is the initial
estimate and E(t) is the estimate at time t. The value of AQ is 0.0 if there is no
adaptation, that is, no change in loudness so that E(t) = E(i); AQ is 1.0 if adaptation is complete with E(t) = 0.0. An AQ of .5, for example, means that loudness
was half as great at time, t, as it was initially. Negative values for AQ mean
that loudness increased. The AQs shown in Fig. 1 are the means of the AQs calculated for each O. The first AQ of 0.0 is for the initial estimate itself, made before the intermittent tone began.

In the control condition, which had no intermittent tone, the loudness decreased about 15% within 90 s and no more after that. (Botte et al. (1982) found
the same mean value of 15%, for 32 Os.) When the tone was presented alone but
decreased 10 dB over 3 min, AQ increased steadily to about .58, a little more than
predicted from the sone function (Scharf, 1978). When the intermittent tone is introduced into the contralateral ear, curves for the continuous tone of unchanging
level look much like that for the physically decreasing tone. The period and duty

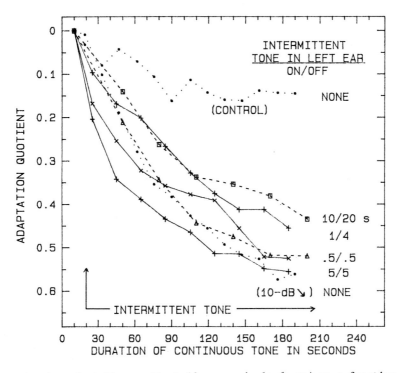

*Fig. 1. Adaptation quotient (decrease in loudness) as a function of duration of a
continuous tone in the right ear. Intermittent tone with various on-off periods
began at 20 s and went to the left ear, except in the control and 10-dB down conditions. Different symbols represent different experiments and Os*

cycle of intermittency make little difference to the amount of adaptation. There
is a suggestion that a 50% duty cycle is optimal, but earlier data (Botte et al.,
1982) did not show a similar trend. Moreover, variability among Os is such as to
render differences less than about .2 non-significant (standard errors are about
.08 to .10 when AQ is maximum). Repeating the sound in the contralateral ear is
necessary since a single 5-s or 10-s burst gave AQs of only .20 and .14. The quality of the tone changes along with the loudness; pitch becomes less clear and the
initially pure tone begins to sound fuzzy.

3. EXPERIMENT II: LOUDNESS REDUCTION AND FREQUENCY SELECTIVITY

     With relatively long on and off periods, it is possible to measure the loud-
ness of the continuous tone while the intermittent tone is off (as in Fig. 1 for
5-s and 10-s off periods) and also while it is on. These last measurements, described in the following section, show that during the on period the loudness of
the continuous tone is greatly reduced for most Os when the frequencies in the two
ears are similar.

     The continuous tone was on in the right ear for 50 s during which O made five
loudness estimates, one while a 10-s tone was on in the left ear. Figure 2 presents the mean AQs from those estimates by 13 Os. The AQ is plotted as a function
of the frequency of the 10-s tone presented to the left ear. But it is the loudness of the 1000-Hz tone that was judged.

     Figure 2 reveals pronounced frequency selectivity with the maximum loudness
reduction caused by 960-Hz and 1000-Hz tones. With those two frequencies loudness

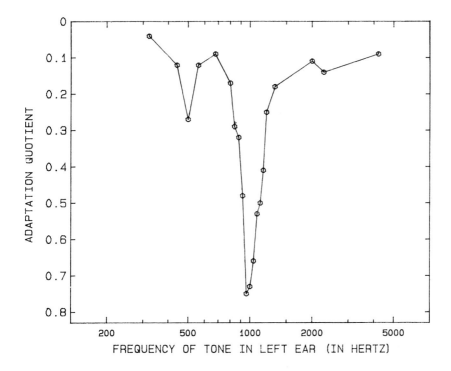

*Fig. 2. Loudness reduction (adaptation quotient) of a 1000-Hz tone in the right
ear caused by tones of different frequencies in the left ear*

went down four fold or 75% (the equivalent of 20 dB on the sone function). Loudness reduction was only about 25% (4 dB) when the frequency was below 840 Hz or above 1160 Hz, except at 500 Hz. Thus, loudness reduction was greatest when the left-ear frequency and the right-ear frequency were within one critical band of each other (approximately 160 Hz at a center frequency of 1000 Hz). Inter-observer variability was also greatest in that range; the standard deviations were often almost 0.40. For example, when both tones were at 1000 Hz, six of the 13 Os reported that the tone in the right ear had disappeared altogether and gave AQs of 1.0, three Os had AQs of .80 or higher, but one O reported no change in loudness and another O reported an increase in loudness in the right ear.

Data at only one test frequency do not permit firm conclusions about the role of frequency selectivity in interaural interaction. However, one reasonable interpretation of these data is that the presentation of the 10-s tone in the left ear initiates interaural funneling. Funneling is the term Bekesy (1958) applied to the inferred neural interaction that results in lateralization of a sound image toward the ear receiving the more intense, temporally leading sound. The resulting sound image captures all the loudness available and is the sum of the loudnesses from both ears, thus leaving the other ear silent. Nearly half our Os did, indeed, report that the right ear was silent (when both tones were 1000 Hz) although the left-ear tone was not more intense and came on 20 s *after* the right-ear tone. However, this unusual funneling was complete only when the tones were the same or nearly the same in frequency. Although we cannot be sure that similar rules apply to interaural interaction at other frequencies, the role of the critical band has been previously demonstrated in central masking (Zwislocki et al., 1958) and at a number of different frequencies in lateralization (Scharf et al., 1976).

Since funneling involves a change in locus as well as in loudness, we need to measure the perceived locus of the sound image but it is almost certain to be toward the left ear for those Os who reported total or large reductions in the loudness in the right ear. As to the loudness in the left ear, Botte et al. (1982) showed that the loudness of the 10-s tone is nearly double that of either tone alone when both are 1000 Hz. From measurements of dichotic summation of loudness (Scharf, 1969), we should expect that the loudness in the left ear would not be increased when the left-ear and right-ear tones are far in frequency.

The loudness of the continuous tone was also measured after the 10-s tone went off. Loudness reduction was much less--from 10 to 30%--than during the on period and showed only weak frequency selectivity. In still other measurements, the 10-s tone was repeated every 30 s resulting in induced loudness adaptation that increased over time (as in Fig. 1 for a 1000-Hz intermittent tone). However, frequency selectivity remained poor, just as Botte et al. (1982) had found with a .5-s intermittent tone repeated every second. Apparently, the loudness reduction during the on period is not based on quite the same mechanism as the loudness adaptation induced during the off periods; the reduction is much stronger and much more frequency dependent.

4. EXPERIMENT III: ADAPTATION INDUCED MONAURALLY AND BINAURALLY

Despite seemingly overwhelming evidence that loudness does not ordinarily adapt (see Scharf, 1983), Hood and his colleagues (Hood and Wade, 1982; Weiler, Sandman, and Pederson, 1981) have attempted to show that loudness really does adapt, even without any kind of interaural interaction. They presented a steady tone to one ear with an increment of 5 or 20 dB every 30 s. Their Os made successive numerical estimates of loudness. Finding that loudness dropped 36 to 53% after 4 min of stimulation, the authors suggested that the increments served as needed references against which to judge the declining loudness of the continuous sound. After repeating and extending these measures, we (Canévet et al., 1983) concluded that the increments served not to reveal loudness adaptation but to induce it. To induce adaptation ipsilaterally, an intermittent tone must be at least 5 dB more intense.

When the increment is 20 dB, adaptation is very strong. Moreover, the duty cycle should be at least 50% and the period long enough to permit O to judge the loudness of the test sound during the off times.

We now describe two new sets of measurements. In the first set, O wore headphones. A 1000-Hz tone was presented monaurally and increased from 50 to 70 dB for 20 s every 30 s. In the second set, O sat in a large anechoic room. A 1000-Hz tone was presented continuously at 50 dB from a loudspeaker at 0° azimuth and was increased to 70 dB every 10 to 30 s for 5 to 25 s.

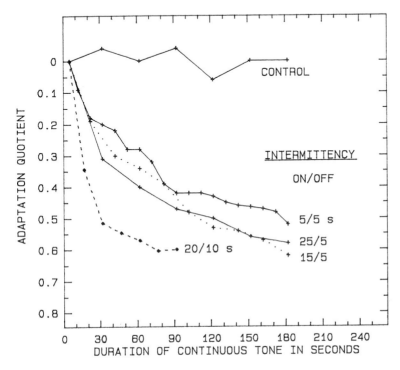

Fig. 3. Adaptation quotient as a function of duration for a 50-dB tone whose loudness was judged during the 5-s intervals separating 20-dB increments in its level. The 20/10 condition was via earphone listening by eight Os; the other conditions were in a sound field with four Os

Figure 3 gives both sets of data, with AQ plotted as a function of the duration of the continuous 50-dB tone. All estimations were made while the increment or more intense tone was off. The control series in the anechoic room showed that loudness did not decline at all for these four Os when the 50-dB tone was presented alone. Introducing a 70-dB tone in the loudspeaker produced a rapid and large decline in the loudness of the 50-dB tone, between 52 and 62% at the end of 3 min or the equivalent of 11 to 14 dB. The loudness drop is impressive for most, but not all, listeners. The duration of the increment made little difference over the range tested. In earphone, monaural listening the adaption was like that in free-field listening over the 90 s tested. We have also performed some preliminary measurements with the continuous tone and its increment coming from two loudspeakers, 90° apart. Adaptation seems to be about the same as shown in Fig. 3.

Other preliminary tests with the 70-dB tone at a different frequency suggest the frequency difference will matter, probably more than in interaurally induced adaptation but less than in the loudness reduction shown in Fig. 2.

Because the intermittent tone is more intense then the continuous tone and goes to the same ear or ears, consideration must be given to a possible role for fatigue in the demonstrated loudness drop. We believe that fatigue plays a negligible role for several reasons. Preliminary data suggest that loudness adaptation is much less when a 1-s silent interval separates the increment from the onset of the weaker tone. Recovery from fatigue is unlikely to be so rapid. Even if the more intense tone caused some threshold increase (TTS), as is likely, it would cause little if any loudness decrease (Botte and Scharf, 1980). Although we reject fatigue as a likely explanation of the data in Fig. 3, we do not have a satisfying alternative to offer. Elsewhere we have suggested that loudness adaptation is avoided, except at low levels, by inherent fluctuations in neural activity in the auditory system. Intermittent tones may disrupt those normal fluctuations through such active processes as funneling in interaural stimulation and, possibly, self-inhibition in monaural or binaural stimulation. Whatever its origins, induced loudness adaptation must be an important, if heretofore unrecognized, aspect of hearing.

Acknowledgements. We thank Alain Marchioni, Ramakrishna Karedla, and Barbara Passarelli for help in these experiments. Research supported by grants from NATO and from the National Institutes of Health, U. S. Public Health Service (2R01NS07270 and RR07143).

REFERENCES

Békésy, G. von (1958). Funneling in the nervous system. *J. Acoust. Soc. Am.* __30__, 399 - 412.

Botte, M.-C., Canévet, G., Scharf, B. (1982). Loudness adaptation induced by an intermittent tone. *J. Acoust. Soc. Am.* __72__, 727 - 739.

Botte, M.-C., Scharf, B. (1980). La sonie. Effets simultanés de fatigue et de masque. *Acustica.* __46__, 99 - 106.

Canévet, G., Scharf, B., Botte, M.-C. (1983). Loudness adaptation, when induced, is real. *Brit. J. Audiol.* __17__ (January).

Hood, J.D., Wade, P. (1982). Loudness adaptation: real or illusory. *Brit. J. Audiol.* __16__, 9 - 15.

Scharf, B. (1969). Dichotic summation of loudness. *J. Acoust. Soc. Am.* __45__, 1193 - 1205.

Scharf, B. (1978). Loudness. In: *Handbook of Perception*, Eds. E.C. Carterette and M.P. Friedman, pp. 187 - 242, New York, Academic Press.

Scharf, B. (1983). Loudness adaptation. In: *Hearing Research and Theory*, Vol. 2, Eds. J.V. Tobias and E.D. Schubert, New York, Academic Press.

Scharf, B., Botte, M.-C., Canévet, G. (in press). Récupération après adaptation induite de sonie. *Année Psychologique.*

Scharf, B., Florentine, M., Meiselman, C.H. (1976). Critical band in auditory lateralization. *Sensory Processes.* __1__, 109 - 126.

Stevens, S.S. (1956). The direct estimation of sensory magnitudes—loudness. *Amer. J. Psychol.* __69__, 1 - 25.

Weiler, E.M., Sandman, D.E., Pederson, L.M. (1981). Magnitude estimates of loudness adaptation at 60 dB SPL. *Brit. J. Audiol.* __15__, 201 - 204.

Zwislocki, J.J., Damianopoulos, E.N., Buining, E., Glantz, J. (1967). Central masking: Some steady-state and transient effects. *Percept. and Psychophys.* 2, 59 - 64.

GENERAL DISCUSSION

RAKOWSKI:
Is it possible that the continuous-tone adaptation at very low levels was due to
the subjects using their threshold of hearing as a reference, while this threshold
was steadily elevating due to the influence of the continuous tone? Did you make
any measurements of the pitch strength of the adapting tone? Is it not possible
that the subjects may subconsciously use the memory of loudness of the intermittent tones as a reference in loudness estimations? The representation of an intermittent tone used actually as a reference in the moment of making a decision may
be distorted due to the time error. This time error (in the presence of a continuous tone) is probably not known. If loudness of this supposed standard is increased in comparison with the "real" loudness of intermittent tone and the subject
assumes it has not changed, then he would judge the loudness of a continuous tone
lower.

SCHARF:
Unlike that adaptation is measured at low levels because threshold serves as reference for several reasons. a) A beating tone set 10 dB above threshold shows no
adaptation. A noise at 10 dB shows much less adaptation than a pure tone. In both
cases threshold could serve as reference. b) In measurements of recovery from interaurally induced adaptation, we have found full recovery for a 60 dB tone (after
a 30 s silent interval) followed ba a readaptation, in the absence of an intermittent sound. Thus we can measure adaptation at a level well above threshold. c) As
shown in Fig. 1 (10-dB decrease), listeners can track with numerical estimations
a tone that decreases slowly from 60 to 50 dB. We have not yet attempted to measure changes in pitch or pitch strength, but we have observed a reduction in pitch
strength that accompanies the loudness decline. The originally pure tone becomes
dull or perhaps noise-like. Some of our subjects have volunteered such observations, and all who showed loudness adaptation did report a pitch change when asked
about it. The weakening of pitch seems to be similar in the various kinds of loudness adaptation. The time-order error, which is of the order of 0.5 dB, is too
small to account for our data. However, it is true that a contralateral intermittent tone increases in loudness, but the increase is very rapid and then remains
constant, while the loudness of the steady sound continues to decrease over time.
More important, however, is our finding that even when the intermittent tone comes
on every 30 s for 10 s, we still find a loudness drop measured during the 20 s
that the steady sound is unaccompanied by a contralateral sound. Furthermore, when
the steady sound is a broad-band noise in one ear and the intermittent sound is
also a broad-band noise in the contralateral ear, we find no loudness adaptation
with on-off periods of 5s/5s. (We believe that the absence of adaptation is due to
the fluctuations in the continuous noise.)

ACCOUNTING FOR THE LOUDNESS OF A SINUSOID IN NOISE

B. J. O'Loughlin

*Department of Psychology, Monash University,
Clayton, Victoria, 3168, Australia*

1. INTRODUCTION

The strong evidence for lateral suppression in hearing suggests that an excitation pattern (EP) model capable of taking into account suppression effects might have value. In this paper, predictions for the loudness of a sinusoid in a broadband noise of variable level are presented from a working model. Experimental data, which are shown to be consistent with previous work, are given. The results are then discussed in the light of some relevant physiological and psycho-acoustical studies.

The model is based quantitatively on the work of Verschuure (1978), which utilised pulsation threshold data, and is intended purely as a means of tying together psychoacoustical and physiological data along the way. The model predicted well the results of a related experiment, which examined the loudness of a sinusoid in a bandreject noise of variable notchwidth, especially when the effects of suppression were taken into account (O'Loughlin and Moore, 1982).

2. METHOD

The loudness standard was a 10 ms 2 kHz sinusoid of 45, 60 or 75 dB SPL. All stimuli had 10 ms cosine-squared rise/fall envelopes. The standard's peak level occurred 20 ms before the offset-completion of a 500 ms broadband noise (0.4-3.6 kHz). The independent variable was the level of the broadband noise, and had values of −2, −4, −6, −9, −12, −16, −20, −25, −35*, and −45* dB relative to the level at which the standard was just masked (*where possible). The dependent variable was the subject-controlled level of a comparison 10 ms 2 kHz sinusoid which was varied to match the loudness of the standard for a given noise level. The comparison's level was changed by computer in 6 dB steps until after the second reversal, when the step size became 2 dB; the levels at the eight reversals following the change in step size were averaged to produce the loudness-match estimate. The order of the standard and comparison sinusoids and the default direction of tracking were counterbalanced, with the standard and comparison always separated by 1 second. The stimuli were presented monaurally through a Sennheiser HD414X headphone, which had been calibrated with a probe-tube microphone at the entrance to the ear canal.

Data for a 45 dB SPL forward-masked sinusoid are also presented but, being less representative of the individual subject's results, are not discussed. The mean of eight loudness matches formed each datum for the individual subjects.

3. PREDICTIONS FROM THE MODEL

It was assumed that EPs exist immediately before the suppression stage reflected in IHCs (e.g., Sellick and Russell, 1979), and that loudness is proportional to the area under the EPs which may be modified by suppression.

The EPs were stylized as asymmetric triangles on log frequency-place/ dB excitation axes, with the parameter dB SPL. Log frequency has often been used in EP models (e.g., Verschuure, 1978; Johnson-Davies and Patterson, 1979). Here, the abscissa is called log frequency-place to make more explicit the assumed relationship for a given sinusoid between the point of maximal excitation and the CF of cn neurones. Rose *et al.* (1971), among others, indicate that the distribution of CFs of individual cn neurones along the BM is approximately logarithmic

for mid to high frequencies. Such an abscissa has a number of advantages. It
should still produce EPs of approximately constant shape, but avoids the need
for a critical band rate scale (e.g., Zwicker and Scharf, 1965). (Following
Rose *et al.*, 1971, a linear frequency scale might be used for low frequencies,
although a better overall fit might be achieved with a power function: Greenwood,
1961; Liberman, 1982.) If a scale derived from the critical band is not used, cn
and HC data can be more directly interpreted in terms of the model. Although
responses measured neurally can be suppressed by a component which does not at the
same time excite (e.g., Javel, 1981), and in this sense the neurone has a bigger
"catchment area" (or, in a limited sense, "integration area") than is implied by
an EP, it may be more profitable to consider this in terms of the ambit of suppression (e.g., Geisler and Sinex, 1980), rather than in terms of the critical
band.
      The EPs were calculated from Verschuure's (1978) model, with average values
at 2 kHz estimated from his Fig. 19 and an assumed threshold of 15 dB SPL. The
high frequency slope, however, was held constant at 125 dB/oct beneath 40 dB SPL.
One difficulty in using Verschuure's model is that it may reflect the self-supp-
ression of a single sinusoid (e.g., Houtgast, 1974a; Moore and Glasberg, 1982).
However, the basic predictions of EP models tend to be relatively insensitive to
changes in slope parameters *per se* over wide ranges (see RESULTS). Verschuure's
model provides a reasonable starting point.
      For each level of the standard stimulus, the EP was plotted and an estimate
was made of the area left uncovered as the level of the noise decreased. For
simplicity, it was assumed that the excitation level of the noise equalled that
of the apex of the standard's EP at masked threshold (see DISCUSSION). Then,
assuming that at equal loudness the area under the EP of the comparison sinusoid
would match that uncovered in the standard, it was possible to interpolate into
the EP family and produce SPL predictions from the areal functions. The predicted matching levels for the noise levels used in the experiment are shown to the
left of Fig. 1, and are essentially straight lines.

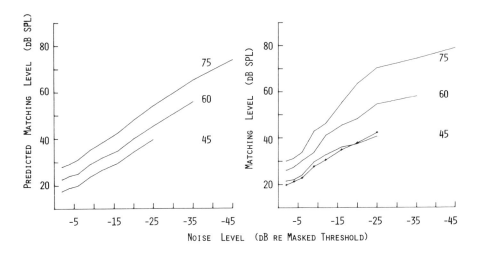

Fig. 1. LHS: *Matching levels predicted from the EP model for 45, 60 and 75 dB SPL
sinusoids as a function of relative noise level. The functions for the 60 and 75
dB SPL sinusoids have been shifted vertically by 5 and 10 dB respectively. RHS:
Actual results (N=3) from both simultaneous and forward masking (crosses). The
noise levels in forward masking were chosen to give the same masking effect as
those used in simultaneous masking. The functions for the two higher level sinusoids have also been shifted vertically*

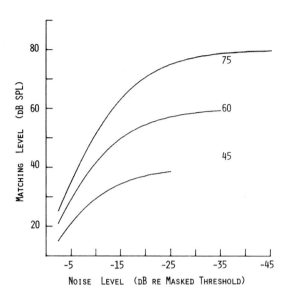

Fig. 2. Results of Stevens and Guirao (1967: Fig 7) from a similar paradigm, fitted with the model of Pavel and Iverson (1981), and replotted to enable comparison with this study. The parameter has been changed from absolute noise level to masked sinusoid level. An effective threshold of 15 dB SPL has been assumed, as in Stevens and Guirao. The curves for the 60 and 75 dB SPL sinusoids have been shifted vertically by 5 and 10 dB respectively, as in Fig. 1, and all curves have been moved 2.5 dB to the right

4. RESULTS

The actual mean results obtained are shown to the right of Fig. 1, with the forward masking results indicated by crosses. The principal difference between the predicted results and those for simultaneous masking is that the obtained results grow more quickly towards their unmasked loudness value; this is especially noticeable for the higher level standards. The rapid increase in loudness as a masking noise's level decreases has also been observed by others (e.g., Houtgast, 1974b: Fig. 7), and is consistent with the more extensive data of Stevens and Guirao (1967: Fig 7) which may be compared with the results of this study. In order to give a more complete picture, their data were fitted with Pavel and Iversons' (1981) model, which has been shown to describe well a large number of loudness matching results. The fitted functions were then used in plotting the data in a comparable form: Fig 2. Despite differences ascribable to experimental details, the pattern of results in Fig. 2 agrees well with those in Fig. 1 (RHS). The rate of growth of loudness with decreasing noise level in simultaneous masking is greater than predicted by a consideration of the EPs alone. (Zwicker and Scharf, 1965, came across a similar problem with their model, although their EPs were derived from simultaneous masking data.) Further, the rate of growth of loudness increases with standards of greater level. Stevens and Guirao (1967) spoke of the effects of inhibition in their results, while Houtgast (1974a,b) argued that lateral suppression - the presently more favoured term - was implicated in his data.

5. DISCUSSION

The loudness of a sinusoid in noise should be strongly related to the responses of individual neurones. Although it has typically been assumed that loudness is proportional to the rate of discharge (e.g., Fletcher, 1940), recent evidence suggests that the auditory system might more readily be able to utilise the sorts of information represented by synchrony measures, which reflect a combination of rate and periodicity (e.g., Sachs *et al.*, 1980).

Neurophysiological results similar to those of Abbas in Fig. 3 (LHS), which show a steep increase in response to a CF sinusoid with decreasing relative noise level, have also been observed by others using rate measures (e.g., Geisler and Sinex, 1980). The rapidity of the rise has typically been attributed to suppression. Abbas' data closely resemble the psychoacoustical results in Figs. 1 and 2, and could be well fitted by Pavel and Iversons' (1981) model. While Abbas'

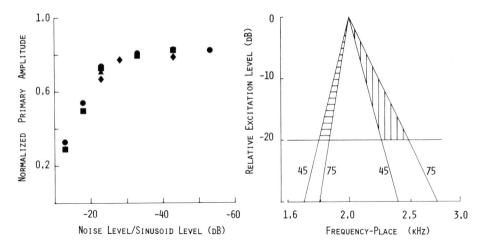

Fig. 3. LHS: *Primary Fourier component response of a single cn unit to a CF sinusoid/broadband noise combination at different levels (after Abbas, 1981). As the relative noise level reduces, the unit's response changes similarly for sinusoids of different absolute levels: 50 (circles), 60 (squares), 70 (triangles) and 80 (diamonds) dB SPL. RHS: EPs predicted by the model for 45 and 75 dB SPL sinusoids, with the relative noise level at -20 dB on masked threshold (horizontal line). With increasing level, the low frequency slope of the sinusoidal EP grows sharper and the high frequency slope becomes shallower. The amount of change is indicated by horizontal and vertical stripes respectively*

results suggest that the form of the loudness functions in Figs. 1 (RHS) and 2 might be established at a very peripheral level, they are not compatible in isolation with the faster rate of growth of loudness for higher level sinusoids. His data show that, to a first approximation, it is the relative levels of the sinusoid and noise which determine the response, irrespective of the absolute levels. However, Abbas' data were only obtained with a sinusoid at CF (or, in terms of the model, with CF corresponding to the EP's apex). Neurones with CF at the EP's apex might be relatively unaffected by changes with level at other frequency-places (see Fig. 3, RHS).

When taking the effects of suppression into account, two major modifications might have to be made to the model. First, the absolute excitation level of the sinusoid may be depressed by suppression from the noise (Houtgast, 1974b). Secondly, and perhaps more importantly for considering the growth of loudness after the initial stages, the noise excitation may need to be complexly represented. Only the second point will be considered in detail in this paper.

Take, for instance, the EP for the 45 dB SPL sinusoid. Javel (1981) has noted the strong resemblance in form between suppression contours and those of excitation. If the sinusoid is considered as F2, and the noise is thought of as a series of sinusoids which we might call F1, then Javel (1981) has shown that suppression will be maximal for fibres having CF corresponding to F2 (the apex of the sinusoid's EP). Suppression will drop off more quickly for fibres with CF below F2 (the low frequency flank of the EP) than it does for fibres with CF above F2 (the high frequency flank of the EP). The pattern of suppression created by the sinusoid will look like the EP (although it may not be as great in extent: Javel, 1981). In terms of the model, this might be represented by placing an asymmetric gap, with a similar form to the EP but inverted, in the noise's EP. For a given F2, the pattern of suppression of the noise excitation, once established, would not be expected to change as the noise level varied, since given a particular F2 the amount of suppression is independent of the level and frequency of F1 (Javel, 1981). With decreasing relative noise level, the effect of having an asymmetric "notch" in the noise's EP should be similar to increasing the width of a notch in a bandreject noise of constant level. (One major difference is that the noise away from the sinusoidal EP's apex should continue to suppress the sinusoid for longer in the latter experiment, being at a constant level: the loudness of a sinusoid should grow more gradually.) The form of the results for the two experiments is in fact very similar, with loudness growing less rapidly in the notched noise experiment. (The notched noise experiment was reported in detail by O'Loughlin and Moore, 1982).

Higher levels of the sinusoid, however, should lead to a change in the pattern of suppression. Javel (1979, 1981) has consistently found that the rate of growth of suppression decreases as F2 goes from below CF in frequency to above CF. In terms of the model, suppression growth will be greater for neurones with CF above the sinusoidal EP's apex. But, since the relative levels of the noise were the same for the different level sinusoids, it is the relative growth of suppression that is of importance. The rate of growth of suppression is less than 1.0 for F2 above CF, 1.0 at CF and greater than 1.0 for F2 below CF (Javel, 1979). The high frequency side of the inverted suppression gap in the noise's EP will drop as the sinusoid's level increases, in much the same way as the high frequency flank of the sinusoid's EP will get shallower.

The spread of suppression to higher frequency-places with increasing level, in a similar way to the spread of excitation, is consistent with the frequently observed, very powerful, effects of a low frequency suppressor at higher levels (e.g., Sachs and Hubbard, 1981). This effect is preserved, at least qualitatively, in the psychoacoustical results (e.g., Houtgast, 1974a).

It is suggested, therefore, that as the level of the sinusoid is increased from 45 to 75 dB SPL, a major effect will be a greater spread of excitation, accompanied by a greater spread of suppression, to higher frequency-places. As the noise level decreases, there will be at each level more neurones strongly responding to the higher level sinusoid (Fig. 3, RHS) and, because of the increased suppression, the threshold of response to the sinusoid will be reached earlier for many neurones. For neurones at CF, suppression will neither relatively increase or decrease (see Fig. 3, LHS). For neurones with CF below the sinusoid's nominal frequency, the model predicts a lesser spread of excitation for higher level sinusoids and, in a similar way, the relative amount of suppression should decrease, since the rate of growth of suppression will be less than 1.0 (Javel, 1979). The effect of level on the high frequency side of the sinusoid's EP is probably sufficient to explain the level-dependent loudness growth with decreasing relative noise level, although, for want of space, a number of major issues remain undiscussed.

Acknowledgements. *The work reported was carried out in the Department of Experimental Psychology, University of Cambridge. I am grateful to Brian Moore, Roy Patterson and the other members of the Cambridge hearing group for earlier discussions, and to Anna Bodi, John Bradshaw, Ross Day and Joe Tong for comments on a version of this paper.*

REFERENCES

Abbas, P.J. (1981). Auditory-nerve responses to tones in a noise masker. *Hearing Research* 5, 69-80.

Fletcher, H. (1940). Auditory patterns. *Rev. Mod. Phys.* 12, 47-61.

Geisler, C.D., and Sinex, D.G. (1980). Responses of primary auditory fibers to combined noise and tonal stimuli. *Hearing Research* 3, 317-334.

Greenwood, D.D. (1961). Critical bandwidth and the frequency coordinates of the basilar membrane. *J. Acoust. Soc. Am.* 33, 1344-1356.

Houtgast, T. (1974a). Lateral suppression in hearing. Ph.D. Thesis, (Free University, Amsterdam).

Houtgast, T. (1974b). Lateral suppression and loudness reduction of a tone in noise. *Acustica* 30, 214-221.

Javel, E. (1979). Two-tone suppression in the auditory nerve of the cat: Suppression thresholds and rate of growth. *J. Acoust. Soc. Am.* 66, S48.

Javel, E. (1981). Suppression of auditory nerve responses. I. Temporal analysis, intensity effects and suppression contours. *J. Acoust. Soc. Am.* 69, 1735-1745.

Johnson-Davies, D., and Patterson, R.D. (1979). Psychophysical tuning curves: Restricting the listening band to the signal region. *J. Acoust. Soc. Am.* 65, 765-770.

Liberman, M.C. (1982). The cochlear frequency map for the cat: Labeling auditory-nerve fibers of known characteristic frequency. *J. Acoust. Soc. Am.* 72, 1441-1449.

Moore, B.C.J., and Glasberg, B. (1982). Interpreting the role of suppression in psychophysical tuning curves. *J. Acoust. Soc. Am.* 72, 1374-1379.

O'Loughlin, B.J., and Moore, B.C.J. (1982). Relationship between excitation patterns, loudness and the auditory filter. *J. Acoust. Soc. Am.* 71, S73-74.

Pavel, M., and Iverson, G.J. (1981). Invariant characteristics of partial masking: Implications for mathematical models. *J. Acoust. Soc. Am.* 69, 1126-1131.

Rose, J.E., Hind, J.E., Anderson, D.J., and Brugge, J.F. (1971). Some effects of stimulus intensity on response of auditory nerve fibers in the squirrel monkey. *J. Neurophysiol.* 34, 685-699.

Sachs, M.B., and Hubbard, A.E. (1981). Responses of auditory-nerve fibers to characteristic-frequency tones and low-frequency suppressors. *Hearing Research* 4, 309-324.

Sachs, M.B., Young, E.D., Schalk, T.B., and Bernardin, C.P. (1980). Suppression effects in the responses of auditory-nerve fibers to broadband stimuli. In: *Psychophysical, Physiological and Behavioural Studies in Hearing* (G. van den Brink and F.A. Bilsen, eds.). Delft University Press, Delft.

Sellick, P.M., and Russell, I.J. (1979). Two-tone suppression in cochlear hair cells. *Hearing Research* 1, 227-236.

Stevens, S.S., and Guirao, M. (1967). Loudness functions under inhibition. *Percept. and Psychophys.* 2, 459-465.

Verschuure, J. (1978). Auditory excitation patterns. Ph.D. Thesis (Erasmus University, Rotterdam).

Zwicker, E., and Scharf, B. (1965). A model of loudness summation. *Psych. Rev.* 72, 3-26.

THE ROLE OF MODULATION IN HEARING

R. Plomp

*Institute for Perception TNO, P.O.Box 23, 3769 ZG Soesterberg, and
Faculty of Medicine, Free University, Amsterdam, The Netherlands*

There is a long tradition in hearing research of exploring the auditory system by means of sinusoidal stimuli, usually called pure tones. Single pure tones are used to investigate just-noticeable differences in frequency and sound-pressure level, absolute and masked hearing thresholds, equal-loudness contours etc. Combinations of two or more tones have come to be applied more and more in recent years in order to study pitch phenomena, the ear's frequency-resolving power, the creation of combination tones, the effect of lateral suppression, timbre perception, etc. Without doubt, our knowledge of the hearing mechanism has increased considerably by these approaches.

It seems to me, however, that other approaches should also have our attention. Just as speech research has gained very much by paying more attention to how speech sounds are perceived by the ear, it may be worthwhile, in studying the ear, to pay more attention to how the speech signal is composed and by what parameters speech intelligibility is determined.

Speech can be considered to be a wide-band complex signal modulated continuously in time in three different respects: (1) the vibration frequency of the vocal cords is modulated, determining the pitch variations of the voice, (2) the temporal envelope of this signal is modulated by narrowing and widening the vocal tract locally by means of the tongue and the lips, and (3) the tongue and the lips in combination with the cavities of the vocal tract determine the sound spectrum of the speech signal, which may be considered as a modulation along the frequency scale.

For each of these three ways of modulation, it is of interest to study the modulations present in the speech sound radiated from the mouth, the extent to which these modulations are preserved on their way from the speaker to the listener, and the ability of the ear to perceive them. The modulations can be studied by considering how they are composed of sinusoidal components. By means of Fourier analysis we are able to describe the properties of the voice and the ear in terms of frequency-response characteristics for the modulation frequencies. In this short contribution I will restrict myself to the temporal and spectral modulations, that is the horizontal and vertical axes of the speech spectrogram, leaving frequency variations of the fundamental out of the discussion.

1. MODULATION IN TIME

a) *The temporal envelope of speech*

Data on the modulation frequencies included in the temporal envelope of connected discourse were collected by Steeneken and Houtgast (1983). To obtain the modulation index as a function of frequency for an octave band of speech centred at, for example, 1000 Hz, essentially the following measuring procedure was used. The output of this frequency band was squared and low-pass filtered (cut-off frequency 30 Hz) to obtain the intensity envelope for that octave band of speech. By means of a computer, this envelope, with components up to 30 Hz, was speeded up 400 times, resulting in a fluctuating signal with components up to 12 kHz. This signal was analysed with a set of one-third octave band-pass filters. For each band-filter the output value, multiplied by $\sqrt{2}$ and divided by the long-term average value of the intensity envelope, represents the modulation index m for speech components present in the octave band centred at 1000 Hz.

In Fig. 1 some results are reproduced. The curves represent average envelope spectra or one-minute speech fragments of connected discourse from ten male speakers who read the same text; the parameter is the centre frequency of the audio

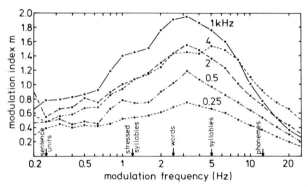

Fig. 1. _Average envelope spectra in terms of the modulation index for one-minute_
connected discourse from ten male speakers. The number of sentence units, stressed
syllables etc. per second is indicated. The parameter is the centre frequency of
the 1/3-oct audio-frequency band

band. We see that the envelope spectrum, except for its absolute position, is
largely independent of audio frequency, and has a maximum at about 4 Hz. For a
group of ten female speakers, and for other texts, almost the same spectra were
found.

b) _The transfer between speaker and listener_
    The extent to which the modulations present in the temporal envelope of
speech are preserved on their way from the speaker to the listener can be expressed by the temporal modulation transfer function (TMTF). For an input signal (band
of noise) at the position of the speaker with a sinusoidally varying intensity
$\bar{I}_i(1 + \cos 2\pi Ft)$, with F = modulation frequency, the output signal at the listener's ear can be described by

$$\bar{I}_0 \ [1 + m \cos(2\pi Ft - \theta)], \tag{1}$$

with m = modulation index; m as a function of F is defined as the TMTF. For communication channels with noise, band limitations, non-linear distortion etc. a technique has been developed (Steeneken and Houtgast, 1980) by which TMTF can be measured. From the TMTF a single measure, STI (Speech Transmission Index), can be derived which has been shown to be an excellent predictor of speech intelligibility
scores for Western languages (Houtgast and Steeneken, 1983).
    In enclosures, the transfer of speech signals is determined by two factors:
(1) the sound reaches the ear not only directly, but also via a great many different transmission paths, each including one or more reflections; the differences in
path length, and therefore in time of arrival, result in attenuation of fast modulations; (2) ambient noise will also reduce the modulation index, but independently from modulation frequency.
    For the case of a listener at a large distance from both the speaker and the
noise source(s) in a room with a diffuse indirect sound field, the TMTF is given
by the simple equation (Houtgast, Steeneken, and Plomp, 1980)

$$m(F) = \frac{1}{1 + I_N/\bar{I}_0} \cdot \frac{1}{\sqrt{1 + 0.207F^2T^2}}, \tag{2}$$

where F = modulation frequency in Hz;
      T = reverberation time in sec;
      I_N = intensity of the noise at the listener's position;
      $\bar{I}_0$ = mean intensity of the speaker's voice at the listener's position.

This equation shows that the TMTF is the product of two independent terms, deter-

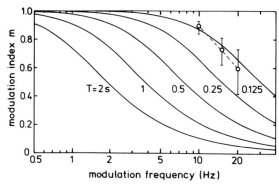

Fig. 2. Temporal modulation transfer function in the diffuse sound field with the reverberation of the room as the parameter. The data points (mean value and standard deviation for 50 subjects) represent the TMTF of the auditory system for 1000 Hz

mined by the signal-to-noise ratio and the product FT, respectively. In Fig. 2 the TMTF without noise is plotted as a function of F, with T as the parameter. For non-diffuse sound fields, the usual situation, algorithms have been developed to compute the TMTF from the geometric and acoustic properties of the room (see Plomp et al., 1980; Wattel et al., 1981; van Rietschote et al., 1981).

c) *The temporal modulation transfer function of the ear*
      Usually the ear's sensitivity to temporal modulation is studied by measuring the just-noticeable amplitude modulation as a function of modulation frequency (see review with references by Viemeister, 1979). Only in a few cases was the peak-to-valley ratio of an (almost) 100% intensity-modulated noise band investigated (Rodenburg, 1977; Festen et al., 1977; Festen and Plomp, 1981; Festen, 1983). In these experiments the threshold of a short probe tone is measured; in one condition this probe tone coincides in time with the maximum of the modulated signal, in the other with the minimum. The difference between these thresholds as a function of modulation frequency can be interpreted as a measure of the ear's TMTF.
      In the experiment by Festen and Plomp (1981) the masker was white noise with a peak-to-valley ratio of 20 dB, low-pass filtered with a cut-off frequency of 4000 Hz. This noise was modulated sinusoidally in intensity with a modulation frequency of 10, 15, or 20 Hz. In a two-alternative forced-choice procedure the detection threshold of a 0.4-msec click, octave filtered with a centre frequency of 1000 Hz, was measured. From the difference in threshold levels at the peaks and the valleys, ΔL, the TMTF of the auditory system is given by

$$\Delta L = 10 \ \log \frac{1 + m}{1 - m} , \text{or} \ m = \frac{10^{\Delta L/10} - 1}{10^{\Delta L/10} + 1} . \tag{3}$$

The data points in Fig. 2 represent the mean values for 50 normal-hearing subjects, with the standard deviation calculated for ΔL.

d) *Discussion*
      It is of interest to compare the cut-off modulation frequencies for speech and hearing presented in Figs. 1 and 2. Taking the frequencies for which the value of m is half its peak value as determining the bandwidth, we may say that, roughly, the modulation frequencies in speech cover a range from 0.3 Hz up to 15 Hz. The cut-off modulation frequency of the ear is, on the average, 25 Hz. This shows that the ear is able to follow the fast fluctuations present in running speech. If the interindividual spread is taken into account, more than 85% of the subjects had a cut-off frequency above 15 Hz. Apparently, in terms of temporal resolution, the capacity of the auditory system is well adapted to human speech.

Fig. 2 also shows the effect of reverberation. Roughly, the data points compare with a reverberation time of 0.12 to 0.15 sec. Since in most cases the reverberation time of rooms and halls is over 0.5 sec, we may conclude that in everyday situations the enclosure is the limiting factor.

2. MODULATION ALONG THE FREQUENCY SCALE

a) *The spectral envelope of speech*
It is more difficult to decide upon the modulation frequencies present in the envelope of the sound spectrum of the human voice than upon those present in its temporal envelope. The frequency range relevant to speech is, compared with the modulation frequencies to be expected, too small to permit application of a reliable Fourier analysis to the spectral envelope.

An alternative way is the following. Instead of analysing the entire audio range, we focus our attention on the lower two formants, F_1 and F_2, of speech vowels. We may expect that the modulation frequency has to be sufficiently high to resolve these two peaks in the envelope spectrum. Klein, Plomp, and Pols (1970) studied vowel spectra by means of one-third octave band-filter analysis, showing that the characteristic differences among vowels are preserved in these spectra. From the average spectra of 50 speakers, the depth of the valley between the F_1 and F_2 peaks is plotted in Fig. 3 as a function of frequency difference between the two formant frequencies.

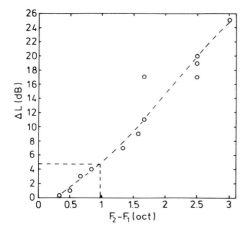

Fig. 3. Mean depth for 50 male speakers of the valley between F_1 and F_2 as a function of $F_2 - F_1$ in octaves

b) *The transfer between speaker and listener*
The fact that, in a room, sounds reach the ear of the listener via a great many transmission paths, not only has influence on the temporal modulations present in the speech signal at the listener's position, but also on the envelope of its spectrum. For steady-state pure tones the sound-pressure level at a large distance from the speaker in a diffuse sound field has a theoretical uncertainty with a standard deviation of 5.57 dB (Schroeder, 1954). Measurements at a great many locations in a concert hall have confirmed this value (Plomp and Steeneken, 1973). This uncertainty is inherent in the vectorial addition of sound waves with random phases and cannot be reduced by acoustical measures.

Since this phenomenon should be regarded as a source of variance introduced by the room, we can compare its effect with the variance present in vowel sounds. From the experiments by Klein, Plomp, and Pols (1970) we know that, measured with one-third octave band-filters, the variance for the same vowels pronounced by different speakers is about 270 dB^2 (speaker-dependent correction included). It is reasonable to require that the room reverberation should not introduce more variance than this value. For a fundamental frequency of 250 Hz, comparable with F_0 for the female voice, the variance due to the room (also with one-third octave bands) does not differ much from this 270 dB^2. Therefore, we may conclude that the effect of the room on vowel spectra is just tolerable.

c) *The spectral modulation transfer function of the ear*

In recent years comb-filtered noise has been introduced for measuring auditory bandwidth (Houtgast, 1974). Comb-filtered noise is easily made by adding noise and the same noise with delay τ; its intensity is sinusoidally modulated in frequency (period $1/\tau$). By measuring the peak-to-valley difference for a probe tone as a function of modulation frequency, we obtain the spectral modulation transfer function (SMTF) of the auditory system.

In a battery of tests applied by Festen and Plomp (1981) to 50 normal-hearing subjects not only the ear's temporal resolution (see Fig. 2) but also its frequency resolution at 1000 Hz was investigated with comb-filtered noise. The experiments were performed in simultaneous masking as well as in forward masking with the probe tone presented immediately after the noise bursts. The results are plotted in Fig. 4. The difference between the two SMTF curves reflects the effects of lateral suppression included in forward masking but not in simultaneous masking (cf. Plomp, 1976).

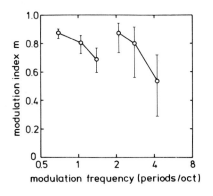

Fig. 4. Spectral modulation transfer function (mean value and standard deviation for 50 subjects) of the auditory system for 1000 Hz. The left-hand curve holds for simultaneous masking, the right-hand curve for forward masking

d) *Discussion*

In the same way as in section 1d, we can compare the results obtained in sections 2a through 2c. Taking a modulation index m = 0.5, corresponding to a peak-to-valley ratio of 4.77 dB, as a criterion of the highest modulation frequency present in vowel sounds, Fig. 3 indicates an upper limit of about 1 period/oct. According to Fig. 4, the ear is able to follow spectral modulations up to a limit of, on the average, about 4 periods/oct (data including the effect of lateral suppression which seems to be the more realistic estimate). Taking the large inter-individual spread into account, we see that more than 85% of the listeners were able to trace spectral modulations up to about 3 periods/oct. We may conclude that the frequency-resolving power of the ear meets the spectral modulations present in speech quite well.

With respect to the influence of the multiple reflections of sound in rooms, I can refer to the finding (see section 2b) that its effect in terms of variance is comparable with the interindividual differences of speakers pronouncing the same vowel.

CONCLUSION

We may conclude that both for the temporal and the spectral modulations the auditory system is able to follow adequately the modulations present in speech. The finding that the frequency-resolving power of the ear is substantially larger than required for perceiving the spectral modulations of speech supports the view that this power's main challenge is to discriminate speech from interfering sounds as good as possible.

REFERENCES

Festen, J.M. *et al.* (1977). Relations between interindividual differences of auditory functions. In: *Psychophysics and physiology of hearing* (E.F. Evans and J.P. Wilson, eds.). pp. 311-319. London, Academic Press.
Festen, J.M., Plomp, R. (1981). Relations between auditory functions in normal hearing. *J. Acoust. Soc. Am.* 70, 356-369.
Festen, J.M. (1983). Studies on relations among auditory functions. Doctoral dissertation, Free University, Amsterdam.
Houtgast, T. (1974). Lateral suppression in hearing. Doctoral dissertation, Free Unversity, Amsterdam.
Houtgast, T., Steeneken, H.J.M., Plomp, R. (1980). Predicting speech intelligibility in rooms from the Modulation Transfer Function. I. General room acoustics. *Acustica* 46, 60-72.
Houtgast, T., Steeneken, H.J.M. (1983). A multi-language evaluation of the RASTI method for estimating speech intelligibility in auditoria. *Acustica*, in press.
Klein, W., Plomp, R., Pols, L.C.W. (1970). Vowel spectra, vowel spaces, and vowel identification. *J. Acoust. Soc. Am.* 48, 999-1009.
Plomp, R., Steeneken, H.J.M. (1973). Place dependence of timbre in reverberant sound fields. *Acustica* 28, 50-59.
Plomp, R. (1976). Aspects of tone sensation. Chapter 1. London, Academic Press.
Plomp, R., Steeneken, H.J.M., Houtgast, T. (1980). Predicting speech intelligibility in rooms from the Modulation Transfer Function. II. Mirror image computer model applied to rectangular rooms. *Acustica* 46, 73-81.
Rietschote, H.F. van, Houtgast, T., Steeneken, H.J.M. (1981). Predicting speech intelligibility in rooms from the Modulation Transfer Function. IV. A ray-tracing computer model. *Acustica* 49, 245-252.
Rodenburg, M. (1977). Investigation of temporal effects with amplitude modulated signals. In: *Psychophysics and physiology of hearing* (E.F. Evans and J.P. Wilson, eds.). pp. 429-437. London, Academic Press.
Schroeder, M. (1954). Die statistischen Parameter der Frequenzkurven von grossen Räumen. *Acustica* 4, 594-600.
Schroeder, M.R. (1981). Modulation transfer functions: Definition and measurement. *Acustica* 49, 179-182.
Steeneken, H.J.M., Houtgast, T. (1980). A physical method for measuring speech-transmission quality. *J. Acoust. Soc. Am.* 67, 318-326.
Steeneken, H.J.M., Houtgast, T. (1983). The temporal envelope spectrum of speech and its significance in room acoustics. To be published in Proc. 11th ICA, Paris 1983.
Viemeister, N.F. (1979). Temporal modulation transfer functions based upon modulation thresholds. *J. Acoust. Soc. Am.* 66, 1364-1380.
Wattel, E., Plomp, R., van Rietschote, H.F., Steeneken, H.J.M. (1981). Predicting speech intelligibility in rooms from the Modulation Transfer Function. III. Mirror image computer model applied to pyramidal rooms. *Acustica* 48, 320-324.

GENERAL DISCUSSION

HAGGARD:
The qualitative point made in your Fig. 2 is a valuable and valid one overall, but the argument behind it should be used with caution. For example, the serial stages in a communication channel have multiplicative effects on modulation. As a consequence, two listeners with a temporal modulation transfer function (TMTF) respectively equivalent to 0.125 s and 0.25 s reverberation time (RT) would not, as your argument appears to imply, experience equivalent lack of difficulty from a preced-

ing stage with an equivalent RT of 1 s. Rather the total system's modulation transfer at the important modulation frequencies for speech intelligibility (4-16 Hz) is what counts. There may be some critical value of modulation transfer for a given combination of speech audio band with modulation-frequency band below which the intelligibility contribution drops away rapidly to zero. If this were about $m = 0.1$, then the tails of the functions for a long reverberation times (1s, 2s) put the speech modulation spectrum into a vulnerable zone. Any further degradation in the listener (for example a listener whose TMTF had an equivalent RT of about 0.35 s) could make a critical difference at these important modulation frequencies, depressing the product of the indices for the serial stages below 0.1. This product, rather than the displacement along the abscissa of the equivalent RT function for the worst stage in the communication channel, is the important determining consideration in adequacy of communication. However, this is not a criticism of your approach. Rather it justifies, indeed predicts, your final comment that the apparent "reserve" capacity of the auditory system is concerned with difficult conditions such as noise and reverberation, which reduce or mask the modulation spectrum. By the foregoing argument, this is precisely when the serial effect of the listener would become critical. An analogous argument can be made for frequency resolution, and with the frequency changes in speech, the frequency bandwidth in the listener can also affect his TMTF.

ON THE PERCEPTION OF SPECTRAL MODULATIONS

T.M. van Veen and T. Houtgast

Institute for Perception TNO
3769 DE Soesterberg, The Netherlands

Auditory stimuli are often considered in terms of a spectral shape, an excitation pattern or related concepts. For the perception of complex stimuli, especially if it concerns differences in spectral sharpness, it may be convenient to describe a spectral shape in terms of sinusoidal spectral modulations. For a linear frequency scale, this is closely related to the autocorrelation of a stimulus. In view of the properties of the ear, in this paper a log-frequency scale has been used to define the spectral modulations. Spectral shapes (on a log-frequency scale) are thus described in terms of ripple spectra. According to this approach two experiments are described. The first experiment is concerned with the relation between changes in spectral sharpness of vowel sounds and the resulting perceptual changes. The second experiment deals with the detection thresholds of spectral modulations.

1. EXPERIMENT I

In a triadic-comparison experiment, subjects had to compare stimuli that differed in spectral sharpness, and give a judgement about their similarity. These results will be related to the physical differences between the stimuli.
Stimuli: The stimuli were synthetic vowels. Smoothing of their spectra was

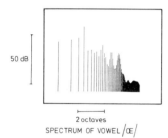

50 dB

2 octaves
SPECTRUM OF VOWEL /œ/

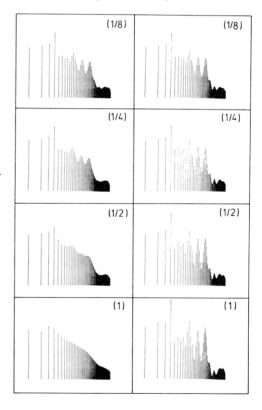

(1/8)   (1/8)

(1/4)   (1/4)

(1/2)   (1/2)

(1)   (1)

Fig. 1. Example of nine different versions of the vowel /œ/. Above: the original vowel. Filter bandwidth (in oct.) applied for smoothing and sharpening (see text) is given between parentheses

done by convolution with Gaussian-shaped filters with a constant bandwidth on a log-frequency scale. The convolution was applied to log-intensities. The sharpened versions were obtained by subtracting the smoothed spectrum from twice the original spectrum. An example of the nine versions of one vowel is shown in Fig. 1. The Fourier transforms ("ripple transfer functions") of the applied filters are shown in Fig. 2.
Loudness, fundamental frequency and duration were kept constant at (ap-

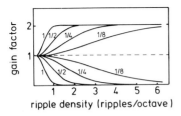

gain factor

ripple density (ripples/octave)

Fig. 2. Ripple transfer functions corresponding to the applied filter functions

proximately) 55 dB SL, 123.5 Hz and 100 msec, respectively.

Procedure: All triads of the set of nine stimuli were successively available, in random order. For each triad, subjects had to respond which pair was most similar and which pair was most dissimilar. The responses were accumulated in a similarity matrix: one point for the most similar and minus one for the most dissimilar pair. The matrix values $M(i,j)$ are supposed to be monotonely related to the perceptual differences between pairs (i,j).

Data analysis: The physical difference $D(i,j)$ between stimuli i and j can be expressed as a weighted difference between the corresponding ripple spectra $S_i(\rho)$ and $S_j(\rho)$:

$$D(i,j) = \left\{ \int H^2(\rho) \, [S_j(\rho) - S_i(\rho)]^2 \, d\rho \right\}^{\frac{1}{2}} \qquad (1)$$

$S(\rho)$ is the Fourier transform of the (log-intensity versus log-frequency) vowel spectrum with ρ as ripple density. $H(\rho)$ is a weighting function. Our goal is to find that weighting function which gives the best fit (along a third-order polynomial) between the spectral differences $D(i,j)$ and similarity values $M(i,j)$. $H(\rho)$ is assumed to be Gaussian, with two parameters: its width (σ) and the position (shift) of its maximum along the ρ-scale.

The analysis is performed on the average data obtained for three subjects and five nine-stimuli sets (based on five different vowels).

The best fit is obtained for $\sigma = 1.3$ ripples/octave and the maximum located at 1.9 ripples/octave. Fig. 3 shows the relation between the perceptual and weighted spectral differences. Fig. 4 shows the standard deviation as a function of the shift of the maximum of $H(\rho)$.

Fig. 3. Dissimilarity values as a function of weighted physical differences for a Gaussian-shaped ripple-weighting function $H(\rho)$ (width = 1.3 and max. at 1.9 ripples/oct.)

DISCUSSION

The obtained weighting function with a maximum at about 2 ripples/octave corresponds to a filter function with negative lobes, with maximal "suppression" at a distance of 1/4 octave from the filter's nominal frequency. This agrees with data concerning lateral suppression (Houtgast, 1974).

The results suggest, that the region around 2 ripples/octave plays an important role in the enhancement or preservation of the contrast in a spectral excitation pattern. One might expect, that this region of ripple densities is also relevant for the detection of stimuli masked by noise. In the next experiment attention is focussed on this aspect of the perception of spectral modulations.

Fig. 4. Standard deviation of similarity values with regard to a best fitting third-order polynomial as a function of the shift along ρ of $H(\rho)$. Width is constant ($\sigma = 1.3$)

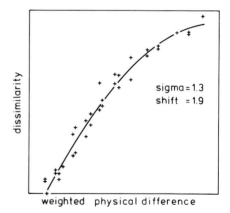

dissimilarity

sigma = 1.3
shift = 1.9

weighted physical difference

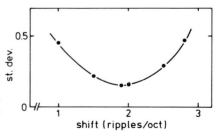

st. dev.

0.5

0

1   2   3

shift (ripples/oct)

2. EXPERIMENT II

In this experiment the detection thresholds of spectral modulations of computer-generated noise were determined in a 4-AFC paradigm.

The modulations were either sinusoidal or had a rectangular ripple spectrum, with either ripple density or cut-off ripple density as independent variables. The rectangular ripple spectra were either "low-pass" or "high-pass", representing two rather extreme cases in terms of spectral modulations. As a log-frequency has been used, the sinusoidal modulations are different from "traditional" ripple noise (e.g. Bilsen, 1968; Yost and Hill, 1978).

Stimuli: The reference stimulus had a flat spectrum and consisted of 160 components spaced at 1/46 octave. The phases were random but fixed. The target stimuli $M(f)$ can be written as:

$$M_1(f) = 1 + A_1 \cos(\rho x) \qquad (2)$$

$$M_2(f) = 1 + A_2 \rho \sin(\rho x)/\rho x \qquad (3)$$

$$M_3(f) = 1 + A_3 \{C \delta(f-f_0) - \rho \sin(\rho x)/\rho x\} \qquad (4)$$

with $x = 2\pi \cdot {}^2\log(f/f_0)$, ρ is ripple density or cut-off ripple density, A^{-1} is the attenuation, and C is a normalisation factor for having a zero ripple amplitude below the cut-off ripple density for $M_3(f)$.

The target was obtained by the (attenuated) addition of the fully modulated reference to the reference. Examples of spectra and the corresponding ripple spectra are given in Fig. 5.

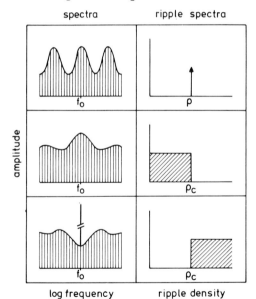

spectra   ripple spectra

amplitude

f_0 ρ

f_0 ρ_c

f_0 ρ_c

log frequency   ripple density

Fig. 5. Schematic representation of spectra and corresponding ripple spectra

The frequencies composing the stimuli ranged from 233 Hz to 2644 Hz. The loudness was approximately 55 dB SL. In order to insure that detection was based on spectral shape, stimulus level was randomized ($\pm$ 2 dB). The duration was 375 msec, with 200 msec intervals.

Procedure: Each trial consisted of 4 stimulus bursts of which a random one was the target. The modulated part was attenuated 4 dB after each correct response until the first incorrect response occurred. Then a two-up one-down procedure (Levitt, 1971) was followed with a stepsize of 1 dB. The last 8 out of 10 reversals of a run were used for computation of the threshold value. Typically eight runs were applied for each condition. Three subjects participated.

Results: Fig. 6 shows the attenuation at threshold as a function of ρ for the sinusoidal modulations. In view of the data analysis in the next section, for $M_2(f)$ and $M_3(f)$ the attenuation factors (A_2^{-1} and A_3^{-1}) at threshold are given in Fig. 7.

Data analysis: As one possible way of interpreting the present data, we propose the following. When supposing that threshold conditions are associated with a constant difference between the peak intensity (at f_0) and the average intensity, the underlying filter function or ripple transfer function $H(\rho)$, can be derived. As for small modulation depths the distinction between intensity modulation and amplitude modulation is not relevant (the proper corrections are applied) this

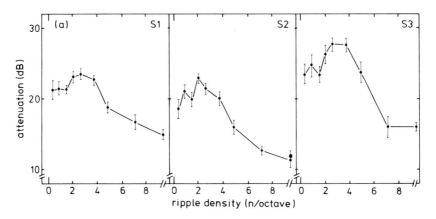

Fig. 6. Attenuation of the sinusoidal modulations as a function of ripple density (thresholds for three subjects). Vertical bars represent standard errors.

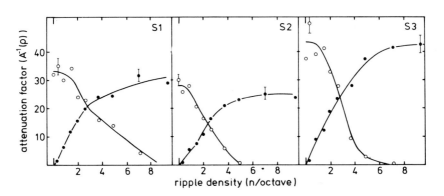

Fig. 7. Attenuation factors of modulations according to "low-pass" (closed circles) and "high-pass" rectangular ripple spectra as a function of cut-off ripple density (threshold values for three subjects). Typical standard errors are shown for the highest values only (vertical bars).

implies that, for the three kinds of modulations, threshold is reached for:

$$A_1(\rho) \int_\rho \delta(\rho-\rho') \, H(\rho') \, d\rho' = \text{constant} \qquad (5)$$

$$A_2(\rho) \int_0^\rho H(\rho') \, d\rho' = \text{constant} \qquad (6)$$

$$A_3(\rho) \int_\rho^\infty H(\rho') \, d\rho' = \text{constant} \qquad (7)$$

As the detection criterion might depend on the features to be detected (Martens, 1982) the possibility of different ripple transfer functions is accepted. It is then easily verified that:

$$H_1(\rho) = A_1^{-1}(\rho) \qquad (8)$$

$$H_2(\rho) = \frac{d}{d\rho} A_2^{-1}(\rho) \qquad (9)$$

$$H_3(\rho) = -\frac{d}{d\rho} A_3^{-1}(\rho) \qquad (10)$$

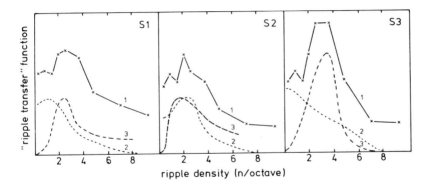

Fig. 8. Ripple transfer functions obtained for three different types of modulations (see text).

To obtain the derivatives needed for eqs. (9) and (10) a smooth curve has been drawn by hand through the datapoints of Fig. 7.

The resulting ripple transfer functions are shown in Fig. 8. The scale for $H_1(\rho)$ is arbitrary with respect to $H_2(\rho)$ and $H_3(\rho)$.

DISCUSSION

Not surprisingly, for the simple detection criterion as assumed here, the different kinds of modulations reveal quite different ripple transfer functions. Possibly, another detection criterion might lead to more similar curves. However, it is reasonable to suppose, that for such a wide range of signals, different features and detection criteria are involved. For instance, for a global change of a spectrum it is likely that detection is based on other processes than the detection of a tone in noise. For higher ripple densities where the peak of $M_2(f)$ becomes rather narrow, the difference between $H_2(\rho)$ and $H_3(\rho)$ might be related to differences in the temporal structure of both modulations. For the sinusoidal modulations as well the temporal structure as the number of spectral peaks may have an influence on the detection threshold. Further experiments are needed for investigating these possibilities.

Acknowledgements: This research was supported by the Netherlands Organization for the Advancement of Pure Research (ZWO).

REFERENCES

Bilsen, F.A. (1968). On the interaction of a sound with its repetitions. Doctoral dissertation. University of Technology, Delft.
Houtgast, T. (1974). Lateral suppression in hearing. Doctoral dissertation. Free University, Amsterdam.
Levitt, H. (1971). Transformed up-down methods in psycho-acoustics. J. Acoust. Soc. Am. 44, 467–477.
Martens, J. (1982). A new theory for multitone masking. J. Acoust. Soc. Am. 72, 397–405.
Yost, W.A. and Hill, R. (1978). Strength of the pitches associated with ripple noise. J. Acoust. Soc. Am. 64, 485–492.

FLUCTUATION STRENGTH OF MODULATED TONES AND BROADBAND NOISE

H. Fastl

*Institute of Electroacoustics, Technical University München, D-8000 München 2
F.R. Germany*

1. INTRODUCTION

Modulation of a sound elicits one of two different kinds of auditory sensation, depending on the speed of modulation. In the case of low modulation frequencies (typically less than about 20 Hz) the resultant sensation is called *fluctuation strength* (see Terhardt, 1968). Faster modulation of sounds leads to the perception of *roughness* (v. Békésy, 1935). As yet, fluctuation strength has received considerably less attention than roughness. Terhardt (1968) and Schöne (1979) studied the dependence of fluctuation strength on some essential signal parameters, using sinusoidally amplitude modulated pure tones. We have recently repeated and extended these earlier observations, to include investigations of the fluctuation strength of AM-broadband noise (Fastl, 1982a) and of FM-tones.

The present paper describes the dependence of the fluctuation strength of sinusoidally amplitude modulated broadband noise (AM BBN), sinusoidally amplitude modulated pure tones (AM SIN) and sinusoidally frequency modulated pure tones (FM SIN) on the following stimulus parameters: modulation frequency, sound pressure level, modulation depth, and frequency deviation. The fluctuation strength elicited by AM BBN, FM SIN, and AM SIN at different frequencies is compared directly and related to the fluctuation strength produced by an unmodulated narrow band noise (NBN).

2. PROCEDURE

The test stimuli were presented monaurally through an electrodynamic earphone (Beyer DT 48) with a free-field equalizer (Zwicker and Feldtkeller, 1967, p. 40). The subjects sat in a sound-isolated booth. Experiments with AM BBN, AM SIN, and FM SIN were performed by six, eight, and seven subjects, respectively. All subjects had normal hearing and were between 25 and 37 years old. A method of magnitude estimation was applied. The modulated sounds, switched on and off at the minima of the modulation, were presented in pairs. The first sound of a pair was assigned a number (e.g. 100), representing the magnitude of its fluctuation strength. Relative to this standard, the subject had to scale the fluctuation strength of the second sound within each pair (e.g. 20 for a decrease in fluctuation strength by a factor of five). For each stimulus parameter, two sets of experiments were performed: one with a standard eliciting large fluctuation strength (assigned the number 100) and another with a standard of small fluctuation strength (assigned the number 10). During a session, each combination of standard and comparison was presented four times in random order. On the average, the corresponding four numbers, assigned to identical stimuli, differed by less than ± 10, indicating only small intra-individual differences. For each comparison, the responses of all subjects were compiled, leading to a total of 24, 32, and 28 datapoints respectively. From these data, medians and interquartiles were calculated and normalized relative to the maximal median within each figure (for further detail see Fastl, 1982a). In all figures the standards are indicated by filled symbols. The broadband noise used was actually "uniform masking noise" (Zwicker and Feldtkeller, 1967, p. 58).

3. RESULTS AND DISCUSSION

    The dependence of fluctuation strength of modulated sounds on modulation
frequency is displayed in Fig. 1. The left panel shows the results for amplitude
modulated broadband noise (AM BBN), the middle panel for AM-tones and the right
panel for FM-tones. The stimulus parameters are given in the legend to the figure; the abbreviations of physical parameters are listed in Table I.

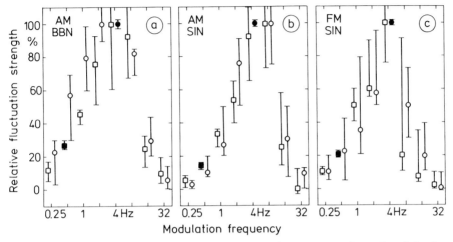

*Fig. 1. Fluctuation strength of modulated sounds as a function of modulation
frequency. (a) Amplitude-modulated broadband noise (AM BBN) L = 60 dB, Δf_N =
16 kHz, d = 40 dB. (b) Amplitude-modulated pure tone (AM SIN) L = 70 dB, f =
1000 Hz, d = 40 dB. (c) Frequency modulated pure tone (FM SIN) L = 70 dB, f =
1500 Hz, Δf = 700 Hz*

    The results plotted in Fig. 1 demonstrate that the fluctuation strength of
modulated sounds shows a bandpass characteristic as a function of modulation frequency. The bandpass seems to be somewhat more sharply tuned for modulated tones
than for modulated broadband noise, and the maximum of fluctuation strength tends
to occur at a higher modulation frequency for AM SIN than for AM BBN and FM SIN.
However, these differences can only be properly evaluated when the magnitudes of
the interquartiles are accounted for. These are extremely large for FM SIN, due
to interindividual differences. Note in addition, that the results for different
sounds were produced by different groups of subjects. Taking all this into consideration, it is reasonable to assume that the fluctuation strength of modulated sounds shows a bandpass characteristic as a function of modulation frequency
with a maximum around 4 Hz, irrespective of the bandwidth of the modulated sound
and the type of modulation.
    For AM SIN and $f_{mod} \geq 5$ Hz our results are in excellent agreement with data
of Terhardt (1968). Terhardt measured fluctuation strength of AM-tones only for
modulation frequencies down to 5 Hz. He found that a low-pass characteristic
with 13 Hz cut off accounted nicely for his data. However, for very slow fluctuations a bandpass characteristic provides a more adequate description. As discussed earlier (Fastl, 1982a), the upper slope of the bandpass can be ascribed
to the inertia of the ear, while the lower slope may be related to short-term
memory limitations. These memory effects account also for the increase of modulation threshold at extremely low modulation frequencies (Zwicker, 1952).
    Fig. 2 shows the dependence of fluctuation strength of modulated sounds on
sound pressure level. In order to present sounds with relatively large fluctuation strength, a modulation frequency of 4 Hz was used throughout. The results
plotted in Fig. 2 suggest that fluctuation strength of modulated sounds increases

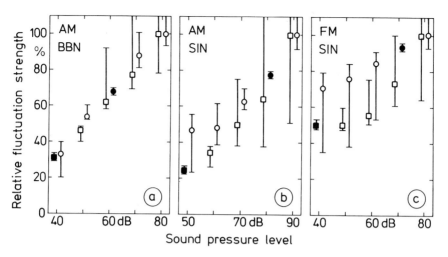

Fig. 2. Fluctuation strength of modulated sounds as a function of sound pressure level. Stimulus parameters same as in Fig. 1 but modulation frequency f_{mod} = 4 Hz

with increasing sound pressure level. The increase seems to be more pronounced for AM BBN and AM SIN than for FM SIN. Results for modulated *tones* - in particular FM-tones - depend somewhat on the standard used and show larger interquartile ranges due to inter-individual differences. This effect was also reported by Terhardt (1968) for AM-tones. In accordance with his data it can be stated that for an increase of 40 dB in SPL, fluctuation strength of modulated sounds increases by a factor of between 3 and 1.7. For AM BBN the increase of fluctuation strength with SPL could be traced back to an increase in the depth of the temporal masking pattern (Fastl, 1982a). For AM SIN and FM SIN, the spread of the masking pattern along the critical band rate scale must also be taken into account (Fastl, 1982b, p. 26).

Fig. 3 shows the dependence of fluctuation strength of AM sounds on both modulation depth d and modulation factor m, which are related according to the formula: $d = 20lg\{(1+m)/(1-m)\}$. Fluctuation strength is zero until about 4 dB modulation depth, after which it increases approximately linearly with the logarithm of modulation depth. For the

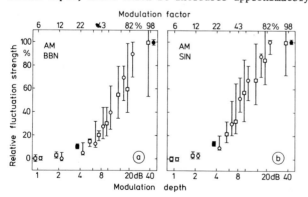

Fig. 3. Fluctuation strength of amplitude-modulated sounds as a function of modulation depth as well as modulation factor. (a) AM BBN with L = 60 dB, Δf_N = 16 kHz, f_{mod} = 4 Hz. (b) AM SIN with L = 70 dB, f = 1 kHz, f_{mod} = 4 Hz

maximal fluctuation strength of AM BBN a modulation depth of 40 dB is necessary, while for AM SIN the maximal value of fluctuation strength is almost reached at a modulation depth of 20 dB. The results for AM SIN are mostly in agreement with data of Terhardt (1968) and Schöne (1979). However, for 20 dB modulation depth Schöne got only 62 % relative fluctuation strength, while Fig. 3 indicates some 92 %. This difference in results is presumably due to sinusoidal versus trapezoidal modulation. If the modulation depth is increased from 20 dB to

40 dB, the depth of the temporal masking pattern increases considerably more for trapezoidal modulation (as used by Schöne) than for sinusoidal modulation as used in our experiments (see also Fastl, 1982b, p. 23).

Fig. 4 shows the dependence of fluctuation strength of a FM-tone on frequency deviation. Fluctuation strength starts to be perceived at about 20 Hz frequency deviation and increases approximately linearly with the logarithm of frequency

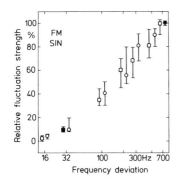

deviation. This result applies for a FM-tone at 1500 Hz with 70 dB SPL and 4 Hz modulation frequency. For such a tone, the JND for FM is about 4 Hz frequency deviation (Zwicker, 1982, p. 55). Significant values of fluctuation strength (say 10 % relative fluctuation strength) are achieved for frequency deviations larger than about ten times the magnitude of the JND. This rule seems to apply also for AM-sounds: The modulation depth at which 10 % relative fluctuation strength is reached (see Fig. 3) is about ten times larger than the JND for amplitude of 0.4 dB for a 70 dB AM-tone and 0.7 dB for AM BBN as reported by Zwicker (1982, p. 69).

Fig. 4. Fluctuation strength of frequency-modulated tones as a function of frequency deviation. L = 70 dB, f = 1500 Hz, fmod = 4 Hz

Fig. 5 enables the comparison of fluctuation strength of eleven different sounds, the physical data of which are listed in Table I. The largest fluctuation strength is produced by an FM-tone with large frequency deviation followed by AM broadband noise. AM-tones (sounds 3 to 9) elicit almost the same fluctuation strength irrespective of their carrier frequency, except at

8000 Hz were fluctuation strength is somewhat smaller. As expected from results plotted in Fig. 4, the FM-tone with small frequency deviation (sound 10) produces only about one tenth of the fluctuation strength produced by sound 1.

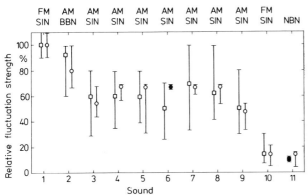

The fluctuation strength elicited by the unmodulated narrow band noise (sound 11) can be estimated as follows: In a very first approximation the narrow band noise can be regarded as an AM-tone at 1000 Hz with 6.4 Hz modulation frequency (see Fastl, 1975). Assuming an effective modulation factor of 40 % for narrow band noise (Fleischer, 1982), according to Fig. 3b, the fluctuation strength of NBN should be about a factor of 2.5 smaller than the fluctuation strength of AM-tones with 98 % modulation factor. However, Fig. 5 shows that the fluctuation strength of AM SIN and NBN differs by a factor of four to five. It is appa-

Fig. 5. Fluctuation strength of sounds with different bandwidth, frequency and different type of modulation. For stimulus parameters see Table I

rently the periodic rather than statistic amplitude fluctuation of AM-tones that enhances the perceived fluctuation strength.

The large fluctuation strength of AM BBN and FM SIN (sound 2 and 1) may be correlated with the large extent of the masking patterns along the critical band rate scale. It is postulated that fluctuation strength is summed up across critical bands. This concept was successfully applied to the description of roughness in FM-tones (Fastl, 1982b, p. 26). It is also expected to hold for fluctuation strength.

Table I. Physical data of sounds 1 through 11.

Sound	1	2	3	4	5	6	7	8	9	10	11
Abbreviation	FM SIN	AM BBN	AM SIN	AM SIN	AM SIN	AM SIN	AM SIN	AM SIN	AM SIN	FM SIN	NBN
Frequency, f in Hz	1500		125	250	500	1000	2000	4000	8000	1500	1000
Level, L in dB	70	60	70	70	70	70	70	70	70	70	70
Modulation-frequency, f_{mod} in Hz	4	4	4	4	4	4	4	4	4	4	–
Modulation depth, d in dB	–	40	40	40	40	40	40	40	40	–	–
Frequency deviation, Δf in Hz	700	–	–	–	–	–	–	–	–	32	–
bandwidth, Δf_N in Hz	–	16000	–	–	–	–	–	–	–	–	10

4. SUMMARY

Slowly modulated sounds produce an auditory sensation called fluctuation strength. For AM broadband noise, AM tones and FM tones, the dependence of fluctuation strength on relevant stimulus parameters was investigated. As a function of modulation frequency, fluctuation strength shows a bandpass characteristic with a maximum around 4 Hz. For an increase in level of 40 dB, fluctuation strength increases by a factor of 1.7 to 3. For modulation depths larger than 4 dB and frequency deviations larger than 20 Hz, fluctuation strength increases approximately linearly with the logarithm of modulation depth and frequency deviation, respectively. The largest fluctuation strength is produced by FM-tones with large frequency deviation and by AM broadband noise. The maximal fluctuation strength of AM-tones is a factor of about 1.7 smaller, almost independent of carrier frequency. Unmodulated narrow band noise elicits a fluctuation strength four to five times smaller than fluctuation strength of AM tones. The dependence of fluctuation strength on stimulus parameters is rather similar for sounds of different bandwidth (BBN vs. SIN) and different type of modulation (AM vs. FM).

REFERENCES

Békésy, G.v. (1935). Über akustische Rauhigkeit. *Z. Techn. Phys.* 16, 276-282.
Fastl, H. (1975). Loudness and masking patterns of narrow noise bands. *Acustica* 33, 266-271.
Fastl, H. (1982a). Fluctuation strength and temporal masking patterns of amplitude-modulated broadband noise. *Hear. Res.* 8, 59-69.
Fastl, H. (1982b). *Beschreibung dynamischer Hörempfindungen anhand von Mithörschwellen-Mustern.* Hochschul Verlag, Freiburg.
Fleischer, H. (1982). Calculating psychoacoustic parameters of amplitude modulated narrow noise bands. *Biol. Cybern.* 44, 177-184.
Schöne, P. (1979). Messungen zur Schwankungsstärke von amplitudenmodulierten Sinustönen. *Acustica* 41, 252-257.
Terhardt, E. (1968). Über akustische Rauhigkeit und Schwankungsstärke. *Acustica* 20, 215-224.
Zwicker, E. (1952). Die Grenzen der Hörbarkeit der Amplitudenmodulation und der Frequenzmodulation eines Tones. *Acustica* AB, 125-133.
Zwicker, E. (1982). *Psychoakustik.* Hochschultext, Springer, Berlin.
Zwicker, E. and Feldtkeller, R. (1967). *Das Ohr als Nachrichtenempfänger.* Hirzel-Verlag, Stuttgart.
ACKNOWLEDGEMENT. This work was supported by the Deutsche Forschungsgemeinschaft, SFB 204, Gehör, München.

GENERAL DISCUSSION

RAKOWSKI:
The perceived fluctuation strength and roughness are qualitatively different sensations but they are both related to the effect of the so-called "psychoacoustic
dissonance" which is of great importance for music. Helmholtz, who first investigated this effect, made a somewhat arbitrary assumption that the sensation of dissonance is due to roughness. Some later investigators followed his line and spoke
of a dissonance while looking for maximum roughness. However, as it appeared from
the experiments that we performed in Warszaw Academy of Music, this is not true
for low musical tones. For these tones musical dissonance sensation is rather dependent on perceived fluctuation strength than on roughness. Therefore Dr. Fastl's
results are relevant for music.

FASTL:
I agree completely with Dr. Rakowski that both fluctuation strength and roughness
are of great importance for the perception of musical sounds.

PICK:
Possibly your results might be influenced by problems associated with categorial
perception. The most obvious category boundary might occur between 'roughness'
and 'fluctuation strength'. Have you investigated whether category boundaries can
be shifted by adaption?

FASTL:
There is no clear cut boundary between fluctuation strength and roughness. Rather,
sounds with modulation frequencies around 20 Hz may elicit both fluctuation
strength and roughness. We did not try to shift the frequency range in which both
hearing sensations show up by adaption.

SCHARF:
Since you ascribe increasing fluctuation strength, at least in part, to excitation
over a larger number of critical bands, would you not expect a band stop noise to
reduce markedly the dependence of strength on level?

FASTL:
We have not yet performed such an experiment. The problem in these experiments is
the large loudness difference between the sounds to be compared. However, we
could show that high-pass noise maskers reduce the roughness of AM-tones considerably. Since fluctuation strength and roughness are closely related, we can expect
that masking sounds like bandstop noise also reduce the perceived fluctuation
strength and its dependence on level.

TERHARDT:
When a fluctuating sound is heard, the following conditions can be reasonably
distinguished (as a function of fluctuation frequency): Very slow fluctuations
(<2 Hz) are usually well perceived; but these are by many subjects not called
"fluctuations". The "fluctuation strength" assigned to them is small. Fluctuations
in the range 2 Hz ... 25 Hz actually are typical. As Fastl shows, their maximal
subjective strength is achieved around 4 Hz. Fluctuations more rapid than about
25 Hz produce constant loudness and may be perceived as "roughness".

EVANS:
Like others I am confused by the meaning of "fluctuation strength". I would have
said that AM at 0.4 Hz modulation rate had the greatest "strength of fluctuation".
Is there a semantic confusion here? Likewise, could the reduction in fluctuation
strength with increasing f_{mod} beyond 4-8 Hz in your Fig. 1 simply be due to subjects now calling "fluctuation strength", "roughness"? In other words, are we
really referring to two separable phenomena (which I think do have physiological
correlates) or merely using different linguistic labels to describe different
parts of a single continuum?

FASTL:
The subjects were asked to scale the "Schwankungsstärke" of the sounds. This German term was translated into "fluctuation strength" (Terhardt, 1968). In fact, the subjects can separate fluctuation strength and roughness as being different hearing sensations which might have physiological correlates.

EVANS:
Does the German word translated "fluctuation strength" mean something more specific? To the English ear, the translation implies perceived depth of modulation rather than change or rate of change, which appears to be the intended meaning.

TERHARDT:
In reply to the terminological questions raised by Evans, I may point out that in our experiments on roughness subjects throughout produced reasonable results in terms of distinguishing between "fluctuation strength" and "roughness". Therefore that distinction may be considered as more or less "natural". These findings are in accordance with those found much earlier by von Helmholtz and von Békésy.

HAFTER:
I wonder if it might be useful to consider the use of a different term for the independent variable in your experiments. Even though the parameter is modulation, the problem is that the very low modulation-frequency tuning that Schreiner reported (this volume) for cortical cells and that you have found with listeners is well outside of the range of modulation frequencies that dominate pitch or lateralization. For example, lateralization of the envelope delay falls off drastically for modulation frequencies below 50 Hz. Perhaps a word that reflects your adjustment parameter would be better, referring to the stimuli as amplitude or frequency "fluctuation".

FASTL:
Dr. Hafter's comment refers to a comparison of physiological and psychoacoustic results. As far as the hearing sensation fluctuation is concerned, it has to be pointed out that fluctuation strength can be scaled irrespective of the type of modulation.

MONAURAL PHASE EFFECTS IN MASKING WITH MULTICOMPONENT SIGNALS

S. Mehrgardt and M.R. Schroeder

*Drittes Physikalisches Institut, Universität Göttingen, Bürgerstrasse 42-44
D-3400 Göttingen, Federal Republic of Germany*

The human ear has considerable sensitivity to certain phase differences. Phase differences are either detectable because of amplitude variations of combination-tones (caused by mechanical nonlinearities) or can be perceived on account of signal envelope differences. Although phase effects have been demonstrated with two-component maskers (Raiford and Schubert, 1971, and others), more detailed investigations of the perceptive relevance of signal envelopes must be carried out with multicomponent maskers.

1. SYNTHESIS OF MULTICOMPONENT SIGNALS WITH "SILENT" INTERVALS OF DIFFERENT DURATIONS

Masking properties of multicomponent signals depend considerably on the length of the "silent" intervals occurring in the signal envelope. Let us consider a signal composed of 30 harmonics with Hamming-weighted amplitudes and zero phases. This signal, shown in the upper curve of Fig. 1, has long "silent" intervals between consecutive pulses. Even for a fixed amplitude spectrum, these intervals can be shortened by selecting different phases: The second and third curve show signals with phase angles according to

$$\varphi_n = \pi\, n^2\, Q$$

where n is the harmonic number and Q a parameter determining the "silent"-interval duration. Finally gapless ("random") signals can be obtained (bottom curve) for a proper choice of Q. A general formula, yielding signals with low peak amplitudes for arbitrary spectra, was given by Schroeder (1970).

Our experimental results show that the ear uses time-windows to detect even very weak test tones during short "silent" intervals. By contrast gapless maskers without any "silent" intervals will yield very high thresholds.

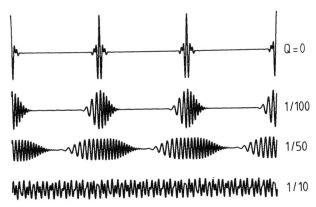

Fig. 1. Four signals with identical power spectrum but different phase spectra. The signals are composed of 30 harmonics with Hamming-weighted amplitudes. Phases according to the formula given in the text. Phase parameter Q determines length of signal pulses

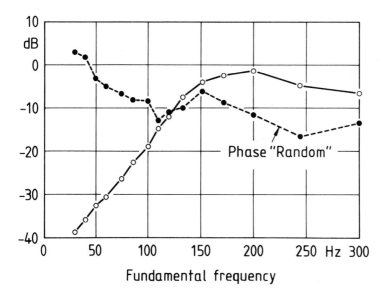

Fundamental frequency

Fig. 2. Threshold of a test tone (1200 Hz), masked by a harmonic complex. Amplitudes of harmonics proportional to 1/f, phases constant (o) or "random" (●). Fundamental frequencies are chosen to be submultiples of 1200 Hz

2. MASKED THRESHOLD OF A CONTINUOUS TEST TONE

In our first experiment we use harmonic tone-complex maskers with 1/f amplitude spectrum, bandlimited to about 6 kHz. Fundamental frequencies vary between 30 Hz and 300 Hz, and they are restricted to submultiples of the test frequency (1200 Hz). The harmonics have either constant phase or "random" phases. The absolute detection threshold of a 1200-Hz test tone is determined using an adaptive 3-alternative-forced-choice experiment. (Similar measurements were published by Duifhuis, 1970 and Martens, 1981, but only on maskers with zero-phase harmonics.)

Figure 2 shows the masked threshold of a 1200-Hz tone. Let us first consider the result with "random" masker (●): Decreasing fundamental frequency from 300 Hz to 30 Hz yields an increase in threshold, caused by more and more masking harmonics falling into the critical band of the test tone.

Threshold with constant-phase masker (o) shows a quite contrary behavior. The threshold remains nearly constant, as fundamental frequency is lowered from 300 Hz to 150 Hz. But further decrease of the fundamental frequency now results in a considerable *decrease* of threshold. At a fundamental frequency of 30 Hz the threshold of a constant-phase masker is 40 dB (!) below the threshold of a "random"-phase masker. This amazing masking difference between two maskers of identical power spectrum will be shown to be a consequence of the "silent" intervals in the maskers envelopes.

As an interesting second-order effect, we observed in our experiments that the pitch of masked test tones differed considerably from the pitch of unmasked test tones. This pitch shift depends critically on test-tone phase. Detailed investigations (Mehrgardt, 1982) show that the pitch shifts of test tones, having the same phase as the corresponding masker-harmonic, are approximately proportional to the test frequency, an effect well-known from noise-maskers.

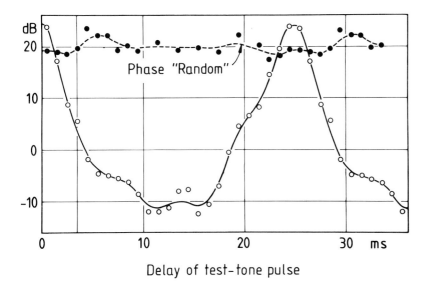

Fig. 3. *Threshold of a test-tone burst (1600 Hz, 5 ms) as a function of the test-tone delay. Masker as described in Fig. 2, fundamental frequency 40 Hz. Phases of harmonics are constant(o) or "random" (●)*

3. MASKING PERIOD PATTERNS OF MULTICOMPONENT MASKERS

Perceptive relevance of "silent" intervals can be demonstrated by using short test-tone pulses instead of continuous test tones. Varying the position of a test-tone pulse within the masker period yields a pattern that is believed to reflect, approximately, the envelope of basilar membrane motion at the place corresponding to the test frequency (Schroeder, Mehrgardt, 1982). In experiments with multicomponent maskers this technique was also used by Duifhuis (1971) and Zwicker (1976) in measuring time resolution of the ear.

Our measurements are carried out with 5-ms test-tone pulses of 1600 Hz. Maskers have a fundamental frequency of 40 Hz, and either constant or "random" phases of the harmonics are used. Figure 3 shows the results.

A random masker (●) yields high threshold levels, nearly independent of the test-tone delay. This reflects an approximately constant signal envelope of random maskers. By contrast a constant-phase masker (o) results in thresholds strongly dependent on the test-tone delay. Threshold maxima occur when the test tone is centered on a masker-pulse (i.e. a delay of 0 ms, 25 ms), whereas the test tone is best perceived (corresponding to a threshold minimum) when it is centered in a "silent" interval between consecutive masker pulses (delay ca. 12.5 ms). At this optimum position the threshold is 30 dB below values obtained with the random masker.

As Fig. 3 suggests, thresholds of *continuous* test tones (Fig. 2) are reflected in the threshold *minima* of the test-tone pulses because only these minima show threshold differences between constant-phase and random-phase maskers as high as are found with continuous test tones. Our next experiment gives further support to this conjecture: We measure threshold minima of test-tone pulses for various fundamental frequencies and compare these with the thresholds of continuous test tones.

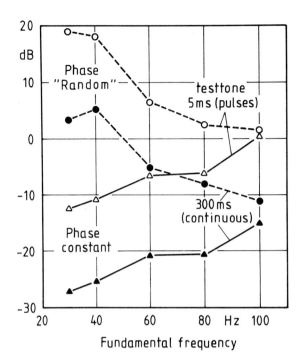

<u>Fig. 4.</u> *Comparison of thresholds of continuous test tones (300 ms, filled sym-
bols) with threshold minima of test-tone pulses (5 ms, open symbols). These measurements are carried out by varying test-tone position within the masker period,
until the lowest threshold results. Test frequency is 1600 Hz. Masker as described in Fig. 2, with fundamental frequencies between 30 Hz and 100 Hz (abscissa). Phases of harmonics are constant (triangles) or random (circles)*

     Results are shown in Fig. 4. The figure shows threshold minima of test-tone
pulses (open symbols) and thresholds of continuous test tones (filled symbols).
Maskers had either random phases (circles) or constant phases (triangles).
     Let us first consider results with continuous test tones. We again find (see
also Fig. 2) that lowering of the fundamental frequency yields decreasing thresholds with constant-phase maskers, whereas random maskers cause increasing values.
Curves of very similar shape are now obtained by threshold minima of test-tone
pulses. These curves show a considerable shift towards higher thresholds, reflecting the ear's ability to integrate signals within certain time intervals for the
continuous test tone.
     A more accurate comparison of the results confirms this conjecture. Consider
for example thresholds obtained with constant-phase maskers (triangles): Independent of fundamental frequency, the threshold of test-tone pulses (open triangles) is exactly (within 1 dB) 15 dB above the threshold of the continuous test
tones (filled triangles). This close correlation between the two curves suggests
that the ear has the ability to use short time windows in analyzing signals.

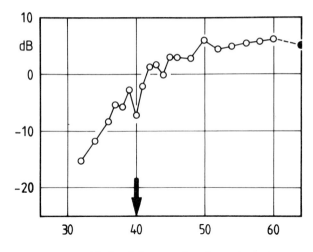

Fig. 5. *Threshold of a 1600-Hz tone masked by a lowpass harmonic complex as function of the cutoff frequency. Masker as described in Fig. 2. Fundamental frequency is 40 Hz and harmonics have random phases. The arrow marks the position of the test tone*

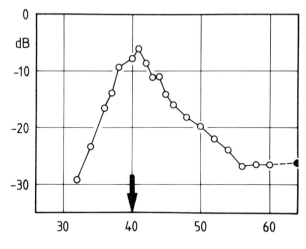

Highest harmonic of masker

Fig. 6. *Same as Fig. 5, but with constant phase of the masking harmonics*

4. THRESHOLD MEASURMENTS WITH LOWPASS MASKERS

Another impressive phase effect obtained with multicomponent maskers is
shown in Figs. 5 and 6. These figures represent threshold measurements of a 1600-
Hz test tone, masked by lowpass signals. The cutoff frequency is given by the
number of the highest harmonic contained in the masker (abscissa). The fundamental frequency is 40 Hz.

Let us first consider the results with random maskers (Fig. 5). Starting with
low fundamental frequencies, low threshold values are found because the cutoff
frequency of the masker lies considerably below the test frequency. Increasing
the cutoff frequency first increases the threshold, as more harmonics of the masker fall into the critical band of the test tone. Finally, a nearly constant
threshold level is obtained because further harmonics outside the critical band
of the test tone have no additional masking effect.

The result with constant-phase masker (Fig. 6) shows a similar behavior, as
long as the cutoff frequency is below the test frequency. But adding more *higher*
harmonics surprisingly yields a considerable *decrease* of threshold: A cutoff at
harmonic 60 of the masker (corresponding to 2400 Hz) yields a threshold more than
30 dB below the curve with random masker in Fig. 5. This astounding decrease is
again due to a better definition (or lengthening) of the "silent" intervals by
the addition of higher harmonics.

5. CONCLUSION

Masking experiments with maskers composed of many harmonics are described.
Maskers with identical (1/f) amplitude spectrum, and two extreme phase spectra
are used: 1) Constant phase of the harmonics, resulting in maskers with long
"silent" intervals between consecutive pulses, and 2) "random" phases yielding
nearly constant signal envelopes. Threshold of test tones differed as much as 40
dB between both types of masker.

Experiments with short test-tone pulses confirm the assumption that the ear
uses short time-windows in analysing these signals. The ear seems to be able to
make use of the "silent" intervals occurring in constant-phase maskers, leading
to the very low threshold values found in the experiments.

Our last experiment with lowpass maskers demonstrates the importance of "silent" intervals even more clearly: *Adding* masking harmonics *lowers* the threshold of a test tone by as much as 20 dB. This unmasking effect is also explained
by the occurrence of "silent" intervals.

REFERENCES

Duifhuis, H. (1970). Audibility of High Harmonics in a Periodic Pulse.
    J. Acoust. Soc. Amer. 48, 888-893.
Duifhuis, H. (1971). Audibility of High Harmonics in a Periodic Pulse. II. Time
    Effect. J. Acoust. Soc. Amer. 49, 1155-1162.
Martens, J.-P. (1981). Audibility of harmonics in a periodic complex.
    J. Acoust. Soc. Amer. 70, 234-237.
Mehrgardt, S. (1982). Die subjektive Tonhöhe fehlender Teiltöne in harmonischen
    Komplexen. In: Fortschritte der Akustik - FASE/DAGA '82, pp. 1231-1234,
    Göttingen.
Raiford, C.A., Schubert, E.D. (1971). Recognition of Phase Changes in Octave
    Complexes. J. Acoust. Soc. Amer. 50, 559-567.
Schroeder, M.R. (1970). Synthesis of Low-Peak Factor Signals and Binary Se-
    quences With Low Autocorrelation. IEEE Trans. on Information Theory IT-16,
    85-89.
Schroeder, M.R., Mehrgardt, S. (1982). Auditory masking phenomena in the percep-
    tion of speech. In: The representation of speech in the peripheral auditory
    system (R. Carlson and B. Granström, eds.). pp. 79-87. Amsterdam, Elsevier
    Biomedical Press.
Zwicker, E. (1976). Masking period patterns of harmonic complex tones.
    J. Acoust. Soc. Amer. 60, 429-439.

GENERAL DISCUSSION

ZWICKER:
The term "unmasking" may be misleading. Masking depends on both the temporal and on the spectral distribution of the masker. Do you see any effects in your data besides what is already known of the dependence of masking on the temporal and spectral characteristcs of the masker?

MEHRGARDT:
In contrast to classical forward-backward masking experiments, we need to know not only the excitation patterns (amplitude distributions), but also require precise knowledge of phase values. For example, the effect shown in Fig. 6 (a decrease of the masked threshold by 20 dB caused by an addition of energy in the masker) could hardly be predicted without actually carrying out the experiment. Additionally, we found interesting discrepancies in the dynamic behaviour of the ear in the experi- mets with constant-phase maskers compared to noise-like maskers. One example is the difference in (parallel) shifts in Fig. 4 between test-tone pulses and contin- uous test-tones.

MOORE:
Your idea that the differences in threshold for phases constant and phases "random" depends upon the presence of "silent" intervals is consistent with our own work on gap detection (Shailer and Moore, submitted). In your Fig. 2 differen- ces start to appear for a fundamental around 120 Hz, corresponding to intervals of about 8-9 ms. This is close to the threshold we found for gap detection at the signal frequency you used (1200 Hz).

DECAY OF PULSATION THRESHOLD PATTERNS

J. Verschuure, J.N. Kroon, M.P. Brocaar

Dept. of Otolaryngology, Erasmus University Rotterdam
P.O. Box 1738, 3000 DR Rotterdam, the Netherlands

1. INTRODUCTION

The functioning of the auditory system can be described as performing with a certain time constant, a frequency analysis of the incoming signals. Such an analysis means that frequency selectivity and time resolution are closely linked. It has led in practice to the use of narrow-band signals for the determination of the frequency selectivity and of wide-band signals (noise or clicks) for the determination of the temporal acuity. The use of suchs signals avoids the interactions as much as possible and makes it difficult to determine the effects of frequency selectivity and temporal resolution on each other.

One of the ways to determine the time resolution, is the measurement of the aftereffects of a stimulus. Many authors have described post masking experiments for a variety of masker and probe signals in which masked thresholds were determined as a function of the time delay between masker and probe. The probe level is thought to represent the level of activity or sensitivity caused by the masker that is still present after the specific time delay. A decay or recovery curve can thus be estimated.

Some authors have used tone bursts for the two signals in order to restrict the frequency region. Spectral splatter may affect the measurements and the interpretation of the data may be affected by cueing phenomena (Terry and Moore, 1978; Moore, 1980) and off-frequency listening (Verschuure, 1981; Johnson-Davies and Patterson, 1979). Most authors use the same frequency for masker and probe. The measured patterns show the decay at that particular frequency, but not how frequency selectivity and time resolution interact. The interaction can be seen in postmasking patterns, measured for various time delays (Fastl, 1979; Bechly and Fastl, 1982).

It is the purpose of this paper to determine the interaction between frequency selectivity and time resolution by measuring pulsation patterns with silent intervals inserted between pulsator and probe. The advantage of the technique is the relatively long probe duration, which minimizes the splatter, the absence of cueing and the fact that Verschuure (1981) has established a relationship between pulsation patterns and the underlying excitation pattern. We therefore know when off-frequency listening is of importance.

2. METHODS

We determined input and output pulsation threshold patterns (Verschuure, 1981) with silent intervals inserted between pulsator and probe. The duration of pulsator and probe was always kept constant at 125 ms. The signals were switched with smoothing envelopes. It is a gaussian amplitude evelope with a time constant of 3.55 ms. The duration of signals and gaps is defined as the time between the half-amplitude points. The equipment has been described by Verschuure *et al.*(1976).

Four experienced observers participated in the experiments, but none of them did all the experiments. Data will be shown on individual observers. The validity of the data is checked by others who did not do the extensive measurement.

The rationale behind the experiment is the same as the one presented by Plomp (1964). The pulsator evokes a distribution of activity in the auditory system. This excitation pattern will decay after the pulsator is switched off. It is not importa at this point whether it is a decay of activity or a recovery of sensitivity. The probe builds up another excitation pattern. It is assumed that the probe is heard as continuous only if there is no significant drop in activity level in any channel stimulated by the probe, during the time the probe is off (Houtgast, 1974;

Verschuure, 1981). This means that the excitation pattern of the probe must be fully contained within the decayed excitation pattern of the pulsator. This interpretation takes off-frequency listening into account and the nonlinearity with level. The use of various gap durations will show how the excitation pattern decays, both with the course of time and in the frequency domain.

3. RESULTS AND DISCUSSION

a) *Pattern of decay*

Observer MB measured input and output extension patterns at 0.5, 1.0 and 2.0 kHz for different pulsator levels and for a number of gap durations. An example of an input extension pulsation pattern at 1.0 kHz for a level of 65 dB SPL is given in fig. 1 for gap durations of 0, 20, 40, 50 and 60 ms.

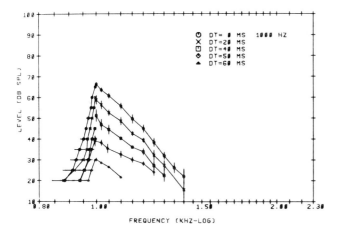

Fig. 1. Input extension pulsation patterns at 1 kHz, 65 dB SPL. Patterns are measured for silent intervals between pulsator and probe stimulus of 0, 20, 40, 50 and 60 ms

Three frequency regions have to be distinguished:
- In the upper high-frequency region a parallel downward shift of the pulsation pattern is found.
- The shift in the lower high-frequency region is characterized by a gradual reduction of the slope of the shallow edge to the pattern. In certain instances this has even led to a shift of the maximum probe level to a higher frequency than the pulsator frequency. This is particularly found for the very high pulsator levels of about 80 dB.
- The decay of the low-frequency edge results again in a more or less parallel shift of the pulsation patter.
Postmasking patterns of Fastl (1979) can be interpreted in very much the same way except that the parallel shift in the upper high-frequency region is not clear because data points are not available in this region. The patterns of Bechly and Fastl (1982) for gaps longer than 20 ms are very similar to ours.
Verschuure (1981) has shown that the high-frequency edge to the pulsation pattern represents the high-frequency edge to the excitation pattern. Off-frequency detection could not take place because the slope of the excitation patterns gets less steep with level. This means that the high-frequency edge to the excitation level of the probe is less steep. It implies that the high-frequency edge to the pulsation patterns of fig. 1 reflects the edge to the excitation pattern. The observed pattern change reflects a change in the distribution of auditory activity. The low-frequency edge to the pulsation patterns does not reflect the excitation pattern. This slope gets steeper with level so the slope of the probe excitation

pattern is less steep than the slope of the pulsator excitation pattern, resulting
in off-frequency detection. It implies that the observed parallel shift of the low-
frequency edge does not necessarily represent a parallel shift of the excitation
pattern. Conclusions on the shape of the excitation pattern in this region cannot
be drawn.

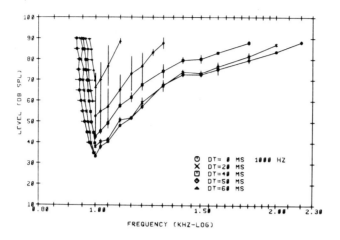

Fig. 2. Output extension pulsation patterns at 1 kHz, 35 dB SPL. Patterns are
measured for silent intervals between pulsator and probe stimulus of 0, 20, 40, 50
and 60 ms

     In fig. 2 we present output extension patterns, resembling the psychophysical
tuning curves (Small, 1959; Zwicker, 1974). The description of the decay distinguishes three regions:
- The low-frequency edge to the patterns shows again a more or less parallel shift,
but interpretation is complicated because of the strong nonlinearity involved
(Verschuure, 1981).
- The part of the high-frequency edge just above the pulsator frequency, now seems
to steepen with gap duration.
- The decay of the more remote part of the pattern cannot be seen from the figures
because the levels rapidly approach the maximum level.
     Restricting ourselves to the part just above the pulsator frequency, we see
that input and output patterns seem contradictory. The slope of the input pattern
gets less steep with gap duration and the slope of the output pattern gets steeper.
Rephrased in pattern terms, a "blunting" of the input pattern is linked with a
"sharpening" of the tip of the output pattern. The contradiction can be explained
by the nonlinear decay pattern that is described in the Section 3 b. It will be
shown that at lower pulsator levels (a condition met near the tip) the effective
decay is much slower than at higher pulsator levels (a condition met further up
the curve). All this implies that input patterns reflect the change in auditory
tuning, while output patterns reflect strongly the nonlinear decay pattern.
This fact proves once again that the idea that tuning curves represent the auditory tuning is not justified. The method is very sensitive to the level nonlinearity (Verschuure, 1981) and can thus lead to false conclusions.
     The above described effects may have their consequences for postmasking
determinations of auditory tuning. In all these experiments, short tone burst are
presented some 20 ms after the masker has been switched off. The delay is long
enough to show signs of decay and thus a change of apparent tuning, particularly
if tuning is determined by psychophysical tuning curves. The data of Fastl (1979)
and Bechly and Fastl (1982) even suggest that the post masking patterns show a
larger decay after 20 ms than found in pulsation patterns.

Concluding, we see that the decay of the patterns is not a simple parallel shift (multiplicative factor) nor a gradual flattening of the excitation pattern. The decay is linked with a change in frequency selectivity.

b) *Time constants*
    The figs. 1 and 2 show the change in shape of pulsation patterns and reflect the decay of the excitation pattern at the high-frequency side. They do not give a clear picture of the time pattern of the decay. This is shown in fig. 3, where the probe level at 1100 Hz is given as a function of the gap duration for a pulsator at 1000 Hz (observer JK). The frequency combination was chosen in order to avoid problems of pulsator and probe identification which occur when they are close in frequency. We plotted the decay in three different ways: level vs time, level vs log time and log level vs time. The last plot gave the best interpretable results and we use this way of presentation in fig. 3.

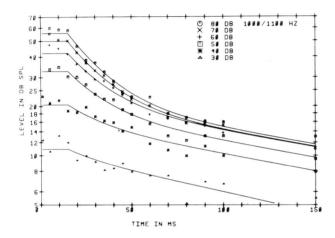

Fig. 3. *Decay of pulsation for pulsator of 1000 Hz and probe of 1100 Hz. Decay patterns of obs. JK are shown for pulsator levels of 80, 70, 60, 50. 40 and 30 dB SPL*

    The use of the logarithm of the level is not common. Its use can be argued by assuming a decay process that is related to a neural proces like a change in sensitivity. We have to realise that stimulus levels are transformed into neural activity levels in the peripheral auditory system. The transformation is logarithmic, justifying the use of dB scales. If we further assume that the change in the neural process can be described by an exponential function with time, such a process will manifest itself as a linear process if we take the logarithm of activity, thus the log level.
    Fig. 3 shows that the pulsation levels start to fall after a time delay of about 10 to 15 ms. Between this delay and a delay of about 60 ms, we observe a substantial drop in pulsation level. The curves for different levels seem to converge to one point. For gaps longer than 60 ms, we observe a set of almost parallel curves, pointing to a decay with a level independent time constant.
    The two linear parts seen in fig. 3, suggest that the decay can be described by the function:

$$I(t)=I_1.\exp(-(t-t_0)/\tau_1)+I_2.\exp(-(t-t_0)/\tau_2)+M$$

with M is threshold of hearing to the time delay at which decay starts I_1, I_2, τ_1 and τ_2 the parameters of the function.
We assessed the four parameters for each level with the aid of the MLAB computer program (Knott and Reece, 1972). The data of one observer at the frequencies 0.5, 1.0 and 2.0 kHz are given.

We first assumed that the long time constant τ_2, related to the data points for gap durations longer than 60 ms, does not depend on level. The best fit functions showed that the short time constant τ_1 depended only slightly on level. The time constant seemed to be almost constant for higher levels and it was somewhat larger for lower levels. At these levels, however, the level associated with the faster decaying part (I_1) gets small and the estimate of the time constant rather unreliable. We therefore decided to try and make a fit with two time constants that are independent of level. The time constants obtained from the best fitting functions in the least-mean-square sense, are shown in table I.

Table I. Time constants for pulsation decay.

frequency (kHz)	0.5	1.0	2.0
τ_1 (ms)	21.3	20.2	22.5
τ_2 (ms)	132	299	285

The table shows a frequency-independent short time constant of about 20 ms and a frequency-dependent long time constant, although the values at 1 and 2 kHz do not seem to vary anymore.

We were very puzzled by the fact that the short time constant was level independent, while fig. 3 seems to suffest a clear dependence. The level independence can be understoot if one realizes that the parts of the curve between delay time t_0 and about 60 ms is the superposition of two exponential functions. The long time constant can easily be assessed from the longer gap durations where the contribution of the first exponential is neglisible. The short time constant can only be assessed after the effects of the long time constant have been substracted from the measured curve.

The time delay t_0 was taken from plots like fig. 3. It was assumed to be level independent and was taken large enough to exclude any effects of the non-decaying parts of the curve. Its value was 10 ms at 2.0 kHz and 15 ms at 0.5 and 1.0 kHz. Data points for gap durations shorter than t_0 were not included in the fit.

The other parameters are the levels I_1 and I_2. We show their values as a function of dB SL in fig. 4.

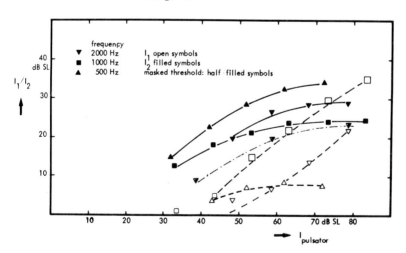

Fig.4. Best fit levels I_1 (open symbols) and I_2 (filled symbols) at different pulsator levels for different pulsator-probe frequency combinations

The figure suggests a great similarity between the levels I_2 related to the long time constant, especially since different ratios have been used of pulsator and probe frequency. Each curve seems to level off at higher stimulus levels and its shape can be described by an exponential function with an asymptote near 25 dB. The function seems to depart from zero for levels over about 20 dB which can be interpreted as the level of the pulsator at which activity appears in the probe channel.

We have found a similar function if we measure the detection threshold of the probe under the same conditions as the pulsation thresholds have been measured. It will be reported elsewhere (Verschuure and Brocaar, 1983) that masked thresholds measured under these conditions, show a similar level nonlinearity as pulsation patterns do, except that the level at the summit of the pattern can be described by an exponential function with an asymptotic value of 25 dB SL. In order to verify the relationship the masked thresholds under identical situations at 2 kHz are plotted as half-filled symbols in fig. 4. There seems to be a difference of about 6 dB. We also measured the decay of the masked thresholds for increasing gap durations and this curve can be described by the same time constant as τ_2. We conclude that I_2 and τ_2 are determined by the masked threshold of the probe.

The levels I_1, related to the short time constant, are shown as open symnols. For 1 and 2 kHz the levels increase rapidly with increasing level; for 0.5 kHz this increase is only small. The differences in the levels are again due to the different frequency ratios of pulsator and probe. However, the curves show that this level becomes important for levels above about 40 dB SL. This is equivalent to the statement that pulsation thresholds deviate from masked thresholds only at levels some 20 dB above threshold. At lower levels the probe will start pulsating as soon as it is above the absolute threshold.

In conclusion we have found that decay of the excitation pattern has consequences for the frequency selectivity. This may lead to false conclusions of the selectivity if measured in post masking. The decay pattern near the summit can be described by a bi-exponential function. The long time constant of 150 to 300 ms is related to masking; the short time constant of 20 ms to continuity perception. Its implications for physiology have to be studied.

REFERENCES

Bechly, M. Fastl, H. (1982). Interaktion der Nachhoerschwellen-Tonheits-Zeitmuster zweier maskierender Schalle. *Acustica* 50: 70-74
Fastl, H. (1979). Temporal masking effects: III. Pure tone masker. *Acustica* 43: 282-294
Houtgast, T. (1974). Lateral suppression in hearing, *Thesis*, VU-Amsterdam
Johnson-Davies, J., Patterson, R.D. (1979). Psychophysical tuning curves: restrictins the listening band to the signal region. *J. Acoust. Soc. Amer.* 79: 765-770
Moore, B.C.J. (1980). Detection cues in forward masking. In: *Psychophysical, Physiological and Behavioural studies in Hearing.* Delft Un. Press
Plomp, R. (1964). Rate of decay of auditory sensation. *J.A.S.A.* 36: 277-282
Small, A.M. (1959). Pure tone masking. *J. Acoust. Soc. Amer.* 31: 1619-1625
Terry, M., Moore, B.C.J. (1977)·"Suppression" effects in forward masking. *J. Acoust. Soc. Am.* 62: 781-784(L)
Verschuure, J. (1981). Pulsation patterns and nonlinearity of auditory tuning. II. Analysis of psychophysical results. *Acustica* 49: 296-306
Verschuure, J., Brocaar, M.P. (1983). Detection thresholds in pulsation measurement, *Proc. 11th ICA,* Paris
Verschuure, J., Rodenburg, M., Maas, A.J.J. (1976). Presentation conditions of the pulsation threshold method. *Acustica* 35: 47-54
Zwicker, E. (1974). On a psychoacoustical equivalent of tuning curves. In: *Facts and Models in Hearing.* Springer Verlag

GENERAL DISCUSSION

JOHNSTONE:
In our laboratory, Cody and Yates have measured recovery after loud tone pips presented to guinea pigs and have shown two time constants which are of comparable time to those shown here. However, we find the time constants are a function of tone per length. Have you noticed any effect of pulsation tone per length on your time constants?

VERSCHUURE:
We haven't investigated the effect of signal (pulsator) duration on the time constants in a direct experiment. In an indirect experiment regarding the detection
threshold of the probe under presentation condition similar to pulsation conditions, the results suggested some change in the long time constant with increasing
pulsation duration, but this change was small.

URBAS:
In single neuron recordings from the medial geniculate body of anaesthetized cats,
I have used a "two-tone" forward masking paradigm where, instead of masker and
probe <u>tones</u>, naturally spoken human speech signals were used (specifically: frica-
tive/ plosive pairs, where the fricative played the role of masker and the plosive
played the role of probe). Plots were then made of the neuron response to the
probe (plosive) as a function of the silent interval between masker (fricative)
and probe. These recovery functions also showed two time-constants which, although
variable from cell to cell, had averaged values of approximately 20 ms and 300 ms.

VERSCHUURE:
Thank you for your additional information.

Section V
Pitch Perception

MUTUAL PITCH INFLUENCE OF COMPONENTS IN A COMPOUND SOUND

G. van den Brink

*Erasmus University Rotterdam, Dept. of Biological and Medical Physics,
P.O. Box 1738, 3000 DR Rotterdam, The Netherlands*

1. INTRODUCTION

It is not generally accepted that the pitch assessed to a residue signal is established by the separate pitch information of the individual components. Neither exists agreement with regard to the relation between the shift of residue pitch due to the presence of other (merely low-frequency) sounds on one hand and the pitch shifts of individual components, due to the same sound, on the other hand.

The results of Van den Brink (1970, 1974, 1975a,b; see also Plomp, 1976), showing similarity between data obtained directly with complex sounds and data calculated from results obtained with pure tones, suggest such a relation. These data seem to be nicely in agreement with Terhardt's (1972) virtual pitch model. Houtsma (1980) and Hall and Soderquist (1982), however, failed to confirm these findings. Their data suggest that such an agreement is too limited to justify Van den Brink's conclusion that the pitch of a complex sound is predictable on the basis of the separate pitches of its components.

The difference between our experimental procedures on one hand and of the authors mentioned on the other hand, is that we determined the pitch as a function of the frequency whereas the other authors chose a limited number of fixed frequency combinations, thereby overlooking a slight, but systematic shift along the frequency scale between measured and calculated data as found by us. This agreement can clearly be seen when pitch shift data are presented as a function of the frequency but can, indeed, be missed when comparison takes place only for fixed separate frequency combinations. Several factors, like the critical band mechanism, the phenomenon of spectral dominance and the existence of combination tones may, or do, play a role in this pattern shift. In the present paper it will be shown that tone-on-tone pitch induction plays a major role in the pitch assessment of individual components of a complex sound.

2. MEASURING PROCEDURE

The experiments have been carried out monaurally by three subjects who are considered to have normal hearing. A test signal, consisting either of a pure tone with frequency f_t together with low pass noise with a cut-off frequency f_n, so that f_t/f_n is a constant factor, or consisting of a harmonic two-component signal, the upper component having a frequency f_t, was presented during 1.6 s. The high-frequency slope of the low-pass noise was 48 dB/octave; the noise levels will be given relative to the level for which the unfiltered noise would just mask the pure tone. The ratio between the frequencies of the two harmonic components was varied between 2:3 and 11:12. After an interval of 0.4 s, a comparison signal consisting of a single pure tone was presented during 0.8 s. The frequency of this comparison signal f_r was adjusted until it had the same pitch as the upper pure tone in the test signal. The subjects were permitted to listen to the signals as often as they needed to make a satisfactory match. The matchings have been carried out as a function of f_t, at a sensation level of about 40 dB. The relative frequency difference between f_r and f_t, necessary for equal pitches, has been plotted as a function of the test tone frequency f_t.

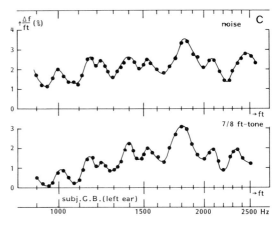

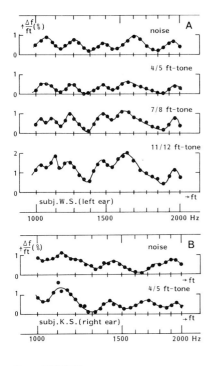

Fig. 1. Examples of pitch-induction by noise and by pure tones as a function of the frequency of the test tone, for three subjects

3.   RESULTS

    Some samples of the results are shown in the Figs. 1a, b and c. The top curves concern the pitch shifts due to the presence of low-pass noise. Cut-off frequencies and levels used by the subjects WS, KS and GB were 0.9 f_r and -12 dB, 0.83 f_r and -10 dB and 0.8 f_r and -5 dB, respectively.
    The remaining curves concern the pitch shifts due to the presence of a lower (harmonic) component. The ratio's between the test frequency f_t and the frequency of the added components are given in the figures.
    A complete set of data with harmonic pure tone induction (GB, right ear) is given in Fig. 2. The frequency interval between the test tone and the comparison signal, varying from 1/13 to 1/2, is the parameter in this set of curves. This figure is the result of a two-dimensional smoothing procedure. The $\Delta f/f$ values in the maxima and the minima, the frequencies for which these values occured and the frequency for which the $\Delta f/f$ values were half-way between the extreme values were plotted separately. Smooth curves were drawn through these points, from which Fig. 2 was constructed.

4.   DISCUSSION

    The most conspicuous result is, that all curves for each of the subjects contain the same frequency-dependent characteristics, independent of the frequency difference between the test tone and the inducing tone and independent of the type of inducing signal used. The maxima and minima occur approximately at the same frequencies in all of them.
The influence of lower frequency energy upon pitch appears to be upwards without any exceptions so far, and depends on the frequency according to a pattern which is very likely related to earlier found frequency-dependent effects like the auditory threshold (Van den Brink, 1970) and various diplacusis-related phenomena (Van den Brink, 1975a and b). There is a general trend of increasing pitch shift with decreasing frequency difference between the inducing signal and the test tone. Although the presented data do not show this, the same effect exists with

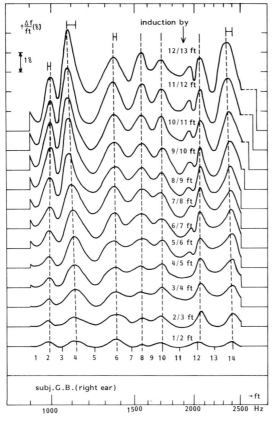

Fig. 2. Pitch induction by different tones with frequencies that have constant ratio's with respect to the test tone. The horizontal distances indicated at the top give the shifts of the maxima along the frequency scale (right ear subject GB)

increasing intensity of the inducing signal.

When the results of the two-tone experiment are plotted as a function of the frequency of the inducing tone instead of as a function of the test tone frequency, the frequency-dependent correspondence, as present in Fig. 2, does not exist. It is justified, therefore, to conclude that the way in which the pitch of a tone with a given frequency is influenced by lower frequency energy is predominantly determined by the properties of the system which are characteristic for the tone itself, and not by those which are characteristic for the induction signal.

Furthermore it is clear that the way in which the pitch changes in dependence of the frequency interval between inducing signal and test tone (and neither in dependence of the intensity of the inducing signal with a given frequency interval) is not the same for all frequencies. The pitch rises more rapidly for one frequency than it does for another frequency.

The simplest mechanism we can imagine to be responsible for all such frequency-dependent phenomena, seems to be a place-dependent irregularity in the mechanical properties along the basilar membrane. If the impedance has place-dependent irregularities, it might account for a threshold fine structure as well as for a non-smooth monaural frequency pitch relation. Non-smooth relations in the two ears account for binaural diplacusis[x].

Places with relatively high impedance might give way less easily to the widening of wave patterns along the basilar membrane with increasing intensity of the inducing sound than places with relatively low impedance. If this is true, the minima in the pitch induction curves should correspond to relatively high impedances and the maxima to relatively low impedances.

The fact that pitch increases more rapidly in the maxima than it does in the minima supports this assumption.

In Fig. 3a and b the values of $\Delta f/f_t$ in, respectively, the maxima and minima, have been plotted as a function of the relative frequency difference between test signal and inducing signal. Assuming a logarithmic relation between place and frequency, the horizontal axis would then represent the distance between the induction frequency and the test frequency along the basilar membrane. The test frequency is in this case located at "1" at the abcissa. The odd and even numbers at the curves refer to the minima and the maxima, respectively, as indicated at the bottom of Fig. 2. The fact that the growing influence of a tone, as it moves toward the test frequency, is not smooth, might be an indication that impedance irregularities in between the locations of test and inducing signal may affect the

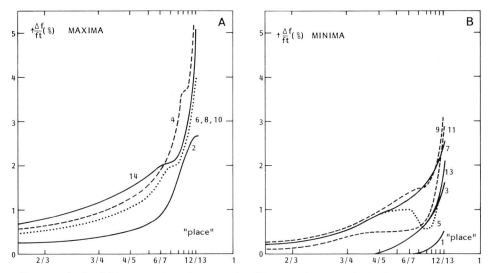

*Fig. 3. Pitch shift as a function of the distance between inducing tone
and test tone for frequencies coinciding with the maxima (a) and the
minima (b), as indicated at the bottom of Fig. 2.*

influence of the inducing signal. A first rough check in this respect seemed to
be confirmative. The fact that the curves in Fig. 3 are different for different
maxima and minima might be the consequence of the existence of local impedance
irregularities and, eventually, of local impedance gradients.

The shift in the locations along the frequency scale where the curves of
Fig. 2 have maxima for different amounts of induction are indicated at the top
part of this figure. This shift varies up to about 5% of the frequency in question
and might be due to the same local impedance conditions.

While a connection appears to exist between impedance irregularities on one
hand and fine-structures that have been found in monaural thresholds, in monaural
frequency-pitch relations and in pitch induction on the other hand, it is very
tempting to seek as well for a relation with stimulated acoustic emission, or
echo's, as have been found by Kemp (1978). Given the assumed relation between
echo's and threshold fine-structure and given a relation between this structure
and the existing irregularities in frequency-pitch relations and in induction
phenomena, a relation between the latter phenomena and echo's is bound to exist
as well. The long delay between stimulus and echo, however, is often used as an
argument for the assumption that echo's are not being caused by direct reflections
but that they are the result of some active process, presumably at the
level of the haircells. If the above mentioned relations exist, it might be
necessary to look for other causes of these long delays.

In that respect, it must be realized that Von Békésy (1960) observed
"paradoxal waves" in his pendulum model[**], that are generated at locations where
an impedance step is present. These waves move in the opposite direction. It must
be realized too, that the building up of travelling waves as well as of paradoxal
waves is an extremely slow process. Considering these facts, the question could
be reconsidered whether these paradoxal waves are related to echo's and whether
the building up of these waves is a sufficiently slow process to account for the
relatively long delays.

If these facts are proven to be correct, or when it appears that the assumed
active processes are accompanied by (apparent) local changes of the impedance, the
assumption of a relation between echo's and threshold fine-structure (and other
phenomena as well) would have a more solid base.

5. CONCLUSIONS

The influence of a lower-frequency signal upon the pitch of a test tone is always upward and increases with decreasing frequency difference between inducing signal and test tone and with increasing intensity of the inducing signal.

The influence depends dominantly on the frequency of the test tone and less (or not at all) on the frequency of the inducing signal. There are several maxima within an octave.

Induced pitch shifts measured so far, are up to about 5%. They are of the same order as previously reported pitch deviations and seem to be related to those.

The locations of the maxima and minima along the frequency scale are different from person to person but are nearly constant per person, regardless the type of induction signal and regardless the intensity, in the same way as is the case for threshold and diplacusis fine structures.

The present phenomena as well as the other phenomena mentioned, might be due to irregularities in the course of the impedance along the basilar membrane.

A relation between echo's on one hand and threshold and pitch fine-structures on the other hand, is likely to exist.

In a private discussion on this matter, J. Tonndorf mentioned the existence of small blood vessels in the bony part along the basilar membrane, penetrating slightly into the membrane itself. He suggested that these vessels might account for such small impedance irregularities.

**A film of about an hour, made by Von Békésy, demonstrating his models of basilar membrane travelling waves is available to be shown during the meeting.*

REFERENCES

Von Békésy, G. (1960). Experiments in hearing. McGraw-Hill, New York. (And the demonstration film of the pendulum model by Von Békésy.)

Brink, G. van den (1970). Two experiments on pitch perception. *J. Acoust. Soc. Amer.* 48, 1355-1365.

Brink, G. van den (1974). Monotic and dichotic pitch matchings with complex sounds. In: *"Psychophysical Models and Physiological Facts in Hearing"*, E. Zwicker and E. Terhardt (eds.). Springer, Berlin/Heidelberg/New York.

Brink, G. van den (1975a). The relation between binaural diplacusis for pure tones and for complex sounds. *Acustica* 32, 159-165.

Brink, G. van den (1975b). Monaural frequency-pitch relations. *Acustica* 32, 166-174.

Hall, J.W. and D.R. Soderquist (1982). Transient complex and pure tone pitch change by adaptation. *J. Acoust. Soc. Amer.* 71, 665-670.

Houtsma, A.J.M. (1980). Influence of masking noise on the pitch of complex tones. In: *Psychophysical, Physiological and Behavioural Studies in Hearing"*, G. van den Brink and F.A. Bilsen (eds.), Delft University Press.

Houtsma, A.J.M. (1981). Noise-induced shifts in the pitch of pure and complex tones. *J. Acoust. Soc. Amer.* 70, 1661-1668.

Kemp, D.T. (1978). Stimulated acoustic emission from within the human auditory system. *J. Acoust. Soc. Amer.* 64, 1386-1391.

Plomp, R. (1976). Aspects of tone sensation. *Academic Press*, London/New York/San Francisco.

Terhardt, E. (1972a). Zur Tonhöhenwahrnehmung von Klangen I. Psychoakustische Grundlagen. *Acustica* 26, 173-186.

Terhardt, E. (1972b). Zur Tonhöhenwahrnehmung von Klangen II. Ein Funktionsschema. *Acustica* 26, 187-199.

Terhardt, E. (1979). Calculating virtual pitch. *Hear. Res.* 1, 155-182.

MONOTIC AND DICHOTIC PITCH JND'S COMPARED

F.A. Bilsen and J. Raatgever

Applied Physics Department,
Delft University of Technology, the Netherlands

1. INTRODUCTION

In the peripheral auditory system, complex sounds are decomposed into a series
of sinusoidal frequency components. These components can give rise to individual
pitches, or to a low pitch if a more or less harmonic relation exists between them.
Information on these components, either spectral (place) or temporal, is carried on
to the central nervous system and constitutes the "central spectrum". Modern pitch
theories (Goldstein, 1973; Terhardt, 1972; Wightman, 1973) have in common that the
central pitch processor performs an operation on this central spectrum.
    Reviewing the pitches of monotic and dichotic noise signals, Bilsen (1977) in-
dicated that parsimony of pitch processing calls for utmost three ways in which
a central spectrum is generated: (a) directly from the spectral information at
either of the cochleae (internal, peripheral spectrum), (b) directly from the spectral information of both cochleae together (Houtsma and Goldstein, 1972), and (c)
after binaural processing on the temporal information from left and right cochlea
(Bilsen and Goldstein, 1974). Here, we are faced with important questions about the
relative rôle of temporal versus spectral coding, and about the limitations on processing set by the auditory system.
    Pertinent to these issues is the accuracy of pitch perception as expressed in
the just noticeable difference of pitch (JND). Therefore, in the present paper, the
JND is compared for different types of signals, viz. monotic signals like the periodic pulse (PP) and comb filtered noise (COMB) and dichotic signals like multiple-
phase-shifted noise (MPS). It will appear possible to predict the MPS-JND from the
COMB-JND by considering the shape of the internal spectrum as measured psychophysically, its internal modulation depth M_{int} in particular.

2. HYPOTHESES

In order to compare the JND's of monotic and dichotic signals and to predict
one from the other, hypotheses, some of which have been tested already, have to be
made, viz.:
- Signals with similar (internal) power spectrum evoke the same pitch (much evidence available; compare e.g. Bilsen, 1977).
- Signals with similarly shaped (internal) power spectrum having the same peak-
  valley difference, i.e. modulation depth M_{int} (dB), give the same JND.
- The internal spectrum of dichotic noise signals can be found from appropriate
  BMLD-measurements (compare Raatgever and Bilsen, 1977).
- The M_{int} (dB) of COMB-signals is equal to $M_{acoust.}$ (dB) for the first harmonics
  (compare Houtgast, 1977).

3. SIGNAL DESCRIPTION

The use of a periodic pulse (PP) as a test stimulus in the JND experiments
being sufficiently familiar, COMB-noise and MPS-noise require further explanation.
    COMB-noise is a monaural stimulus. It is the result of feeding white gaussian
noise into a delay line with feed-back of a fraction g of the output. This results
in a comb-like power spectrum with peaks at harmonic frequencies n/τ as indicated
in Fig. 1b, where τ represents the delay (n=0,1,2...). The figure shows normalized
power spectra of COMB-noise for two values of the feed-back factor g. It clearly
demonstrates the influence of g on the modulation depth, characteristic for COMB-
noise. Theoretically, the peaks in the power spectrum have the value $1/(1-g)^2$,
whereas the minimal values in between are given by $1/(1+g)^2$.

MPS-noise is a dichotic stimulus in the sense that no spectral information is present at the separate ears but the desired spectral patterns arise due to binaural interaction. Although detailed knowledge is necessary to predict the internal spectra from their dichotic signal conditions, we use some essential simplifications to illustrate the spectral patterns involved (Raatgever, 1980). We consider the perceptual image of such dichotic noise stimuli, lateralized in the centre of the head, to be the result of a perfect addition of the signals at both ears, under preservation of their time structures. The, in this way idealized, internal signals with their specific spectral properties are assumed to constitute the spectral inputs for the pitch extracting mechanism in an analogous way as assumed for monaural signals like PP and COMB-noise. In the dichotic stimuli, moreover, the spectral information is subject to imperfections of the binaural interaction mechanism.

MPS-noise is, like COMB-noise, the result of white gaussian noise passing a delay line with feed-back of a signal fraction g. In order to obtain a flat frequency spectrum a negative fraction of the input $-g/(1-g^2)$ is added to the output

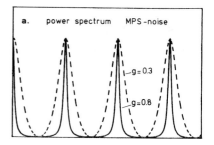

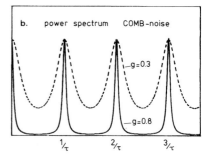

Fig. 1. Normalized power spectra (linear scale) of MPS-noise (a) and COMB-noise (b) for g=0.3 and 0.8

(Bilsen, 1976). The signal at the contralateral ear is the original noise, balanced for equal power at both ears. Due to the specific phase relation between the signals at the ears, the resulting internal power spectrum of MPS-noise has peaks at harmonic frequencies n/τ as shown in Fig. 1a (n=0,1,2...). In this figure the supposed normalized power spectrum of MPS-noise is shown for two values of g. Theoretically, the peaks are given by $4/(1-g)^2 (1+g)^2$. For frequencies just in between, the power equals zero for every g. This difference between the internal power spectra of COMB-noise and MPS-noise is reduced by the imperfect, noisy, operation of the binaural system, effectively reducing the modulation depth.

4. EXPERIMENTAL PROCEDURE

Two sets of JND-experiments have been carried out. These experiments concerned the monotic COMB-noise at one hand and the dichotic MPS-noise at the other. Both sets of experiments have been performed using four normal hearing subjects. Two of the subjects took part in all experiments.

In all cases a two-alternative forced-choice procedure has been used to measure the JND of pitch. The JND thus obtained corresponds to a 75% correct discrimination in f_0. For COMB-noise as well as for MPS-noise the JND is defined as: JND=$\Delta f_0/f_0$ (%). Here, $f_0(=1/\tau)$ is the frequency of the fundamental in the spectrum and τ is the basic delay used in the generation of the signals (section 3). JND-measurements were based on the detection of τ. For JND-measurements, in general, the condition $\Delta\tau \ll \tau$ is valid, so in that case: JND$\approx \Delta\tau/\tau$ (%).

Subjects, seated in a sound-proof booth, were presented with stimuli with an average sensation level of 40 dB. TDH 39 headphones have been used. The signals always consisted of two properly shaped stimuli of 500 ms duration.

The subjects had to respond to a number of series of maximally 12 pairs of randomized stimuli with fixed $\Delta\tau$. Each series resulted in a positive score if at least 75% of the responses were correct. During the monotic experiments these scores have been recorded systematically as a function of $\Delta\tau$, i.e. the spectral difference to be detected. The JND's have been estimated from the average reversal from positive to negative scores. For the dichotic experiments a computer-controlled adaptive method has been used to determine the JND of dichotic pitch from the positive and negative scores in the same way. In both experiments the 90%-confidence limits have been computed.

5. RESULTS

a) *JND of COMB-noise*

The JND of COMB-noise was measured as a function of f_p (=1/τ), for three values of g, by four subjects. The results of two subjects which also participated in the dichotic JND-measurements, are represented in Fig. 2. The bars in the figures indicate the 90%-confidence limits. The other two subjects showed similar results. For f_0=200 Hz (τ=5 ms), the JND is replotted as a function of g for these four subjects in Fig. 4.

Note that for g=0.85 the JND is independent of f_0 and that the average value for the four subjects amounts to 0.3%. For smaller values of g, the JND increases and becomes dependent on f_0.

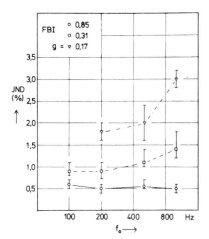 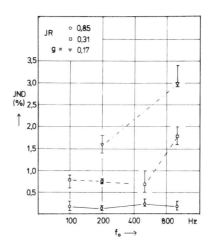

Fig. 2. The just noticeable difference in pitch (JND) of COMB-noise as a function of f_0(=1/τ) for three values of g and two subjects

b) *JND of MPS-noise*

The results of the JND-experiments for MPS-noise are plotted in Fig. 3 for g=0.8 and two subjects. The figures show the relative JND as a function of f_0(=1/τ). The 90%-confidence limits are indicated in the figures.

For both subjects we see minimal JND's for frequencies of the fundamental around 200 to 250 Hz and around 500 Hz. The minimal JND is 0.75% for observer JR and 1% for FB. Maximal JND's of about 2.3% are found for both observers at frequencies around 350 to 400 Hz. These two observers took also part in the monaural experiments. The other two subjects, not presented here, showed a similar behaviour, although one had significantly higher JND's.

The shape of the JND-curves presented here is different from the monaural data. It seems that JND's of dichotic pitch are minimal if the fundamental or its second harmonic is in the range of 500 Hz.

JND-measurements have also been performed with an extra interaural delay resulting in a lateralized pitch image of MPS-noise. The results, not presented here, show strikingly little effect on the JND's.

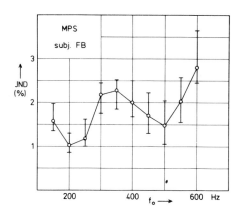
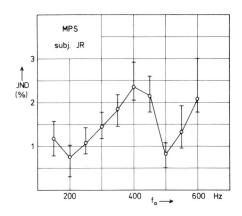

Fig. 3. The just noticeable difference in pitch (JND) of MPS-noise as a function of $f_o(=1/\tau)$ for g=0.8 and two subjects

6. DISCUSSION

The following differences between the JND's of the (monotic) COMB-noise and the (dichotic) MPS-noise can be observed. First, for g=0.8 the 200 Hz-JND's differ by about a factor 3 on the average. This, apparently, is in accordance with the general observation that monotic pitch is more easily perceived than dichotic pitch. Secondly, for this value of g, the MPS-JND is not independent of f_o as is the COMB-JND. As noticed in section 5, both subjects show minimum JND's for f_o=200 Hz and 500 Hz. This is probably due to the general fact that, different from monotic pitch, dichotic pitch shows a strong dominance effect for the frequency region around 500 to 600 Hz. This dominance is also observed for other binaural phenomena like lateralization and BMLD (compare Bilsen and Raatgever, 1973; Raatgever, 1980). For f_o=200 to 250 Hz the second harmonic of the MPS-spectrum is in the dominance region. For f_o=500 Hz it is the fundamental itself.

According to the hypotheses (section 2) the MPS-JND is expected to be predictable from the COMB-JND, in first order approximation. The following reasoning applies: For the MPS-signal the internal spectrum is reflected by appropriate BMLD-measurements. Thus, the modulation $M_{int.}$(dB) of the internal spectrum can be taken as the average peak-valley difference in dB for the (most pronounced) first and second peak. For f_o=250 Hz and g=0.8, this value amounts to 7 dB for subject JR and 8 dB for subject FB (Raatgever and Bilsen, 1977, Fig. 2). For COMB-noise $M_{int.}$(dB)= $M_{acoust.}$(dB) for the lowest peaks (compare Houtgast, 1977). Using this equality we are able to find the (monotic) COMB-spectrum that shows the same modulation depth as the MPS-signal. With the relation $M_{acoust.}$=10 log{$(1+g)^2/(1-g)^2$} (compare section 3) it follows that g=0.38 for subject JR and g=0.43 for subject FB. Now, in Fig. 4 we read the corresponding JND-values, viz. 0.7% for

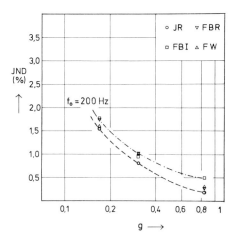

Fig. 4. The just noticeable difference in pitch (JND) of COMB-noise as a function of g for f_o=200 Hz (τ=5 ms) and four subjects

subject JR and 0.8% for subject FB. Comparing these values with the values actually measured, viz. 0.75% for subject JR and 1% for subject FB, there appears to be a good correspondence.

Further, it is interesting to compare the JND-data of COMB-noise with the JND of a periodic pulse (PP). Recent measurements in our lab. (Wittkämper, unpublished results) using exactly the same experimental procedure resulted in an average JND of about 0.3% for f_0=200 Hz. Realizing that a PP has a line spectrum, while COMB-noise has a continuous spectrum (the lines have, in fact, undergone a certain broadening), we conclude that COMB-noise with g=0.85 has "optimum sharpness of peaks", i.e. increasing the steepness of the spectral peaks by increasing g above 0.85 does not improve the JND in pitch.

7. CONCLUSIONS

- The COMB-JND is independent of f_0 and equal to 0.3% on the average, if g=0.85
- The MPS-JND is dependent on f_0. Minimum values of 0.9% on the average were obtained for f_0 about equal to 250 Hz and 500 Hz. This is attributed to the dominance phenomenon.
- The MPS-JND can be predicted from the COMB-JND by considering the modulation depth M_{int} of the (psychophysically measured) internal spectra of the signals.
- The internal modulation depth M_{int} of (dichotic) MPS-noise with g=0.8 is comparable to M_{int} of (monotic) COMB-noise with a g-factor of about 0.4
- For g=0.85 the COMB-JND is equal to the PP-JND.

Acknowledgements.
The MPS-JND-measurements formed part of a master-thesis by J.W. Müller.
The COMB-JND-measurements formed part of a master-thesis by F.W. Wittkämper.

REFERENCES

Bilsen, F.A., and Raatgever, J. (1973). Spectral dominance in binaural lateralization. *Acustica* 28, 131-132.

Bilsen, F.A., and Goldstein, J.L. (1974). Pitch of dichotically delayed noise and its possible spectral basis. *J.Acoust.Soc.Am.* 55, 292-296.

Bilsen, F.A. (1976). Pronounced binaural pitch phenomenon. *J.Acoust.Soc.Am.* 59, 467-468.

Bilsen, F.A. (1977). Pitch of noise signals: Evidence for a "central spectrum". *J.Acoust.Soc.Am.* 61, 150-161.

Goldstein, J.L. (1973). Optimum processor theory for the central formation of the pitch of complex tones. *J.Acoust.Soc.Am.* 54, 1496-1516.

Houtgast, T. (1977). Auditory filter characteristics derived from direct-masking data and pulsation-threshold data with a rippled-noise masker. *J.Acoust.Soc. Am.* 62, 409-415.

Houtsma, A.J.M., and Goldstein, J.L. (1972). The central origin of the pitch of complex tones: evidence from musical interval recognition. *J.Acoust.Soc.Am.* 51, 520-529.

Raatgever, J. and Bilsen, F.A. (1977). Lateralization and dichotic pitch as a result of spectral pattern recognition. In: *Psychophysics and physiology of hearing* (E.F. Evans and J.P. Wilson Eds.), pp. 443-453, London, Academic Press.

Raatgever, J. (1980). On the binaural processing of stimuli with different interaural phase relations. *Doctoral dissertation*, Delft University of Technology.

Terhardt, E. (1972). Zur Tonhöhewahrnehmung von Klängen. *Acustica* 26, 173-199.

Wightman, F.L. (1973). The pattern-transformation model of pitch. *J.Acoust.Soc.Am.* 54, 407-416.

ADDENDUM by RAATGEVER and BILSEN:

For a better understanding of the (idealized) central-spectrum patterns of comb-noise and MPS noise, mathematical descriptions are presented here.

COMB-noise is a monotic stimulus. It is the result of white noise passing a delay-line (delay τ) with feed-back of a signal fraction g. It can therefore be characterized in the spectral domain by:

$$A_C(\omega) = \frac{\exp{-j\omega\tau}}{1-g \ \exp{-j\omega\tau}} \ .$$ (1)

So the corresponding power-spectrum is given by:

$$\left| A_C(\omega) \right|^2 = \frac{1}{1-2g \ \cos\omega\tau+g^2} \ .$$ (2)

It has maxima: $\frac{1}{(1-g)^2}$ if $\cos\omega\tau=1$ or $\omega=n\frac{2\pi}{\tau}$

and minima: $\frac{1}{(1+g)^2}$ if $\cos\omega\tau=-1$ or $\omega=(2n+1)\frac{\pi}{\tau}$.

MPS-noise is a dichotic stimulus. The spectral pattern in the very centre of the binaural activity pattern corresponds to the dichotic pitch image that is lateralized in the centre of the head. It is the result of the interaction of the (undelayed) information from both ears. The signal at one ear is the result of white noise passing a delay-line (delay τ) with feed-back of a signal fraction g. To the output is also added a negative fraction $-g/(1-g^2)$ of the input signal. The signal at the contralateral ear consists of the input noise signal multiplicated by a factor $1/(1-g^2)$. Do we suppose the interaction process to be an addition, then the central spectrum can be characterized by:

$$A_M(\omega) = \frac{1+\exp{-j\omega\tau}}{(1+g)(1-g \ \exp{-j\omega\tau})} \ .$$ (3)

The corresponding power-spectrum is then given by:

$$\left| A_M(\omega) \right|^2 = \frac{2+2 \ \cos\omega\tau}{(1+g)^2(1+g^2-2g \ \cos\omega\tau)} \ .$$ (4)

It has maxima: $\frac{4}{(1+g)^2(1-g)^2}$ if $\cos\omega\tau=1$ or $\omega=n\frac{2\pi}{t}$

and minima: 0   if $\cos\omega\tau=-1$ or $\omega=(2n+1)\frac{\pi}{\tau}$.

Combining eq. (2) and (4) we see that the power spectra of COMB-noise and MPS-noise are related as follows:

$$g\left| A_M(\omega) \right|^2 + \frac{1}{(1+g)^2} = \left| A_C(\omega) \right|^2 \ .$$ (5)

In other words: The power-spectrum of COMB-noise is a factor g less modulated and lifted over a constant factor $1/(1+g)^2$ with respect to the corresponding power-spectrum of MPS-noise.

PITCH DISCRIMINATION AND MUSICAL INTERVAL RECOGNITION
IN BACKWARD MASKING

A. Rakowski

Department of Music Acoustics, Frederic Chopin Academy of Music
00-368 Warszawa, Poland

1. INTRODUCTION

In recent years several authors have studied the interfering effect of a
sound appearing later than a probe tone on the exact estimation of a pitch or
timbre quality of that probe. Various terms have been introduced to describe this
effect, such as "informational masking" (Pollack, 1975), "Backward interference"
(Loeb and Holding, 1975) or "temporal interference" (Yost, Berg and Thomas,
1976). The amount of this interference is not critically dependent on the intensity ratio of interfering and probe tones.
     The most controversial issue concerning the backward-interference effect is
the length of time in which it is effective. Massaro (1970, 1975) employing various procedures determined this time length as being of the order of 200 msec.
The reliability of his results was questioned by Leshowitz and Cudahy (1973) and
Loeb and Holding (1975). Yost et al. (1976) found substantial backward interference of a 500-msec, 800-Hz tone with the pitch recognition at a 20-msec probe
tone. The probe tone terminated 5 msec before the onset of the 800-Hz interfering tone and its frequency was either slightly higher (correct recognition:
"high") or slightly lower (correct recognition: "low") than 800 Hz.
     The main objection that may be raised against the reliability of most of
these and other authors' results is the possible side effect of the interference
tone taken by the subjects as a template in pitch comparison tasks. As a typical
example see the above description of Yost et al.'s "single interval recognition"
experiment.
     In the course of experiments described below the following was intended:
- to investigate the backward interference effect in pitch discrimination and
recognition using 2AFC and single-interval recognition procedures, with tonal
backward maskers not constituting reference points for pitch comparisons,
(though remaining in a common critical band with the probe tone),
- to investigate the performance in backward-interference tasks of some particularly sensitive musical listeners with several years' intensive practice in pitch
discrimination and recognition experiments,
- to use relative and absolute musical pitch memory of selected musical listeners in order to employ multi-alternative pitch-recognition procedures.

2. EXPERIMENTS I AND II: PITCH DISCRIMINATION

a) Method
     Four musicians aged 22-26 with 2-5 years' experience in psychoacoustic ex-
periments concerning pitch discrimination participated as subjects. 2AFC procedure was used. Test trials were presented through a loudspeaker in series of 50
trials each. The subjects were seated in a sound isolated booth and tested in individual sessions not exceeding two hours (with 3-4 breaks).
     Each trial consisted of a trail of two 50-msec test tones followed by a
100-msec masking sound. The test tones were separated by a 700-msec silent interval. The time interval between the termination of a masker and the beginning of
the next trial was 3000 msec. In this time a subject was to decide if the second
test tone was "higher" or "lower" in pitch, and push the appropriately labelled
button. No information as to the correctness of the answer was supplied to the
listeners. The frequency of the first test tone was always 1000 Hz. The frequency

of the second test tone was either 997 Hz or 1003 Hz; both versions were equally likely.

In Experiment I, with three subjects participating, the time interval Δt between the termination of the second test tone and the masker onset was 800, 600, 400, 300, 200, 100, 50, and 10 msec in consecutive sessions. In the first part of this experiment white noise was used as a masker. The noise was presented at 73 dB SPL, while all tones in both parts of the Experiment I were presented at 40 dB (linear ramps). The subjects were tested with one 50-trial test series at each value of Δt. Prior to each test series a 20-trial sample of it was presented for practicing. Prior to the first test series (with Δt equal 800 msec), an introductory series was presented with the masker excluded. No additional training was considered necessary for the subjects, as each of them had been participating in similar experiments (though without backward masking) for more than a hundred hours.

In the second part of the Experiment I, a 960-Hz tone was used as a masker. Subjects were tested with four 50-trial series at each value of Δt from 800 msec to 50 msec. Measurements at Δt equal 20 and 10 msec were not accomplished as the results appeared to be at a chance level.

In Experiment II the time interval Δt between the second test tone and the masker was held constantly at 100 msec, but the masker frequency f_M was being changed. All the stimuli were presented at 40 dB SPL. The experiment was conducted with the participation of two subjects. One of them (AM) had already participated in the first experiment; the other one did not have this particular experience, however, his general experience in similar tasks was outstanding. Both subjects were given a training of at least 500 trials at each experimental condition before the data was recorded. At each of the masker frequencies of 550, 660, 960, and 1000 Hz as well as the "no masker" conditions, five 100-trial test series were conducted with each of the subjects. Subject LK was additionally tested at f_M=780, 840, and 930 Hz with the same number of trials. Test series with various masker conditions were presented in chance order throughout the experiment after the training of the listeners had been completed.

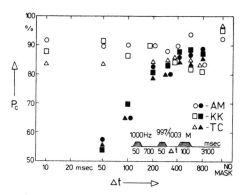

Fig. 1. Percentage of correct responses in 2AFC frequency-discrimination procedure as a function of the time interval Δt between the second test tone and the masker. Subjects: AM, KK, and TC. Open symbols: wide band-noise masker, closed symbols: tone masker 960 Hz

b) *Results and discussion*

The results of Experiment I are presented in fig. 1. It may be noted that application of a white-noise backward masker (open symbols) did not influence markedly the subjects' performance in pitch discrimination.

Still more important, this performance was not in the slightest way dependent upon the time distance between the second test tone and the masker.

A quite different situation arose when a tonal masker was applied (filled symbols). Here, the performance of all three subjects decreased markedly for Δt smaller than 200 msec and fell to a chance level at Δt smaller than 50 msec. The largest dispersion (not represented in the figure) among the results obtained by the individual subject in four consecutive series performed at a given time distance Δt were 22% and 24%. (Subject AM, Δt=100 msec and Δt=50 msec). The average dispersion for all the data points was 10.1%.

The frequency of a masker (960 Hz) was chosen in such a way as to remain in a common critical band with frequencies of the test tones (1000±3 Hz). The variable pitch distance between the second test tone and the masker could not have been used by the subjects as additional cue in pitch discriminations for the following reasons:

When the second test tone was "higher" than the first one (1000 Hz), the frequency interval between the masker and the second test tone was 1003/960 or 73 cents.

When the second test tone was "lower" than the first one, the frequency interval between the masker and the second test tone was 997/960 or 63 cents. The difference between the two intervals specified above was smaller than the JND for frequency ratio (Moran and Pratt, 1926). Incidentally, this would not have been the case if frequency differences between the test tones had been substantially larger. Consequently, it may be claimed that an unusual subjects' sensitivity for frequency discrimination tasks was used in the present experiments as a safeguard against some of the possible mistakes in the procedure.

The results of Experiment II are presented in fig. 2. They show how the subjects' performance changes with the changing relation between the test tone and the masker's frequency. It may be concluded that the largest decrease in performance concerns the situation in which the masker and the test tone remain in the same critical band. This conclusion however, is not very obvious because of the very large dispersion of the results at individual data points (about twice as large as in Experiment I).

It should be remembered that in contrast to the situation in the previous experiment the subjects in Experiment II were very carefully trained in each test situation.

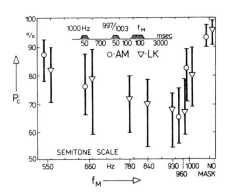

Fig. 2. Percentage of correct responses in 2AFC frequency-discrimination procedure as a function of the masker frequency. Subjects: AM and LK. Mean value and total dispersion of results in five 100-trial series for each individual subject are represented at each measuring point

The explanation of this fact is rather difficult. It may be argued, however, that at a very high level of the subjects' concentration and efficiency in performing the tasks, the interfering effect of backward tonal masking may be at times overcome to a large degree. Such a conclusion is consistent with the fact that subject AM, while participating in Experiment I, showed unusually great dispersion of results in the two final experimental arrangements.

Particular attention should be drawn to the results obtained at masker frequency 1000 Hz. At this experimental arrangement, both subjects reached considerably higher level of performance than at other masker frequencies within the same critical band. However, this particular arrangement may be taken as a good example of the situation with the possibility of using the masker as a template in pitch comparisons. Here, unlike in all other arrangements, the frequency of the masker is "central" in relation to both possible versions of the second test tone's frequency (997 or 1003 Hz). The subjects' decision (second tone "higher" or "lower" than the first tone) may be easily based upon comparing the pitch of the second tone with that of the masker, rather than with the memorized pitch of the first tone (as in all the other arrangements).

3. EXPERIMENT III: MUSICAL INTERVAL RECOGNITION

a) Method

Four musicians aged 20-26 participated as subjects. One of the subjects (AM) significantly exceeded the remaining three as far as their previous experience in similar tasks was concerned. He had participated in various psychoacoustic experiments for more than 5 years. He had also taken part in Experiment I and Experiment II of the present series. The other three subjects were selected out of a large group of music students as performing exceedingly well in pitch and timbre discrimination tests. All four subjects acquired great skill in the tasks concerning the immediate recognition of the musical intervals.

The subjects were tested in individual sessions not exceeding 2 hours (with 3-4 intermissions). Test trials were presented in series of a 100 trials each. All stimuli were presented through a high quality loudspeaker at 80 dB SPL while subjects were seated in a sound isolated booth. Each trial consisted of a 50-msec test stimulus followed by a 500-msec masker. The time interval Δt between the test stimulus and the masker was 300, 100, 50, 20, 12, 3 or 1 msec. The time interval between the termination of the masker and the beginning of the next trial was 5000 msec. Rise and decay times of all stimuli were 2 msec (linear ramps).

Each test stimulus was composed out of pure tones, their frequencies forming a tempered musical interval. The lower frequency of a tone pair was always set at 932 Hz, higher was set at 1175, 1245, 1319, 1397 or 1480 Hz. Accordingly, five musical intervals were formed; a major third, a perfect fourth, a tritone, a perfect fifth, and a minor sixth. The noise band with central frequency 1326 Hz and 300 Hz bandwidth was used as a masker. In a 100-trial test series each of the five musical intervals appeared 20 times. The subjects' task in each trial was to recognize a test stimulus as one out of five musical intervals equally likely to appear. When not being able to decide, they had to guess. The answer had to be taken down within 5 sec after the termination of the masker. (No psychological feedback was supplied.)

The subjects were given a training of 3 test series at each experimental arrangement before the data was collected. In the course of training it was found out that the subjects could more easily recognize the smallest and the largest interval of the set (i.e. a major third and a minor sixth) than the remaining three intervals. It was concluded that in these recognitions, the subjects were probably using some additional cues apart from their long-term musical memory. The results of the recognitions of these two skirt intervals were therefore excluded from the final computations. The results presented concern only correct recognitions of 3 intervals in 60-item series of trials. Five test series were presented for each value of Δt. The order of the presentations was random.

b) Results and discussion

The results of the experiment are presented in fig. 3. As may be seen in this figure the performance of the three subjects (TR, KS, and EZ) was under the strong effect of backward recognition masking of a noise-band masker. This effect was particularly evident in the results obtained by KS and EZ. At very short time intervals between the test stimulus and the masker, the percentage of correct recognitions by subjects KS, EZ, and TR was next to chance level (33%). The substantial influence of backward masking on these results may be seen for time intervals shorter than 50 msec (KS, EZ) and 12 msec (TR).

The performance of the subject AM was strongly contrasted to that of the remaining three subjects. He seemed to be able to overcome the effect of backward interference at all time arrangements used in the present experiment. At this point attention should be drawn towards the amount of practice acquired by individual subjects. Subjects KS, EZ, and TR had been chosen out of a large group of musicians as the best scoring ones in preliminary tests, and had later received an adequate training in actual conditions of the present experiment. They definitely may be treated as experienced subjects. Their results seem to be reliable,

Fig. 3. Percentage of correct re-
cognitions of the test stimulus as
one of three musical intervals: a
fourth, a tritone and a fifth, in
dependence on the time distance
between the test stimulus and
the noise-band masker. Subjects:
AM, KS, TR, and EZ. Mean value
and total dispersion of results
of five 60-trial series for each
individual subject are represent-
ed at each measuring point

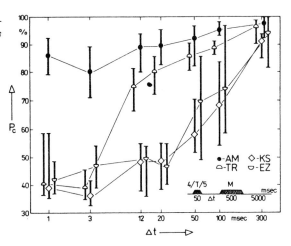

as showing not too great intra-subject and inter-subject variability. Nevertheless, these results appear not to reflect adequately the human auditory faculties. To estimate these faculties still more practice and concentration on the
part of the subjects are required. In the present experiment such extreme requirements happen to have been met by the subject AM.

4. EXPERIMENT IV: ABSOLUTE PITCH RECOGNITION

a) Method
        Two musicians aged 25 and 30 participated. They both possesed excellent per-
manent memory of twelve within-octave pitch standards of contemporary music (so-
called "absolute pitch"). They also had a significant, several years' experience
in participating as subjects in various psychoacoustic tests concerning absolute
pitch. They listened to the test stimuli according to similar procedure as the
subjects in Experiment III. The differences in test arrangements were following:
1) Five tone frequencies were used (Bb_5 – 932 Hz, B_5 – 988 Hz, C_6 – 1047 Hz, $C_{\#6}$
– 1109 Hz, D_6 – 1175 Hz) rather than five musical intervals. 2) The masker was
composed of nine pure tones (frequencies 831–1245 Hz in 8 semitone steps) rather
than of noise. 3) Time arrangements were as presented in fig. 4. 4) The test
stimulus and the masker were both presented at the loudness level 75 phones.
5) Correct recognitions of all five tones were computed; the procedure applied
may be called "Single-Interval, 5 Alternative Recognition". 6) Two 100-trial series were presented to each subject at all measuring points. No preliminary training was applied but the tests were presented in a growing order of difficuly (decreasing Δt).

b) Results and discussion
        The results are shown in fig. 4. Contrary to previous experiments the proce-
dure adopted in Experiment IV allowed to introduce test stimuli of shorter duration (10 msec rather than 50 msec) without unduly increasing the level of stimulus
uncertainty. Consequently, the effect of backward interference at short time intervals between the masker and test stimuli could be studied with greater precision. It appears from these results that backward recognition masking is effective
only at the time intervals shorter than 50 msec. This finding may be used as a
partial explanation of the inconsistency of results obtained in some previously
described experiments in which 50-msec test stimuli were used.

Fig. 4.   Percentage of correct frequency recognitions by two absolute pitch possessors, in backward recognition masking. Single-interval 5-alternative recognition tasks; frequencies 932, 988, 1047, 1109, and 1175 Hz

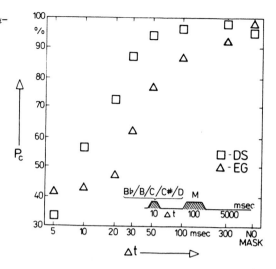

Acknowledgement. Support of the work was provided by the Polish Academy of Sciences (Program MRI - 24).

REFERENCES

Leshowitz, B. and Cudahy, E. (1973). Frequency discrimination in the presence of another tone. *Percept. Psychophys.* 54, 882-887.

Loeb, M. and Holding, D.H. (1975). Backward interference by tones or noise in pitch perception as a function of practice. *Percept. Psychophys.* 18, 205-208.

Massaro, D.W. (1970). Perceptual auditory images. *J. Exp. Psychol.* 77, 411-417.

Massaro, D.W. (1975). Backward recognition masking. *J. Acoust. Soc. Am.* 58, 1059-1065.

Moran, H. and Pratt, C.C. (1926). Variability of judgements on musical intervals. *J. Exp. Psychol.* 9, 492-500.

Pollack, I. (1975). Auditory informational masking. *J. Acoust. Soc. Am.* 57, Suppl. 1, s.5.

Yost, W.A., Berg, K., and Thomas, G.B. (1976). Frequency recognition in temporal interference tasks: A comparison among four psychophysical procedures. *Percept. Psychophys.* 20, 353-359.

THRESHOLD DURATION FOR MELODIC PITCH

Roy D. Patterson, Robert W. Peters and Robert Milroy

MRC Applied Psychology Unit
15 Chaucer Road, Cambridge CB2 2EF

Broadly speaking, the pitch of sinusoidal stimuli becomes indistinct to the point of unusable when the duration of the stimulus is less than five complete cycles. The pitch of the voices of many men and some women is at and even below 100 Hz. At first sight this suggests that it takes more than 50 ms to acquire the pitch of each vowel in the speech of these people. Whereas, in point of fact, listeners can follow changes in the pitch of speech almost on a cycle-to-cycle basis. Of course, the explanation for this apparent paradox is that the pitch of the voice is mediated by the residue pitch mechanism which extracts the low pitch of a sound from its higher harmonics – harmonics that complete 25 or more cycles in 50 ms. This suggested to us that one of the important advantages of the residue pitch mechanism is that it enables the listener to extract the low pitch associated with the fundamental of a sound much faster than would be possible if the information had to be extracted from the fundamental alone. This paper presents our attempt to determine the relative advantage of the residue-pitch mechanism for acquiring low melodic pitch.

Ritsma and Cardozo (1963) reported that no residue pitch is perceived when the stimulus duration is below about four complete cycles. The data of Metters and Williams (1973) indicate a lower limit for three-tone complexes of about three cycles. Pollack (1967) found that his listeners could detect a minimal pitch with two to three cycles of a pulse train. Thus, for residue stimuli with pitches in the region of 100 Hz, these studies suggest a threshold for pitch of 25-40 ms. None of the studies, however, employed a melodic pitch task.

1. MELODIC PITCH THRESHOLD

Since our primary interest was in stimuli that give rise to a definite pitch perception, we chose to use a melodic pitch paradigm rather than a frequency discrimination paradigm. Initially, we assembled a set of ten familiar melodies that had no rhythmic information (e.g. Yankee Doodle) and performed a melody recognition experiment in which the listeners simply matched the melody names to the tunes as they were played. The average note value for each melody (or its mean pitch in Hz) was set to 100 Hz. (There is no ambiguity about the pitch of the residue stimuli used in this experiment, and since the paper is concerned with musical pitch, we have adopted the musical convention and describe the pitch in terms of the frequency, in Hz, of the fundamental of the set of components.) The 16 notes of the melody were played over 6 sec. For residue stimuli with five adjacent harmonics, we found that listeners could identify the individual melodies when the duration of the individual notes was less than 10 ms -- at which point the notes sounded like little more than "ticks" and "tocks". The listeners said that although the notes had no real pitch, they could determine the melody by just listening to the overall contour and comparing the vague impression it conveyed with the contours of the melodies of the set. Dowling (1978) has argued that memory for melodies involves two components; memory for a specific musical scale and memory for a contour presented via that scale. The melody recognition task emphasises the contour aspect of this memory, and de-emphasises the musical scale component. Listeners' ability to use melodic contours in the absence of musical scales has also been demonstrated by Moore and Rosen (1979) who used multi-component residue stimuli, 200 ms in duration. They compressed or expanded the musical scale so that the octave bore a ratio of 1:1.3 or 1:4 instead of 1:2. This preserves the contour of the melody but changes

the scale to a non-standard size. The compression resulted in slightly worse
performance than the expansion but in both cases the listeners were still able to
identify the melodies.

To avoid reliance on contours alone, we have used a random melody task in
which the listener hears a short melody and then identifies which note has
changed when the melody is replayed. To make the task as musical as possible we
(a) chose the notes from the diatonic scale, (b) presented the tonic of the scale
at the start of each trial, and (c) presented all of the notes in a strict
rhythm. A diagram of the sequence of events in each trial appears in Fig. 1.
Following a warning light, the listener was presented with what can be thought of
as four bars of music, and then a response interval. The basic time interval, or
beat, was 2/3 of a second; each interval had either one or no notes and the note
started at the beginning of the interval independent of its duration. In the
first bar the listener was presented with two beats of the tonic (doh) followed
by two silent beats. The second interval contained a four note melody; each
note was chosen at random from the notes doh, ray, me, fah, soh of the diatonic
scale. The third bar was entirely silent. The fourth bar contained a repeat of
the melody, except that one of the notes (chosen at random) was moved up or down
(at random) by one step on the diatonic scale. In the example, the second note
is moved down from soh to fah. The listeners had a four-button response panel on
which to indicate which note had changed, and threshold was taken to be the
duration that supported 62.5% correct identification in this four-alternative,
forced-choice task. We used four-note melodies as it is a common bar length and
minimises the short-term memory load. We have, then, defined melodic pitch
threshold as the stimulus duration required to know which member of a four-note
melody has been changed by one note on the second presentation of the melody.

2. GENERAL METHOD

The melody was played using either a sinusoidal stimulus or a multi-harmonic
stimulus that produced a low residue pitch. The fundamental of the harmonic
series determines the note value, that is, the pitch of the note in Hz. The
stimuli were computer generated and the output of the digital-to-analogue
converter was lowpass filtered at 1.5 kHz. For the note me of the scale, the
fundamental was 100 Hz and the sampling rate was 10 kHz. The fundamental was
varied to obtain the other notes by adjusting the sampling rate.

Performance with these residue stimuli was compared with that obtained
using sinusoids; the me of the scale was set to one of four separate frequencies
ranging from 100 to 900 Hz. The stimulus duration was varied from 10 to 80 ms.
The total energy of the stimuli was held constant; thus stimulus power was halved
when stimulus duration was doubled, and the sinusoidal stimuli had n times the
power of each component of a residue stimulus with n components.

The stimuli were presented binaurally over headphones and there was feedback
as to which note had changed at the end of every trial. Blocks of 50 trials
were run with fixed signal type and duration, and all of the durations
associated with one signal type were run before proceeding to another signal
type. The basic measure was the percent correct in a block of 50 trials. Each
condition was replicated 4-8 days after it was first run. Beyond the first day,
which was given over to practice, there were no obvious learning effects.

There were 4 listeners (HM, EL, RM, WW) ranging in age from 24 to 44 years,
all of whom had normal hearing in the range 0.25 to 8 kHz. All four participated in the second experiment; HM was not in the first experiment. One of the
listeners was author RM. The youngest and oldest listeners had no musical
training; the remaining listeners were amateur musicians. The pattern of
results was the same for all of the listeners, although the musically trained
produced slightly higher scores.

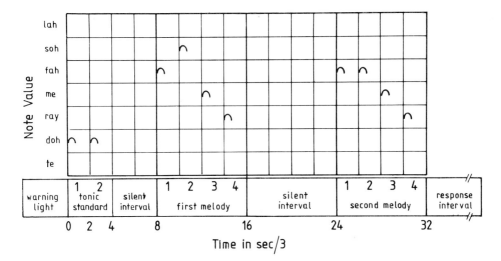

Fig. 1. *Trial Sequence for the Melodic Pitch Experiment: The strip at the bottom shows the order and timing of events in a trial. The time unit is 0.66 sec. The upper portion shows the possible note values and a typical trial*

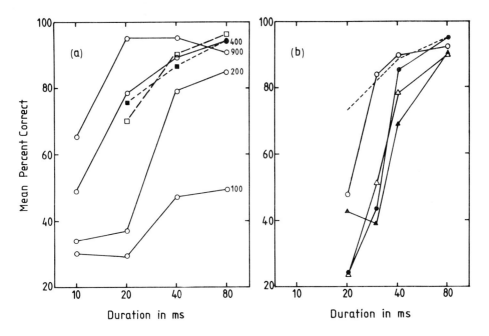

Fig. 2. *Performance versus duration in two melodic pitch experiments: a) Residue stimuli with five harmonics (squares) versus sinusoidal stimuli (circles) with frequencies of 100, 200, 400 or 900 Hz, b) Residue stimuli presented in a notched noise; circles and triangles for split-cosine and complete-cosine on/off ramps, filled and open symbols for ramps starting on or between waveform peaks*

3. EXPERIMENT I

a) *Specific Methodological Details*

In this experiment the residue stimulus was a set of five adjacent harmonics, either harmonics 2-6 or harmonics 7-11. The individual components were presented at about 50 dB SPL. Both the residue and sinusoidal stimuli were gated on and off with 5 ms raised-cosine ramps; the 10 ms stimuli, then, had no steady-state section. The stimuli were presented over a broadband noise, lowpass filtered at 2.0 kHz. Its level was set approximately 25 dB below the point where it would mask the stimuli.

b) *Results*

The data from Experiment I are shown in Fig. 2(a) for the sinusoidal and residue stimuli by circles and squares respectively. The circles show that melodic pitch is extracted from high frequency sinusoids much faster than from low frequency sinusoids. If threshold is taken to be the duration that supports 62.5% correct, then it takes about 7 cycles of a sinusoidal stimulus to support melodic pitch - a value that is not much above that required for minimal pitch perception. The two residue producing stimuli (open and filled squares) produce performance which is roughly comparable to that which can be obtained with a 400 Hz sinusoid. The 100 Hz pitch associated with the fundamental is acquired in under 20 ms, whereas that of the 100 Hz sinusoid takes in excess of 80 ms. The low pitch of the residue stimuli is not, however, acquired as quickly as the high pitch associated with a high frequency tone, even though both of the residue stimuli contain high frequency tones. If one could listen separately to the highest component of the lower residue stimulus or the lowest component of the higher residue stimulus, performance should have been better than was achieved with either of these stimuli.

This experiment, then, suggests that low pitch in the region of 100 Hz can be extracted from a set of harmonics about 4 times as fast as from the corresponding low-frequency sinusoid. Furthermore, harmonics 7-11 which are only poorly resolved by the auditory system transmit the musical pitch as well as harmonics 2-6.

4. EXPERIMENT II

In the previous experiment all of the components of the residue stimulus moved together when the note value changed. Thus it is not clear whether the listeners were using temporal or spectral information. Specifically, one might use the edges of the spectrum to perform the task. In the second experiment a residue producing stimulus was masked by a broadband noise that had a notch in the region 0.2 to 1.4 kHz. This prevents the listeners from using the edges of the signal spectrum to determine the pitch of the stimulus and forces them to use the central section of the stimulus which is quite flat for brief stimuli.

a) *Specific Methodological Details*

The second experiment employed the same procedure for measuring melodic pitch. The only differences were in the masking noise and the residue-producing stimuli; there were no sinusoidal stimuli in this second experiment.

The residue stimulus was composed of 20 harmonics of a fundamental in the region of 100 Hz, and it was lowpass filtered at 1.5 kHz. All of the components started in cosine phase, so producing a peaked waveform. The gating function was either a split cosine as before, wherein the onset and offset ramps were each 5 ms independent of the stimulus duration, or the gate was a complete cosine wherein the onset and offset ramps were half the duration of the stimulus. In addition, the phase of the gate relative to the signal was varied: in one condition waveform peaks occurred at the beginning and end of the interval; in the other condition the gate began and finished mid-way between two peaks. These two variables, gate shape and gate phase, produce small differences in the resolution of the harmonics in the spectrum of the stimulus when the signal duration is short (under 40 ms). The split-cosine gate starting between peaks

produces the best resolution; at 30 ms the peak-to-valley ratio for components
in the centre of the spectrum is about 20 dB. At 30 ms the remaining gate and
phase combinations all produce approximately the same peak-to-valley ratios
(7 dB). Signal duration was varied from 20 to 80 ms.

The masker was a broadband noise which had a notch in the region 0.2 to 1.4
kHz. Below the lower cutoff the spectrum level of the noise was 48 dB, above
the upper edge the spectrum level was 46 dB; the level of the signal components
fell from 56 to 54 dB across the width of the notch. The floor of the notch was
30 dB down and so the residue stimulus was clearly audible.

b) Results

The psychometric functions for this experiment are shown in Fig. 2(b); the
circles and triangles show the data associated with the split-cosine and
complete-cosine conditions respectively. The filled and open symbols show conditions in which the gate began on a pulse or mid-way between two pulses,
respectively. In every case, melodic pitch is acquired from these harmonic
stimuli in under 40 ms, less than half the time taken to acquire the corresponding low pitch from a sinusoid. And when the gate is a split cosine and begins
midway between two pulses, performance is as good as it would be in the absence
of the notched-noise masker, down to a duration of 30 ms. Thus, low melodic
pitch can be extracted from this type of stimulus even when the listener cannot
make use of the edges of the signal spectrum.

The spectra of the residue stimuli are very flat when the duration is 20 ms
and in this condition performance is above chance (25%) for several of the
stimuli. This may indicate that timing information can be used to extract
melodic pitch. However, by the time performance rises convincingly above chance
at 30 ms, the stimuli already show peak-to-valley ratios around the harmonics of
6 or more dB and so we cannot rule out the possibility that spectral cues are
used to derive the low melodic pitch.

*Acknowledgement. The authors are grateful to D.M. Green for setting out the
effects of cosine gates on short-term power spectra, and to B.C.J. Moore for
comments on an earlier version of the paper.*

REFERENCES

Dowling, W.J. (1978). Scale and Contour: two components of a theory of memory
    for melodies. *Psychological Review* 85, 341-354.

Metters, P.J. and Williams, R.P. (1973). Experiments on tonal residues of
    short duration. *Journal of Sound and Vibration* 26, 432-436.

Moore, B.C.J. and Rosen, S.M. (1979). Tune recognition with reduced pitch and
    interval information. *Quarterly Journal of Experimental Psychology* 31,
    229-240.

Pollack, I. (1967). Number of pulses required for minimal pitch. *Journal of
    the Acoustical Society of America* 42, 895.

Ritsma, R.J. and Cardozo, B.L. (1963). The perception of pitch. *Philips
    Technical Review* 25, 37-43.

GENERAL DISCUSSION

PICK:
There might be some interesting findings to be made from examining the fine detail of response. Three possibilities occur to me: 1) By using notes selected from an eight-tone scale, some of your intra-trial note changes will be semitone changes, and some whole-note changes. Are the whole-note changes more likely to be detected? 2) In order to make use of all available information, subjects might be using relative interval information, as well as pitch information. Then, one might expect a higher probability of a correct response for the second and third notes of the melody, where two intervals are available to provide useful information.
3) If interval information is being used, one might obtain more errors displaced by just a single tone, than otherwise expected.

PATTERSON:
1) We have not examined the fine details of the responses, but I expect that you are correct in your postulate that errors on whole-tone changes are less likely. Since natural music employes a mix of whole- and half-tone changes, we thought it best to include both. We did not want to use a chromatic scale, as it implies that 12-tone music is equivalent to diatonic music and this is clearly not the case. 2) and 3) Indeed, the listeners might have been using interval information, and the distribution of half-tone errors across response positions may be non-uniform - although I doubt it would have the simple pattern implied by this pair of questions. The important point, however, is that the design of the experiment means that these cognitive factors are unlikely to have affected the pattern of results and the demonstration that the residue mechanism extracts a low pitch much faster than the equivalent sinusoidal processor.

DE BOER:
1) One should try to avoid imprinting of pitches on memory. Hence: why didn't you vary the tonic (doh) from trial to trial? 2) I noticed that the performance for a single 100-Hz component is very poor at 80 ms duration (Fig. 2a of the paper). At what duration does it become normal?

PATTERSON:
1) We wanted to keep the task as much like music as possible, and simple music does not change tonic every few seconds. However, I agree that the results might have had somewhat greater generalisability if we had changed the tonic every 10 or 20 trials. I do not feel it would have affected the pattern of results, however. 2) Performance with the 100-Hz sinusoid was normal at 160 ms; unfortunately we did not gather data between 80 and 160 ms. I also feel that the procedure of using 50-trial blocks may have produced a slightly pessimistic estimate of performance for the 100-Hz tone at 80 ms. An adaptive procedure might have shown performance as high as threshold (62.5%) at 80 ms.

TYLER:
What would happen to performance if the 100-Hz component were added to the other harmonics, particularly for the longer durations? I'm wondering what importance it has in natural speech.

PATTERSON:
In all probability the addition of the 100-Hz component to our 5-component residue stimuli would not have changed the results, as it would have been quite close to the listeners' absolute threshold. With respect to natural speech, the fundamental is often weak in vowels. Thus, when a speaker with a low-pitched voice speaks at a moderate level, the fundamental will often be at, or below, absolute threshold. In our experiments we omitted the fundamental to ensure that our harmonic stimuli were processed by the residue pitch mechanism.

PITCH OF SINUSOIDS AND COMPLEX TONES ABOVE 10 kHz

Edward M. Burns

Purdue University, W. Lafayette, IN 47907, USA

Lawrence L. Feth

University of Kansas, Lawrence, KS 66045, USA

1. INTRODUCTION

Pitch, although seemingly straightforward in its everyday usage, is quite difficult to define precisely. For example, the ANSI (1960) definition of pitch, "...that attribute of auditory sensation in terms of which sounds may be ordered on a scale extending from high to low," requires only ordinal proper- ties. Certain aspects of timbre (e.g. "sharp-dull") also comply with this def- inition. This possible pitch-timbre confusion is also inherent in operational definitions of pitch based on "pitch-matching" or forced-choice frequency-dis- crimination procedures. The aspect of pitch which would seem to uniquely de- fine it, and which is most closely related to its everyday usage, is the aspect known variously as "tonality," "chroma," and "musical pitch," i.e. that aspect which carries melodic information. This aspect involves the ability of obser- vers to utilize precise frequency-ratio information. It is manifest in the ability of musically-naive observers to recognize familiar melodies, and in the ability of musically-trained observers to produce and recognize specific musi- cal intervals (frequency ratios).

This apparent dichotomy between "musical pitch" and "ordinal pitch" has been linked to the tonotopic-temporal duality of neural encoding of frequency information. It has been suggested (e.g. Schouten, 1970; Attneave and Olson, 1971; Moore, 1977) that musical pitch is coded by temporal information and "or- dinal pitch" by tonotopic information. The primary evidence for this view is the apparent loss of musical pitch for pure tones above about 5 kHz (e.g. Ward, 1954; Attneave and Olson, 1971). A correlate of this viewpoint is that frequen- cy discrimination above 5 kHz is based on tonotopic information (Moore, 1977). However, it is not clear from these limited data whether there is a complete absence of, or merely a degradation of, musical pitch information at high fre- quencies. For example, Ward's (1954) study indicated that the upper limit for the ability to adjust "octave above" was highly dependent on the observer's familiarity with high-frequency sinusoids. The Attneave and Olson results seem to indicate a large increase of variability, rather than a complete loss of mus- ical pitch information, above 5 kHz. Furthermore, Goldstein and Srulovicz (1977) have recently demonstrated that there is sufficient temporal information in eighth-nerve firing patterns to explain psychophysical frequency DL's at high frequencies. It is not necessary, therefore, to postulate that a separate (tonotopic) mechanism mediates discrimination above 5 kHz. In light of these results we have studied musical-pitch perception for pure-tone frequencies above 10 kHz using three paradigms: open-set recognition of familiar melodies by naive observers, and musical interval adjustment and melodic dictation by musically-trained observers.

Another pitch phenomenon which is relevant to the temporal-tonotopic coding question is the pitch associated with rapid frequency modulation. One example is the apparent pitch differences associated with relative amplitude differ- ences between the two components of unresolved two-component complex tones (Helmholtz, 1862; Feth, 1974; Feth *et al.*, 1982). The long term spectra of these stimuli are, of course, exceedingly simple and the pitch differences can be best explained in terms of a weighted average of instantaneous frequency (WAIF) model. Since this type of model is more compatible with temporal encod-

ing of pitch information than with tonotopic encoding (Stover and Feth, 1983),
we have also made a preliminary study of the pitch associated with the unresolved two-component complex tones for frequencies above 10 kHz.

2. MUSICAL PITCH OF HIGH-FREQUENCY PURE TONES

The three paradigms used to investigate musical pitch perception above 10
kHz are similar to those used previously to investigate the pitch of SAM noise
(Burns and Viemeister, 1981) and are described more completely in that publication. For these experiments the stimuli were pure tones generated by a pro-
grammable frequency synthesizer, high-pass filtered at 8 kHz and presented monaurally to the left ear via Audio-Technica ATH-7 headphones. These headphones
showed a virtually flat ($\pm$2 dB) response from 8 kHz to 20 kHz on a flat plate
coupler. In real and artificial (KEMAR) ears there were, of course, substantial resonances and no attempt was made to correct for these resonances. A
lowpass (8 kHz) noise at 40 dB SL was presented along with the high frequency
tones. The tones were presented at a level which corresponded to 70 dB SPL as
measured in the flat-plate coupler.

a) Experiment 1: Open-Set Melody Recognition. Observers with no previous listening experience were asked to identify melodies from a set of twelve melodies. The twelve melodies comprising the set were composed of the first four
bars of familiar melodies (e.g. children's songs, Christmas carols, etc.) modified where necessary so that each was composed of 16 quarter notes (300 msec
tone plus 200 msec silent interval). The melodies were chosen such that the
range of notes in each melody did not exceed a major sixth and were presented
such that the lowest note in each melody had a frequency of 10 kHz. Prior to
beginning the experiment, observers were tested to insure that they could hear
all of the tones contained in the melodies at the 70 dB SPL presentation level.
After the observers completed identification of the 10-kHz melodies, the set
was repeated with a lowest-note frequency of 1 kHz to determine the observer's
actual set size. No prior information on the melody set was provided other
than that "the tunes should be easily recognizable if played with real tones."
A total of fourteen observers participated. The average number of melodies
identified at 10 kHz was 2.9 and the average number identified at 1 kHz was 8.3.
The averages are somewhat misleading in that there was a large disparity among
subjects in their ability to identify the 10 kHz melodies. For example, three
subjects identified 10, 9 and 8 melodies respectively, while four other subjects
were unable to identify any. Although factors other than exact interval information, e.g. contour, do come into play in melody perception, interval information is critically important for recognition of familiar melodies (Dowling,
1982). Therefore we can conclude that at least some of the observers are obtaining substantial musical-pitch information from the high-frequency tones.

b) Experiment 2: Melodic Dictation. This experiment and the following experiment were performed by three musically-trained observers. Two of these observers had participated in other pitch-perception experiments in our laboratory,
some of which involved pure-tone stimuli, but none had been exposed to pure-tone
frequencies above 4 kHz. The observers were presented with four-note melodies
where the notes were defined by pure-tone frequencies relative to a nominal
reference frequency (tonic) of 10 kHz. The actual reference frequency was randomized over a range of $\pm$ 1 semitone to prevent the subjects from using anomalous
intensity differences in one or more of the notes as perceptual anchors. The
upper frequency for which the subjects could detect a tone at 70 dB SPL was determined for each subject and ranged from 17.1 kHz to 18.8 kHz. Therefore, the
range of melodies was limited to a musical fifth (maximum frequency of about
16 kHz). The observers were told that the melodies were in the key of C major
and were told the first note of the melody. Each of the subsequent three notes
was chosen at random from the five possibilities. The observers were given the
opportunity to listen to each melody three times (a trial) and were asked to
write the melody in musical notation on staff paper. All of the observers were

able to perform this task, essentially without error, when the nominal reference frequency was 1 kHz.

The results of the melodic dictation are presented in Figure 1 in a format

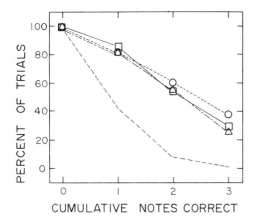

Fig. 1. Percentage of trials for which cumulative number of notes indicated on abscissa were identified correctly. The data for observers 01, 02, and 03 are denoted by circles, triangles, and squares, respectively. Dashed line without data points denotes chance performance assuming intervals identified independently

used by Houtsma (1983) in a similar melodic dictation experiment which assessed the ratio properties of various stimuli. The symbols (connected for clarity) show the proportion of trials for "all three notes correct," "at least two notes correct," and "at least one note correct" for each subject based on 100 trials. The dashed line without symbols represents chance performance under the assumption that each interval judgment is independent. Perfect performance would plot as a horizontal line at 100 percent. It is seen that the performance of all three observers is well above chance and virtually identical. However performance is clearly much poorer than for low frequency stimuli where performance is essentially perfect. As pointed out by Houtsma, observers could theoretically utilize ordinal information, in which case interval judgments would not be independent and chance performance would be higher than shown in Figure 1. For example, if the first note were given as E and the observer noted that the second note was higher, chance identification of the second note would be one in two, rather than one in five. However, trials which started on C (in which case the second note could only be the same or higher) were analyzed separately and performance was found to be virtually identical, implying that ordinal information is playing a relatively small role. Another way of analyzing the results is to assume that the less than perfect performance is basically the result of an ambiguity (or variability) in the pitch of individual notes. Since the observers know that the melody is in a major key, they would be as likely to make wholetone as semit errors. An analysis of the total number of notes correct, and the degree of error of incorrect notes, shows that, for observers 01, 02, and 03: the total percentage of notes correct (over 100 trials) was 60, 54, and 57, respectively; the percentage of notes with either a semit or a wholetone error was 33, 29, and 35 percent, respectively; and therefore the total percentage of notes correct within a wholetone was 93, 83, and 92 percent, respectively. These results imply that all three observers are obtaining musical pitch information from the high-frequency melodies, but that this information is significantly degraded relative to low frequencies.

c) Musical Interval Adjustment. The same three observers who participated in the melodic dictation experiment also participated in this experiment. A standard method of adjustment paradigm was employed. The observers were presented with sequences of tone pairs, a reference tone and a variable tone, and asked to adjust the frequency of the variable tone until it formed a specific musical interval relative to the reference tone. The durations of the tones were 500 msec, the tones within a pair were separated by 500 msec and 1 sec intervened between stimulus pairs. The observer was given unlimited time to perform an ad-

justment. The frequency of the reference tone was varied randomly over a range
of ± 1 semit around a nominal value between runs. The tones were presented monaurally in the left ear except for Observer 1, who performed adjustments in both
ears.

Table I. *Means and standard deviations (in cents) of musical interval adjust-*
ments of three observers at nominal reference frequencies of 1 kHz and 10 kHz.
Average SD's do not include unison adjustments. All data for left ear except
where indicated for Observer 1.

Interval	1 kHz			10 kHz			
	01	02	03	01	01(RE)	02	03
Fifth	702.5	717.4	693.3	691.9	698.8	800.2	709.3
	(16.3)	(7.7)	(43.6)	(59.3)	(57.7)	(87.9)	(68.4)
Tritone	599.7	652.3	623.0	643.4	644.9	720.7	663.2
	(29.0)	(20.0)	(20.9)	(26.3)	(37.4)	(88.1)	(127.2)
Fourth	509.6	541.3	503.8	519.7	507.9	537.4	504.6
	(14.1)	(13.7)	(23.6)	(119.6)	(107.9)	(98.9)	(131.8)
Major third	406.1	411.0	400.7	417.2	400.9	443.5	399.6
	(23.6)	(17.4)	(23.5)	(77.8)	(71.1)	(87.4)	(69.9)
Minor third	321.3	312.7	299.3	361.2	348.8	361.5	289.3
	(19.4)	(17.2)	(19.0)	(66.9)	(90.9)	(62.6)	(75.7)
Major second			185.3				225.9
			(11.0)				(58.8)
Minor second			97.6				174.6
			(18.3)				(40.6)
Unison	1.6	0.7	2.7	29.1	30.5	6.0	29.9
	(1.9)	(1.0)	(4.5)	(26.0)	(43.4)	(8.5)	(23.2)
Avg. SD	(20.5)	(15.2)	(22.8)	(70.0)	(73.0)	(83.8)	(81.8)

The results, in cents re reference frequency, for reference frequencies of
1 kHz and 10 kHz are shown in Table I. The numbers in the columns represent the
means and standard deviations for adjustments by three observers and are based
on at least 10 adjustments for the 1-kHz reference-frequency and at least 20 adjustments for the 10-kHz reference-frequency conditions. At the bottom of each
column are given the average standard deviations (SD's) over all intervals with
the exception of unison. The SD's for unison give an estimate of frequency DL's
at those reference frequencies; however, the possibility exists that intensity
differences may be influencing the results at 10 kHz either as cues in themselves, or by inducing pitch shifts. The average SD's for interval adjustments
are on the order of 3.5 to 5.5 times larger at 10 kHZ than at 1 kHz, but this
is less of an increase in variability than is seen in the SD's for unison adjustments. The standard (equal-tempered) values of the intervals in Table I are
100 through 700 cents for the intervals minor second through fifth. However,
individual subjects in interval adjustment experiments often show consistent
variations from these values. In particular, most subjects show a significant
"stretch" of the wider intervals at frequencies above 1 kHz (Ward, 1954). The
average values of interval adjustments at 10 kHz in this experiment are, given
the variability, well within the expected range in most cases. Only one observer (02), however, shows the amount of subjective stretch of the scale which
would be expected from extrapolation of "octave stretch" data at lower frequencies (Ward, 1954). The results of this experiment imply that these observers are able to obtain ratio information from pure tones with frequencies
above 10 kHz, but that this information is degraded by a factor of about 5
relative to ratio information at low frequencies.

3. PITCH OF UNRESOLVED TWO-COMPONENT COMPLEX TONES

Feth (1974) has shown that under certain conditions observers are able to discriminate between complementary unresolved two-component complex (UTCC) pairs. A UTCC signal is composed of two sinusoidal components separated in frequency by a small Δf and in amplitude by a small ΔI. The complement of a given UTCC is a signal with the same component frequencies but opposite amplitude ratio. If observers are required to discriminate UTCC complementary pairs with a fixed ΔI, and with Δf variable, psychometric functions obtain in which discrimination performance increases with increasing Δf, reaches a plateau of 100% discrimination for a range of Δf's, and then decreases again with increasing Δf as the two tones become resolved. The initial portion of the psychometric function can be fairly well predicted from the WAIF model which assumes that observers are basing their discrimination on pitch differences (Feth *et al.*, 1982). The breakpoint, or threshold of discrimination, at larger Δf's provides estimates of the auditory critical bandwidth (Feth and O'Malley, 1977).

We have obtained preliminary data for two observers on the discrimination of UTCC complementary pairs in the region of 10 kHz along with estimates of pure-tone frequency DL's in the region of 10 kHz. Pure-tone frequency DL's were estimated from the P(C) = 75% point of the psychometric functions obtained using a 2AFC discrimination procedure. The standard frequency was randomized across runs over a range of ±1% around 10 kHz to minimize possible intensity cues associated with different comparison frequencies. Psychometric functions for discrimination of complementary UTCC pairs with an intensity difference of 3 dB were obtained as a function of component separation, Δf, with a 2AFC procedure, and DL's estimated from the P(C) = 75% points. The frequency of the lower component of the UTCC complex was randomized over a range of ±5% around 10 kHz. The psychometric functions for increasing Δf showed the same form as those obtained at lower frequencies, i.e. performance increasing with increasing Δf, plateauing, then decreasing again at large Δf's. The DL's for pure-tones (DLF) and for UTCC component separation (DLDF) are given in Table II for the two observers. Also given is the equivalent pure tone DL (EDLF). This was obtained by transforming the Δf values in the UTCC discrimination psychometric functions to equivalent pure tone frequency differences using the WAIF model and estimating the equivalent frequency difference for P(C) = 75%. It is clear from Table II that the accuracy with which the two observers are able to discriminate complementary UTCC signals in the region of 10 kHz is consistent with their accuracy in discriminating pure tone frequency differences in this region (the WAIF model also predicts somewhat smaller EDLF's at lower frequencies). The extremely small pure-tone DL's for Observer 02 are also consistent with his small SD's for unison adjustments at 1 kHz and at 10 kHz (.05% and 0.5% respectively) obtained in experiment 3 in the previous section.

Table II. Difference limen (in Hz) for pure tones (DLF) and for component separation of UTCC tones (DLDF) in the region of 10 kHz. Also shown is the equivalent pure-tone difference limen derived from the WAIF model (see text).

Observer	DLF	DLDF	EDLF
02	33	68	25
04	115	220	80

4. CONCLUSIONS

We have investigated two pitch phenomena which are commonly assumed to be coded by temporal information: musical pitch and the pitch of UTCC tones. The results of our experiments on the musical pitch of pure tones at frequencies above 10 kHz imply that observers are able to obtain musical pitch information at these frequencies but that it is significantly degraded relative to musical pitch information at low frequencies. However, the degree of degradation of musical pitch at high frequencies does not appear to be any greater than the loss of pure tone frequency information as revealed by the increase of pure tone frequency DL's at high frequencies. Similarly, our preliminary results on the discrimination of complementary UTCC tones at 10 kHz indicate that discrimination performance is degraded to the same extent as pure-tone frequency-discrimination performance. Goldstein and Srulovicz (1977) have recently shown that the fall-off of frequency discrimination acuity at high frequencies is well predicted by a model based on the use of temporal information from eighth-nerve firing patterns. Our results are thus not incompatible with a temporal basis for all three phenomena.

Acknowledgement. This research was supported by a grant from NINCDS.

REFERENCES

American National Standards Institute (1960). *USA Standard Acoustic Terminology*. S1.1-1960.

Attneave, F. and Olson, R.K. (1971). Pitch as a medium: A new approach to psychophysical scaling. *Am. J. Psychol.* 84, 147-166.

Burns, E.M. and Viemeister, N.F. (1981). Played-again SAM: Further observations on the pitch of amplitude-modulated noise. *J. Acoust. Soc. Am.* 70, 1655-1660.

Dowling, W.J. (1982). Melodic information processing and its development. In: *The Psychology of Music*. (D. Deutsch, ed). pp 413-429. New York, Academic Press.

Feth, L.L. (1974). Frequency discrimination of complex periodic tones. *Percept. & Psychophys.* 15, 375-378.

Feth, L.L. and O'Malley, H. (1977). Two-tone auditory spectral resolution. *J. Acoust. Soc. Am.* 62, 940-947.

Feth, L.L., O'Malley, H. and Ramsey, Jw. (1982). Pitch of unresolved, two-component complex tones. *J. Acoust. Soc. Am.* 72, 1403-1412.

Goldstein, J.L. and Srulovicz, P. (1977). Auditory-nerve spike intervals as an adequate basis for aural frequency measurement. In: *Psychophysics and Physiology of Hearing*. (E.F. Evans and J.P. Wilson, eds). pp 337-346. London, Academic Press.

Helmholtz, H.L.F. (1862). *On the Sensations of Tones*. New York, Dover (2nd English Edition, 1954).

Houtsma, A.J.M. (1983). Pitch salience of various complex sounds. *Music Perception* (in press).

Moore, B.C.J. (1977). *An Introduction to the Psychology of Hearing*. London, Academic Press.

Schouten, J.F. (1970). The residue revisited. In: *Frequency Analysis and Periodicity Detection in Hearing*. (R. Plomp and G. Smoorenburg, eds). pp 41-53. Leiden, A.W. Sijhoff.

Stover, L. and Feth, L.L. (1983). Pitch of narrow band signals. *J. Acoust. Soc. Am.* (in press).

Ward, W.D. (1954). Subjective musical pitch. *J. Acoust. Soc. Am.* 26, 369-380.

GENERAL DISCUSSION

EVANS:
There are two ways in which it has been suggested that neural temporal information could be used in mediating the pitch of the residue (for example). The first is the more obvious coding of the pitch in the preferred intervals in fibres whose CFs correspond to the dominant frequency region. The second is the attractive notion of Goldstein and Srulowicz (1977, see Burns and Feth, this volume) that the place information required for pattern recognition 'place' models, is conveyed by the temporal pattern of discharges in the fibres (rather than by their mean rate). Which mode of use of the temporal information do you have in mind?

BURNS:
The second, but for pure-tone pitch perception there is no essential difference.

TERHARDT:
In spite of increased JND's at high frequencies, one can hardly doubt that psychophysical pitch as such is perceived well even beyond 10 kHz. I am thus inclined to
believe that limitation of melody recognition performance in that frequency region
is essentially caused by reduced ability to recognize and process pitch relationships (such as musical intervals). This would mean that it is "central processes"
rather than pitch formation from the stimulus (by what mechanism soever) which determine performance on subjects.

BURNS:
Given the facility of musicians in transposing frequency-ratio information at
"musically normal" frequencies, we would like to assume that their relative in-
ability to obtain this information at very high frequencies is the result of the
lack of the relevant cues at the peripheral level. However, the possibility that
this reflects a deficit at a more central level (e.g. in their "ratio processor"),
as you suggest, certainly exists.

NEURONAL MECHANISMS FOR A PERIODICITY ANALYSIS IN THE TIME DOMAIN

G. Langner

Institut für Zoologie, Technische Hochschule Darmstadt
D-6100 Darmstadt, Germany

1. INTRODUCTION

Periodic acoustic signals are vital components in most biological communication systems, e.g. vowels and voiced consonants in human speech. The main reason may be that these signals are easily produced by various types of acoustic sources. Such periodic signals are composed of harmonics, i.e. the frequencies are multiples of the fundamental frequency.

The first step of processing in the auditory system, at least of mammals and birds, is the peripheral frequency analysis in the cochlea which is comparable to a filter bank analysis. For a periodic signal the output of each activated frequency channel is either a single harmonic, or - due to the limited resolving power of the cochlea - a superposition of several harmonics. The periods of the channel outputs including the periods of the output envelopes are equal to the fundamental period whenever two or more adjacent harmonics are processed in the same frequency channel. Otherwise multiples of the periods correspond to the fundamental period. In a normal acoustic environment this periodicity information may be necessary for an orderly combination of the channel outputs.

There are many evidences that periodicity information is coded in the auditory nerve (Wever, 1949) and that the nervous system makes use of a periodicity analysis in the time domain (Rutherford, 1886, Schouten, 1940a, 1970). A delay line or a neuronal clock were considered as possible mechanisms for such an analysis (Whitfield, 1970). The data presented in this paper suggest a correlation analysis of the second type, with phase coupled oscillations as a time reference.

2. PERIODICITY CODING IN THE MIDBRAIN OF THE GUINEA FOWL

Neuronal coding of periodicity was studied in 420 single units in the auditory midbrain nucleus MLD of the Guinea fowl. Amplitude modulated sine waves (AM) were used as simple models for signals with periodic envelopes. The level of the signals was normally kept to 65 dB SPL. About 20 % of the analysed units showed preferences for AM with certain combinations of the modulation frequency f_m and the carrier frequency f_c (Langner, 1978). In the range of these preferred frequencies an empirical equation describes the variation of the optimal modulation period τ_m with the carrier period τ_c:

$$m \cdot \tau_m + n \cdot \tau_c = 1 \cdot \tau_1,$$

where each m, n and 1 stands for some small integers typical for a given unit. The responses of the investigated units may be interpreted with $\tau_1 = 0.4$ ms as a time constant. In consequence the periodicity equation was interpreted as a coincidence condition of neuronal activity phase coupled to the modulation frequency, i.e. to the signal envelope, and to the carrier frequency including clock type delay mechanisms.

Fig. 1 is a point plot presentation (every point stands for one spike) of the responses of unit N 93 to 50 repetitions of AM with constant f_c. On the y-axis f_m was stepped from 100 Hz to 1000 Hz with equal steps of the period τ_m. The signals were presented from -5 to +55 ms of the given time axis with ramps of 5 ms at the beginning and at the end. However, the periodic modulations started at time zero and stopped at 50 ms of the scale. The amplitude fluctuations at the beginning but also every zero crossing of the envelope triggered in this unit oscillatory responses with intervals of 0.8 - 0.9 ms (about $2 \cdot 0.4$ ms). For f_m being 800 Hz

N 93, AM:

$f_C = 2.8\,kHz, \; f_m = 100 - 1000\,Hz$

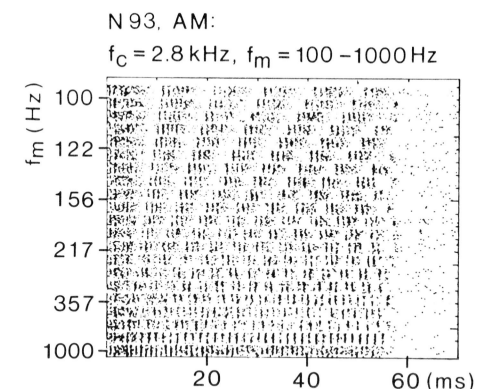

Fig. 1. _Intrinsic oscillations triggered by amplitude fluctuations (from Langner, 1983)_

these oscillations changed into coupled oscillations with one spike per envelope cycle. Note that f_m is not a spectral component of the AM-signal. Thus the oscillations could only be triggered by amplitude fluctuations, which are as discussed above a consequence of the limited resolving power of the frequency channel in the range of f_c.

3. COINCIDENCE EFFECTS

When a unit is stimulated with AM, the optimal f_m is defined by coincidence of phase coupled and oscillatory neuronal activities. An example is demonstrated in fig. 2. The point plots represent the first 30 ms of the responses of unit N 163 to 100 repetitions of AM-signals with two constant f_c's and varying f_m. Several oscillations in response to the onset of the signals are visible. The coincidences of these oscillations (marked by arrows) with the responses to the following modulation cycles resulted in phase shifts indicated by lines. Without the coincidence effects these lines were expected to be straight. As another result of the coincidence the response strength is enhanced for those (optimal) f_m's where periods parallel the intrinsic oscillations.

Note that as a consequence of different f_c's in these two experiments the intrinsic oscillations and the optimal f_m's are different. This effect is described by the periodicity equation. Due to the coincidence in experiments with varying f_c and constant f_m the medium phase delay of the responses shift proportional to certain multiples of τ_c (Langner, 1981). The present model explain these results by an input with intervals corresponding to certain multiples of τ_c (interval multiplier).

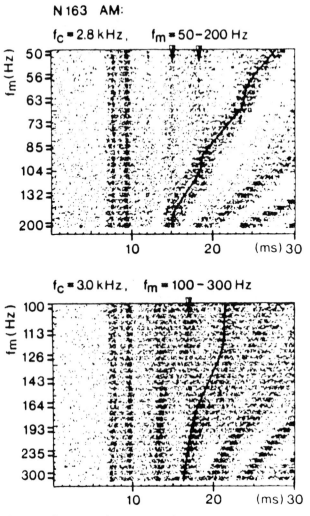

Fig. 2. Phase coupling to AM determined by coincidence effects (from Langner, 1983)

4. A CORRELATION MODEL

A component of a hypothetical neuronal correlation network together with 4 realizations of the periodicity equation is presented in fig. 3. It was taken into account that the optimal periods τ_m are defined by the stimulus periods τ_c of the carriers as well as by the periods of the intrinsic oscillations.

In each of the 4 cases in fig. 3 τ_m is identical and τ_c is different. It is assumed that the interval multiplier sums up 6 periods of the carrier and that the period of the intrinsic oscillations is $2 \cdot \tau_1 = 0.8$ ms, resp. $4 \cdot \tau_1 = 1.6$ ms. If both, the oscillations and the multiplied τ_c-intervals are synchronized by the zero crossings of the envelope, the periodicity equation is fulfilled in each case with different parameters m, n and l.

The neuronal model at the right side proposes some mechanisms for an oscillator, an interval multiplier and a coincidence unit, which is thought to be located at the recording site in the auditory midbrain. The correlation constant τ_1 is

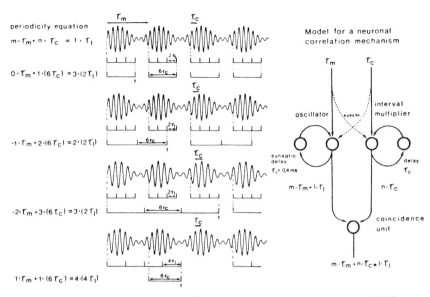

Fig. 3. Mechanisms for a periodicity analysis (from Langner, 1983)

realized by a synaptic delay of 0.4 ms. The illustrated oscillator would produce an oscillation period of $2 \cdot \tau_1$, longer periods would require more units.

In contrast to the oscillator units the two units of the interval multiplier activate each other *below* threshold. Thresholds are reached by additional inputs phase coupled to the carrier. The postulated mechanisms would produce multiples of τ_c depending on the involved time constants and τ_c. The coincidence unit is activated only when the inputs from the oscillator and the multiplier coincide. Because of a synchronizing mechanism (stippled lines) this is the case when the periodicity equation is fulfilled.

5. PITCH OF PERIODIC SIGNALS

To a first approximation the residual pitch of an AM-signal corresponds to a pitch evoked by the modulation frequency alone. This fits in with the hypothesis that the period of the envelope of periodic signals is the relevant parameter for pitch perception. However, Schouten (1940b) observed that pitch varies with the carrier frequency in spite of a constant envelope period. In consequence the idea of the envelope period as pitch parameter was given up and no theory of pitch perception in the time domain could comply with this effect.

The prominent modern pitch theories (Wightman, 1973, Goldstein, 1978, Whitfield 1980, Terhardt et al., 1982) postulate processing of the resolved frequency pattern somewhere in the auditory system. These theories do not contradict the basic concept of the place principle of von Helmholtz (1863), since the pitch of each frequency component may be related to a certain place of activation on the basilar membrane.

If the correlation mechanisms presented in this paper are relevant for pitch perception, they contradict the place principle as well as the theories assuming a pattern recognition in the frequency domain. They correspond partly to the duplex-theory of Licklider (1951) and also to the envelope coding in the residue theory of Schouten (1940a). The main new steps are the indroduction of oscillator and multiplier mechanisms in the correlation analysis.

6. EVIDENCES FOR PITCH PERCEPTION IN THE TIME DOMAIN

Many pitch effects described in the auditory literature may be explained by
a neuronal correlation analysis in the time domain (de Boer, 1956, van den Brink
et al., 1976). It seems, however, that these effects may as well be explained by
a spectral analysis.

The described neuronal correlation mechanisms may be adequate for a pitch
analysis. The variation of the units optimal modulation frequencies with the
carrier frequencies could correspond to the psychophysical effect of pitch shift
with the carrier frequencies observed by Schouten (1940b). The periodicity equation suggests that the period τ_p of a pure tone with the same pitch as the residual
pitch of an AM-signal may be described as a linear function of the carrier period
τ_c:

$$\tau_p = a \cdot \tau_c + b.$$

With this approximation in about 50 % of 60 measured pitch curves the values a
were found to be integers - as expected by the periodicity equation - and the
values b were found to be multiples of 0.4 ms (Langner, 1981). This may also be
expected from the periodicity equation, if one assumes that the synaptic delays in
the auditory systems of the species of man and Guinea fowl are optimized. An additional evidence for the same time constant and hence for the corresponding neuronal mechanisms are steps found in the pitch curves of some persons where the
values of τ_p were multiples of 0.4 ms (see fig. 4).

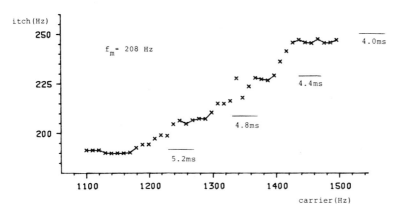

Fig. 4. Steps in a psychophysical measurement of the pitch of AM-signals (from
Langner, 1981)

Acknowledgement. This study was supported by the Deutsche Forschungsgemeinschaft
(SFB 45). I wish to thank Mrs. M. Hansel and Mrs. U. Körner for the preparation
of the figures, Mr. M. Camargo for computer support, Prof. Dr. H. Scheich for
support of experiments.

REFERENCES

Boer, E. de (1956). On the residue in hearing. *Academisch Proefschrift*, Universi-
      teit van Amsterdam.
Brink, G. van den, Sintnicolaas, K., Stam, W.S. van (1976). Dichotic pitch fusion.
      J. Acoust. Soc. Am. 59, 1471-1476.
Goldstein, J.L. (1978). Mechanisms of signal analysis and pattern perception in
      periodicity pitch. *Audiology* 17, 421-445

Helmholtz, H.L.F. von (1863). Die Lehre von den Tonempfindungen als psychologische
    Grundlage für die Theorie der Musik. F. Vieweg + Sohn, Braunschweig.
Langner, G. (1978). The periodicity matrix. A correlation model for central audi-
    tory frequency analysis. *Verh. Dtsch. Zool. Ges.*, p. 194.
Langner, G, (1981). Neuronal mechanisms for pitch analysis in the time domain.
    Exp. Brain Res. 44, 450–454.
Langner, G. (1983). Evidence for neuronal periodicity detection in the auditory
    system of the Guinea fowl: Implications for pitch analysis in the time domain.
    Exp. Brain Res. (in press).
Licklider, J.C.R. (1951). A duplex theory of pitch perception. *Experientia* 7,
    128–134.
Rutherford, W. (1886). A new theory of hearing. *J. Anat. and Physiol.* 21, 166–168.
Schouten, J.F. (1940a). The residue and the mechanism of hearing. *Proc. Kon.*
    Nederl. Akad. Wetensch. 43, 991–999.
Schouten, J.F. (1940b). The perception of pitch. *Philips Techn. Rev.* 5, 286–294.
Schouten, J.F. (1970). The residue revisited.In: *Frequency analysis and periodicity*
    detection in hearing, Eds. R. Plomp and G.F. Smoorenburg, pp. 41–54, Leiden,
    Sijthoff.
Terhardt, E., Stoll, G., Seewann, M. (1982). Pitch of complex signals according to
    virtual pitch theory-tests, examples, and prediction. *J. Acoust. Soc. Am.* 71,
    671–678.
Wever, E.G. (1949). *Theory of hearing*, New York, Wiley.
Whitfield, I.C. (1970). Central nervous processing in relation to spatio-temporal
    discrimination of auditory pattern. In: *Frequency analysis and periodicity*
    detection in hearing, Eds. R. Plomp and G.F. Smoorenburg, pp. 136–147, Leiden,
    Sijthoff.
Whitfield, I.C. (1980). Auditory cortex and the pitch of complex tones. *J. Acoust.*
    Soc. Am. 67, 644–647.
Wightman, F.L. (1973).The pattern transformation model of pitch. *J. Acoust. Soc.*
    Am. 54, 407–416.

GENERAL DISCUSSION

EVANS:
Your model requires two inputs: one, the intervals of which correspond to the
period of the envelope; the other corresponding to the carrier period. At the
cochlear nerve level in the cat, I have not seen this: only fibres with CFs in the
region of the stimulus components, having intervals corresponding to the pitch
heard, including the important "pitch-shift" case where neither the pitch nor the
intervals correspond to the envelope period (Evans, Audiol. 17, 369, 1978). I have
never encountered envelope synchronized periodicities in fibres with CFs corresponding to the envelope frequency, although a report of this effect has appeared
(Boerger and Gruber, in: Plomp and Smoorenburg, Frequency Analysis and Periodicity
Detection in Hearing, Leiden, 1970, p. 148-149). How does your model deal with the
pitch shift case, if the major neural periodicity in its input corresponds only to
the envelope and carrier periods?

LANGNER:
The model does not really require input intervals corresponding to the envelope
period. The only condition is that the oscillator is triggered by the envelope as
indicated in Fig. 1. I also did not observe synchronized responses to the envelope
of units with CFs corresponding to f_m, however, I did observe synchronized responses of those units with CFs corresponding to the carrier frequencies. The pitch
shift effects are explained in my model by the coincidence mechanisms which compare certain multiples of the carrier period not with the modulation period but,
due to oscillations, to the modulation period plus some multiples of 0.4 ms.

DE BOER:

Your Fig. 4 shows effects that differ from what everybody else has found. In what
respect do these experiments differ?

LANGNER:
It is known that the residual pitch is ambiguous as expressed in my pitch equation
by several possibilities for the integer parameters n and 1. However, nobody has
observed before steps in the pitch curves, where 'pitch periods' correspond to a
multiple of 0.4 ms.

NARINS:
Have you found a correlate for the 0.4 ms intrinsic time constant that you describe for the guinea fowl?

LANGNER:
The first time I postulated a synaptic delay of 0.4 ms (Langner, 1978), I was
criticised by several physiologists because they assumed that synaptic delays must
be greater than 0.8 ms. Now I know several reports about synaptic delays of about
0.4 ms in the auditory system of the cat and of the chick (Clark and Dunlop, Exp.
Neurology 20, 31, 1968; Guinan et al., Intern. J. Neurosci. 4, 101, 1972;
Hackett, Neuroscience 7, 1455, 1982).

BIALEK:
Your suggestion that synaptic delay provides a time scale in the extraction of
pitch suggest that the residue phenomenon should be temperature dependent.
Although biological oscillators are sometimes temperature-compensated, typically
this occurs for multi-step, long term cycles such as the circadian rythm; in no
case is the temperature compensation fully understood. For a single synaptic delay,
temperature dependence seems to be unavoidable. I suggest that Prof. Klinke's experiments on perfect pitch at various body temperatures (Emde and Klinke, in:
Inner Ear Biology, Portmann and Aran, Eds., INSERM, Paris, 1977, p. 145) be extended to the residue, and that if significant effects are not observed then the
synaptic-delay theory be discarded.

PICKLES:
If I understand your model correctly, the "oscillator" neurons of Fig. 3 should
fire in a sustained manner at a high rate (1250/sec in that case). Have you seen
such neurons? They should be very obvious because of their extraordinarily high
sustained firing rate.

LANGNER:
The oscillator does not fire in a sustained manner; it is instead triggered by
amplitude fluctuations of the acoustic signals. However, the shortest oscillation
period is 0.8 ms corresponding to an upper limit of about 1250 Hz for envelope
coupled responses.

BURNS:
We are unable to replicate the steplike microstructure of your psychophysical
pitch-shift results using a paradigm similar in all respects except that we changed carrier frequency in a random fashion from trial to trial rather than continuously. Could you explain why you feel that this difference is crucial for obtaining your results?

LANGNER:
This effect of pitch steps could be obtained from some persons in some experiments
with continuous variations of the carrier from low to high frequencies or reverse.
It was, however, never observed using your paradigm changing the carrier frequency
in a random way. I ascribe this effect to the neuronal oscillators envolved in the
pitch analysis. Such entrainments like the magnet effect described by v. Holst
would not be expected for random variations of the stimulus frequencies.

LINDEMANN:
Do you have any physiological hints for the width of the coincidence window of the
coincidence detection units?

LANGNER:
In most coincidence units it was observed that for modulation frequencies below
the optimal frequency the phase coupling improved during 30-50 ms after stimulus
onsets. In contrast, the phase coupling broke down after about 20-30 ms for higher

modulation frequencies. This effect may be explained by the different transients
of the phase delays which indicate that the oscillatory inputs to the coincidence
units scan through coincidence windows with a size of 0.4-0.5 ms. These windows
had constant latencies relative to zero crossings of the envelopes and are attributed to a second synchronized input to the coincidence units.

KIM:
What effects of anaesthesia have you observed in your experiments?

LANGNER:
Effects of anaesthesia were not observed, since all neurophysiological experiments
were performed on awake animals.

Section VI
Speech and Hearing Impairment

AUDITORY-NERVE REPRESENTATION OF VOICE PITCH

M. I. Miller and M. B. Sachs

Department of Biomedical Engineering
Johns Hopkins University School of Medicine
Baltimore, Maryland 21205 USA

INTRODUCTION

In a recent series of papers (Sachs and Young, 1979; Young and Sachs, 1979; Voigt *et al.*, 1983; Sachs *et al.*, 1983; Miller and Sachs, 1983a) we have considered the encoding of vowels and stop consonants in the firing patterns of populations of auditory-nerve fibers. In those papers we have emphasized the encoding of speech features related to vocal tract configuration; e.g., formant frequencies and general spectral shape. In this paper we will emphasize aspects of our experimental results which relate to the encoding of the fundamental frequency of glottal excitation, i.e., voice pitch. The mechanisms underlying the perception of the pitch of complex sounds has long been a focus for auditory physiology and psychoacoustics (see de Boer, 1976 for review). Our discussion here will relate to auditory-nerve correlates of two mechanisms which have received most attention. The present study was done with anesthetized cats (Nembutal).

TEMPORAL REPRESENTATION OF PITCH

Figure 1 shows the particular stimulus we will use as an example and illustrates the stimulus feature underlying the first of these mechanisms. All of the data to be presented here come from auditory-nerve fiber responses to the consonant-vowel syllable /da/, generated by a digital representation of a cascade of tuned circuits (Klatt, 1980). The temporal waveform of this syllable is shown in Fig. 1A. The regularly spaced major peaks which occur about every 8.3 msec during the first 50 msec correspond to the periodic pitch excitation of 120 Hz. During the last 50 msec of the stimulus the pitch frequency decreases linearly from 120 to 116 Hz, so that the interval between major peaks increases slightly. The exponentially decaying impulse response of the resonators modelling the vocal tract is seen between the peaks. During the first 50 msec of the stimulus the first three formant frequencies (resonances) changed

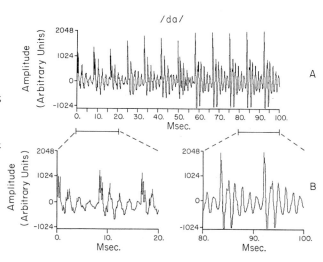

Fig. 1. Waveform of synthesized /da/. (Redrawn from Miller and Sachs, 1983a)

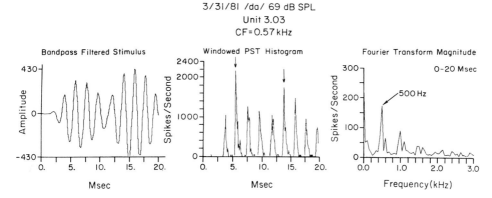

3/31/81 /da/ 69 dB SPL
Unit 3.03
CF=0.57 kHz

Fig. 2. Left: First 20 msec of filtered /da/; filter models basilar membrane tuning at 0.57 kHz. Center: PST histogram of first 20 msec response to /da/ of a fiber with CF equal to 0.57 kHz. Right: Fourier transform of the PST histogram. (Redrawn from Miller and Sachs, 1983a)

linearly from 500, 1580 and 2680 Hz to 700, 1200 and 2400 Hz, respectively.

Figure 1B shows the first and last 20 msec segments of the stimulus on an expanded scale. During the first 20 msec there are four prominent peaks in each 8.3 msec pitch period; these peaks reflect the large energy in the stimulus at 480 Hz which is the harmonic of the 120 Hz fundamental frequency (pitch) nearest to the first formant frequency. During the last 50 msec there are 6 peaks in each pitch period reflecting the 700 Hz first formant during the steady vowel segment. In 1940, Schouten proposed that in determining the pitch of a complex stimulus such as this, the auditory system would measure the intervals between the major pitch-related peaks. Specifically, Schouten (1940) and Plomp (1966) show hypothesized outputs from cochlear filters in response to a multicomponent stimulus (a periodic pulse train). For filters with high enough center frequencies so that a number of stimulus harmonics fall within the filter passband, the filter output has a periodic envelope modulation whose period equals the period of the stimulus fundamental. Figure 2 shows that such envelope modulations are indeed present in the outputs of cochlear filters, i.e., in the discharge patterns of single auditory-nerve fibers. The left panel shows a filtered version of the first 20 msec segment of the stimulus waveform, obtained by filtering the speech waveform with a linear bandpass filter which models basilar membrane tuning (Duifuis, 1973; Goldstein *et al.*, 1971; Siebert, 1968). The center frequency of the filter was chosen to match the characteristic frequency of the fiber illustrated in the figure. This model cochlear filter output demonstrates the pitch periodic envelope modulations discussed by Schouten (1940) and Plomp (1966).

The center panel of Fig. 2 shows a post-stimulus time histogram (PST) of responses of a single fiber whose characteristic frequency was 0.57 kHz. This histogram was computed using only spikes occurring during the first 20 msec of the stimulus (the same interval as depicted in the model output at left). This histogram shows considerable similarity to the filtered stimulus waveform shown at left. Its envelope has peaks separated by intervals equal to the period of the 120 Hz pitch frequency (arrows). The intervals between the more closely spaced peaks are about 2 msec, the reciprocal of the frequency of the first formant during this 20 msec stimulus segment. The Fourier transform of the PST histogram (right panel) shows a peak at 500 Hz and a smaller peak at 600 Hz. Note that the resolution of the Fourier transform based on a 20 msec histogram is 50 Hz; thus 500 Hz is the closest transform frequency to 480 Hz, the fourth harmonic of the pitch. If the data are analyzed with 25 msec histograms (40 Hz

resolution) then the peaks
occur exactly at harmonics
of the pitch (see Miller
and Sachs, 1983b). It is
the combination of these
response components at the
pitch harmonics which leads
to the pitch-related en-
velope modulation in the
PST histogram. Similar envelope modulations have
been demonstrated by
Delgutte (1980).

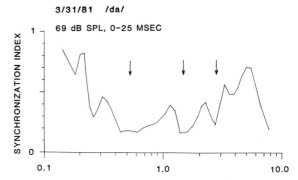

We have previously
shown that such pitch-re-
lated envelope modulations
occur for units with CFs
across the population of
auditory-nerve fibers.

Fig. 3. Synchronization index at 120 Hz plotted versus characteristic frequency. (Redrawn from Miller and Sachs, 1983b)

(Miller and Sachs, 1983b). Exceptions occur, as Delgutte (1980) has shown, for units tuned very close to the first and second formant frequencies or very near the lower harmonics of the pitch. Units which show no envelope modulations are those whose responses are dominated by a single stimulus harmonic (Miller and Sachs, 1983b). Synchronization index (Johnson, 1980) at the pitch frequency provides a good measure of the pitch-related envelope modulation of PST histo-grams (Miller and Sachs, 1983b). Figure 3 shows synchronization index at 120 Hz plotted versus CF for a population of fibers studied on 3/31/81. Synchroniza-tion index was computed from PST histograms for fiber responses over the first 25 msec of the stimulus shown in Fig. 1. Arrows point to the formant frequencies of the stimulus. Synchronization index at 120 Hz, and hence pitch-related en-velope modulation, is relatively large among units with CFs greater than the third formant frequency, near the pitch frequency and between the formant fre-quencies.

For a time varying stimulus such as the consonant-vowel syllable used here, as the formant frequencies change the locations of fibers in the population show-ing envelope modulations will also change (Miller and Sachs, 1983b). As stimulus level increases, the degree of envelope modulation decreases even among fibers with CFs between the formant frequencies (Miller and Sachs, 1983b; Delgutte, 1980). Considerable modulation remains, even at the
highest levels used, for
fibers with CFs above the
third formant. Finally,
Fig. 4 shows that pitch-
related envelope modula-
tions, as reflected in synchronization index at the
pitch frequency, are de-
creased in the presence of
background noise. The
figure shows synchroniza-
tion index at 120 Hz plotted
versus CF for the first 25
msec of /da/ presented alone
(solid line) and in the
presence of broadband noise
(dashed line). Signal-to-
noise ratio (measured in

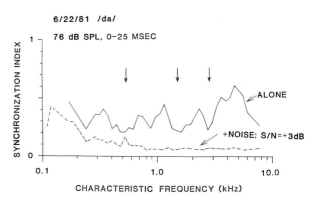

Fig. 4. Synchronization index at 120 Hz plotted versus CF for /da/ presented alone and in background noise. (Redrawn from Miller and Sachs, 1983b)

the 0-3000 Hz band) was +3 dB. Synchronization to 120 Hz is decreased throughout the population, the greatest reductions being in the high frequency region.

SPECTRAL REPRESENTATION OF PITCH: PHASE-LOCKED MEASURES

    Figure 5A shows the stimulus feature which underlies the second pitch mech-
anism to be considered here. The plot shows the spectrum of the first 25 msec of
the /da/ stimulus. The spectrum has a rapidly varying component with peaks at
the harmonics of the pitch frequency (arrows) superimposed on a smooth envelope
which has peaks at the formant frequencies. Goldstein (1973) and others have
suggested that the determination of pitch is based on the harmonic structure of
the spectra of complex stimuli such as that illustrated in Fig. 5A. We have
shown previously that this harmonic structure is maintained in the population of
auditory-nerve fibers (Miller and Sachs, 1983a). The responses of single fibers,
such as the one illustrated in Fig. 2, are dominated by components at harmonics
of the pitch. Fibers with highly envelope-modulated PST histograms will show responses at a number of consecutive pitch harmonics. However, at high stimulus
levels or in noise where pitch-related envelope modulations become small or
disappear, the harmonic structure is lost at the single unit level. In these
situations, each unit's response is usually dominated by a single pitch harmonic. Nonetheless, it is possible to extract pitch from the harmonic structure
of the responses of the population of fibers as follows:
    The responses to any harmonic of the pitch are largest among fibers whose
CFs are close to the fre-
quency of that harmonic.
Thus, as we have previously
argued (Young and Sachs,
1979), it makes sense to
take as a measure of the
population response to any
harmonic the amplitude of
the response to that har-
monic, averaged across
fibers tuned near the harmonic. We therefore de-
fined such a measure (average localized synchronized
rate, ALSR) at any fre-
quency as the average value
of the amplitude of the
Fourier transform component
(synchronized rate, ex-
pressed in spikes/second)
at that frequency; the
average is computed over
all fibers whose CFS are
within ± 0.25 or ± 0.125
octaves of the frequency.
The ALSR reflects both
place and temporal information about the population
response to a frequency:
place because only fibers
tuned near that frequency
are included in the aver-
age; temporal because the
measure averaged is
synchronized rate. Figure
5B shows the ALSR plotted

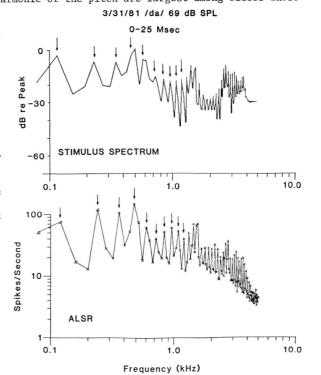

Fig. 5. Top: *Stimulus spectrum for first 25 msec of
/da/. Bottom: Average localized synchronized rate
for population of auditory-nerve fibers. Arrows
point to first 10 harmonics of 120 Hz pitch. (Redrawn from Miller and Sachs, 1983b)*

versus frequency for re-
sponses from a population
of auditory-nerve fibers to
the stimulus whose spectrum
is shown in Fig. 5A. The
similarity between the ALSR
and the stimulus spectrum
is clear. Specifically,
the ALSR shows the peaks at
harmonics of the pitch
(arrows) and troughs be-
tween. We have demonstra-
ted previously (Miller and
Sachs, 1983a) that pitch
can be computed very pre-
cisely from this ALSR
measure. Furthermore, this
spectral representation of
pitch is quite resistant
to changes in stimulus
level or to the addition
of background noise
(Miller and Sachs, 1983b).

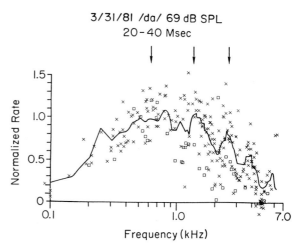

Fig. 6. *Normalized average discharge rate plotted
versus CF. Solid line is average of data points. Xs
show units with spontaneous rate greater than 1/sec;
open squares are units with lower spontaneous rates.
(Redrawn from Miller and Sachs, 1983a)*

SPECTRAL REPRESENTATION OF PITCH: AVERAGE RATE MEASURE

The ALSR measure is, as we have pointed out, a temporal-place measure. One
could take as a response measure of the fibers of the population average discharge
rate, which discards the temporal or phase-locked information in the unit responses. We have discussed the properties of rate-place representations of formant structure in great detail elsewhere (Sachs and Young, 1979; Miller and Sachs,
1983a). Figure 6 shows normalized discharge rate (defined as discharge rate minus
spontaneous rate, divided by saturation rate minus spontaneous rate, Sachs and
Young, 1979) plotted versus characteristic frequency for units of a population
studied with /da/ as the stimulus. These rates were computed over the interval
20 to 40 msec after stimulus onset. The solid curve is a weighted average of the
data points. Although there are peaks in this average rate profile in the vicinity of the formant frequencies (arrows), there is no indication of any harmonic
structure from which pitch could be extracted.

SUMMARY

Pitch of consonants and vowels can be represented as envelope modulations
of PST histograms of single fibers. However, such modulations decrease with increasing stimulus levels and virtually disappear in background noise. On the
other hand, pitch can also be represented spectrally across the population of
fibers in terms of phase-locked responses which are dominated by harmonics of
the pitch. Such a spectral representation is robust with regard to level
changes and background noise. Finally, we have not found a good representation
of pitch in terms of average discharge rate.

*Acknowledgement. This work was supported by a grant from the National Institute
of Neurological and Communicative Disorders and Stroke. Michael I. Miller is a
trainee of the Institute of General Medical Sciences.*

REFERENCES

Delgutte, B. (1980). Representation of speech-like sounds in the discharge patterns of auditory-nerve fibers. *J. Acoust. Soc. Am.* 68, 843-857.

de Boer, E. (1976). On the "residue" and auditory pitch perception. In: *Handbook of Sensory Physiology, Vol. V: Auditory System, part 3: Clinical and Special Topics* (W. D. Keidel and W. D. Neff, eds), New York, Springer-Verlag.

Duifhuis, H. (1973). Consequences of peripheral frequency selectivity for non-simultaneous masking. *J. Acoust. Soc. Am.* 54, 1471-1485.

Goldstein, J. L. (1973). An optimum processor theory for the central formation of the pitch of complex tones. *J. Acoust. Soc. Am.* 54, 1496-1516.

Goldstein, J. L., Baer, T. and Kiang, N. Y. S. (1971). A theoretical treatment of latency, group delay and tuning characteristics for auditory-nerve responses to clicks and tones. In: *Physiology of the Auditory System* (M. B. Sachs, ed), pp. 133-142, Baltimore, National Educational Consultants.

Johnson, D. H. (1980). The relationship between spike rate and synchrony in responses of auditory-nerve fibers to single tones. *J. Acoust. Soc. Am.* 68, 1115-1122.

Klatt, D. (1980). Software for a cascade/parallel formant synthesizer. *J. Acoust. Soc. Am.* 67, 971-995.

Miller, M. I. and Sachs, M. B. (1983a). Representation of stop consonants in the discharge patterns of auditory-nerve fibers. *J. Acoust. Soc. Am.* (in press).

Miller, M. I. and Sachs, M. B. (1983b). Temporal and spectral representation of voice pitch in the auditory nerve. *Hearing Research* (submitted).

Plomp, R. (1966). Experiments on tone perception. Academic thesis, Utrecht.

Sachs, M. B. and Young, E. D. (1979). Encoding of steady-state vowels in the auditory nerve: representation in terms of discharge rate. *J. Acoust. Soc. Am.* 66, 470-479.

Sachs, M. B., Voigt, H. F. and Young, E. D. (1983). Auditory nerve representation of vowels in background noise. *J. Neurophysiol.* (in press).

Schouten, J. F. (1940). The residue and the mechanism of hearing. *Proc. Kon. Acad. Wetensch* (Neth) 43, 991-999.

Siebert, W. M. (1968). Stimulus transformations in the peripheral auditory system. In: *Recognizing Patterns* (P. A. Kolers and M. Eden, eds). pp. 104-133, Cambridge, M.I.T. Press.

Voigt, H. F., Sachs, M. B. and Young, E. D. (1982). Representation of whispered vowels in discharge patterns of auditory-nerve fibers. *Hearing Research* 8, 49-58.

Young, E. D. and Sachs, M. B. (1979). Representation of steady-state vowels in the temporal aspects of the discharge patterns of populations of auditory-nerve fibers. *J. Acoust. Soc. Am.* 66, 1381-1403.

GENERAL DISCUSSION

DE BOER:
A PST histogram is closely related to the signal that drives a unit but rectified. Hence the FT of the histogram is confounded by quadratic distortion products. How do you avoid that?

MILLER:
The rectifier distortion products are at harmonics of the primary. In generating our synchronized rate estimate at 1 kHz for example, we add the DFT coefficients of neurones whose characteristic frequencies are within 1/4 octave of 1 kHz. If there were large rectifier distortion products at 1 kHz in the DFTs of the population, they would be in neurones showing large primary responses to 125 Hz, 250 Hz or 500 Hz. These neurones would have CFs well below 1/4 octave of 1 kHz and there-

fore their distortion components would not confound our estimates of the 1 kHz response. We have talked extensively about rectifier distortion in a previous paper (Young and Sachs, J.A.S.A. 66, 1381, 1979).

HARRISON:
You present average discharge versus CF data in which the stimulus level is 69 dB SPL. Most fibres are thus operating at or near to the saturation region of their mean rate versus intensity functions. How much better would the stimulus frequency components be resolved in terms of mean rate at lower stimulus levels? For the comparison of average rate data with synchronized rate data, a similar i.e. log rate ordinate may be more appropriate.

MILLER:
We have looked at onset spectra of the consonant-vowel syllable as low as 45 dB SPL (Miller and Sachs, 1983a). During the onset, when average rate has its largest dynamic range (Smith and Brachman, Brain Res. 184, 499, 1980; Miller and Sachs, 1983a), the first three formant components in the stimulus are well represented. However, we could not find a representation of the harmonic structure corresponding to the fundamental frequency of voicing in the average rate measure at any sound level. We have plotted the average rate on a linear scale, since it has much less dynamic range than the synchronized rate measure. Therefore a log plot compresses the information. Our strategy has always been to present the data so that features are most evident.

MOORE:
Your average localized synchronized rate measure (Fig. 5) shows better resolution of the higher harmonics than is found psychophysically. This might mean that human observers cannot extract temporal responses to single components when in fact several components are exciting the same neurones. In other words, your Fourier Transform may extract more information from the temporal patterns of firing than people can. Nevertheless, I like your general approach very much.

BIALEK:
Although the authors do not explicitly attempt to do so, it is tempting to interpret these neural observations rather directly in terms of psychophysical data (e.g. resolution of partials as mentioned by Dr. Moore). I must emphasize the difficulty of doing this from average measures of neural response. As began by Siebert, Goldstein, Colburn et al., and shown also by Duifhuis at this meeting, comparisons between physiology and behaviour can be based only on the application of rigorous detection theory to a statistical characterization of the neural response. It is clear, for example, from Duifhuis' representation that seemingly obvious interpretations of the neural data need not survive such rigorous analysis. The data of Miller and Sachs are the first necessary step toward understanding the neural basis of psychophysical discrimination performance, but complete understanding requires theoretical developments which allow application of detection theory to the full body of statistical information which can be extracted from such experiments (interval distributions, correlations among successive intervals, etc.), and not just to simple models of these data such as the Poisson process. Any connection between physiology and behaviour is tentative without such a theory, and particularly when the best current methods (based on the Poisson model) have not been used to calculate the reliability of the information carried in the spike train.

GUMMER:
Remembering that a DFT can extract harmonics which are psychophysically undetectable, have you statistically tested the significance of all these harmonics for each histogram? Because of the possibility of systematic errors, care should be exhibited when making significance conclusions which are based simply on some averaging process across histograms.

MILLER:
Our interest in these studies is describing the characteristics of the temporal
representation of acoustic stimuli in auditory nerve discharge patterns. For that
reason, we have not tried to model any sort of psychophysical process when analyzing the data. Our phase-locking estimates are based on averaging responses to several stimulus presentations, enough to get at least 400 spikes in each histogram.
This is sufficient to provide statistically stable estimates of phase-locking.
The applicability of our results to speech perception depends on estimation of the
variance of response measures. We can, of course, estimate variance from our data
and have begun to analyze the data from this point of view.

EVANS:
I think there is now more convergence of views. Your ALSR 'maps' are analogous to
a phase-locked amplifier analysis - providing you average for long enough, you
will get all the resolution of the stimulus spectrum you could wish for. But the
nervous system clearly cannot do this. We agree that some measure is required,
better than rate (setting aside the uncertainty about the possible role played by
the low spontaneous rate units), and "worse" than the ALSR. Perhaps measures such
as autocorrelations may be a neuronally realizable bet.

MILLER:
We generate PST responses by temporal averaging across several stimulus presentations. The CNS would instead generate an ensemble average via convergence of neurones all close in characteristic frequency. Spectral estimates derived from autocorrelations functions are equivalent to those we derive from PST histograms,
since we discard phase information and use only power spectral components.

GHITZA:
Regarding the comments of B. Moore, B. Bialek and T. Evans on the possible discrepancy between the ALSR measure and the psychophysical responses, the ALSR scheme
is equivalent to the central spectrum suggested by Goldstein and Srulovicz (in:
Psychophysics and Physiology of Hearing, Evans and Wilson, Eds., London, 1977,
pp. 337-346), the only difference being that Miller and Sachs have decided to use
spectral estimates derived from PST histogram rather than those derived from interspike interval histograms. Goldstein has shown that the auditory precision with
which the central processor may measure components of a complex stimulus using the
central spectrum does correspond to the performance of psychophysically trained
subjects performing the task (see Fig. 1, Ghitza and Goldstein, this volume).

JNDs FOR THE SPECTRAL ENVELOPE PARAMETERS IN NATURAL SPEECH

Oded   Ghitza and Julius L. Goldstein

*Department of Electronic Communications,
Control and Computer Systems
Tel-Aviv University
Ramat-Aviv, Tel-Aviv 69978, ISRAEL*

1. INTRODUCTION

Flanagan in 1955 performed psychoacoustical experiments to measure the JNDs
for the formant center-frequency (Flanagan, 1955a) and its intensity (Flanagan,
1955b), and thereby determine the precision required in formant vocoder speech
synthesis (Flanagan,1957).   These experiments were performed on steady-state, synthetic speech vowels, yielding the JNDs for formant center-frequency, bandwidth
and intensity, and interformant valley depth, respectively: JNDF = 3% – 5%,
JNDB = 20% – 40%, JNDI = 1dB – 3dB, JNDV = 10dB, (Flanagan, 1970, 1972).
Flanagan and Saslow (1958) also examined the JND for the fundamental frequency of
steady-state synthetic speech sounds and found it to be $JNDf_o$ = 0.3% – 0.5%.

A reasonable question arises about the relevance of these data for the human
ability to discriminate each of these spectrally defined parameters under the dynamic conditions of natural speech. Indeed, Klatt (1973) re-examined the JND for
the fundamental frequency using synthetic speech sounds that modeled the time varying feature of the pitch in natural speech, and found it about an order of magnitude larger than reported earlier.   Is the same tendency to be expected when
re-examining the JNDs of the formant parameters?

Yet another factor needs attention, namely the possible dependence upon frequency of the JNDs for each of the formant parameters. Flanagan's data shows the
range of the possible values for each JND, but the behaviour of the JND upon frequency is unknown. A guide to the unknown dependence can be found in pitch theory
studies. Goldstein (1973) found from human performance in perceiving the fundamental frequency of complex-tone stimuli that the precision in aural measurment of
component frequencies depends upon the frequency, as shown in Fig. 1. We suggest
in Section 2 that this dependence upon frequency also can be expected for the formant JNDs. In Section 3, the necessary experiments are designed, in order to determine the appropriate magnitudes for the various JNDs for natural speech. The
appropriate synthesized speech segments were created by a back-to-back LPC-10 residual excited coder. The required quantization tables were established by applying a novel perceptually-motivated JND-distortion measure, defined in Section 3.B.

2. DEPENDENCE OF JND UPON FREQUENCY: THEORY

Goldstein and his associates (Goldstein, 1973, Goldstein et al, 1978, Gerson
and Goldstein, 1978) comprehensivly described the human perception of periodicity
pitch of complex tones by viewing the auditory system as a maximum a-posteriori
probability receiver that provides an optimal estimate of the pitch, as well as
the harmonic numbers of the stimulus components, on the basis of imprecise auditory measurements of the stimulus frequencies. Fig. 1 shows the relative standard
deviation with which the central processor measures the frequency of a component
tone, as a function of the frequency of the tone (solid line curve). Recall that
JND is defined by the standard deviation of the subject's decisions during the experiment.

This quantified psychophysical model was the basic framework for Goldstein
and Srulovicz's (Goldstein and Srulovicz, 1977, Srulovicz, 1982, Srulovicz and

Goldstein, 1983) physiologically-based model for the perception of the periodicity pitch. Assuming that the central auditory system operates on neural interval times, they provided an excellent physiological explanation for the psychophysical measured component frequency errors. The neural JND curve in Fig. 1 (dashed curve) was calculated on the basis of optimal use of neural interspike intervals from a single auditory nerve fiber; it was also shown that suboptimal processing of the neural intervals brings the physiological curve into closer registration with the psychological curves.

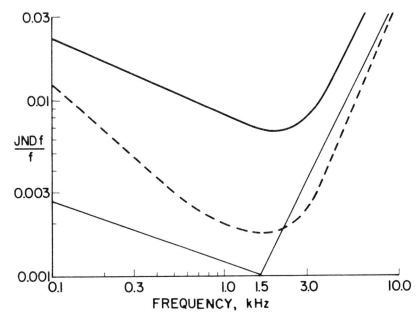

Fig. 1. *Auditory precision in measuring component frequency of complex tone:*
psychophysics (solid), neural timing (dashed), linear approximation

Confirmation of Goldstein and Srulovicz's claim about the essential role of neural timing in auditory central processing was given by Sachs and Young (1979, 1980, Young and Sachs, 1979). Examining physiological data, they found that to estimate the detailed spectral structure of the acoustical input, the timing information in the firing pattern should be processed while processing the average discharge rate is inadequate.

Although the performance curve of their physiologically-based model was calculated for frequency measurement tasks, we suggest that the same trend should exist for other tasks that the auditory central processor must deal with. We base this proposal on the idea that central information in the stimulus spectrum is probably based upon similar temporal-spatial processing of auditory-nerve spike patterns as for the measurement of component frequencies in periodicity pitch (Srulovicz and Goldstein, 1983, Young and Sachs, 1979, Sachs and Young, 1980). Thus, the trend of the performance curve in Fig. 1 is also relevant for auditory measurements of the spectral envelope parameters. In our JND-distortion measure, we used piecewise linear approximation for the curve, as is shown in Fig. 1. To every formant parameter a suitable JND-curve is attached. Their behaviour upon frequency is identical, the difference is in the value of the minimum point, JNDmin. In order to find JNDFmin, JNDBmin, JNDImin and JNDVmin, psychophysical experiments were conducted with natural speech sounds. As a starting point to these experiments, it was necessary to choose some reasonable initial values for the various JNDmin points as defined below.

Definition 2.1: *The JND1-set of curves*   is a set of four JND-curves (JNDF, JNDB, JNDI, JNDV) , their coresponding JNDmin points are the minimum values found by Flanagan for steady-state vowels (Flanagan, 1970, 1972).

Definition 2.2: *The JNDM-set of curves*   is as in the previous definition, except that each curve in the JND1-set is multiplied by M.

Note that the JNDmin values in the JNDM-set of curves are obtained by *simultaneously* multiplying the steaty-state JNDs. When listening to a stimulus defined by a set of parameters with a time-varying features, the JNDs are expected to be larger then in steady-state listening. Because of our assumption of similar neural processing, similar proportions between the corresponding JNDs in the two cases should be maintained.

3. PSYCHOPHYSICAL MEASURMENT OF THE JNDmin POINTS FOR NATURAL SPEECH SOUNDS

3.A Method

As a first step towards the psychoacoustical experiments we create a library of speech segments, containing an original speech segment followed by four synthe-sized speech segments, each of which is a member of a different perceptually-equivalent class of signals representing the original. Each of these four classes is defined by its JNDM-set of curves, M=3,4,5,6. The technique we used to produce each synthesized segment was a special version of a back-to-back

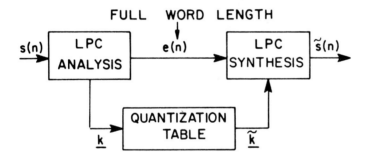

Fig. 2. Residual excited LPC-10 back-to-back coder: a special version, for quality judgement

residual exited LPC-10 coder, shown in Fig. 2.   In this version, the full-precision (16 bit per sample) residual signal excites the recursive filter, defined by the appropriately quantized reflection coefficients. The quantization tables are related to the JNDM-set of curves via the JND-distortion measure which is introduced in Section 3.B.

The procedure for the linear prediction is described in Section 3.C.   It yields both the current reflection coefficients vector $\underline{k}$ and its matched residual signal, e(n). Feeding the full-precision filter (defined by the full-precision vector $\underline{k}$) with the full-precision e(n) yields a synthesized output which is the original input frame itself (with a neglectable truncation error due to the finite word length of the processor). All the synthesized speech segments in our library were produced by feeding this full-precision residual signal into filters with the same structure, but with different $\underline{k}^q$, according to the desired quantization tables. Four quantization tables were used, one for each JNDM-set of curves, M=3,4,5,6.   Two points are to be noted: 1) since e(n) is the full-precision in-verse-filter response to the original speech, it contains the minimum information possible on the spectral envelope; this causes the synthesized speech spectral envelope to be affected mainly by the quantization error in $\underline{k}^q$. 2) only the JNDs for voiced frames were examined since the psychophysical data apply to such sounds, while larger JNDs are expected for unvoiced sounds. Thus, no processing was performed on the non-voiced frames (the V-UNV decision was by energy consider-ations), each unvoiced frame was represented by its original.

3.B The JND-distortion measure

   Previous distortion measures suggested for the speech spectral envelope quantization problem are based, in general, on the *average* spectral error. We argue that a *binary* decision is more appropriate, regarding the auditory system performance. Given the JNDs for the formant center-frequency, bandwidth and in-tensity and interformant valley depth, for natural speech, a deviation from each reflection coefficient is permitted until exceeding any JND boundary, each bounda-ry is perceptually equally weighted. Fig. 3 illustrates the proposed measure;

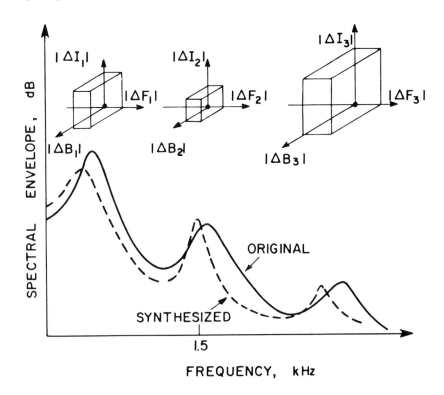

Fig. 3. The JND-distortion measure: illustration

the JNDs are different for each formant, according to their frequencies, the deci-sion is binary OR: either one of all difference vectors emerges from the box- the penalty is '1', otherwise it is '0'.

3.C Database and analysis conditions

   Synthesized speech sounds were generated that were within a JNDM distance from the original. Natural speech consisting of four 6-seconds speech segments, spoken by two males and two females provided the database. High quality FM radio broadcasts of news programs in Hebrew were digitized at 10 K/s sample rate using a 12 bit A-D converter, preceded by a 4th order low-pass filter set at 4 KHz.

A 10th order LPC analysis with the auto-correlation method (Levinson recursion) was then performed on a 25 msec non-overlapped frames (250 sample points) with a Hamming window. No pre-emphasis was used.

The quantization tables for the special version LPC-10 coder were generated empirically, using a large database of speech segments; the JND-distortion measure was applyed in an appropriate single-parameter perturbation-analysis to every reflection coefficient, providing the quantitative basis required for the quantization boundaries and levels computation. Several such perturbation-analysis sessions were carried out, one for each JND-set of curves defining the JND-distortion measure.

3.D Psychophysical procedure and results

The subject is exposed to a two interval forced choice experiment. The two intervals (drawn from the library) are the original segment and one of its synthesized segments which was randomly selected; the order of their appearence is also random. The subject's task is to give a score to the synthesized part, the lowest mark is 1, the highest is 9. Each speech segment in the database was examined by the subject in a 100 trial experiment. Typical scoring versus M is given in Table 1. The abrupt increase in perceived quality at M=4 points to the appropriate JNDmin points for natural speech sounds.

Table 1. Typical quality-scoring results

JNDM	Mean	σ	Mean	σ	Mean	σ	Mean	σ
3	7.10	1.73	6.65	2.06	7.74	1.21	7.63	1.54
4	6.17	1.71	7.00	2.01	6.80	1.43	7.11	1.38
5	3.00	1.44	3.31	1.85	2.92	1.05	3.52	2.05
6	2.06	1.71	2.40	2.15	1.84	1.63	1.73	1.84

4. Conclusions

1. Spectral distortions in synthesized speech sounds corresponding to more than 4 times the steady state JNDs can be tolerated without significant distortion in quality.

2. The quantization tables corresponding to JND4 provides more efficient linear prediction vocoding than standard scalar quantization tables that are based upon heuristic and mathematically convenient distortion measures, modulated by listening experiments (e.g. see review by Markel and Gray, 1980).

REFERENCES

Flanagan, J.L. (1955a) "A difference limen for vowel formant frequency", J. Acous. Soc. Amer., p. 613, May 1955.
Flanagan, J.L. (1955b) "Difference limen for the intensity of a vowel sound", J. Acous. Soc. Amer., p. 1223, Nov. 1955.
Flanagan, J.L. and Saslow, M.G. (1958) "Pitch discrimination for synthetic vowels", J. Acous. Soc. Amer., p. 435, May 1958.
Flanagan, J.L. (1957) "Estimates of the maximum precision necessary in quantizing certain "dimensions" of vowel sounds", J. Acous. Soc. Amer., p. 533, May 1957.
Flanagan, J.L. (1970) *Digital representation of speech signals,* BTL Symposium on Digital Techniques in Communication, Nov. 12 and 13, 1970.
Flanagan, J.L. (1972) *Speech Analysis, Synthesis and Perception* , Springer Verlag, New York, 1972.
Gerson, A. and Goldstein, J.L. (1978) "Evidence for a general template in central optimal processing of pitch of complex tones", J. Acous. Soc. Amer., p. 498, Feb. 1978.

Goldstein, J.L. (1973) "An optimum processor theory for the central formation of the pitch of complex tones", J. Acous. Soc. Amer., p. 1496, Dec. 1973.

Goldstein, J.L. and Srulovicz, P. (1977) "Auditory-nerve spike intervals as an adequate basis for aural spectrum analysis", In Evans, E.F. and Wilson, J.P. (Editors) *Psychophysics and Physiology of Hearing* , Academic-Press, London, p. 337.

Goldstein, J.L., Gerson, A., Srulovicz, P. and Furst, M. (1978) "Verification of the optimal probabilistic basis for aural processing in pitch of complex tones", J. Acous. Soc. Amer., p. 486, Feb. 1978.

Klatt, D.H. (1973) "Discrimination of fundamental frequency contours in synthetic speech: implications for models of pitch perception", J. Acous. Soc. Amer., p. 8, Jan. 1973.

Markel, J.D. and Gray, A.H. (1980) "Implementation and comparision of two transformed reflection coefficient scalar quantization methods", IEEE Trans. Acous., Speech and Signal Proc., ASSP-28, p. 575, Oct. 1980.

Sachs, M.B. and Young, E.D. (1979) "Encoding of steady-state vowels in the auditory nerve: representation in terms of discharge rate", J. Acous. Soc. Amer., p. 470, Aug. 1979.

Sachs, M.B. and Young, E.D. (1980) "Effects of nonlinearities on speech encoding in the auditory nerve", J. Acous. Soc. Amer., p. 858, Sept. 1980.

Srulovicz, P. (1979) "Neural timing as a physiological basis for aural representation of frequency spectrum; the central spectrum", Ph.D. Thesis, Bioengineering Program, School of Engineering, Tel-Aviv University. Supervised by J.L. Goldstein.

Srulovicz, P. and Goldstein, J.L. (1983) "A central spectrum model: A synthesis of auditory-nerve timing and place cues in monaural communication of frequency spectrum", scheduled to appear in J. Acoust. Soc. Amer., March 1983.

Young, E.D. and Sachs, M.B. (1979) "Representation of steady-state vowels in the temporal aspects of the discharge patterns of populations of auditory-nerve fibers", J. Acous. Soc. Amer., p. 1381, Nov. 1979.

GENERAL DISCUSSION

RITSMA:
Did you also look for speech intelligibility apart from the quality scores?

GHITZA:
The JND concept is appropriate only in the context of quality preservation. Therefore, psychophysical discrimination experiments were performed, comparing the synthesized speech segments with the original segment itself. The speech intelligibility problem should be studied within a different context in which much broader distortions of different kinds are to be considered.

STERN:
How does the bit rate needed to transmit vocoded speech quantized according to JND4 compare to the bit rate obtained using conventional methods? Secondly, you weight equally the JNDs for formant amplitude, frequency, intensity, and valley depth in constructing the JNDM measure. Do you think that the quality-scoring results would be very different with some other weighting?

GHITZA:
1) For the representation of the spectral envelope, conventional scalar-quantization methods require around 40 bits per frame, while the JND4 quantization method requires only 25 bits per frame (and complete preservation of quality is still maintained).

2) The JNDmin values in the JNDM-set of curves were indeed obtained by simultaneously multiplying the minimum steady-state JNDs measured by Flanagan (1955). When listening to a stimulus defined by a set of parameters with a time-varying feature, the JNDs are expected to be larger than in steady-state listening. With our assumption of similar neural processsing, similar proportions between the correspond-

ing JNDs in the two cases should be maintained. Nevertheless, if each JNDmin value
were varied separately, I would assume that the quality-scoring results will con-
verge, in the end, to the values around JND4. I should add that in order to verify
our assumption about the dependence of each JND on frequency (shown in Fig. 1) we
also explored the effect of assuming that JND/f is a constant, independent of frequency. The psychophysical experiments clearly indicate that if a quantization
scheme based on constant JND/f with the same number of bits is used, the synthesized speech segments are of much poorer quality.

THE RECEPTION THRESHOLD OF INTERRUPTED SPEECH FOR HEARING-IMPAIRED LISTENERS

J.A.P.M. de Laat and R. Plomp

Faculty of Medicine, Free University, Amsterdam, The Netherlands

1. INTRODUCTION

In previous research in our group (Dreschler & Plomp, 1980; Festen & Plomp, 1983) data on different auditory functions were correlated with the speech-reception threshold (SRT) in quiet and in noise, both for normal-hearing and hearing-impaired listeners. In this paper we will report on experiments in which the speech signal is disturbed by noise discontinuous in time or/and in frequency. Additionally to SRT the auditory bandwidth of the subjects was measured (Houtgast, 1974). This parameter, together with hearing loss, appeared to be the most representative factor with respect to the results of SRT measurements (Festen & Plomp, 1981).

In the past several authors have reported on experiments in which the intelligibility of interrupted speech was investigated, including the effect of added noise. Miller & Licklider (1950) measured the intelligibility of interrupted speech. The interruption rate was an important parameter. The best results were obtained for a rate of about 10 interruptions per second. Huggins (1975) published the results of experiments with speech segmented in time. He, too, found an optimal rate of 10 interruptions per second, as well as an optimal duty cycle of 50%. Powers & Wilcox (1979) experimented with and without intervening noise. They observed that the intelligibility is highest if the interruptions are filled with noise at about the same loudness level as the interrupted speech.

2. EXPERIMENTS

Method

Firstly the pure-tone threshold was measured for 11 frequencies (125 Hz, 250 Hz, 500 Hz, 630 Hz, 800 Hz, 1000 Hz, 1250 Hz, 1600 Hz, 2000 Hz, 4000 Hz and 8000 Hz). We used an adapted Békésy procedure which takes about ten minutes per ear.

Secondly the speech-reception threshold (SRT) for sentences was measured for five different conditions: (1) quiet, (2) continuous noise, (3) interrupted noise, (4) filtered noise, and (5) interrupted and filtered noise. The sentences were presented in an adaptive up-and-down procedure as described by Plomp & Mimpen (1979). The noise had the same spectrum as the long-term average spectrum of the sentences. The level of this noise was 85 dB(A) for the second condition. The amplification factor was not changed by introducing the interruptions and filter combinations. The interruption rate was 10 per sec, with a duty cycle of 50%. In the filtered conditions the noise was present only in the one-third octaves around the frequencies 125 Hz, 250 Hz, 500 Hz, 1000 Hz, 2000 Hz and 4000 Hz. The slopes of the filters are 60 dB per octave.

Thirdly the auditory bandwidth was measured with a 1000 Hz probe tone presented simultaneously with a comb-filtered noise (85 dB(A)). The detection threshold was measured both on the peak and in the valley of the noise signal, with ripple densities of 0.5, 1 and 2 ripples per 1000 Hz. We used an adapted two-alternative forced-choice procedure which takes about thirty minutes per ear.

Apparatus

The experiments were controlled by computer. The subjects were situated in an anechoic chamber and listened monaurally by headphone.

Subjects

The subjects were 20 pupils of a high-school for the hearing impaired. Their age varied from 13 to 17 years. Their hearing loss was sensorineural. As a reference group we used 10 pupils at the same education level as the hearing-impaired subjects.

3. RESULTS

In fig. 1 the results of the first experiment on the pure-tone threshold are plotted, with reference to the mean results of the normal-hearing subjects. As can be seen the group of 20 subjects had a great variability in slope in the audiogram, plotted along the x-axis, as well as in mean audiometric loss, plotted along the y-axis. In the experiments of Dreschler & Plomp (1980) these two parameters appeared to be the most important to describe the audiogram, so we have used them for correlation with the other data.

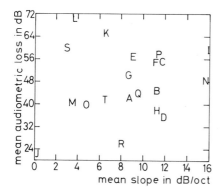

Fig. 1. *Mean slope and mean audiometric loss for the 20 hearing-impaired subjects*

In fig. 2 the SRT values obtained in the second experiment are plotted. In this scatter diagram the threshold difference between SRT in continuous noise and in filtered noise is plotted as a function of the threshold difference between SRT in continuous noise and in interrupted noise, both for the normal-hearing and the hearing-impaired subjects. The reliability coefficient of these data points is above 0.90. If only the energy of the noise is taken into account, a threshold difference for the temporal interruptions of 3 dB (duty cycle 50%) and for the spectral interruptions of 4.7 dB (1/3 octave noise per octave) has to be expected.

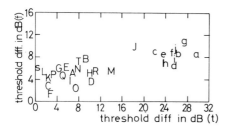

Fig. 2. *Difference between SRT in continuous noise and in filtered noise as a function of difference between SRT in continuous noise and in interrupted noise, both for normal-hearing (under-cast symbols) and hearing-impaired (upper-cast symbols) subjects*

The following comments can be made.

(1) Although the reliability of this test is very high, the data points of the normal-hearing subjects vary over a substantially larger range than in continuous noise: about 5 dB for the temporal interruptions and about 3 dB for the spectral interruptions, whereas the SRT levels in continuous noise vary only about 1 dB (all standard deviations).

(2) The data for the hearing-impaired subjects differ from the data for the normal-hearing subjects significantly only for the temporal interruptions. Apparently the gain of using only 1/3 octave of noise at one octave distances is very poor.

(3) For some of the hearing-impaired subjects the gain is less than the theoretically expected gain (respectively 3 dB and 4.7 dB), so they had no profit of the discontinuities of the noise.

In fig. 3. results from the first and the second experiments are combined. The threshold difference between SRT in continuous noise and in interrupted noise is plotted as a function of the mean audiometric loss.

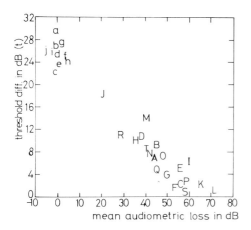

Fig. 3. Difference between SRT in continuous noise and in interrupted noise as a function of mean audiometric loss, both for the normal-hearing (under-cast symbols) and hearing-impaired (upper-cast symbols) subjects

There is a very good correlation between the two parameters, with a correlation coefficient of 0.85. All other combinations of data from the first experiment and data from the second experiment have lower correlation coefficients.

In fig. 4 the results of the third experiment are presented. The logarithms of the bandwidth values are plotted as a function of the SRT in filtered noise relative to the mean results of the normal-hearing subjects. The two parameters correlate quite well (coefficient is 0.70) which means that the ear's frequency selectivity is clearly involved in the SRT measurements with filtered noise.

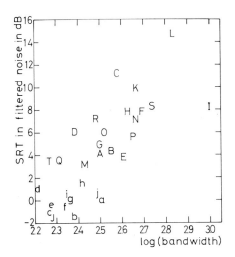

Fig. 4. SRT with filtered noise as a function of the logarithm of the auditory bandwidth, both for the normal-hearing (under-cast symbols) and hearing-impaired (upper-cast symbols) subjects

4. CONCLUSIONS

(1) Normal-hearing subjects vary significantly in their SRT in noise interrupted in time and/or frequency.

(2) The mean audiometric loss correlates quite well with the effect of temporal interruptions of the masking noise on SRT.

(3) The auditory bandwidth correlates well with the SRT in filtered noise.

Acknowledgement. This study is supported by the Netherlands Organization for the Advancement of Pure Research (ZWO).

REFERENCES

Dreschler, W.A. & Plomp, R. (1980), Relation between psychophysical data and speech perception for hearing-impaired subjects (I), J.Acoust.Soc.Am. 68, 1608-1615.

Festen, J.M. & Plomp, R. (1981), Relations between auditory functions in normal hearing, J.Acoust.Soc.Am. 70, 356-369.

Festen, J.M. & Plomp, R. (1983), Relations between auditory functions in impaired hearing, J.Acoust.Soc.Am. 73, scheduled for the february issue.

Houtgast, T. (1974), Lateral suppression in hearing, Ph.D.-Thesis, Academische Pers B.V., Amsterdam.

Huggins, A.W.F. (1975), Temporally segmented speech, Perception & Psychophysics 18, 149-157.

Miller, G.A. & Licklider, J.C.R. (1950), The intelligibility of interrupted speech, J.Acoust.Soc.Am. 22, 167-173.

Plomp, R. & Mimpen, A.M. (1979), Improving the reliability of testing the speech reception threshold for sentences, Audiology 18, 43-52.

Powers, G.L. & Wilcox, J.C. (1977), Intelligibility of temporal interrupted speech with and without intervening noise, J.Acoust.Soc.Am. 61, 195-199.

GENERAL DISCUSSION

TYLER:
It was not clear to me whether you felt this interrupted noise has some analogy to everyday listening situations or whether it was a technique for stressing the auditory system.

DE LAAT:
Indeed, one of our reasons to introduce interruptions both in time and in frequency was to have interfering sounds more representative of everyday listening situations than just steady-state noise. A second argument was to try out speech-reception conditions related to experiments with tone bursts, combfiltered noise, etc.

IMPAIRED FREQUENCY/TIME RESOLUTION
AND ITS EFFECT ON SPEECH INTELLIGIBILITY

W.A. Dreschler

*Department of Clinical Audiology, Academic Medical Centre,
Meibergdreef 9, 1105 AZ Amsterdam, The Netherlands*

1. INTRODUCTION

In subjects with sensorineural hearing impairment many psychophysical functions are deteriorated. However, there is only little knowledge about the impact of these deteriorations on speech intelligibility. Especially the psychophysical correlates of impaired speech intelligibility in background noise are unknown. Some authors suggest a detrimental effect on speech intelligibility due to a reduced frequency resolving power of pathological ears (Evans, 1978; Scharf, 1978). Experimental evidence for this hypothesis is provided by studies of Ritsma et al. (1980) and Festen and Plomp (1983). Others point out the importance of a normal temporal resolution for the perception of speech (Elliott, 1975; Danaher, Wilson and Pickett, 1978). Tyler and Summerfield (1980) found a significant correlation between gap detection and speech intelligibility in noise, indicating a possible relationship. However, in our opinion the relations between speech perception and temporal properties of the ear are underexposed.

In a preliminary study we focused our attention on the relation of speech reception thresholds in quiet and noise and a number of non-temporal psychophysical tests: the audiogram, the critical ratio, the bandwidth as measured with comb-filtered noise and the perception of isolated steady-state vowels (Dreschler and Plomp, 1980; Dreschler, 1980). The deteriorations in speech perception appeared to be correlated with both audiometric data and frequency-resolution parameters. Because of their strong mutual relation, it is difficult to separate the effects of audiogram and frequency-resolving power on speech perception. Humes (1982) even states that most studies obtaining reduced frequency resolution in hearing-impaired subjects are simply a reflection of a - mostly not considered - elevation of the pure-tone thresholds.

In this study we will consider again some of the non-temporal properties mentioned with the experiment extended with several measures of the temporal properties of the ear. Additionally, a relationship is sought with the perception of initial consonants, in which the temporal resolution may be expected to play an important role.

2. SUBJECTS, TESTS AND PROCEDURES

In this study 21 sensorineurally impaired adolescents participated on a voluntary basis. The following tone-perception data were measured:
a) The *audiogram* at octaves from 250 to 4000 Hz.
b) The *uncomfortable loudness level* for 500 Hz, 1 kHz and 2 kHz. The values found were combined with the audiometric thresholds in order to get three measures of the dynamic range of the ear.
c) The *critical ratio* at 500 Hz, 1 kHz and 2 kHz by measuring the masked thresholds of pure tones in white noise with a spectral density of 60 dB/Hz.
d) The *forward and backward masking* thresholds for octave-filtered clicks around 500 Hz, 1 kHz and 2 kHz, presented 30 and 3 ms before the switching-on and 5 and 50 ms after the switching-off of a 60 dB/Hz white-noise burst, 150 ms in duration. From these thresholds the backward- and forward-masking slopes for each frequency were calculated by linear interpolation.

e) The *gap-detection* thresholds for octave-filtered band-pass noises (60 dB/Hz) at 500 Hz, 1 kHz and 2 kHz.

All thresholds in a), c), d) and e) were measured by means of a 2AFC-procedure, using an adaptive up-down strategy. In b) the method of limits was used. The following phoneme-perception data were measured:

f) The dissimilarity matrices of *isolated steady-state vowel segments* by means of the method of triadic comparisons. The resulting matrices were analysed by a 2-dimensional INDSCAL-analysis in order to find individual weightings of the fundamental dimensions used in vowel perception (Carroll and Chang, 1970).

g) The confusion matrices of *initial consonants* in nonsense CVC-syllables, both in quiet and in a speech-shaped background noise. These confusion matrices were symmetrized and considered as similarity matrices. A 3-dimensional INDSCAL-analysis provided the individual weightings – both in quiet and in noise – of the fundamental dimensions used in the perception of initial consonants.

Finally, some speech-perception data have been included:

h) The *speech-reception threshold* for sentences in quiet and at two levels of interfering noise (60 and 80 dB(A)), using the accurate test developed by Plomp and Mimpen (1979). From the fitted curves two parameters emerged: (1) the D-parameter, representing the elevation of the speech-reception threshold in noise relative to normal-hearing subjects. This parameter may be interpreted as a distortion term. (2) the A-parameter, representing the extra elevation of the speech-reception threshold in quiet, interpreted as an attenuation term.

g) The speech-reception thresholds of *low-pass and high-pass filtered* sentences in noise (f_c=1200 Hz). The thresholds found were related to the unfiltered speech-in-noise thresholds, resulting in two parameters indicating the extra elevation of the threshold due to low-pass and high-pass filtering.

All tests were performed monaurally (better ear) with headphones. For the estimation of the accuracy all tests were measured both in test and in retest on separate days.

3. RESULTS

The results of the tone-perception experiments are summarized in Table I. For each parameter the lower quartile, the median, and the upper quartile are presented as an indication of the range of values obtained. As a measure of accuracy the standard error of the measurement has been calculated. The test-retest correlation (r_{tr}) reflects the reliability of each parameter. On behalf of further analyses an abbreviation code has been introduced. The values obtianed show deteriorations of all auditory properties compared to normal-hearing subjects. The reliability proved to be high for all parameters.

The results of the 2-dimensional INDSCAL-analysis on the vowel perception results are presented in Figure 1. In panel a the stimuli are plotted along the fundamental dimensions revealed by the (dis)similarity judgements (object space). These dimensions explain 79.0% of the total variance: 49% by the first dimension, which is related to the position of the first formant (F1) and 30% by the second dimension which is related to the position of the second formant (F2). In panel b the individual weightings of these dimensions are plotted (subject space). The quarter of a circle represents the extreme position of the individual points, reached if all variance is explained by the first two dimensions.

The results of the 3-dimensional INDSCAL-analysis on the initial-consonant results are presented in a comparable way in Figure 2. In a combined analy-

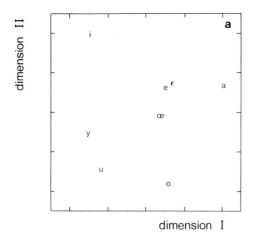

dimension II

dimension I

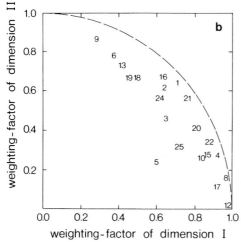

weighting-factor of dimension II

weighting-factor of dimension I

Fig. 1. Results of a two-dimensional INDSCAL-analysis of vowel-dissimilarity matrices. Panel a: object space. Panel b: subject space

sis of the quiet and noise conditions 66.7% of the total variance was explained. From the object space (panel a) it can be seen that the first dimension, which explains 39.5% of the variance, differentiates between nasals, voiced and unvoiced consonants. The second dimension explains 16.6% of the variance and separates the stops /p/, /t/, /b/, /d/, and /k/ from the fricatives /s/, /z/, /v/, /ᵪ/, /f/, /w/ and /h/. The extreme position of /s/, and /z/ also reveals the importance of sibilance. The third dimension explains 10.6% of the variance and shows some relation to the place of articulation, differentiating between the dentals /s/, /z/, /d/ and /t/, the bilabials /w/, /b/ and /p/ and the labiodentals /v/ and /f/. The individual weightings for the quiet conditons are presented in panel b, for the noise conditions in panel c.

The 8-phoneme-perception parameters obtained are summarized in Table II. Due to the measurement error in such experiments it is not suprising that some of the parameters yield a rather low test-retest correlation. In further analysis the role of the F1-weighting and of the place-of-articulation weightings can be neglected. The other parameters, however, have a rather high test-retest correlation.

The speech-perception parameters are summarized in Table III.

4. MUTUAL RELATIONS

The mutual relations between the 30 parameters have been investigated by means of a correlation analysis. In order to visualize the mutual relations between the tests a principal-components analysis has been carried out on the matrix of correlation coefficients. In this analysis directions or factors are determined which explain as much as possible of the total variance. Figure 3(a) shows the percentages of variance explained by the successive factors. In two dimensions 62.0% of the variance could be explained. The correspondence of each test to a certain factor is expressed in the so-called factor-loadings. A plot of the tests according to their factor loadings provides a picture of mutual relations of tests: closely related tests will be recognized as clusters. In Figure 3(b) this plot is shown. In order to situate all tests in the right half plane the polarity of some tests was changed. The circle is reached if all the variance of a certain test is explained by the two factors.

Table I. Summary of tone-perception data

test parameter	abbreviation code	r_{tr}	standard error	lower quartile	median	upper quartile	dimension
audiometric loss							
500 Hz	A1	0.98	3.25	21.1	29.3	46.0	dB
1 kHz	A2	0.98	3.21	26.0	47.4	58.6	dB
2 kHz	A3	0.98	2.83	45.8	53.8	71.4	dB
dynamic range							
500 Hz	D1	0.92	5.73	56.1	62.1	75.1	dB
1 kHz	D2	0.96	5.20	41.2	49.3	66.3	dB
2 kHz	D3	0.88	5.63	31.9	45.8	56.8	dB
critical ratio							
500 Hz	C1	0.88	1.01	17.6	18.7	19.9	dB
1 kHz	C2	0.76	1.46	20.8	21.6	23.3	dB
2 kHz	C3	0.85	1.18	24.5	25.5	27.7	dB
backward masking slope							
500 Hz	B1	0.96	0.12	0.49	0.80	1.14	dB/ms
1 kHz	B2	0.98	0.10	0.63	0.92	1.40	dB/ms
2 kHz	B3	0.98	0.09	0.34	0.91	1.25	dB/ms
forward masking slope							
500 Hz	F1	0.96	0.06	0.29	0.42	0.69	dB/ms
1 kHz	F2	0.96	0.06	0.29	0.35	0.64	dB/ms
2 kHz	F3	0.99	0.03	0.29	0.39	0.58	dB/ms
gap detection threshold							
500 Hz	G1	0.95	1.72	9.3	10.3	13.0	ms
1 kHz	G2	0.95	1.78	6.6	8.3	10.8	ms
2 kHz	G3	0.96	2.12	6.0	6.8	9.1	ms

Tabel II. Summary of the weighting-factors obtained from INDSCAL-analyses on phoneme-perception data

test parameter	abbreviation code	r_{tr}	standard error	lower quartile	median	upper quartile	dimension
isolated vowels							
F1-weighting	f1	0.38	0.159	0.603	0.709	0.873	−
F2-weighting	f2	0.73	0.120	0.271	0.457	0.667	−
initial consonants quiet							
nasality/voicing	q1	0.85	0.108	0.478	0.802	0.890	−
stop/fricative	q2	0.69	0.106	0.103	0.143	0.231	−
place	q3	0.58	0.103	0.107	0.182	0.290	−
initial consonants noise							
nasality/voicing	n1	0.70	0.126	0.253	0.402	0.540	−
stop/fricative	n2	0.66	0.123	0.317	0.483	0.636	−
place	n3	0.15	0.181	0.195	0.308	0.403	−

Table III. Summary of the speech-perception data

test parameter	abbreviation code	r_{tr}	standard error	lower quartile	median	upper quartile	dimension
SHL in noise	D	.90	0.76	1.1	2.5	3.3	dB(A)
ΔSHL in quiet	A	.98	1.71	23.3	31.9	41.2	dB(A)
ΔSHL lp-filtered	ΔDL	.82	1.60	4.1	5.2	7.7	dB(A)
ΔSHL hp-filtered	ΔDH	.94	1.54	6.9	9.6	13.8	dB(A)

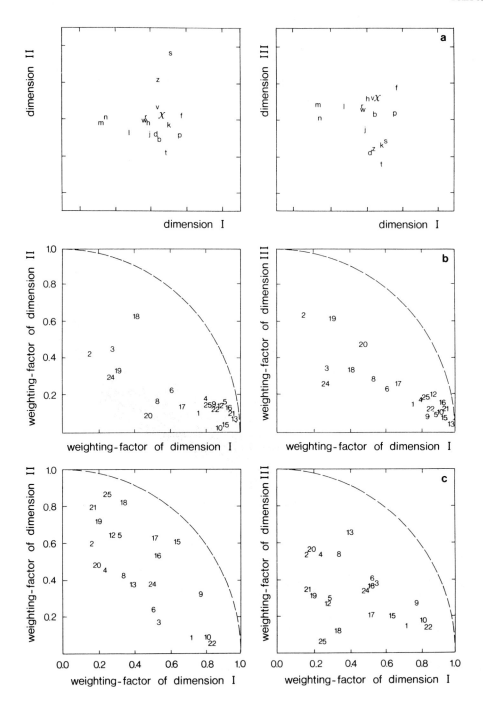

Fig. 2. Results of a three-dimensional INDSCAL-analysis on confusion matrices of initial consonants. Panel a: object space. Panel b: subject space (quiet). Panel c: subject space (noise)

5. DISCUSSION

In Figure 3(b) all tests are positioned reasonably near the circle, with the exception of n3, the test with the lowest test-retest correlation. This indicates that the variance in most tests is rather well represented by the two factors. Concerning the clustering of tests the following remarks can be made:

a) There is a clear dichotomy between tone-perception parameters and phoneme-perception parameters. This indicates that the tone-perception parameters used are not the determinating properties for the perception of phonemes.

b) For the tone-perception parameters there is a clustering per frequency rather than per test: the dynamic range, the critical ratio and the forward and backward masking slopes seem to be closely related to the audiometric loss. For the gap detection thresholds this relation is less clear.

c) The SHL in noise (D) is positioned in the middle of the cluster with 2 kHz-tests. This means that the high-frequency tests are very important for speech perception in noise.

d) The extra elevation of the speech hearing loss in quiet (A) is positioned between the 500 Hz an 1 kHz clusters: in quiet the low-frequency characteristics are important.

e) High-pass filtering causes a shift towards the phoneme-perception parameters in quiet, low-pass filtering towards the phoneme-perception parameters in noise.

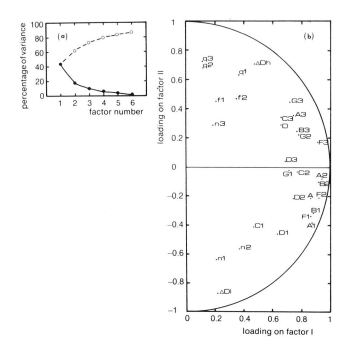

Fig 3. Results of the principal-components analysis.
Panel a: percentage of variance explained by the successive factors.
Panel b: factor loadings of the tests on the first two dimensions

Summarizing, the unfiltered speech-perception data are related mainly to tone-perception data: in quiet to low-frequency and in noise to high-frequency parameters. The phoneme-discrimination data seem to play only a role of secondary importance, which become relevant in cases of filtering. The place of the filtered speech conditions in Figure 3 suggests that the influence of noise on the perception of phonemes is caused by the lower frequency parts of the noise spectrum. This is in agreement with earlier findings (Dreschler, 1983) and it provides a possible explanation for the importance of high-frequency parameters for speech perception in noise.

REFERENCES.

Carroll, J.D. and Chang, J.J. (1970). Analysis of individual differences in in multidimensional scaling via an n-way generalization of the 'Eckart-Young'-decomposition. *Psychometrica* 35, 283-319.

Danaher, E.M. and Wilson, M.P. and Pickett, J.M. (1978). Backward and forward masking in listeners with severe sensorineural hearing loss. *Audiology* 17, 324-338.

Dreschler, W.A. (1980). Reduced speech intelligibility and its psychophysical correlates in hearing-impaired subjects. In: *Psychophysical, physiological and behavioural studies in hearing* (G. v.d. Brink and F.A. Bilsen, eds). pp 466-469. Delft University Press.

Dreschler, W.A. (1983). The effects of presentation level and signal-to-noise ratio on phonemic confusions for hearing-impaired subjects. Submitted for publication in *Audiology*.

Dreschler, W.A. and Plomp, R. (1980). Relation between psychophysical data and speech perception for hearing-impaired subjects. I. *J.A.S.A.* 68, 1608-1615.

Elliot, L.L. (1975). Temporal and masking phenomena in persons with sensorineural hearing loss. *Audiology* 14, 336-353.

Evans, E.F. (1978). Peripheral auditory processing in normal and abnormal ears: physiological considerations for attempts to compensate for auditory deficits by acoustic and electric prosthesis. *Scand. Aud.* suppl. 6, 9-47.

Festen, J.M. and Plomp, R. (1983). Relations between auditory functions in impaired hearing. *J.A.S.A.* (in press).

Humes, L.E. (1983). Spectral and temporal resolution in hearing impaired. *Annals of O.R.L.* (in press).

Plomp, R. and Mimpen, A.M. (1979). Improving the reliability of testing the speech-reception threshold for sentences. *Audiology* 18, 43-52.

Ritsma, R.J. Wit, H.P. and van der Lans, W.P. (1980). Relations between hearing loss, maximal word discrimination score and width of the psychophysical tuning curves. In: *Psychophysical, physiological and behavioural studies in hearing* (G. v.d. Brink and F.A. Bilsen, eds). pp 472-475. Delft University Press.

Scharf, B. (1978). Comparison of normal and impaired hearing. II: frequency analysis, speech perception. *Scan. Aud.* suppl. 6, 81-106.

Tyler, R.S. and Summerfield, A.Q. (1980). Psychoacoustical and phonetic measures of temporal processing in normal and hearing-impaired listeners. In: *Psychophysical, physiological and behavioural studies in hearing* (G. v.d. Brink and F.A. Bilsen, eds). pp 458-465, Delft University Press.

This study was granted by the Netherlands Organization for the Advancement of Pure Research.

GENERAL DISCUSSION

PICK:
You find that high frequency information is more salient for speech perception in
noise, compared with speech perception in quiet. Could this be because your patients have predominantly high-frequency losses, so that, possibly in quiet high-
frequency information in speech might be below threshold, whereas in noise they
might be able to make more efficient use of the high-frequency information in
speech?

DRESCHLER:
As I have shown in one of my slides, the sloping audiograms are not overproportio-
nally represented. So I doubt this effect to be conclusive for our results. Above
this, the audiometric slope is not correlated significantly with speech hearing
loss in noise.

VERSCHUURE:
You have classified the audiometric loss by averaged loss and averaged slope. We
have analysed the hearing of a family with a hereditary progressive hearing impairment starting in the high frequencies. Your two factors (loss and slope) were suggested by the principal component analysis, explaining about 92% of the variance.
The data, however, could be much better described by the slope and the place of
the slope, as the latter relates strongly with the phonemes that can be identified.
Wouldn't you get a better relation between your phoneme results and your audiometric data if you took slope, place of slope and mean loss as variables?

DRESCHLER:
I think the approach you suggest would require more data points than actually measured in this study. Besides, your results may be inherent to the specific form of
audiograms within your group of patients. It may not be appropriate to describe
the audiograms within a rather heterogeneous group as used in this study.

CAP UNMASKING, CAP TUNING AND CAP THRESHOLDS IN HUMANS

W.L.C. Rutten

ENT Dept., Univ. Hospital, 10 Rijnsburgerweg
Leiden, The Netherlands

1. INTRODUCTION

In revealing analytical properties of the human cochlea tuning and two-tone suppression phenomena play an important role. In the compound action potential (CAP) tuning and suppression can be demonstrated by the use of two-tone masking and three-tone (un)masking paradigms respectively (Eggermont, 1977; Harrison et al., 1981, Harris, 1979). Unmasking in man has also been measured by psychophysical methods (Houtgast, 1974; Shannon, 1976).

CAP unmasking is believed to reflect two-tone rate suppression (Harris, 1979), i.e. the phenomenon that the response of an auditory fibre to an excitatory tone may be reduced by a second tone which itself need to be excitatory. It is one aspect of cochlear non-linear behaviour. Non-linear behaviour is susceptible to cochlear pathology in the animal (Dallos et al., 1980; Robertson et al., 1981; Robertson, 1976; Schmiedt and Zwislocki, 1980; Schmiedt et al., 1980) and in man (Leshowitz and Lindstrom, 1977; Penner, 1980; Smoorenburg, 1972). However, the precise dependence on nature, degree and spatial extent of cochlear injury is complicated, as many animal studies indicate (Dallos et al., 1980; Evans, 1980; Robertson and Johnstone, 1981; Schmiedt and Zwislocki, 1980, Schmiedt et al., 1980). For example, different effects of pathology were reported on low- and high-frequency suppression (low- and high with respect to the characteristic frequency of the fibre) (Dallos et al., 1980; Evans, 1980; Schmiedt and Zwislocki, 1980).

As in the normal animal suppression areas flank the tuning curve above and below CF, the suggestion is raised of a relation between suppression and tuning mechanisms and due to their susceptibility to pathology, also of a correlation with threshold elevation. However, it has been demonstrated that the former supposed relation is not a simple one. For example, near-normal tuning can be found together with reduced high-frequency two-tone rate suppression in cochleas damaged by ototoxic agents, noise or oxigen deficit (Dallos et al., 1980; Robertson and Johnstone, 1981; Evans, 1980).

In this study we address ourselves to the interrelation between CAP unmasking, CAP tuning and CAP threshold in normal and pathological human ears. Part of the material can also be found in Rutten and Kuper, 1982.

2. METHODS AND SUBJECTS

Unmasking and tuning data were collected in addition to a clinical transtympanic electrocochleography (ECoG) test-procedure, in which CAP thresholds in response to short tone bursts (trapezoidal envelope, 2 periods rise and fall time, 4 ms plateau) are measured at frequencies of 0.5, 1, 2, 4 and 8 kHz (Eggermont et al., 1974; Rutten and Kuper, 1982).

In the unmasking experiments a test-tone burst, with the same envelope as given above, with frequency f_T was presented. The level was chosen such that a well defined CAP response was elicited, usually at 10-30 dB above threshold. A second tone burst, the masker, was then added in a forward masking configuration, having the same frequency and (usually) the same intensity (in dB SPL during the plateau) as the test tone. Rise and fall time of the masker burst was 5 ms, the plateau length was 100 ms. Setting the masker level equal to the test tone level resulted usually in a 50% reduction of the test tone response. The test tone started 10 ms after the end of the masker. Repetition rate of the masker test-tone combination is 4/sec. A third tone burst, to be called the suppressor, was presented simultaneously with the masker. The frequency of the suppressor f_s was varied between 250 and 12000 Hz.

its level was fixed 20 dB above the masker level. Usually f_T was set at 3 kHz. We will refer to this type of unmasking experiment as $U(\Delta f)$. Test tone, masker and suppressor were generated and attenuated separately, mixed electrically and delivered to the same free-field exponential horn loudspeaker. There was no phase lock between the three tones.

CAP frequency tuning curves (CAPFTC) were measured using a simultaneous masking paradigm. Test-tone level was adjusted 10–40 dB above CAP threshold, Usually f_T was 2 or 3 kHz. The masker was an independently generated and attenuated continuous sinusoid. Frequency and intensity of the masker were varied. At each masker frequency the masker intensity corresponding to 50% reduction of test tone response amplitude was determined. The 50% point was found by interpolation in a response (linear) versus intensity (logarithmic) plot between at least three data points.

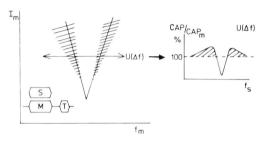

Fig. 1. Left: Schematic plot of tuning curve with flanking suppression areas (hatched). Horizontal arrow indicates how suppression and excitation areas are traversed in a $U(\Delta f)$ experiment, in which only frequency of suppressor f_s varies. In the lower left corner the unmasking paradigm is given, i.e. two simultaneous maskers (masker M and suppressor S) both influence the test tone (T) response in a forward masking configuration

Fig. 1. Right: Schematic qualitative plot of CAP/CAP_m versus f_s, as expected on basis of fig. 1 left. Where the suppressor "crosses" suppression areas, CAP/CAP_m ratios will exceed the 100% reference level, i.e. unmasking is observed (hatched area)

Fig. 1 serves to illustrate schematically how the third tone, the suppressor, "cross-sections" the CAPFTC in an $U(\Delta f)$ experiment. The hatched area in the left part of fig. 1, flanking the CAPFTC indicates the suppression area (Arthur et al., 1971; Harris, 1979; Sachs and Kiang, 1968). It is in this area that we expect the suppressor tone to reduce the masker activity and thus to unmask the test tone response. The right part of fig. 1 sketches the expected course of an $U(\Delta f)$ curve. The hatched area indicates where unmasking is present, i.e. where the CAP response to test plus masker plus suppressor exceeds the CAP_m response to test plus masker alone (the 100% reference level).

Eighteen adult subjects took part in $U(\Delta f)$ (9 subjects) or in the CAPFTC experiments (9 subjects). In two other adult subjects both $U(\Delta f)$ and CAPFTC were measured. In this total of eleven CAPFTC subjects thirteen tuning curves were determined. All subjects were extensively analysed by a conventional audiometric test battery before ECoG. All but two had losses of cochlear origin, two subjects had moderate conduction losses. A majority of the eighteen cochlear loss subjects were diagnosed as Menière patients. However, as we do not know in these and other patients the extent, degree and type of cochlear damage, we shall divide the total group in "normals" and "abnormals" on basis of their CAP "audiograms". "Normals" have an average CAP threshold less than or equal to 25 dB HL. Thus classified, six $U(\Delta f)$ curves belonged to normals, five to abnormals. Seven out of the eleven CAPFTC subjects met the abnormality criterion. CAP thresholds were always within 15 dB equal to pure tone audiometry thresholds.

3. UNMASKING RESULTS

CAP amplitudes obtained from an $U(\Delta f)$ series are plotted in fig. 2 (left part). Amplitudes are expressed as CAP/CAP_m ratios where CAP_m is the response amplitude to test plus masker alone. Values in excess of 100% indicate unmasking (shaded area). Unmasking is clearly to be seen both for $f_s > f_T$ and for $f_s < f_T$, it is maximal (190%) at f_s = 2 kHz. The right part of fig. 2 shows the audiogram of this "normal" subject. The drawn line is the pure tone audiogram, filled circles are the CAP thresholds.

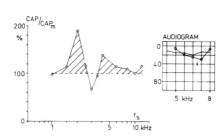

Fig. 2. CAP/CAP$_m$ ratios versus f$_s$ (left). The CAP/CAP$_m$ ratio for the test plus masker alone condition has been chosen as the 100% reference level. Hatched areas indicate unmasking areas. The audiogram is given on the right. Circles denote CAP thresholds; the solid line is the pure-tone subjective audiogram. The plus symbol indicates frequency and level of the test tone. Test tone: 3 kHz, 40 dB HL. Masker: 3 kHz, 40 dB HL; suppressor: 60 dB SPL

Immediate remeasurement of U(Δf) in this and other subjects showed that CAP/CAP$_m$ values could have been changed by at most ± 20%. On the average this intrasubject variation, i.e. the "reproducibility", was about ± 10%.

Although the U(Δf) curve in fig. 2 meets very well our expectations (fig. 1) there are large inter-individual unmasking differences, even in the "normal" group. This is shown in fig. 3 where we plotted U(Δf) curves for six "normals". For better inter-comparison, the horizontal f$_s$ axis has been scaled to the ratio f$_s$/f$_T$. In four cases both low- and high frequency unmasking is present, more or less peaked like the curve of fig. 2. Two subjects show unilateral unmasking. Of these, one subject (drawn curve ——) has only broad, large (maximum 237%) low-f unmasking and a broad sub-reference-level extra masking area. The other curve (—·—·—·) indicates broad, large high-frequency unmasking and almost no sub-reference-level extra masking. Notably in these two unilateral cases, CAP/CAP$_m$ maxima are the highest met across all subjects.

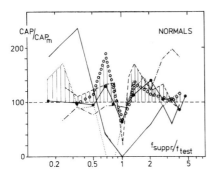

Fig. 3. CAP unmasking in "normals". U(Δf) in six "normal" subjects (mean CAP thresholds less than or equal to 25 dB HL). The suppressor frequency has been scaled by the test tone frequency for better inter-comparison. Four subjects show unmasking for f$_s$/f$_T$ > 1 and f$_s$/f$_T$ < 1, whereas in two subjects unmasking is unilateral (—— and —·—·—·). Vertical hatching indicates unmasking areas across the four "bilateral" subjects

Whereas in the "normal" group the unmasking areas are shaped more or less as expected, in the "abnormal" group (fig. 4) one observes broadening of unmasking. Unmasking is still present at the utmost lowest and/or highest suppressor frequencies. On the contrast, in the "normals" CAP/CAP$_m$ has already returned to about 100% at these extremes (except for the two unilateral cases). However, also in this group, inter-individual differences are large (see also Duifhuis, 1980).

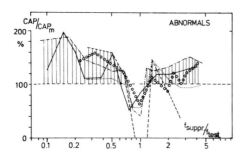

Fig. 4. CAP unmasking in "abnormals" U(Δf) in five "abnormal" subjects (mean CAP thresholds larger than 25 dB HL). As a trend, the subjects show unmasking behaviour up to very low and/or very high f$_s$, in contrast to the "normal" group (except the two unilaterals in fig. 3). Vertical hatching indicates unmasking areas across all five abnormals

In order to detect some correlation with hearing loss we refined our analysis numerically. From the literature the notion appears that non-linear behaviour is reduced by pathology (see Introduction). Taking hearing loss as a gross indicator for pathology one might expect that unmasking will be progressively reduced as a function of increasing hearing loss. One of the determining factors will be the loss at the suppressor frequency. Fig. 5 shows CAP/CAP_m values for each specific f_s versus hearing loss at that specific f_s. As is evident from fig. 5 no correlation can be seen, even not upon considering exclusively the unmasking maxima (filled circles).

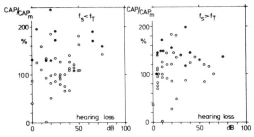

Fig. 5. CAP/CAP$_m$ for specific f$_s$ frequency (from U(Δf) experiments) versus hearing loss at that specific f$_s$. Not included are the f$_s$ = f$_T$ data points.
Left: for frequencies f$_s$ < f$_T$. Unmasking maxima have been drawn as filled circles. Right: as left, but for f$_s$ > f$_T$

4. TUNING RESULTS

With a simultaneous masking technique (see section 2) thirteen 50% iso-reduction curves (CAPFTC's) were determined in eleven subjects. Test-tone frequency was 2 or 3 kHz. In one subject also tuning at 0.5 and 4 kHz was measured. In this paper we focus on the relation between sharpness of tuning Q_{10dB} (i.e. ratio of tip frequency and frequency-width at 10 dB above the tip) and the hearing loss at the tip frequency. Results are shown in fig. 6.

There is a good correlation of Q_{10dB} with hearing losses up to 60 dB. It is tempting to describe the relation by the equation for the regression line (drawn line in fig. 6, correlation coefficient r = 0.93).

$$Q_{10dB} = 8.0 - 0.13 \ L$$

where L is the hearing loss in dB.

It is to be noted that in all thirteen CAPFTC's presented here f_T and tip-frequency coincided within 20%. In CAP tuning work under pathology this is not a very common finding. For example, f_T may differ in some cases from the tip-frequency by one octave or more. In such cases one observes that Q_{10}'s are scattered well beyond the area, confined by the two dashed lines in fig. 6.

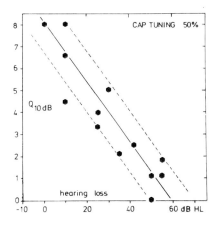

Fig. 6. Quality of tuning Q$_{10dB}$ versus threshold at the tip frequency for thirteen CAPFTC's in eleven subjects. The drawn line is the regression line through all points, except the Q = 4.5/10 dB point. The two dashed lines serve as a guide to the eye

5. DISCUSSION

Unmasking and tuning

It was found in this study that 1) unmasking is not correlated with hearing loss 2) tuning quality is inversely correlated with hearing loss. This seems to point in the direction of a "decoupling" of tuning quality and unmasking (suppression) as it implies no correlation between unmasking and quality of tuning. This becomes still even clearer when performing the experiments, illustrated in fig. 7. In two subjects U(Δf) curves were remeasured after increase of test-tone level (and corresponding increase of masker and suppressor level). The results show an outward shift (referred to CF) of the position of the unmasking areas. This can be understood (see also fig. 1) by assuming 1) that tuning curves shift shape-invariantly, i.e. retaining the same shape in the frequency intensity plane, towards higher level upon increasing the test tone level, and 3) at the same time, the flanking suppression areas do not shift shape-invariantly towards higher levels, but *maintain more or less their absolute position*. These two suppositions being valid, cross-sectioning horizontally the tuning curve at two suppressor levels implies that at the higher level suppression areas will be left and entered at lower and higher frequencies at the low- and high-frequency side of the tuning curve, respectively, compared to the situation at the lower suppressor level. The first supposition seems valid on basis of earlier CAP tuning work (Dallos and Cheatham, 1976) (psychophysically the same was observed by Wightman et al. (1977). We are not aware of reports in the literature about test tone level variation in CAP-unmasking experiments which might offer arguments in favour of or against the second supposition. Thus, our results indicate that in humans CAP suppression areas shift less upward (or not at all) than the CAP tuning does upon increasing the test tone level. Possibly, this means that CAP suppression and tuning measure different aspects of cochlear auditory analysis and will not necessarily be correlated.

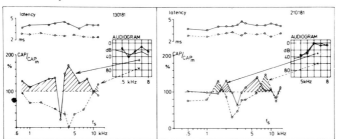

Fig. 7A. As in fig. 2, for two levels of test tone. Solid curves are for the low-level situation (+ symbol in the audiogram, test tone and masker: 3 kHz, 50 dB HL; suppressor: 80 dB SPL). Dashed curves are for the high-level situation (x symbol in the audiogram; test tone and masker: 3 kHz, 75 dB HL; suppressor: 105 dB SPL)

Fig. 7B. As in fig. 7A. Solid curve: low level (test tone and masker: 3 kHz, 30 dB HL; suppressor: 70 dB SPL). Dashed curve: high level (3 kHz, 60 dB HL; suppressor: 90 dB SPL).

In a recent article (Schmiedt, 1981) came independently to the same conclusion. He found single fibre suppression boundaries in the gerbil to be largely independent of the tuning curve, especially below CF. Schmiedt suggests that suppression is a global mechanism, while tuning (being fairly linear as well) is locally determined.

Psychophysical correlates

In two hearing impaired subjects Wightman et al. (1977) observed the absence of unmasking in elevated thresholds regions, accompanied by reduced difference (on the high-frequency side) between forward and simultaneous tuning curves. This leads them to the firm conclusion: the suppression is rendered totally ineffective by the hearing loss", which is obviously in contrast with our CAP findings. Possibly, there are a few reasons why Wightman et al. failed to observe unmasking. For a discussion, we refer to Rutten and Kuper (1982).

Ritsma et al. (1980) investigated psychophysically the relations between hearing loss, tuning quality and maximum word discrimination. They obtained 1) a good correlation between Q_{10} and hearing loss, 2) practically no correlation between Q_{10} and maximal word discrimination. As word discrimination will be dependent (among other factors) on phenomena such as tuning and suppression, we feel that their results are in line with our CAP results.

This work was supported by the Heinsius Houbolt fund and the Dutch Organization for the Advancement of Pure Research (ZWO).

REFERENCES

Arthur, R.M., Pfeiffer, R.R. and Suga, N. (1971). Properties of 'two-tone inhibition' in primary auditory neurones. *J. Physiol.* (London) 212, 593-609.

Dallos, P. and Cheatham, M.A. (1976). Compound action potential (AP) tuning curves. *J. Acoust. Soc. Am.* 59, 591-597.

Dallos, P., Harris, D.M. and Cheatham, M.A. (1980). Two-tone suppression and intermodulation distortion in the cochlea: effect of outer haircell lesions. In: *Psychophysical, Physiological and Behavioural Studies in Hearing*, pp. 242-252. Editors: G. v.d. Brink and F.A. Bilsen. Delft University Press.

Duifhuis, H. (1980). Level effects in psychophysical two-tone suppression. *J. Acoust. Soc. Am.* 67, 914-927.

Eggermont, J.J., Odenthal, D.W., Schmidt, P.H. and Spoor, A. (1974). Electrocochleography. Basic principles and clinical application. *Acta Otolar.* Suppl. 316.

Eggermont, J.J. (1977). Compound action potential tuning curves in normal and pathological human ears. *J. Acoust. Soc. Am.* 62, 1247-1251.

Evans, E.F. (1980). Comment on Dallos et al. (see above).

Harris, D.M. (1979). Action potential suppression, tuning curves and thresholds: comparison with single fiber data. *Hearing Res.* 1, 133-154.

Harrison, R.V., Aran, J.M. and Erre, J.P. (1981). AP tuning curves from normal and pathological human and guinea pig cochleas. *J. Acoust. Soc. Am.* 69, 1374-1385.

Houtgast, T. (1974). Lateral suppression in hearing. *Thesis*, Amsterdam.

Leshowitz, B. and Lindstrom, R. (1977). Measurement of non-linearities in listeners with sensorineural hearing loss. In: *Psychophysics and Physiology of Hearing*, pp. 283-293. Editors: E.F. Evans and J.F. Wilson, Academic Press, London.

Penner, M.J. (1980). Two-tone forward masking patterns and tinnitus. *J. Speech Hearing Res.* 23, 779-786.

Ritsma, R.J., Wit, H.P. and van der Lans, W.P. (1980). Relations between hearing loss, maximal word discrimination score and width of psychophysical tuning curve. In: see under Dallos et al. above in this list, pp. 472-475.

Robertson, D. and Johnstone, B.M (1981): Primary auditory neurons: Non-linear responses altered without changes in sharp tuning. *J.A.S.A.* 69, 1096-1098.

Robertson, D. (1976). Correspondence between sharp tuning and two-tone inhibition in primary auditory neurones. *Nature* (London) 259, 477-478.

Rutten, W.L.C. and Kuper, P. (1982). AP unmasking and AP-tuning in normal and pathologcail human ears. *Hearing Research* 8, 157-178.

Sachs, M.B. and Kiang, N.Y.S. (1968). Two-tone inhibition in auditory nerve fibers. *J. Acoust.Soc. Am.* 43, 1120-1128.

Schmiedt, R.A. and Zwislocki, J.J. (1980). Effects of hair cell lesions on responses of cochlear nerve fibers. II. Single and two-tone intensity functions in relation to tuning curves. *J. Neurophysiol.* 43, 1390-1405.

Schmiedt, R.A., Zwislocki, J.J. and Hamernik, R.P. (1980). Effects of hair cell lesions on responses of cochlear nerve fibres. I. Lesions, tuning curves, two-tone inhibition and responses to trapezoidal wave patterns. *J. Neurophysiol.* 43, 1367-1389.

Schmiedt, R.A. (1982). Boundaries of two-tone rate suppression of cochlear-nerve activity. *Hearing Research* 7, 335-351.

Shannon, R.V. (1976). Two-tone unmasking and suppression in a forward masking situation. *J. Acoust. Soc. Am.* 59, 1460-1470.

Smoorenburg, G.F. (1972). Combination tones and their origin. *J.A.S.A.* 52, 615-632.

Wightman, G., McGee, T. and Kramer, M. (1977). Factors influencing frequency selectivity in normal and hearing impaired listeners. In: see under Leshowith et al. above in this list, pp. 295-308.

GENERAL DISCUSSION

EVANS:
I have similar results from studies mapping two-tone suppression areas in cat cochlear fibres with different types of cochlear pathology e.g. due to anoxia (Evans,
in: Psychophysical, Physiological and Behavioral Studies in Hearing, v. d. Brink
and Bilsen, Eds., Delft, 1980, p. 250) furosemide and local damage. These effects
were studied over a wide range of losses of tuning and CF sensitivity in excess of
40 dB. In these cases, the low frequency two-tone suppression area was surprisingly robust: the high-frequency suppression area shifted upward at about the same
rate as the shift in CF threshold, and may effectively disappear.

HARRISON:
I have previously reported (Harrison et al., JASA 69, 1374, 1981) CAP tuning curve
measures from pathological human and guinea pig cochleas in which two-tone suppression (as estimated from the difference between forward and simultaneous masking curves) is reduced after threshold elevations greater than 50-60 dB, and in
particular in frequency regions above the test frequency. The guinea pigs had
aminoglycoside induced cochlear damage. The patients were of mixed ethiology. Do
you think that your findings of maintained two-tone suppression is restricted to
Ménière's disease?

RUTTEN:
Possibly, our finding of maintained two-tone suppression is indeed restricted to
patients with Ménière symptoms, as our group of patients was rather homogeneous in
this respect. Some findings, reported by Brian Moore during this conference, confirm the presence of suppression in Ménière patients, investigated psychophysically. Future experiments on patients with different ethiology (noise exposure, ototoxic damage) are planned to resolve this issue.

JOHNSTONE:
Some of your results are from measurements with probes at levels near 70 dB. Such
a loud probe may excite a large band of fibres and the results for many subjects
may be critically dependent on the exact level. You may obtain different results
if you change your paradigm to a constant output and vary the input.

RUTTEN:
Your comment pertains to only a small number of the patients (see Rutten and
Kuper, Hear. Res. 8, 157, 1982). Most test-tone probes are near 50 dB. Nevertheless, you are right if you mean that the stimulus parameters should be varied one
by one. In fact, in the above mentioned reference such an attempt was made.

SOME ASPECTS OF SIGNAL PROCESSING IN INDIVIDUALS
WITH RESIDUAL HIGH-FREQUENCY HEARING

Glenis R. Long and John K. Cullen, Jr.

Kresge Hearing Research Laboratory of the South
Department of Otorhinolaryngology, LSU Medical Center
New Orleans, LA 70119, USA

INTRODUCTION

We define residual high-frequency hearing as impairment where pure-tone thresholds in the conventional audiometric frequency range are poor while thresholds for high frequencies are normal or near normal. This type of hearing loss, which has been described by a number of authors (c.f., Böhme, 1978; Osterhammel, 1980; Collins, Cullen and Berlin, 1981) is exemplified by the threshold profiles of Figure 1, shown in contrast to a threshold contour obtained by averaging measures from 6 control listeners. Persons with residual high-frequency hearing generally are bilaterally impaired with histories that indicate their hearing losses existed from birth, or onset at a very young age. What is most remarkable about this group of hearing-impaired individuals is their very good receptive and productive speech capability despite the severity of hearing loss across the range of frequencies one would consider necessary for effective communication.

We have been interested in studying signal processing in persons having residual high-frequency hearing with two broad questions in mind: (1) what are the characteristics of their auditory function that might contribute to their exceptional speech performance, and (2) how good are they at processing high frequency sounds that might be used to advantage in designing hearing aids for these individuals? In this paper, we would like to report on two aspects of signal processing in persons with residual high-frequency hearing central to our two broad questions; first, the degree of frequency resolution obtainable at high frequencies and, secondly, temporal resolution.

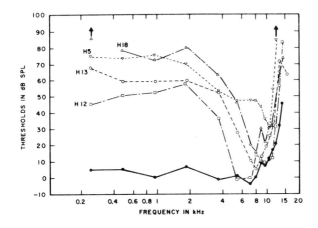

Fig. 1. Threshold profiles from four representative subjects with residual high-frequency hearing contrasted with the mean thresholds of six control subjects (solid line)

We have chosen to measure frequency resolution by estimating difference limens from the detection of frequency modulated sinusoids and by obtaining estimates of "tuning" at high frequencies using a narrowband masking procedure. The frequency modulation detection task was selected to avoid difficulties of "higher-lower" judgments involved in the more conventional estimates of frequency difference limens by comparison of pulsed sine waves of differing frequency. Avoiding these difficulties seemed particularly important since our listeners would be relatively untrained and the pitch quality of signals above 5 kHz (c.f., Ward, 1954; Attneave and Olson, 1978) differs from that of lower frequency signals. The frequency change of a frequency modulated signal are also more analogous to changes in speech and less dependent on sensation level (Zwicker and Feldkeller, 1976). A narrowband masking procedure, using a constant masker, for estimating frequency resolution was selected in favor of the more popular "psychophysical tuning curves" because this procedure eliminates the need for very high intensity maskers. A narrowband noise masker also reduced problems of off-frequency listening and combination-tone detection.

Two tasks were selected to estimate temporal processing: gap detection and "rate-change" detection. Several authors (reviewed in Fitzgibbons and Wightman, 1982; Tyler, Summerfield, Wood, and Fernandes, 1982) have shown that longer time constants are often obtained from persons with more conventional types of sensorineural hearing losses, and Tyler et al. (1982) have shown that this increase correlates with performance on speech discrimination tasks. Gap detection is one of a variety of possible measures of the time constant(s) of the auditory system that may relate to a listener's ability to distinguish between silence- non-silence in speech. The rate-change detection task was selected as a second temporally related measure because we thought that persons with residual high-frequency hearing might be able to use their remaining basal-end fibers to temporally "code" the low frequency characteristics of complex signals.

METHODS

Observations have been obtained from the best ear of nine individuals with residual high-frequency hearing. As we have not yet located a sufficient number of persons with residual high-frequency hearing in the New Orleans region, subjects have been flown to our Laboratory for four-day weekends of testing. We realize that such intensive testing does not provide measures of optimal performance; therefore, we used a similar schedule to test six control subjects whose audiometric thresholds from 0.25-16 kHz are within 10 dB of published norms (c.f., Stelmachowicz, Gorga, and Cullen, 1982).

All testing was done using a computer-controlled, two-interval, forced choice paradigm with immediate feedback. Data were obtained using an adaptive procedure with a 75% criterion (PEST; Taylor and Creelman, 1967) with the exception of the gap detection task. We found that the subjects adapted rapidly to this task and produced stable thresholds. The subjects' task for both threshold and narrowband masking measurements was to determine which interval contained two, 250 msec tone bursts (25-msec rise and decay) separated by 300 msec. The narrowband maskers were 1-sec bursts (25-msec rise and decay) of 100-Hz low pass noise multiplied by the center frequency of the masker. The onset of the first tone followed the onset of the masker by 100 msec so that the tone pulses were centered in the noise. Two masking curves were obtained from each subject -- one at the frequency of best hearing and the other near 4 kHz (i.e., in the region of impaired hearing).

The frequency and rate discrimination measures required the subject to indicate which of two stimuli was changing. In the former, the subject discriminated a 1-sec (25-msec rise and decay) constant-frequency tone from one which was frequency modulated by a 4-Hz sinusoid. Threshold was taken as the rms frequency modulation at threshold to allow for the limited time the tone was at the peak frequencies (Hartman and Klein, 1980). Frequency modulation thresholds were obtained at 40 dB SL at the same two frequencies as the masking functions unless the combination of ear canal resonance and earphone characteristic meant that frequency modulation at these frequencies would be accompanied by significant amplitude modulation. In such cases an adjacent frequency was chosen. Stimuli

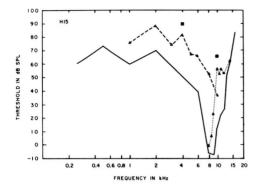

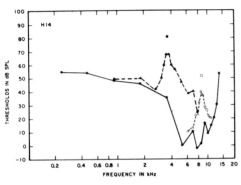

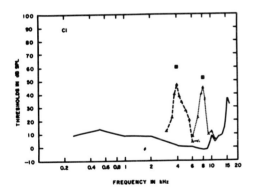

*Fig. 2. Quiet thresholds (solid line)
and masked thresholds (maskers indicated
by squares) for two experimental
subjects (H15, H14) and one control
subject(C1)*

for the rate discrimination task were
1-sec long trains of 30-μsec pulses
high pass filtered at 5 kHz (115
dB/octave, 80 dB rejection ratio)
presented at 79-dB peak sound pressure
level. The subject compared constant
rate stimuli of 50, 100, 200, and 400
Hz with stimuli in which the rate was
incremented in the second 500 msec.
Gap discrimination measures were
obtained using the method of constant
stimuli. The subjects compared a
standard stimulus containing a 0.1-msec
gap in a 65 dB SPL, 5 to 15 kHz band of
noise with stimuli containing gaps of 1
to 16 msec.

Stimuli or maskers were limited to
approximately 90 dB SPL in all
procedures and presentation was via
Koss HV/X earphones. All measures were
referenced to SPL measured by placing a
probe within 3 mm of the tympanic
membrane of each subject (Stelmachowicz
et al., 1982).

RESULTS

Rather than present the narrowband
masking data from all nine subjects
with residual high-frequency hearing
(or average across very disparate
results), we present data from the two
extreme subjects along with
representative data from one control
subject (Fig 2.). All masking
functions obtained at frequencies where
hearing is near normal (8-11 kHz) show
steep, low-frequency slopes and a steep
high-frequency slope where it is not
curtailed by a rapidly increasing
threshold curve (subject H15, Fig. 2).
Q_{10dB} for experimental subjects (except
H15) and control subjects varied
between 7 and 12 at these frequencies,
suggesting normal frequency resolution.
At frequencies within the region of
impaired hearing (3-4kHz), masking
functions from four subjects (H13, H15,
H18, H19) display no true tip and
follow the threshold curve (subject
H15, Fig. 2). One subject (H5) shows
very broad tuning with maximum masking
near the best frequency of the
audiogram, and four subjects (H13, H14,
H16, H17) show broad masking functions
with Q_{10dB} from 2 to 4. The sharpest
tuning can be seen in Fig 2b. Control
subjects display sharp masking
functions with Q_{10dB} of 6 to 8 (Fig.
2c).

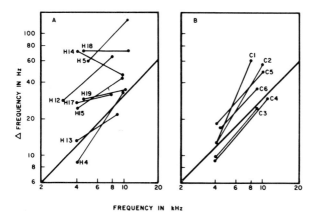

Fig. 3. Frequency modulation detection thresholds as a function of frequency for nine experimental subjects (A) and six control subjects (B). The broad solid line indicates 0.3% discrimination

Frequency-modulation detection thresholds in the control subjects (Fig. 3b) vary somewhat, but in most cases fall near 0.3% at both frequencies, with two subjects showing slightly poorer relative discrimination in the high-frequency region. We see this pattern in only two of the experimental subjects (H12,H14). Three experimental subjects show relative Δfs in the low frequencies that are approximately twice as large as those in the high frequencies. Three subjects (H17,H18,H19) obtain similar absolute Δfs at both frequencies and one subject (H16) gives a larger Δf at 4 kHz than at 10 kHz.

Gap detection thresholds do not appear to differ significantly in the two groups. The 75% correct point on the averaged psychometric function is 2.9 msec for the experimental group and 2.7 msec for the control group.

The residual high-frequency hearing subjects show constant relative rate discrimination near 5% (Fig. 4a) as has been found in other measures of temporal coding (reviewed in Fay, 1982). Our normal hearing subjects do not, however, fit this pattern (Fig. 4b). Three control subjects (C1,C2,C3) perform as expected up to 200 Hz but give a much smaller Δr at 400 Hz. The other three control subjects show either constant Δr or a slight decrease in Δr with increasing frequency. The mean and standard deviation of data from five other subjects (experienced and unexperienced listeners) are also indicated in Fig 4b. All these subjects show a slight decrease in Δr with increasing frequency. The addition of low pass noise (4 kHz cut-off at 40 dB SPL for 3 subjects, and 500 Hz cut-off at 65 dB SPL for two subjects) did not influence the results.

DISCUSSION

Even though persons with residual high-frequency hearing show similar characteristics in terms of threshold profiles, they do not constitute a homogeneous population from the standpoint of auditory-signal processing. This is seen most clearly in the narrowband masking functions. All experimental subjects show sharply defined functions for maskers in the region of good high-frequency hearing. However, this is not the case for low-frequency maskers (i.e., in the frequency region of impaired hearing). Four subjects showed moderate tuning consistent with their elevated thresholds (c.f, Florentine Buus, Scharf, and Zwicker; 1980). Four others showed a broad elevation of threshold with no tuning, indicating little apical cochlear function. One subject (H5) shows broad tuning with a shift in maximum masking toward the frequency of best hearing, suggesting that this individual's total auditory capability is based on the functioning of a very few receptors near the extreme basal end of the cochlea. A similar shift in maximum masking frequency was seen in psychophysical tuning curves obtained in previous testing of this subject.

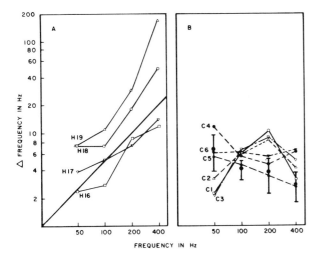

Fig. 4. Rate discrimination thresholds as a function of frequency for 4 experimental subjects (A) and six individual control subjects (B). The means and standard deviation (circles and bars) of five additional normal hearing subjects are also shown. (the broad solid line indicates 5% discrimination)

Frequency difference limens, as measured by frequency modulaton detection indicate two general types of performance. For most of the subjects, relative difference limens for frequency are better in the region of their good high-frequency hearing than in the region of their poorer, low frequency hearing. Three experimental subjects show almost identical absolute frequency difference limens for both high- and low-frequency tones, suggesting identical mechanisms may be involved in frequency discrimination in the two regions. In contrast, control subjects with normal hearing have similar relative frequency difference limens for both high- and low-frequency regions that are close to generally accepted norms. We also note that it is unlikely that the high frequency difference limens for frequency were contaminated by subjects responding to intensity differences (Henning, 1966). Amplitude modulation detection thresholds measured at identical frequencies and sensation level (40 dB) in a separate experiment ranged between 2 and 4 dB -- a larger variation than that of ear canal SPL across the range of frequency change at threshold.

Measures of temporal resolution do not show the diversity of individual performance for the experimental subjects as do the frequency resolution measures. Gap detection appears normal in the experimental subjects. This contrasts with reports of impaired temporal resolution in indiviuals with more conventional hearing losses (reviewed in Fitzgibbon and Wightman, 1982, Tyler et al, 1982), but is consistent with evidence that good temporal resolution is highly frequency dependent (Fitzgibbon and Wightman, 1982; Florentine and Buus, 1982; Tyler et al., 1982).

The rate-change experiment was designed to measure temporal coding of low-frequency information. The performance of the experimental subjects, showing constant relative discrimination, is consistent with previous measures of temporal coding (reviewed in· Fay and Passow, 1982). This contrasts with the performance of our normal hearing subjects who either maintain approximately constant absolute discrimination or show constant relative discrimination to 200 Hz with a reduction in threshold at 400 Hz. We believe that two processes may be operating: one dependent on temporal processing and one on some kind of pitch perception that the subjects with residual high-frequency hearing are not able to use. Experienced listeners report that the higher rates used have a pitch-like quality which differs from that normally associated with the repetition rates used. This "pitch" does not appear to be dependent on frequency components which failed to be eliminated by the 115 dB/octave filter, as addition of low-pass noise does not alter performance.

In summary, the subjects with residual high-frequency hearing we have tested show frequency resolution comparable to normals in their region of good high-frequency hearing. Similarly, their temporal processing is good. These

observations are not sufficient to explain why persons with this type of hearing
loss do so well in speech discrimination. However, their frequency and temporal
resolution do not appear to be limiting factors. Further our data suggest that
mild amplification of high-frequency signal components (to take advantage of the
dynamic range of a region of essentially normal hearing) may prove to be the most
effective approach to aiding individuals with residual high-frequency hearing.

*Acknowledgement. This work was supported in part by NINCDS, NS 11647, Kam's Fund
and the Lions Eye and Ear Foundation of Louisiana.*

REFERENCES

Attneave, F., Olson, R.K. (1971). Pitch as a medium: A new approach to
    psychophysical scaling. *Am. J. Psychol.* 84, 147-166.
Böhme, G. (1978). Hochtonaudiometrie. II. Klinische Ergebnisse. *HNO* 26,
    316-319.
Collins, M.J., Cullen, J.K.,Jr., Berlin, C.I. (1981). Auditory signal processing
    in a hearing impaired subject with residual ultra-audiometric hearing.
    Audiology 20, 347-361.
Fay, R.R. and Passow, B. (1982). Temporal discrimination in the goldfish. *J.
    Acoust. Soc. Am.* 72, 753-760.
Fitzgibbons, P.J., Wightman, F.L. (1982). Gap detection in normal and
    hearing-impaired listeners. *J. Acoust. Soc. Am.* 72, 761-765.
Florentine, M., Buus, S. (1982). Is the detection of a temporal gap frequency
    dependent? *J. Acoust. Soc. Am.* 71, S48.
Florentine, M., Buus, S., Scharf, B., Zwicker, E. (1980). Frequency selectivity in
    normally-hearing and hearing-impaired observers. *J. Speech. Hear. Res.* 23,
    646-669.
Hartman, W.M., Klein, M.A. (1980). Theory of frequency modulation detection for
    low modulation frequencies. *J. Acoust Soc. Am.* 67, 928-934.
Henning, G.B. (1966). Frequency discrimination of random-amplitude tones. *J.
    Acoust. Soc. Am.* 39, 336-339.
Osterhammel, D. (1980). High frequency audiometry. Clinical aspects. *Scand.
    Audiol.* 9, 249-256.
Stelmachowicz, P.G., Gorga, M.P., Cullen, J.K. (1982). A calibration
    procedure for the assessment of thresholds above 8000 Hz. *J. Speech Hear.
    Res.* 25, 618-623.
Taylor, M.M., Creelman, C.D. (1967). PEST: Efficient estimates on probability
    functions. *J. Acoust. Soc. Am.* 41, 782-787.
Tyler, R.S., Summerfield, Q., Wood, E.J., Fernandes, M.A. (1982). Psychoacoustic
    and phonetic temporal processing in normal and hearing-impaired listeners. *J.
    Acoust. Soc. Am.* 72, 740-752.
Ward, W.D. (1954). Subjective musical pitch. *J. Acoust. Soc. Am.* 26, 369-380.
Zwicker, E., Feldkeller, R. (1967). *Das Ohr als Nachrichtenempfänger.* Stuttgart:
    Hirzel-Verlag.

GENERAL DISCUSSION

WILSON:
We have seen one of these "high frequency" subjects (also mentioned after the
paper of Wilson and Sutton, this volume) who came to us as a tinnitus sufferer.
The tinnitus pitches correspond with spontaneous emissions of 8 kHz in both ears.
What was surprising was that we also obtained strong stimulated emissions in this
high frequency region using continuous tone stimulation - a feature that we have
not found in normal hearing subjects. It might be interesting to look for these in
your subjects.

THE RELATIONSHIP BETWEEN PURE-TONE THRESHOLDS AND PSYCHOACOUSTICAL TUNING CURVES
IN THE HEARING IMPAIRED: PRELIMINARY FINDINGS

Richard S. Tyler, Susan J. Holland, Lee A. Harker and Bruce J. Gantz

Department of Otolaryngology - Head and Neck Surgery
University Hospitals
Iowa City, Iowa 52242 USA

Physiological evidence from many studies has infered a close correspondence
between elevated thresholds and a reduction in frequency resolution. Data to support such a relationship is of three types. First, animals with an induced threshold loss exhibit broadened frequency threshold (tuning) curves (FTC) compared to
other animals with normal hearing (e.g. Kiang, Moxon and Levine, 1970). Second,
FTCs measured in auditory nerve fibers show elevated thresholds and broadened
FTCs after cochlear insult (e.g. ototoxicity, noise exposure, mechanical damage)
compared to other nerve fibers recorded from the same animal but before the insult
(e.g. Evans et al.1974). Third, measurements within single fibres have been obtained before and after cochlear insult (e.g. Evans and Klinke, 1974, 1982 a,b;
Robertson and Manley, 1974). The results showed elevated thresholds and broadened
FTCs.

Psychoacoustical studies show less consistency between thresholds and frequency resolution. First, hearing-impaired subjects often display reduced frequency
resolution that accompanies their threshold elevation compared to other normal
subjects (e.g. Pick et al.1977; Tyler, Wood and Fernandes, 1982a). However, exceptions have been observed. For example, Tyler, Fernandes and Wood (1982b) noted
that some hearing-impaired listeners had abnormally large critical ratios in regions of near-normal thresholds. Second, psychoacoustical tuning curves (PTCs)
(Small, 1959; Zwicker, 1974) typically show normal PTCs in regions of normal thresholds but broadened PTCs in regions of elevated thresholds measured in the same
hearing-impaired listeners. However, Tyler, Fernandes and Wood (1980) and Hoekstra
(1981) have noted abnormal frequency resolution in regions of normal thresholds
in hearing-impaired listeners. Third, Pick and Evans (1980) have observed poor
frequency resolution in listeners with normal thresholds between 500-8000 Hz but
poor speech understanding.

In the present report we provide further psychoacoustical evidence that dis-
associates thresholds from PTCs. We present data of three different types. First,
we measured PTCs from regions of near-normal thresholds from the two ears of a
person with a unilateral high-frequency hearing loss. Although thresholds are about
the same at the low-frequency signal frequency, the two PTCs are markedly different.
Second, we show that the drug urea (used like glycerol to reduce endolymphatic hydrops) can produce changes in PTCs without changes in thresholds. Third, we present
data from a patient with active Ménière's syndrome who showed dramatic differences
in PTCs obtained on two separate occasions, which were accompanied by only minimal
changes in thresholds.

1. METHOD

Audiograms were obtained with a 5 dB step size using the procedure recommended
by ASHA. Signal thresholds were remeasured with a 2 dB step size and the signal was
then presented at 10 dB sensation level (SL) and successively pulsed (500 ms duration, 50% duty cycle). PTCs at 500 and 4000 Hz were measured with an ascending method of limits with a 2 dB step size. The level of a continuous pure-tone masker
was slowly increased by the tester until the subject reported that the pulsed signal was no longer audible. 3 replications per condition were obtained which were
typically within 2 - 4 dB of each other. The order of masker frequencies was randomized. For the 500 Hz signal, masker frequencies were 215, 390, 460, 500, 540,
615 and 740 Hz. For the

4000-Hz signal, masker frequencies were 1720, 3120, 3680, 4000, 4320, 4920 and 5920
Hz (after Florentine et al. 1980). Stimulus frequencies were set within 0.5%. The
masker was produced by a Hewlett-Packard 200CD oscillator which was mixed with a
pure tone from a Grason-Stadler 1701 audiometer. The audiometer was used to pulse
the signal, to mix the stimuli, and to control stimulus levels.

2. RESULTS

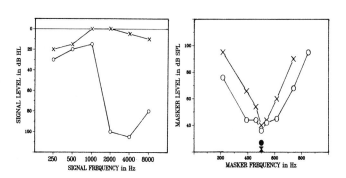

*Figure 1. Subject A.
LEFT: Audiograms
showing absolute
thresholds in left
(crosses) & right
(circles) ears. Non-
test ear masking was
used when appropri-
ate. RIGHT: PTCs
measured at 500 Hz in
the left & right
ears. Filled symbols
here & elsewhere
represent signal
thresholds.*

A. Difference in PTCs between ears. Subject A had a high-frequency hearing loss in
one ear, but near-normal thresholds in the other ear (see Figure 1). The etiology of
this patients' hearing loss is unknown. He has some retrocochlear signs (pronounced tone
decay, absent early and middle latency evoked potentials) in the affected ear, but a
normal bilateral pneumocisternogram. The internal auditory canals appeared relatively
narrow. Notably, this patient has no speech understanding in his impaired ear, despite
near-normal thresholds up to and including 1000 Hz.

Counter to the similar near-normal thresholds in the low-freqeuncy region of the
two ears, the PTC is much broader in the ear with the high-frequency hearing loss.
Similar masker levels in the two ears are required near the signal frequency, but in the
impaired ear lower masker levels are required remote from the signal. Although the
low-frequency thresholds have not been greatly affected by the hearing loss in the
impaired ear, frequency resolution has been reduced. It may be that the abnormal high-
frequency regions can remotely influence freqeuncy resolution at 500 Hz. Alternatively,
there may be physiological abnormalities in the region of 500 Hz that are revealed by
frequency resolution but not by threshold measurements. If frequency resolution is a
precursor to threshold loss in some cases, then this could be used clinically to monitor
the administation of ototoxic drugs, or as a sensitive index to noise exposure (see Humes,
1980).

B. Pre- and Post-administration of Urea. We have also tested two subjects originally
suspected of Ménières disease. PTCs were obtained before and after the oral
administration of urea. As with glycerol, urea is thought to reduce the abnormally high
amount of endolymph surrounding the cochlear partition (e.g. McCabe and Wolsk, 1961;
Babin and Bumsted, 1980).

Subject B had a sudden onset of hearing loss in the left ear (right ear normal).
The etiology is uncertain but is probably not Ménières disease (no tinnitus or dizziness).
Figure 2 shows audiograms and PTCs obtained before and after a 20 mg oral ingestion
of urea. Although the audiograms and speech intelligibility (100 % on W-22s) show
virtually no differences, there are some notable changes in the PTCs. At 500 Hz, the
post-urea PTC required different masker levels to mask the signal at two masker
frequencies compared to the pre-urea PTC.

At 4000 Hz, the changes are more dramatic. The post-urea PTC required lower masker levels on both the low- and high-frequency slope compared to the pre-urea PTC. In the other (normal) ear, signal thresholds were 5 dB different in the pre- and post-urea conditions, and small (0-10 dB) unsystematic changes were seen in the masker levels that did not alter the PTC shape.

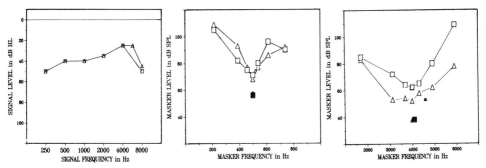

Figure 2. Subject B. LEFT: Audiograms obtained before (squares) and after (triangles) adminstration of urea. CENTER: PTCs at 500 Hz. RIGHT: PTCs at 4000 Hz.

Subject C, also suspected of having Ménières disease, had a unilateral hearing loss for about 4 years which was accompanied with vertigo and nausea. He was tested three times; one week before the urea tests, and the pre- and post-urea tests. Speech intelligibility scores (W-22s) on the three successive tests were 84, 100 and 100%. In Figure 3 compare the initial test results to the pre-urea tests, taken one week apart. The signal threshold at 500 Hz has decreased by 10 dB and the pre-urea PTC requires lower masker levels. The high-freqeuncy region of the audiogram shows minimal threshold changes, but the high-frequency side of the PTC requires lower masker levels. It is much broader and has a minimum at a higher frequency. These changes reflect fluctuations in the hearing loss over a one week interval.

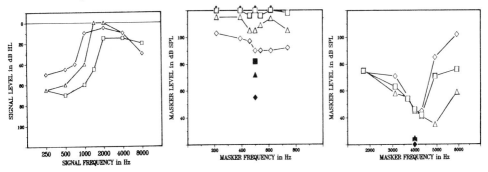

Figure 3. Subject C. LEFT: Initial audiogram (squares), and audiograms taken before (triangles) and after (diamonds) administration of urea (the latter two taken 1 week after the initial test). MIDDLE: 500-Hz PTCs. LEFT: 4000-Hz PTCs.

Now compare the pre- and post-urea results. In the low-freqeuncy region the audiogram shows 15-30 dB improvement in thresholds. What was a W-shaped PTC in the pre-urea test has become a flat PTC in the post-urea test. In the high-frequency region there are minimal changes in threshold, but greater masker levels are required in the PTC, particularly on the high-frequency slope.

Thus, in subject C the administration of urea did not markedly change thresholds at 4000 Hz, but higher masker levels on the high-frequency PTC slope were observed which resulted in a sharpening of the high-frequency PTC slope. Recall in subject B the post-urea 4000 Hz PTC showed a decrease in the masker level. Therefore, our preliminary experience with urea suggests that frequency resolution can be altered without changes in threshold, but the direction of the change in frequency resolution is unclear.

C. Changes in PTCs over time.   We have also measured PTCs in another subject (D) with fluctuating thresholds and Ménières syndrome. He had a bilateral high-frequency hearing loss which was accompanied by a feeling of fullness in the ears, vertigo and nausea. He was seen on two occasions, with about 1 month between visits. Speech intelligibility was near 100 % on both occasions.

Figure 4 shows the results. On his first visit he had flat PTCs at both 500 and 4000 Hz. On his second visit, his audiogram had not changed, but dramatic changes were observed in the PTCs. At 500 Hz, the PTC had become very sharply tuned, and the frequency resolution at 4000 Hz had also improved. Similar results were obtained for the other ear.

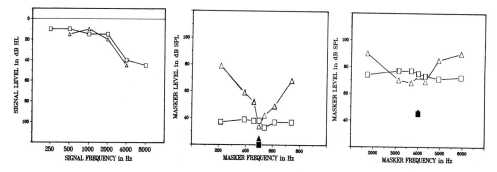

Fig. 4. Subject D. LEFT: Audiograms for right ear taken initially (squares) and then one month later (triangles). MIDDLE: 500 Hz PTCs. RIGHT: 4000 Hz PTCs.

In both subjects C (initial visit compared to pre-urea) and D we noted changes in PTCs obtained at different sessions, while signal thresholds in the frequency region of the PTC were unchanged. In subject C, thresholds were changing in other frequency regions, but in subject D thresholds throughout the audiometric range were stable. It appears that fluctuating hearing loss can manifest itself in fluctuations in frequency resolution and not exclusively in fluctuations in threshold.

3. DISCUSSION

Our results suggest that frequency resolution can be impaired in regions of normal sensitivity. While direct comparisons between PTCs and FTCs are not possible (PTCs represent the responses of many fibers, and are influenced by beats, suppression, combination-tones, and shifting of the auditory filter; e.g. Small and Tyler, 1978; Patterson and Nimmo-Smith, 1980), there is qualitative and quantitative evidence to suggest that both reflect some common sources of peripheral frequency resolution (e.g. Pickles, 1977). Although our comparison of PTCs within subjects would reduce the role of central decision factors, it is know that combination tones (e.g. Smoorenborg, 1972), suppression (e.g. Dallos et al., 1980) and temporal resolution (and therefore possibly beat detection; e.g. Tyler, Summerfield, Wood and Fernandes, 1982) are affected by hearing loss. Although our changes in PTCs may be influenced by these factors, the reason for lack of correspondence between PTCs and FTCs in impaired ears remains unclear.

There is some physiological evidence that does not show a close correspondence between FTCs and thresholds. Dallos and Harris (1978) found that most nerve fibers recorded from regions of threshold loss and outer hair cell damage showed elevated thresholds but approximately normal, sharp FTC tip segments. However, this disassociation is in the opposite direction of what we have reported here. More recently, Harrison and Aran (1982) have observed abnormal high-frequency whole-nerve action potential tuning curves, with normal thresholds in two patients with Ménières syndrome. It is perhaps relevant that others have noted changes in two-tone suppression and distortion-product responses in nerve fibers without changes in FTCs (e.g. Dallos et al., 1980; Robertson and Johnstone, 1981). Our psychoacoustical data provide preliminary evidence that suggests a disassociation between frequency resolution and thresholds in some patients with hearing impairment.

Our preliminary experience with urea is equivocal. Urea might be expected to reduce endolymphatic hydrops and therefore improve frequency resolution. This was observed in Subject C. Subject B, however, showed a *decrease* in the sharpness of the 4000-Hz PTC post-urea. However it is likely Patient B did *not* have endolymphatic hydrops. The urea may have created an abnormal decrease in endolymphatic fluid, or may have created an electrolyte imbalance. We are continuing our investigation on the effects or urea.

In mechanical models of the cochlea, Tonndorf (1957, 1976) noted that increased fluid in the "endolymph" (intended to model properties of Ménières disease) created a bulging in the "basilar membrane" that decreased sensitivity, shifted the envelope of the displacement pattern proximally, and made the displacement pattern asymmetrical. These data support the notion of a change in frequency resolution due to changes in the mechanical properties of the travelling wave that accompany endolymphatic hydrops.

ACKNOWLEDGMENTS. We wish to thank Paul Abbas for his comments and Julie Hanger for her typing.

REFERENCES

Babin, R.W. and Bumsted, R.M. (1980). Urea test and vestibular dysfunction in suspected Ménière's disease. *Journal of Otolaryngol.* 9, 201-206.
Dallos, P. and Harris, D. (1978). Properties of auditory nerve responses in absence of outer hair cells. *J. of Neurophysiology* 41, 365-383.
Dallos, P., Harris, D.M., Relkin, E. and Cheatham, M.A. (1980). Two-tone suppression and intermodulation distortion in the cochlea: effect of outer hair cell lesions. In: *Psychophysical, Physiological and Behavioural Studies in Hearing.* (G. van den Brink and F.A. Bilsen, eds.) Noordwijkerhout, Delft University Press.
Evans, E.F. (1974). The effects of hypoxia on the tuning of single cochlear nerve fibres. *Journal Physiol.* 238, 65-67.
Evans, E.F. and Klinke, R. (1974). Reversable effects of Cyanide and Furosemide on the tuning of single cochlea fibres. *J. Physiol.* 242, 129-131.
Evans, E.F. and Klinke, R. (1982a). The Effects of Intracochlear Cyanide and Tetrodotoxin on the Properties of Single Cochlear Nerve Fibres in the Cat. *J. Physiol.* 331, 385-408.
Evans, E.F. and Klinke, R. (1982b). The Effects of Intracochlear and Systemic Furosemide on the Properties of Single Cochlear Nerve Fibres in the Cat. *J. Physiol.* 331, 409-427.
Florentine, M., Buss, S., Scharf, B. and Zwicker, E.(1980). Frequency selectivity in normally-hearing and hearing-impaired observers. *J. Speech and Hearing Res.* 23, 646-669.
Harrison, R.V. and Aran, J.-M. (1982). Electrocochleographic measures of frequency selectivity in human deafness. *Brit. J. Aud.* 16, 179-188.
Hoekstra, A. (1981). Frequency discrimination and frequency analysis in hearing. Unpublished doctoral dissertation.
Humes, L.E. (1980). Susceptibility to TTS: A review of recent developments. *ASHA Reports* 10, 77-85.
Kiang, N.Y.S., Moxon, E.C. and Levine, R.A. (1970). Auditory-nerve activity in cats with normal and abnormal cochleae. In: *Sensorineural Hearing Loss* (G.E.W. Wolstenholme and J.E.A. Knight, eds). London, Churchill.
McCabe, B. and Wolsk, J. (1961). Experimental inner ear pressure changes. *Ann. Otolaryng.* 70, 541-555.

Patterson, R.D. and Nimmo-Smith, I. (1980). Off-frequency listening and auditory-filter asymmetry. *J. Acoust. Soc. Am.* 67, 229-245.

Pick, G.F., Evans, E.F. and Wilson, J.P. (1977). Frequency resolution in patients with hearing loss of cochlear origin. In: *Psychophysic and Physiology of Hearing.* (E.F. Evans and J.P. Wilson, eds.). London, Academic Press.

Pick, G.F. and Evans, E.F. (1980). Frequency resolution in patients with difficulty in speech perception but with normal audiogram. Paper presented at the meeting of The British Society of Audiology, Nottingham, 7-8 July.

Pickles, J.O. (1977). Neural correlates of the masked threshold. In: *Psychophysics and Physiology of Hearing.* (E.F. Evans and J.P. Wilson, eds.). London, Academic Press Inc., Ltd.

Robertson, D. and Manley, G.A. (1974). Manipulation of frequency analysis in the cochlea ganglion of the guinea pig. *J. Comp. Physiol.* 91, 363-375.

Robertson, D. and Johnstone, B.M. (1980). Primary auditory neurons: nonlinear responses altered without changes in sharp tuning. *J. Acoust. Soc. Am.* 69, 1096-1098.

Smoorenburg, G.F. (1972). Combination tones and their origin. *J. Acoust. Soc. Am.* 52, 615-632.

Small, A.M. (1959). Pure-tone masking. *J. Acoust. Soc. Am.* 31, 1619-1625.

Small, A.M. and Tyler, R.S. (1978). Additive masking effects of noise bands of different levels. *J. Acoust. Soc. Am.* 63, 894-904.

Tonndorf, J. (1957). The mechanism of hearing loss in early cases of endolymphatic hydrops. *Annals of Oto.Rhino and Laryng.* 66, 766.

Tonndorf, J. (1976). Endolymphatic hydrops: mechanical causes of hearing loss. *Arch. Oto-Rhino Laryng.* 212, 293-299.

Tyler, R.S., Fernandes, M. and Wood, E.J. (1980). Masking, temporal integration and speech intelligibility in listeners with noise-induced hearing loss. In: *Disorder of Auditory Function III.* I. Taylor and A. Markides, eds). London, Academic Press.

Tyler, R.S., Wood, E.J. and Fernandes, M. (1982). Frequency resolution and hearing loss. *Brit. J. of Audiology* 16, 45-63.

Tyler, R.S., Fernandes, M. and Wood, E.J. (1982) Masking of pure tones by broadband noise in cochlear pathology. *J. Speech Hearing Res.* 25, 117-124.

Tyler, R.S., Summerfield, Q., Wood, E.J. and Fernandes, M.A. (1982). Psychoacoustic and phonetic temporal processing in normal and hearing-impaired listeners. *J. Acoust. Soc. Am.* 72, 740-752.

Zwicker, E. (1974). On a psychoacoustical equivalent of tuning curves. In: *Facts and Models in Hearing.* (E. Zwicker and E. Terhardt, eds). Berlin, Springer-Verlag.

GENERAL DISCUSSION

TEN KATE:
Do you think that remote masking (interference effect in microphonics) cause the broad bandwidth of the PTC in Fig. 1 from the right ear of subject A? May a non-simultaneous masking procedure reveal whether the distortion waves from clipping in the high-frequency region were present or not?

TYLER:
I do not know how the effects you mention contribute to these results. When I suggested remote effects from the high-frequency region, I was thinking of some changes (perhaps in an active mechanism) which would alter some aspect of travelling wave motion.

HORST:
Do you have any reports about subjective changes? Is there any indication that in those cases where tuning was improved, the speech perception was also improved?

TYLER:
Our subjects with fluctuating hearing loss report subjective changes but we didn't see the patients frequently enough to compare these to objective measurements. We did not notice changes in our word intelligibility test in quiet.

VERSCHUURE:
1) Patients sometimes do not understand what one expects them to do. Did you check their performance and did you assess the reliability of the adjustments? 2) You mentioned that you were aware of problems such as combination tones etc. Did you ask the patients for their observations of combination tones, beats etc., and did you try to include these effects by the use of masking noise band?

TYLER:
1) Masker frequencies were chosen randomly with three replications, and all three masker levels for each condition were usually within 2-4 dB. Subject B had normal PTCs in the opposite ear which virtually overlapped before and after urea. 2) We did not ask the patients for their subjective impression of the quality of the stimulus. These tests were obtained in the clinic and we did not have the capability of doing forward masking or introducing noise bands at that time.

JOHNSTONE:
It appears that simultaneous masking PTC's are defining the two-tone suppression bounderies. Our basilar membrane measurements indicate that suppression is a function of basilar membrane displacement. Thus in hydrops the basilar membrane is presumably somewhat displaced and hence partial suppression is already present. This would lead to a spread of the inhibitory sidebands and so a flatter PTC. Urea by reducing the hydrops and so the "static masking", would give a sharper PTC. However, a mixed pathology could give a confusing picture.

FESTEN:
The dissociation between frequency resolution and hearing loss demonstrated here for 4 subjects, and also dealt with by Pick and Evans (this volume), is in close agreement with recently published data on 22 sensorineurally hearing-impaired subjects (Festen and Plomp, J.A.S.A. 73, 652, 1983). In a study on relations among auditory functions we applied a battery of tests focused on the 1000-Hz frequency region. Apart from the audiogram we selected tests on frequency resolution measured in simultaneous and in nonsimultaneous masking, on temporal resolution, and on speech perception. In a principal-components analysis on the matrix of correlations it appeared that tests on frequency resolution form a cluster closely related to hearing loss for speech in noise and approximately independent of audiometric loss.

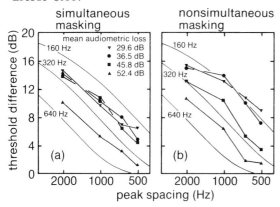

Threshold-level difference between peak and trough of comb-filtered noise (20 dB modulation, 1000 Hz probe tone). Subjects (5 or 6 resp.) divided in four subgroups on the basis of their mean loss. Smooth curves: calculated threshold difference for a Gaussian-shaped filter.

However, as the fig. shows, for frequency resolution measured in non-simultaneous masking the situation is different. While in simultaneous masking there is no relation with audiometric loss, in nonsimultaneous masking the correlation coefficient is o.71. Moreover, in contrast to normal hearing where bandwidths for the two masking paradigms differ by almost a factor of 2 due to lateral suppression (Houtgast, Dissertation, 1974), this difference is much smaller for our hearing-impaired group. As this indicates reduced lateral supression with hearing loss (cf. Wightman et al. in: Psychophysics and Physiology of Hearing, Evans and Wilson, Eds., London, 1977, pp 295 - 306; Leshowitz and Lindstrom, ibid. pp 283 - 292; Dallos et al. in: Psychophysical, Physiological and Behavioural Studies in Hearing, v.d.Brink and Bilsen, Eds., Delft 1980, pp 242 - 249), it is obvious to presume the same origin for the correlation between hearing loss and frequency resolution in nonsimultaneous masking. These conclusions, however are in disagreement with CAP measurements by Rutten (this volume).

TYLER:
Although we show exceptions here, our general experience is that threshold elevations correlate with poor frequency resolution. Your lack of correlation using
simultaneous masking is surprising. Since your frequency resolution results are
presumably obtained with the auditory filter <u>centered</u> at the 1000-Hz place, it
seems appropriate to relate this to the threshold loss at the 1000-Hz place not
the average audiometric loss.

HARRISON:

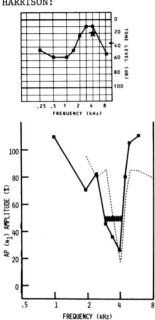

I have made physiological measures of cochlear frequency selectivity from the CAP (using a two-tone
suppression paradigm: Harrison and Aran, British J.
Audiol. <u>16</u>, 179, 1982) in Ménière's patients before
and up to two hours after administration of glycerol.
This is, like urea, an hyperosmotic agent assumed to
modify the putative endolymphatic hydrops. In 5 patients, an improvement in frequency selectivity, by
a factor of 1.5 - 2.5, was observed. In two subjects
there was a deterioration. In 3 subjects there were
no significant changes. The changes that I observe
occur about 30 mins. after glycerol. What is the
time course of changes in your observations?
In the figure, the pre-glycerol CAP iso-intensity
suppression curve is shown by the continuous curve.
The bandwidth measure at 50% CAP suppression is 0.5
oct. The dashed curve was obtained 65 mins. after
oral glycerol. Bandwidth has narrowed to 0.33 oct.
No changes in CAP threshold occurred at 4 kHz. The
4 kHz test tone level is shown by the star symbol in
the audiogram. Suppression tone level is indicated
by the arrow on the right ordinate.

TYLER:
We have not yet followed the time course of this effect. Our measurements were
made about 3 - 6 hours after the drug administration.

RUTTEN:
We occasionally observed on CAP-tuning curves, obtained by forward masking, bad
quality of tuning, while CAP thresholds were normal. Also, pure tone thresholds
and speech audiograms were normal.

EVANS:
Similar physiological evidence of dissociations between tuning and threshold have
been reported by Comis et al.(Bumetanide poisoning, Scand.Audiol.Suppl.<u>14</u>,85,1981).

PICKLES:
I was interested to see your results in Fig. 1 because I often see exactly similar
effects in guinea pig auditory nerve fibres. (i) A small, 10 dB or less increase
in threshold at the tip of the FTC, (ii) a widening of the FTC on the lower side,
and (iii) I have the impression that such fibres are mainly seen when the cochlea
is in the process of deterioration, (e.g. due to hypoxia) and a hearing loss is
sweeping down from the high frequency end, but thresholds in the FTC region are
still unaffected.

TYLER:
Subject A did have a progressive threshold loss from high to low frequencies.

DISSOCIATION BETWEEN FREQUENCY RESOLUTION
AND HEARING THRESHOLD

G.F. Pick[*] and E.F. Evans[**]

Department of Postgraduate Medicine[*]*, and*[**]
Department of Communication and Neuroscience[**]*,*
University of Keele, Keele, Staffordshire, ST5 5BG, U.K.

1. INTRODUCTION

In measurements of the frequency threshold curves (FTCs) of single cochlear-nerve fibres in animal with acute pathological conditions of the cochlea deter-ioration in the FTC bandwidth is generally directly related to CF-threshold elev-ation (e.g. Evans, 1975). Our early studies of such changes in chronic pathol-ogical conditions (kanamycin poisoning), however, suggested that on occasion, deterioration in tuning bandwidth could occur without substantial change in threshold. In our own psychoacoustical investigations, and those of others, on patients with hearing loss of cochlear origin, substantial deviations from this direct relationship have also been found. In these latter studies, although im-paired frequency resolution *is* correlated with absolute threshold elevation, most studies report correlation coefficients in the range 0.4 to 0.8 (e.g. Pick *et al.*, 1977, Dreschler, 1980, Ritsma *et al.*, 1980, and Tyler *et al.*, 1982). It would seem that not all of this variance can be ascribed to poor experimental design. This belief is substantiated by two additional observations: a) Pick (1980a) reported evidence which suggested that poor frequency resolution can be dissoc-iated from threshold in TTS, and b) more recently, clear physiological evidence has been obtained that FTC bandwidths in guinea pig can be impaired, without substantial elevation of threshold, after chronic or acute administration of oto-toxic diuretics (Pratt and Comis, 1982, and Comis *et al.*, 1981).

In the present clinical study, we have specifically sought for cases of im-paired frequency resolution dissociated from elevation in threshold. We have chosen the small group of patients who complain of difficulty in understanding speech in noisy environments, but who proved to have normal audiometric thresh-olds. In these cases it was not possible to attribute the cause to psychological or central, neurological problems. Our aim was to investigate whether these pat-ients, for whom there was no reasonable explanation for their hearing difficulty, suffered from impaired frequency resolution.

2. PATIENT SELECTION

Eleven members of the Midlands Otological Society agreed to select patients for us. They sent us copies of relevant medical-test results, and if we consid-ered them to be suitable we invited the patient to take part in our study (travel and meal expenses were paid). Of the 17 patients that we have tested, one showed clearly different symptoms and results. Her hearing was impaired, subjectively and objectively, by sounds at frequencies below 100 Hz. Her results have been excluded from this study. After obtaining a relevant medical history from the patients, detailed pure-tone audiograms were obtained (Bekesy-tracking, contin-uous-frequency 0.1 to 10 kHz in 10 minutes). The results of these preliminary investigations were used as a basis for selection of ear and frequency for subsequent testing. Frequency resolution was measured using gated tones and a simultaneous comb-filtered noise (CFN) masker as described by Pick *et al.* (1977) and Pick (1980b). The effective bandwidth of the auditory filter at the tone frequency was derived from an integral transform of the function describing the progressive reduction in the resolution of the gated tone in the presence of CFN as a function of successively higher relative peak density (examples of this

function are shown in Fig. 1). When time allowed, frequency resolution was
tested in both ears. In most cases frequency resolution was tested in one ear at
1 and 4 kHz, using a 25-40 dB SPL spectrum-level, CFN masker. Speech perception
for two subjects was measured using free-response taped word lists (Boothroyd,
1967), in quiet and in the presence of a white-noise masker. In an attempt to
improve precision the remaining patients were tested using a two-alternative,
forced-choice consonant test (Grose and Pick, 1977) aimed specifically at detect-
ing consonant confusions common in patients with cochlear losses. For these
tests, the competing noise was provided by a six-speaker babble at 87 dB SPL.
The aim of these tests was to determine the level at which 75% of consonant
choices were correctly reported. In some cases, it was not always possible accurately to specify this level, and results from such patients have been excluded
from the analysis.

3. THE PATIENTS

Frequency resolution was measured in 22 ears from 16 patients. The patients
were within the age range 18-39 years (10 male, 6 female). All but one patient
are native English speakers. MK is Turkish, but speaks fluent English (he is a
postgraduate student).

4. RESULTS

a) *Medical History*
There was no indication of a common history of hearing pathology, and no abnormal familial hearing problems. The only factor which was revealed was that
eleven patients had received regular exposure to moderate or fairly high levels
of noise during the period that they noticed that their hearing had deteriorated.
Most commonly, this arose from regular attendance (once or more a week) at rock
concerts or discos (MA, DC, SI, SK, MM, RS, BW). Other reported noise exposures
were of industrial origin (FK - tile making, and EM - auto assembly), shooting
(MA, SI, BW), or drag racing (JH). SF suffered a hemorrhaged tympanic membrane
after exposure to a low-frequency pressure wave. Often, post-exposure TTS and/or
tinnitus had been noticed. All felt that their ability to understand speech,
especially in noisy surroundings, had deteriorated over a period of several
months.

b) *Audiograms*
Typical results are illustrated in Fig. 1. In general the continuous-
frequency audiograms were within normal limits, although high-frequency notches
were often apparent. Three patients had rather deeper notches: MA (40 dB HL),
PA (35 dB HL), and JP (40 dB HL), centred at 2.8, 5.0, and 5.4 kHz respectively.
The patient population could not be differentiated statistically from normal on
the basis of their audiograms (e.g. at 1 kHz: mean HL = 2.1 dB, s.e. = 1.1 dB,
at 4 kHz: mean HL = 6.3 dB, s.e. = 2.5 dB).

c) *Frequency Resolution*
The derived frequency-resolution bandwidths are summarised in Fig. 2. The
mean of the effective bandwidths was significantly worse than normal at 4 kHz
(t = 3.11, df = 30), but not at 1 kHz (t = 0.07, df = 30). Variations in threshold could not statistically account for the variance in frequency-resolution
bandwidth (e.g. at 1 kHz: F = 2.11, df = 1,19; at 4 kHz: F = 0.76, df = 1,19).

d) *Speech perception in quiet*
Speech perception results are summarised in Fig. 3. Speech perception in
quiet was significantly[1] worse than normal (t = 2.23, df = 33). A number of

---

1 *The threshold for statistical significance is the 5% level. The statistical
modelling should be interpreted with caution, however, as in most models, one
dependent variable is used to attempt to explain variance in another dependent
variable.*

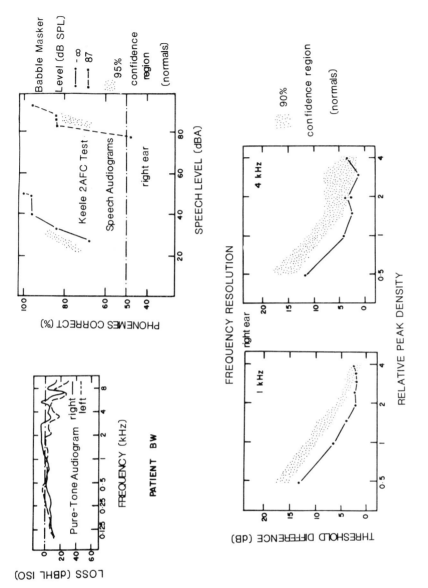

Fig. 1. Results from patient BW. Top-left: smoothed-tracing from the Bekesy-tracking audiogram. Top-right: speech audiograms in quiet and noise background. Bottom: frequency-resolution function

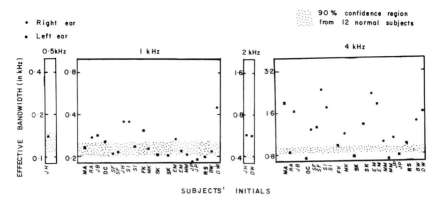

<u>Fig. 2.</u> *Frequency resolution bandwidth from all patients in comparison with the*
normal range

parameters were used in an attempt to model the variance in the speech measures,
either singly, or in justifiable combinations using a generalised, linear, statistical model (Nelder and Wedderburn, 1972). These parameters were:
    Threshold at 1 and 4 kHz (T1, and T4);
    Frequency-resolution at 1 and 4 kHz (BW1 and BW4);
    Logarithm of BW1 and BW4 (LBW1 and LBW4);
    Slope of frequency-resolution function (as in Fig. 1) at 1 and 4 kHz (SL1
    and SL4);
    Intercept of frequency-resolution function with 0 dB at 1 and 4 kHz (IN1 and
    IN4).
The only parameter to make a significant contribution to the reduction of variance was T4 (F = 6.9, df = 1,13). However, if only patients with a history of
noise exposure were included in the model, then BW4 became a very significant
parameter (F = 14.1, df = 1,8 - the only parameter to reach the 1% significance
level).

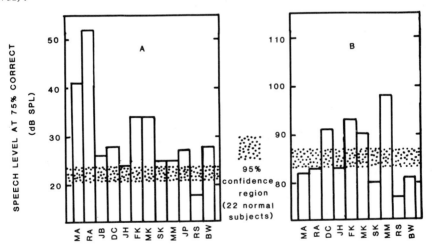

<u>Fig. 3.</u> *Speech reception threshold in quiet and noise, in comparison with*
normal range

e) *Speech perception in noise*
     Speech perception in noise was not significantly different from normal (t = 1.49, df = 32). Speech perception in quiet explained very little of the variance (F = 0.17, df = 1,11). The only significant parameters were the various measures of frequency resolution at 1 kHz (most significant were IN1+SL1: F = 6.9, df = 2,9), a result which was not affected by including only those patients with a noise history. This finding is particularly interesting, as neither the speech nor frequency-resolution results at 1 kHz were significantly different from normal for the patient sample.

5. DISCUSSION AND CONCLUSIONS

     In a random sample of patients presenting with difficulty in understanding speech, yet with clinically normal audiometry, frequency resolution was significantly impaired at 4 kHz. This deterioration in frequency resolution can account statistically for some of their difficulty with speech perception, paradoxically, at least in quiet.
     The history of noise exposure shared by most of the patients suggests the hypothesis that measures of frequency resolution might be a more sensitive indicator of noise-induced hearing impairment than absolute threshold. Pal'gov and Tereschenko (1973) have reported the possibly related result that patients with noise-induced losses exhibit abnormal critical ratios even at frequencies at which threshold is nearly normal. Another result which might be related is the finding of Young and Wilson (1982) that subjects show deterioration in speech perception in noise after ingestion of large quantities of acetylsalicylic acid without deterioration of threshold or speech perception in quiet.
     Our inability to find in our study significant deterioration in speech scores in noise is a paradox. It is possible that conventional speech audiometry, including our own 2AFC test, may not be sufficiently sensitive to confirm the subjective difficulty in speech perception.
     The underlying dissociation between frequency resolution and threshold cannot yet be clearly understood from current models of cochlear processes. In addition to the findings of Comis and colleagues, cited above, Carlier and Pujol (1982) have reported some loss of CAP tuning in cat and rat without threshold elevation, after transection of the efferent bundle. Many current models of the mechanisms underlying normal cochlear frequency resolution (e.g. Pick, 1980c) suggest that frequency resolution is achieved with the aid of intracochlear nonlinear feedback. If cochlear pathology can be considered to introduce attenuation in the feedback path, then it is likely that the strength of the linkage between frequency resolution and threshold will depend on the position of the attenuation in the feedback loop.

Acknowledgement. *The research was supported by the U.K. Medical Research Council. We are grateful to the following otologists for their willing cooperation in referring patients: R.J. Bennett, N.L. Crabtree, G.A. Dalton, A.R. Gupta, T.R. Kapur, J.T. Little, I.W. Mackie, A.L. Pahor, P.M. Shenoi, D.W. Stuart, and D.P.C. Williams. Drs. J.P. Wilson, S.R. Pratt, and D.J. Parker made useful comment on the manuscript. Technical assistance from Mr. J.B. Ruscoe, and typing by Ms. M. Hodgson.*

REFERENCES

Boothroyd, A. (1967). Developments in speech audiometry.
     Int. Audiol. 6, 136-145.
Carlier, E., Pujol, R. (1982). Sectioning the efferent bundle decreases cochlear frequency selectivity. *Neurosci. Letters* 28, 101-106.
Comis, S.D., Leng, G., Pratt, S.R. (1981). The effects of frusemide, bumetanide and Piretanide on the guinea-pig cochlea and auditory nerve.
     Scand. Audiol. Suppl. 14, 85-94.
Dreschler, W.A. (1980). Reduced speech intelligibility and its psychophysical correlates in hearing-impaired subjects. In: *Psychophysical, Physiological*

& *Behavioural Studies in Hearing*. (G. van den Brink & F.A. Bilsen, eds.).
     pp 466-469. Delft University Press.
Evans, E.F. (1975). Normal and abnormal functioning of the cochlear nerve.
     Symp. Zool. Soc. Lond. **37**, 133-165.
Grose, J., Pick, G.F. (1979). The calibration and validation of a two-
     alternative forced-choice test for evaluating hearing loss of cochlear
     origin. *Proc. Inst. Acoust.* 13-16.
Nelder, J.A., Wedderburn, R.W.M. (1972). Generalised linear models.
     J. Roy. Statist. Soc. A, **135**, 370-384.
Pal'gov, V.I., Tereshchenko, V.N. (1973). Effectiveness of critical bands as
     indicator of the damage to the auditory system. *Biophysics* **18**, 773-780.
Pick, G.F., Evans, E.F., & Wilson, J.P. (1977). Frequency resolution in
     patients with hearing loss of cochlear origin. In: *Psychophysics &
     Physiology of Hearing*. (E.F. Evans & J.P. Wilson, eds.). pp 273-281.
     London, Academic Press.
Pick, G.F. (1980a). Comment on 'Relations between hearing loss, maximal word
     discrimination score and width of psychophysical tuning curves'. (R.J.
     Ritsme, *et al.*). In: *Psychophysical, Physiological & Behavioural Studies
     in Hearing*. (G. van den Brink & F.A. Bilsen, eds.). p. 476. Delft
     University Press.
Pick, G.F. (1980b). Level dependence of psychophysical frequency resolution and
     auditory filter shape. *J. Acoust. Soc. Amer.* **68**, 1085-1095.
Pick, G.F. (1980c). Theoretical dependence of cochlear-fibre discharge rate
     versus intensity function on frequency evidence for basilar-membrane non-
     linearity? *Hearing Research* **2**, 559-564.
Pratt, S.R., Comis, S.D. (1982). Chronic effects of loop diuretics on the
     guinea-pig cochlea. *Brit. J. Audiol.* **16**, 117-122.
Ritsma, R.J., Wit, H.P., van der Lans, W.P. (1980). Relations between hearing
     loss, maximal word discrimination score and width of psychophysical tuning
     curves. In: *Psychophysical, Physiological & Behavioural Studies in Hearing*.
     (G. van den Brink & F.A. Bilsen, eds.). pp 472-475. Delft University Press.
Tyler, R.S., Wood, E.J., Fernandes, M. (1982). Frequency resolution and hearing
     loss. *Brit. J. Audiol.* **16**, 45-64.
Young, L.L., Wilson, K.A. (1982). Effects of acetylcalicylic acid on speech
     discrimination. *Audiol.* **21**, 342-349.

GENERAL DISCUSSION

HAGGARD:
You have done a useful service in showing that parameters at 4 kHz, despite being "within the normal range", contribute to difficulties with speech in quiet.
There are quite probably other non-peripheral and even non-auditory features
contributing to the definition of this group of semi-patients, but it is good to
know that measurable yet mild noise-related aspects of hearing do contribute.
It is not too surprising that the correlated factors shift as you change the
S/N ratio ($-\infty$ to about nominal -7) as this is a general finding. In particular
one would predict that as the noise knocks out the higher frequency region for
most of the subjects, the important spectral region shifts downwards, so the
variance at low to mid frequencies contributes to the variance in the speech-in-
noise task. Again the lack of a significant difference between the two groups on
speech-in-noise simply reflects the high within-group variability that makes the
foregoing correlations possible, and this poses no paradox. Both experimental and
correlational evidence are useful but we may have to choose which to concentrate
on. For subtle effects it is necessary to design subtle tests. For example with
the Four Alternative Auditory Feature (FAAF) test sensitised by filtering out the
normally important mid-frequencies, we have succeeded in showing effects of the
ototoxic anti-cancer agent displatinum upon the otherwise relatively redundant
high frequencies, where an unfiltered version showed no difference.

TEN KATE:
Should it not be valuable to study the existence of a dissociation between threshold and frequency resolution when using a non-simultaneous masking procedure
with cosine noise instead of a simultaneous one (see comment of J.M. Festen on
paper of R.S. Tyler et al.). Does the slope SL_4 in your statistical model give
extra information above what the bandwidth BW_4 at 4 kHz gives us? Do you obtain
a correlation between SL_4 and BW_4?

PICK:
I agree that a study of frequency resolution in forward masking might well elicit
fresh phenomena.
Without referring back to the results of my statistical modeling, I cannot give
definitive answers to the second part of your question. Usually, however, in our
studies, we have found a strong correlation between SL_4 and BW_4.

VERSCHUURE:
Could you clarify the selection of patients? You state that they were selected
on their complaints of bad speech intelligibility in noise and nevertheless most
of your patients show near normal or better than normal speech reception in noise!

PICK:
All of the patients visited their general practitioner complaining of difficulty
in understanding speech exacerbated in noise. They were then sent to an ENT con-
sultant, and these consultants referred these patients to us. We invited all
patients to be tested.
Hence it was somewhat surprising to us that they gave normal speech perception
in noise. Possibly, the test that we used was not typical of the conditions under
which their difficulties occurred.

This book may be kept